Basic Physiology for Anaesthetists

Second Edition

Dr David Chambers is a Consultant Neuroanaesthetist at Salford Royal NHS Foundation Trust, Salford, UK. His interests include anaesthesia for awake craniotomy, total intravenous anaesthesia and postgraduate anaesthetic training. He co-organises the North West Final FRCA exam practice course.

Dr Christopher Huang is Professor of Cell Physiology at Cambridge University. His research interests have covered signalling processes in skeletal myocytes and osteoclasts, cellular electrolyte homeostasis, cerebral cortical spreading depression and cardiac arrhythmogenesis. He was editor of the *Journal of Physiology, Monographs of the Physiological Society* and *Biological Reviews*.

Dr Gareth Matthews is a National Institute of Health Research Academic Clinical Fellow in Cardiology at Cambridge University Hospitals NHS Foundation Trust. He is also a Fellow in Medicine at Murray Edwards College, University of Cambridge, where he supervises undergraduate physiology. His research interest is the pathophysiology of cardiac arrhythmia.

Basic Physiology for Anaesthetists

Second Edition

David Chambers
Salford Royal NHS Foundation Trust

Christopher Huang
University of Cambridge

Gareth Matthews
University of Cambridge

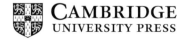
CAMBRIDGE
UNIVERSITY PRESS

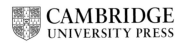

Shaftesbury Road, Cambridge CB2 8EA, United Kingdom

One Liberty Plaza, 20th Floor, New York, NY 10006, USA

477 Williamstown Road, Port Melbourne, VIC 3207, Australia

314–321, 3rd Floor, Plot 3, Splendor Forum, Jasola District Centre,
New Delhi – 110025, India

103 Penang Road, #05–06/07, Visioncrest Commercial, Singapore 238467

Cambridge University Press is part of Cambridge University Press & Assessment,
a department of the University of Cambridge.

We share the University's mission to contribute to society through the pursuit of
education, learning and research at the highest international levels of excellence.

www.cambridge.org
Information on this title: www.cambridge.org/9781108463997
DOI: 10.1017/9781108565011

First published 2015
Second edition 2019 (version 2, May 2023)

Printed in the United Kingdom by TJ Books Limited, Padstow Cornwall

A catalogue record for this publication is available from the British Library.

Library of Congress Cataloging-in-Publication Data
Names: Chambers, David, 1979- author. | Huang, Christopher, 1951- author. |
    Matthews, Gareth, 1987- author.
Title: Basic physiology for anaesthetists / David Chambers, Christopher
    Huang, Gareth Matthews.
Description: Second edition. | Cambridge, United Kingdom ; New York, NY :
    Cambridge University Press, 2019. | Includes bibliographical references
    and index.
Identifiers: LCCN 2019009280 | ISBN 9781108463997 (pbk. : alk. paper)
Subjects: | MESH: Physiological Phenomena | Anesthesiology–methods
Classification: LCC RD82 | NLM QT 104 | DDC 617.9/6–dc23
LC record available at https://lccn.loc.gov/2019009280

ISBN 978-1-108-46399-7 Paperback

....

DC:

To Sally, for not vetoing this second edition.

CH:

To friends and teachers: Charles Michel, Morrin Acheson, Richard Adrian, Sir David Weatherall and John Ledingham. *In memoriam absentium, in salutem praesentium.*

GM:

To my wife, Claire, and our beautiful baby daughter, Eleanor. I also remain indebted to Professor Christopher Huang for fostering my original interest in physiology, as well as supporting me throughout my career.

Contents

Foreword

This second edition of *Basic Physiology for Anaesthetists* has carried forward the style, depth and content that made the first edition such a great success. It covers all aspects of human physiology that are essential for the art and science that is modern anaesthesia. Patients need to be reassured that their anaesthetists are well informed of the workings of the human body in health as well as disease.

The authors are both expert physiology scientists and clinicians – this combination is clearly seen in the book's structure. Each chapter explains the physiology and is followed by the clinical applications relevant to the speciality. The illustrations are simple line drawings that are easy to follow and, importantly for trainee anaesthetists, easy to recall or even reproduce

in the exam setting. Not only should this book be essential reading for those new to the speciality or those preparing for exams, but established specialists and consultants should have access to a copy to give structure to their teaching, as well as to rekindle fading knowledge. Those sitting anaesthesia exams can be confident that many of those responsible for testing their knowledge will themselves have consulted this book!

Dr Russell Perkins FRCA
Consultant Anaesthetist, Royal Manchester
Children's Hospital
Member of Council and Final FRCA Examiner,
Royal College of Anaesthetists

Preface to the Second Edition

'Why are you writing a second edition? Surely nothing in classical physiology ever changes?' One of us (DC) has been asked these questions several times. It is true that many of the fundamental physiological concepts described in this second edition of *Basic Physiology for Anaesthetists* remain the same. What does change, however, is how we apply that physiological knowledge clinically. In the four years since we wrote the first edition of this book, high-flow nasal oxygen therapy has revolutionised airway management, cancer surgery has become the predominant indication for total intravenous anaesthesia and new classes of oral anticoagulants have emerged, to name but a few developments. All of these changes in daily anaesthetic practice are underpinned by a thorough understanding of basic physiology.

To that end, in addition to thoroughly revising and updating each chapter, we have added six new chapters, including those on the physiology of the eye and upper airway and on exercise testing. We have also sought to include more pathophysiology, such as cardiac ischaemia and physiological changes in obesity. We have tried to remain true to the principles with which we wrote the first edition, keeping the concepts as simple as possible whilst remaining truthful and illustrating each chapter with points of clinical relevance and easily reproducible line diagrams. In response to positive feedback, the question-and-answer style remains to best help readers prepare for postgraduate oral examinations.

Preface to the First Edition

An academically sound knowledge of both normal and abnormal physiology is essential for day-to-day anaesthetic practice, and consequently for postgraduate specialist examinations.

This project was initiated by one of us (DC) following his recent experience of the United Kingdom Fellowship of the Royal College of Anaesthetists examinations. He experienced difficulty locating textbooks that would build upon a basic undergraduate understanding of physiology. Many of the anaesthesia-related physiology books he encountered assumed too much prior knowledge and seemed unrelated to everyday anaesthetic practice.

He was joined by a Professor in Physiology (CH) and a Translational Medicine and Therapeutics Research Fellow (GM) at Cambridge University, both actively engaged in teaching undergraduate and postgraduate physiology and in physiological research.

This book has been written primarily for anaesthetists in the early years of their training, and specifically for those facing postgraduate examinations. In addition, the account should provide a useful summary of physiology for critical care trainees, senior anaesthetists engaged in education and training, physician assistants in anaesthesia, operating department practitioners and anaesthetic nurses.

We believe the strength of this book lies in our mixed clinical and scientific backgrounds, through which we have produced a readable and up-to-date account of basic physiology and provided links to anaesthetic and critical care practice. We hope to bridge the gap between the elementary physiology learnt at medical school and advanced anaesthesia-related texts. By presenting the material in a question-and-answer format, we have aimed to emphasize strategic points and give the reader a glimpse of how each topic might be assessed in an oral postgraduate examination. Our numerous illustrations seek to simplify and clearly demonstrate key points in a manner that is easy to replicate in an examination setting.

Abbreviations

ACA	anterior cerebral artery		DNA	deoxyribonucleic acid
ACE	angiotensin-converting enzyme		DOAC	direct-acting oral anticoagulant
ACh	acetylcholine		DRG	Dorsal respiratory group
AChE	acetylcholinesterase		ECF	extracellular fluid
ACI	anterior circulation infarct		ECG	electrocardiogram
AChR	acetylcholine receptor		EDPVR	end-diastolic pressure-volume relationship
ACom	anterior communicating artery		EDV	end-diastolic volume
ADH	antidiuretic hormone		EEG	electroencephalogram
ADP	adenosine diphosphate		EF	ejection fraction
AF	atrial fibrillation		EPO	erythropoietin
AGE	alveolar gas equation		ER	endoplasmic reticulum
AMP	adenosine monophosphate		ESPVR	end-systolic pressure-volume relationship
ANP	atrial natriuretic peptide		ESV	end-systolic volume
ANS	autonomic nervous system		ETT	endotracheal tube
APTT	activated partial thromboplastin time		FAD	flavin adenine dinucleotide
ARDS	acute respiratory distress syndrome		FEV_1	forced expiratory volume in 1 s
ARP	absolute refractory period		F_iO_2	fraction of inspired oxygen
ATP	adenosine triphosphate		FRC	functional residual capacity
AV	atrioventricular		FTc	flow time corrected
BBB	blood–brain barrier		FVC	forced vital capacity
BMR	basal metabolic rate		GABA	γ-amino butyric acid
BNP	brain natriuretic peptide		GBS	Guillain–Barré syndrome
BSA	body surface area		GCS	Glasgow coma scale
CA	carbonic anhydrase		GFR	glomerular filtration rate
C_aO_2	arterial oxygen content		GI	gastrointestinal
CBF	cerebral blood flow		Hb	haemoglobin
CC	closing capacity		HbA	adult haemoglobin
CCK	cholecystokinin		HbF	foetal haemoglobin
CI	cardiac index		HCN	hyperpolarisation-activated cyclic nucleotide gated
CMR	cerebral metabolic rate		HFNO	High-flow nasal oxygen
CNS	central nervous system		HPV	hypoxic pulmonary vasoconstriction
CO	cardiac output		HR	heart rate
CoA	coenzyme A		ICA	internal carotid artery
COHb	carboxyhaemoglobin		ICF	intracellular fluid
COPD	chronic obstructive pulmonary disease		ICP	intracranial pressure
CPET	cardiopulmonary exercise test		IRI	ischaemic reperfusion injury
CPP	cerebral perfusion pressure		IVC	inferior vena cava
CRPS	complex regional pain syndrome		LA	left atrium
CSF	cerebrospinal fluid		LBBB	left bundle branch block
C_vO_2	venous oxygen content		LMA	laryngeal mask airway
CVP	central venous pressure		LOH	loop of Henle
CVR	cerebral vascular resistance		LOS	lower oesophageal sphincter
DASI	Duke activity status index		LV	left ventricle
DBP	diastolic blood pressure		LVEDP	left ventricular end-diastolic pressure
DCML	dorsal column-medial lemniscal		LVEDV	left ventricular end-diastolic volume
DCT	distal convoluted tubule		LVESV	left ventricular end-systolic volume
DHPR	dihydropyridine receptor			

LVF	left ventricular failure
MAC	minimum alveolar concentration
MAO	monoamine oxidase
MAP	mean arterial pressure
MCA	middle cerebral artery
MET	metabolic equivalent of a task
MetHb	methaemoglobin
MG	myasthenia gravis
MI	myocardial infarction
MPAP	mean pulmonary artery pressure
MW	molecular weight
N_2O	nitrous oxide
NSTEMI	non-ST elevation myocardial infarction
NAD^+	nicotinamide adenine dinucleotide
NMDA	N-methyl-D-aspartate
NMJ	neuromuscular junction
OER	oxygen extraction ratio
OSA	obstructive sleep apnoea
PAC	pulmonary artery catheter
P_aCO_2	arterial tension of carbon dioxide
P_aO_2	arterial tension of oxygen
P_B	barometric pressure
PCI	percutaneous coronary intervention
PCT	proximal convoluted tubule
PCA	posterior cerebral artery
PCom	posterior communicating artery
PCWP	pulmonary capillary wedge pressure
PE	pulmonary embolism
PEEP	positive end-expiratory pressure
$PEEP_e$	extrinsic positive end-expiratory pressure
$PEEP_i$	intrinsic positive end-expiratory pressure
PEFR	peak expiratory flow rate
PNS	peripheral nervous system
PPP	pentose phosphate pathway
PRV	polycythaemia rubra vera
PV	peak velocity
PVA	pressure-volume area
PT	prothrombin time
PTH	parathyroid hormone
PVR	pulmonary vascular resistance
RA	right atrium
RAA	renin–angiotensin–aldosterone

RAP	right atrial pressure
RBC	red blood cell
RBF	renal blood flow
RMP	resting membrane potential
RNA	ribonucleic acid
ROS	reactive oxygen species
RR	respiratory rate
RRP	relative refractory period
RSI	rapid sequence induction
RV	right ventricle
RVEDV	right ventricular end-diastolic volume
RVF	right ventricular failure
RyR	ryanodine receptor
SA	sinoatrial
S_aO_2	arterial haemoglobin oxygen saturation
SBP	systolic blood pressure
SD	stroke distance
SR	sarcoplasmic reticulum
SSEP	somatosensory evoked potential
STEMI	ST elevation myocardial infarction
SV	stroke volume
SVC	superior vena cava
SVI	stroke volume index
SVR	systemic vascular resistance
SVT	supraventricular tachycardia
SVV	stroke volume variation
TF	tissue factor
TIMI	thrombolysis in myocardial infarction
TLC	total lung capacity
TOE	trans-oesophageal echocardiography
$\dot{V}/\dot{Q}$	ventilation–perfusion
$\dot{V}_A$	alveolar ventilation
V_A	alveolar volume
VC	vital capacity
V_D	dead space volume
$\dot{V}_E$	minute ventilation
V_T	tidal volume
VF	ventricular fibrillation
VRG	ventral respiratory group
VT	ventricular tachycardia
VTI	velocity-time integral
vWF	von Willebrand factor

General Organisation of the Body

Physiology is the study of the functions of the body, its organs and the cells of which they are composed. It is often said that physiology concerns itself with maintaining the status quo or 'homeostasis' of bodily processes. However, even normal physiology is not constant, changing with development (childhood, pregnancy and ageing) and environmental stresses (altitude, diving and exercise). Physiology might be better described as maintaining an 'optimal' internal environment; many diseases are associated with the disturbance of this optimal environment.

Anaesthetists are required to adeptly manipulate this complex physiology to facilitate surgical and critical care management. Therefore, before getting started on the areas of physiology that are perhaps of greater interest, it is worth revising some of the basics – this chapter and the following four chapters have been whittled down to the absolute essentials.

How do the body's organs develop?

The body is composed of some 100 trillion cells. All life begins from a single totipotent embryonic cell, which is capable of differentiating into any cell type. This embryonic cell divides many times and, by the end of the second week, gives rise to the three germ cell layers:

- **Ectoderm**, from which the nervous system and epidermis develop.
- **Mesoderm**, which gives rise to connective tissue, blood cells, bone and marrow, cartilage, fat and muscle.
- **Endoderm**, which gives rise to the liver, pancreas and bladder, as well as the epithelial lining of the lungs and gastrointestinal (GI) tract.

Each organ is composed of many different tissues, all working together to perform a particular function. For example, the heart is composed of cardiac muscle, conducting tissue, including Purkinje fibres, and blood vessels, all working together to propel blood through the vasculature.

How do organs differ from body systems?

The organs of the body are functionally organised into 11 physiological 'systems':

- **Respiratory system**, comprising the lungs and airways.
- **Cardiovascular system**, comprising the heart and the blood vessels. The blood vessels are subclassified into arteries, arterioles, capillaries, venules and veins. The circulatory system is partitioned into systemic and pulmonary circuits.
- **Nervous system**, which comprises both neurons (cells that electrically signal) and glial cells (supporting cells). It can be further subclassified in several ways:
  - Anatomically, the nervous system is divided into the *central nervous system* (CNS), consisting of the brain and spinal cord, and the *peripheral nervous system* (PNS), consisting of peripheral nerves, ganglia and sensory receptors, which connect the limbs and organs to the brain.
  - The PNS is functionally classified into an *afferent limb*, conveying sensory impulses to the brain, and an *efferent limb*, conveying motor impulses from the brain.
  - *The somatic nervous system* refers to the components of the nervous system under conscious control.
  - *The autonomic nervous system* (ANS) regulates the functions of the viscera. It is divided into *sympathetic and parasympathetic nervous systems.*
  - *The enteric nervous system* is a semiautonomous system of nerves that control the digestive system.
- **Muscular system**, comprising the three different types of muscle: skeletal, cardiac and smooth muscle.

- **Skeletal system**, the framework of the body, comprising bone, ligaments and cartilage.
- **Integumentary system**, which is essentially the skin and its appendages: hairs, nails, sebaceous glands and sweat glands. Skin is an important barrier preventing invasion by microorganisms and loss of water (H_2O) from the body. It is also involved in thermoregulation and sensation.
- **Digestive system**, including the whole of the GI tract from mouth to anus and a number of accessory organs: salivary glands, liver, pancreas and gallbladder.
- **Urinary system**, which comprises the organs involved in the production and excretion of urine: kidneys, ureters, bladder and urethra.
- **Reproductive system**, by which new life is produced and nurtured. Many different organs are involved, including the ovaries, testes, uterus and mammary glands.
- **Endocrine system**, whose function is to produce hormones. Hormones are chemical signalling molecules carried in the blood that regulate the function of other, often distant cells.
- **Immune system**, which is involved in tissue repair and the protection of the body from microorganism invasion and cancer. The immune system is composed of the lymphoid organs (bone marrow, spleen, lymph nodes and thymus), as well as discrete collections of lymphoid tissue within other organs (for example, Peyer's patches are collections of lymphoid tissue within the small intestine). The immune system is commonly subclassified into:

  - *The innate immune system*, which produces a rapid but non-specific response to microorganism invasion.
  - *The adaptive immune system*, which produces a slower but highly specific response to microorganism invasion.

The body systems do not act in isolation; for example, arterial blood pressure is the end result of interactions between the cardiovascular, urinary, nervous and endocrine systems.

What is homeostasis?

Single-celled organisms (for example, an amoeba) are entirely dependent on the external environment for their survival. An amoeba gains its nutrients directly from and eliminates its waste products directly into the external environment. The external environment also influences the cell's temperature and pH, along with its osmotic and ionic gradients. Small fluctuations in the external environment may alter intracellular processes sufficiently to cause cell death.

Humans are multicellular organisms – the vast majority of our cells do not have any contact with the external environment. Instead, the body bathes its cells in extracellular fluid (ECF). The composition of ECF bears a striking resemblance to seawater, where distant evolutionary ancestors of humans would have lived. Homeostasis is the regulation of the internal environment of the body to maintain a stable, relatively constant and optimised environment for its component cells:

- **Nutrients** – cells need a constant supply of nutrients and oxygen (O_2) to generate energy for metabolic processes. In particular, plasma glucose concentration is tightly controlled, and many physiological mechanisms are involved in maintaining an adequate and stable partial pressure of tissue O_2.
- **Carbon dioxide (CO_2) and waste products** – as cells produce energy in the form of adenosine triphosphate (ATP), they generate waste products (for example, H^+ and urea) and CO_2. Accumulation of these waste products may hinder cellular processes; they must be transported away.
- **pH** – all proteins, including enzymes and ion channels, work efficiently only within a narrow range of pH. Extremes of pH result in denaturation, disrupting the tertiary or quaternary structure of proteins or nucleic acids.
- **Electrolytes and water** – the intracellular water volume is tightly controlled; cells do not function correctly when they are swollen or shrunken. As sodium (Na^+) is a major cell membrane impermeant and therefore an osmotically active ion, the movement of Na^+ strongly influences the movement of water. The extracellular Na^+ concentration is accordingly tightly controlled. The extracellular concentrations of other electrolytes (for example, the ions of potassium (K^+), calcium (Ca^{2+}) and magnesium (Mg^{2+})) have other major physiological functions and are also tightly regulated.

- **Temperature** – the kinetics of enzymes and ion channels have narrow optimal temperature ranges, and the properties of other biological structures, such as the fluidity of the cell membrane, are also affected by temperature. Thermoregulation is therefore essential.

Homeostasis is a dynamic phenomenon: usually, physiological mechanisms continually make minor adjustments to the ECF environment. Following a major disturbance, large physiological changes are sometimes required.

How does the body exert control over its physiological systems?

Homeostatic control mechanisms may be intrinsic (local) or extrinsic (systemic) to the organ:

- **Intrinsic homeostatic mechanisms** occur within the organ itself through autocrine (in which a cell secretes a chemical messenger that acts on that same cell) or paracrine (in which the chemical messenger acts on neighbouring cells) signalling.

For example, exercising muscle rapidly consumes O_2, causing the O_2 tension within the muscle to fall. The waste products of this metabolism (K^+, adenosine monophosphate (AMP) and H^+) cause vasodilatation of the blood vessels supplying the muscle, increasing blood flow and therefore O_2 delivery.

- **Extrinsic homeostatic mechanisms** occur at a distant site, involving one of the two major regulatory systems: the nervous system or the endocrine system. The advantage of extrinsic homeostasis is that it allows the coordinated regulation of many organs and feedforward control.

The vast majority of homeostatic mechanisms employed by both the nervous and endocrine systems rely on negative feedback loops (Figure 1.1). Negative feedback involves the measurement of a physiological variable that is then compared with a 'set point', and if the two are different, adjustments are made to correct the variable. Negative feedback loops require:

(a) Negative feedback loop:

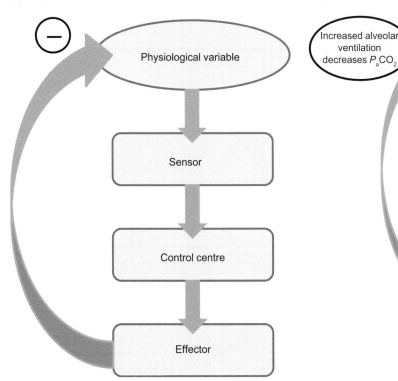

(b) Negative feedback loop for P_aCO_2:

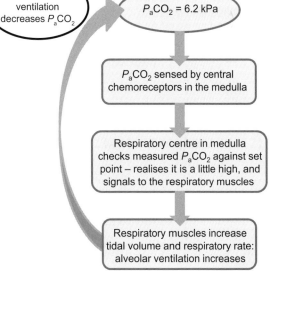

Figure 1.1 (a) Generic negative feedback loop and (b) negative feedback loop for arterial partial pressure of CO_2 (P_aCO_2).

- **Sensors**, which detect a change in the variable. For example, an increase in the arterial partial pressure of CO_2 (P_aCO_2) is sensed by the central chemoreceptors in the medulla oblongata.
- **A control centre**, which receives signals from the sensors, integrates them and issues a response to the effectors. In the case of CO_2, the control centre is the respiratory centre in the medulla oblongata.
- **Effectors**. A physiological system (or systems) is activated to bring the physiological variable back to the set point. In the case of CO_2, the effectors are the muscles of respiration: by increasing alveolar ventilation, P_aCO_2 returns to the 'set point'.

What is positive feedback?

In physiological terms, positive feedback is a means of amplifying a signal: a small increase in a physiological variable triggers a greater and greater increase in that variable (Figure 1.2). Because the body is primarily concerned with homeostasis, negative feedback loops are encountered much more frequently than positive feedback loops, but there are some important physiological examples of positive feedback:

- **Haemostasis.** Following damage to a blood vessel, exposure of a small amount of subendothelium triggers a cascade of events, resulting in the mass production of thrombin.
- **Uterine contractions in labour.** The hormone oxytocin causes uterine contractions during labour. As a result of the contractions, the baby's head descends, stretching the cervix. Cervical stretching triggers the release of more oxytocin, which further augments uterine contractions (Figure 1.2). This cycle continues until the baby is born and the cervix is no longer stretched.
- **Protein digestion in the stomach.** Small amounts of the enzyme pepsin are initially activated by decreased gastric pH. Pepsin then activates more pepsin by proteolytically cleaving its inactive precursor, pepsinogen.
- **Depolarisation phase of the action potential.** Voltage-gated Na^+ channels are opened by depolarisation, which permits Na^+ to enter the cell, which in turn causes depolarisation, opening more channels. This results in rapid membrane depolarisation.
- **Excitation–contraction coupling in the heart.** During systole, the intracellular movement of Ca^{2+} triggers the mass release of Ca^{2+} from the

(a) Positive feedback loop:

(b) Positive feedback loop for oxytocin during labour:

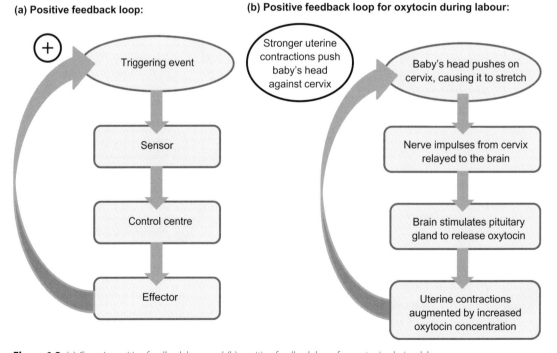

Figure 1.2 (a) Generic positive feedback loop and (b) positive feedback loop for oxytocin during labour.

sarcoplasmic reticulum (an intracellular Ca^{2+} store). This rapidly increases the intracellular Ca^{2+} concentration, facilitating the binding of myosin to actin filaments.

Where positive feedback cycles do exist in physiology, they are usually tightly regulated by a coexisting negative feedback control. For example, in the action potential, voltage-gated Na^+ channels inactivate after a short period of time, which prevents persistent uncontrolled depolarisation. Under certain pathological situations, positive feedback may appear as an uncontrolled phenomenon. A classic example is the control of blood pressure in decompensated haemorrhage: a fall in arterial blood pressure reduces organ blood flow, resulting in tissue hypoxia. In response, vascular beds vasodilate, resulting in a further reduction in blood pressure. The resulting vicious cycle is potentially fatal.

Further reading

L. S. Costanzo. *Physiology, 6th edition.* Philadelphia, Elsevier, 2018.

W. F. Boron, E. L. Boulpaep. *Medical Physiology, 3rd edition.* Philadelphia, Elsevier, 2017.

B. M. Koeppen, B. A. Stanton. *Berne and Levy Physiology, 7th edition.* Philadelphia, Elsevier, 2017.

Chapter 2

Cell Components and Function

Describe the basic layout of a cell

Whilst each cell has specialist functions, there are many structural features common to all (Figure 2.1). Each cell has three main parts:

- **The cell surface membrane**, a thin barrier that separates the interior of the cell from the extracellular fluid (ECF). Structurally, the cell membrane is a phospholipid bilayer into which are inserted glycoproteins akin to icebergs floating in the sea. The lipid tails form a hydrophobic barrier that prevents the passage of hydrophilic substances. The charged phosphate-

containing heads of the lipids are hydrophilic and thereby form a stable lipid–water interface. The most important function of the cell membrane is to mediate and regulate the passage of substances between the ECF and the intracellular fluid (ICF). Small, gaseous and lipophilic substances may pass through the lipid component of the cell membrane unregulated (see Chapter 4). The transfer of large molecules or charged entities often involves the action of the glycoproteins, either as channels or carriers.

- **The nucleus**, which is the site of the cell's genetic material, made up of deoxyribonucleic acid

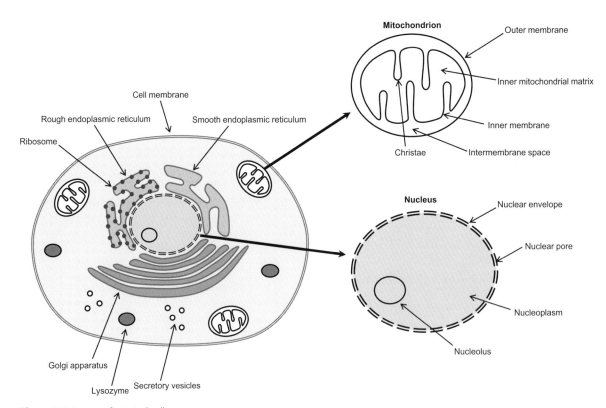

Figure 2.1 Layout of a typical cell.

(DNA). The nucleus is the site of messenger ribonucleic acid (mRNA) synthesis by transcription of DNA and thus coordinates the activities of the cell (see Chapter 3).

- **The cytoplasm**, the portion of the cell interior that is not occupied by the nucleus. The cytoplasm contains the cytosol (a gel-like substance), the cytoskeleton (a protein scaffold that gives the cell shape and support) and a number of organelles (small, discrete structures that each carry out a specific function).

Describe the composition of the cell nucleus

The cell nucleus contains the majority of the cell's genetic material in the form of DNA. The nucleus is the control centre of the cell, regulating the functions of the organelles through gene – and therefore protein – expression. Almost all of the body's cells contain a single nucleus. The exceptions are mature red blood cells (RBCs; which are anuclear), skeletal muscle cells (which are multinuclear) and fused macrophages (which form multinucleated giant cells).

The cell nucleus is usually a spherical structure situated in the middle of the cytoplasm. It comprises:

- **The nuclear envelope**, a double-layered membrane that separates the nucleus from the cytoplasm. The membrane contains holes called 'nuclear pores' that allow the regulated passage of selected molecules from the cytoplasm to the nucleoplasm, as occurs at the cell surface membrane.
- **The nucleoplasm**, a gel-like substance (the nuclear equivalent of the cytoplasm) that surrounds the DNA.
- **The nucleolus**, a densely staining area of the nucleus in which RNA is synthesised. Nucleoli are more plentiful in cells that synthesise large amounts of protein.

The DNA contained within each nucleus contains the individual's 'genetic code', the blueprint from which all body proteins are synthesised (see Chapter 3).

What are the organelles? Describe the major ones

Organelles (literally 'little organs') are permanent, specialised components of the cell, usually enclosed within their own phospholipid bilayer membranes. An organelle is to a cell what an organ is to the body – that is, a functional unit within a cell. Organelles found in the majority of cells are:

- **Mitochondria**, sometimes referred to as the 'cellular power plants', as they generate energy in the form of ATP through aerobic metabolism. Mitochondria are ellipsoid in shape and are larger and more numerous in highly metabolically active cells, such as red skeletal muscle. Unusually, mitochondria contain both an outer and an inner membrane, which creates two compartments, each with a specific function:
  - *Outer mitochondrial membrane.* This is a phospholipid bilayer that encloses the mitochondria, separating it from the cytoplasm. It contains porins, which are transmembrane proteins containing a pore through which solute molecules less than 5 kDa (such as pyruvate, amino acids, short-chain fatty acids) can freely diffuse. Longer-chain fatty acids require the carnitine shuttle (see Chapter 77) to cross the membrane.
  - *Intermembrane space*, between the outer membrane and the inner membrane. As part of aerobic metabolism (see Chapter 77), H^+ ions are pumped into the intermembrane space by the protein complexes of the electron transport chain. The resulting electrochemical gradient is used to synthesise ATP.
  - *Inner mitochondrial membrane*, the site of the electron transport chain. Membrane-bound proteins participate in redox reactions, resulting in the synthesis of ATP.
  - *Inner mitochondrial matrix*, the area bounded by the inner mitochondrial membrane. The matrix contains a large range of enzymes. Many important metabolic processes take place within the matrix, such as the citric acid cycle, fatty acid metabolism and the urea cycle.

As all cells need to generate ATP to survive, mitochondria are found in all cells of the body (with the exception of RBCs, which gain their ATP from glycolysis alone). Mitochondria also contain a small amount of DNA, suggesting that the mitochondrion may have been a microorganism in its own right prior to its evolutionary incorporation into larger cells. The cytoplasm and hence mitochondria are exclusively acquired from the mother, which underlies the maternal inheritance of mitochondrial diseases.

- **Endoplasmic reticulum** (ER), the protein- and lipid-synthesising apparatus of the cell. The ER is an extensive network (hence the name) of vesicles and tubules that occupies much of the cytosol. There are two types of ER, which are connected to each other:

  - *Rough ER*, the site of protein synthesis. The 'rough' or granular appearance is due to the presence of ribosomes, the sites where amino acids are assembled together in sequence to form new protein. Protein synthesis is completed by folding the new protein into its three-dimensional conformation. Rough ER is especially prominent in cells that produce a large amount of protein; for example, endocrine and antibody-producing plasma cells.

  - *Smooth ER*, the site of steroid and lipid synthesis. Smooth ER appears 'smooth' because it lacks ribosomes. Smooth ER is especially prevalent in cells with a role in steroid hormone synthesis, such as the cells of the adrenal cortex. In muscle cells, the smooth ER is known as the sarcoplasmic reticulum, an intracellular store of Ca^{2+} that releases Ca^{2+} following muscle cell-membrane depolarisation.

- **Golgi apparatus**, responsible for the modification and packaging of proteins in preparation for their secretion. The Golgi apparatus is a series of tubules stacked alongside the ER. The Golgi apparatus can be thought of as the cell's 'post office': it receives proteins, packs them into envelopes, sorts them by destination and dispatches them. When the Golgi apparatus receives a protein from the ER, it is modified through the addition of carbohydrate or phosphate groups, processes known as glycosylation and phosphorylation respectively. These modified proteins are then sorted and packaged into labelled vesicles into which they can be transported. Thus, the vesicles are transported to other parts of the cell or to the cell membrane for secretion (a process called 'exocytosis').

- **Lysosomes** are found in all cells, but are particularly common in phagocytic cells (macrophages and neutrophils). These organelles contain digestive enzymes, acid and free radical species and they play a role in cell housekeeping (degrading old, malfunctioning or obsolete proteins), programmed cell death (apoptosis) and the destruction of phagocytosed microorganisms.

Further reading

B. Alberts, D. Bray, K. Hopkin, et al. *Essential Cell Biology, 4th edition*. Oxford, Garland Science, 2013.

Genetics

In 2003, the completion of the Human Genome Project resulted in the sequencing of every human gene and subsequently heralded the 'age of the genome'. Whilst the knowledge of genetics has revolutionised medicine, the phenotypic significance of most genes remains poorly understood. This will be a major focus of physiological research in the future.

What is a chromosome?

An individual's genetic code is packed into the nucleus of each cell, contained in a condensed structure called chromatin. When the cell is preparing to divide, chromatin organises itself into thread-like structures called chromosomes; each chromosome is essentially a single piece of coiled deoxyribonucleic acid (DNA). In total, each cell contains 46 chromosomes (23 pairs), with the exception of the gamete cells (sperm and egg), which contain only 23 chromosomes.

There are two main types of chromosome:

- **Autosomes**, of which there are 22 pairs.
- **Allosomes** (sex chromosomes), of which there is only one pair, XX or XY.

Both types of chromosome carry DNA, but only the allosomes are responsible for determining an individual's sex.

What is DNA?

DNA is a polymer of four nucleotides in sequence, which is usually bound to a complementary DNA strand and folded into a double helix (Figure 3.1). The DNA strand can be thought of as having two parts:

- **A sugar–phosphate backbone**, made of alternating sugar (deoxyribose) and phosphate groups. The sugars involved in the DNA backbone are pentose carbohydrates, which are produced by the pentose phosphate pathway (PPP; see Chapter 77).

- **Nucleobases**, four different 'bases' whose sequence determines the genetic code:
    - Guanine (G);
    - Adenine (A);
    - Thymine (T);
    - Cytosine (C).

The nucleobases are often subclassified based on their chemical structure: A and G are purines, whilst T and C are pyrimidines.

The double-helical arrangement of DNA has a number of features:

- **Antiparallel DNA chains**. The two strands of DNA run in antiparallel directions.
- **Matching bases**. The two strands of DNA interlock rather like a jigsaw: a piece with a tab cannot fit alongside another piece with a tab – nucleotide A does will not fit alongside another nucleotide A. The matching pairs (called complementary base pairs) are:
    - C matches G;
    - A matches T.

Therefore, for the two DNA strands to fit together, the entire sequence of nucleotides of one DNA strand must match the entire sequence of nucleotides of the other strand.

- **Hydrogen bonding**. The two strands of DNA are held together by hydrogen bonds (a particularly strong type of van der Waals interaction) between the matching bases.

What is RNA? How does it differ from DNA?

The amino acid sequence of a protein is encoded by the DNA sequence in the cell nucleus. But when the cell needs to synthesise a protein, the code is anchored in the nucleus, and the protein-manufacturing apparatus (the endoplasmic reticulum (ER) and Golgi

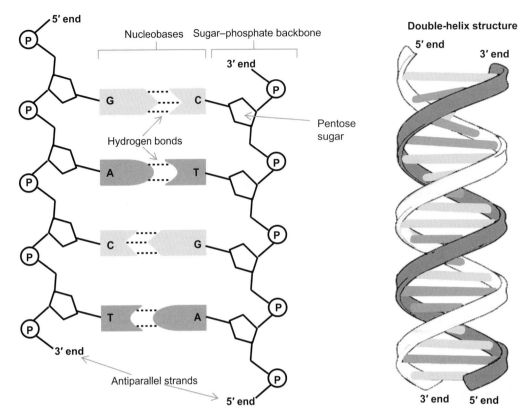

5' end

Nucleobases   Sugar–phosphate backbone

3' end

Double-helix structure

5' end

3' end

Hydrogen bonds

Pentose sugar

3' end

Antiparallel strands

5' end

3' end   5' end

Figure 3.1 Basic structure of DNA.

apparatus; see Chapter 2) is located within the cytoplasm. RNA overcomes this problem: RNA is produced as a copy of the DNA genetic code in the nucleus and is exported to the cytoplasm, where it is used to synthesise protein.

In some ways, RNA is very similar to DNA. RNA has a backbone of alternating sugar and phosphate groups attached to a sequence of nucleobases. However, RNA differs from DNA in a number of ways:

- RNA sugar groups have a hydroxyl group that DNA sugars lack (hence 'deoxy'-ribonucleic acid).
- RNA contains the nucleobase uracil (U) in place of thymine (T).
- RNA usually exists as a single strand; there is no antiparallel strand with which to form a double helix.

There are three major types of RNA:

- **Messenger RNA** (mRNA). In the nucleus, mRNA is synthesised as a copy of a specific section of DNA – this process is called transcription. mRNA then leaves the nucleus and travels to the

ribosomes of the rough endoplasmic reticulum (ER), the protein-producing factory of the cell.
- **Transfer RNA** (tRNA). In the cytoplasm, the 20 different types of tRNA gather the 20 different amino acids and transfer them to the ribosome, ready for protein synthesis.
- **Ribosomal RNA** (rRNA). Within the ribosome, rRNA aligns tRNA units (with the respective amino acids attached) in their correct positions along the mRNA sequence. The amino acids are joined together and a complete protein is released.

What is a codon?

A codon is a small piece of mRNA (a triplet of nucleosides) that encodes an individual amino acid. For example, GCA represents the amino acid alanine. tRNA also uses codons; as tRNA must bind to mRNA, the codons are the 'jigsaw match' of the mRNA codons (called anticodons). For example, CGU is the complementary anticodon tRNA sequence to GCA. CGU tRNA therefore binds alanine.

Clinical relevance: gene mutations

Errors may occur during DNA replication or repair. This abnormal DNA is then used for protein synthesis: transcribed mRNA incorporating the error is exported to the ribosome and translated into an abnormal protein. Common types of error are:

- **Point mutations**, where a single nucleoside is incorrectly copied in the DNA sequence.
- **Deletions**, where one or more nucleosides are accidentally removed from the DNA sequence.
- **Insertions**, where another short sequence of DNA is accidentally inserted within the DNA sequence.

Deletions and insertions are far worse than point mutations as frame shift may occur, with the ensuing DNA encoding a significantly altered protein. The resulting abnormal proteins have clinical consequences. For example:

- **Sickle cell disease** results from a point mutation in the DNA code for the β-chain of haemoglobin (Hb) on chromosome 11. Instead of the codon for the sixth amino acid of the DNA sequence reading GAG (which encodes glutamic acid), it reads GTG (which encodes valine). The substitution of a polar amino acid (glutamic acid) for a non-polar amino acid (valine) causes aggregation of Hb, and thus a change in the shape of the erythrocyte, under conditions of low O_2 tension.
- **Cystic fibrosis** results from mutations in the cystic fibrosis transmembrane conductance regulator (*CFTR*) gene, which encodes a transmembrane chloride (Cl^-) channel. The abnormal *CFTR* gene is characterised by reduced membrane Cl^- permeability and therefore reduced water movement out of cells. The clinical result is thickened secretions that prevent effective clearance by ciliated epithelium, resulting in blockages of small airways (causing pneumonia), pancreatic ducts (which obstructs flow of digestive enzymes) and vas deferens (leading to incomplete development and infertility in males). There are over 1000 different point mutations described in the *CFTR* gene. The most common is the ΔF508 mutation, where there is a deletion of three nucleotides (i.e. an entire codon, one that encodes phenylalanine, F) at the 508th position.
- **Huntington's disease** is a neurodegenerative disorder caused by the insertion of repeated segments of DNA. The codon for the amino acid glutamine (CAG) is repeated multiple times within the Huntington gene on chromosome 4. This is known as a 'trinucleotide repeat disorder'.

The resulting region of DNA becomes unstable, resulting in increasing numbers of trinucleotide repeats with each generation. For this reason, with each generation, Huntington's disease may appear at progressively younger ages or with a more severe phenotype. This is known as 'anticipation'.

What are the modes of Mendelian inheritance? Give some examples

Almost all human cells are diploid, as they contain 46 chromosomes (23 pairs). Gamete cells (sperm or egg) are haploid, as they contain 23 single chromosomes. When the gametes fuse, their chromosomes pair to form a new human cell with 23 pairs of chromosomes. During the formation of the gametes (a process known as 'meiosis'), separation of pairs of chromosomes into single chromosomes is a random process. Each person can therefore theoretically produce 2^{23} genetically different gametes, and each couple can theoretically produce 2^{46} genetically different children!

A trait is a feature (phenotype) of a person encoded by a gene. A trait may be a physical appearance (e.g. eye colour) or may be non-visible (e.g. a gene encoding a plasma protein). Each unique type of gene is called an allele (e.g. there are blue-eye alleles and brown-eye alleles). Every individual has at least two alleles encoding each trait, one from each parent. It is the interaction between alleles that determines whether an individual displays the phenotype (has a particular trait). Dominant alleles (denoted by capital letters) mask the effects of recessive alleles (denoted by lower-case letters).

Common Mendelian inheritance patterns of disease are:

- **Autosomal dominant.** For an individual to have an autosomal dominant disease, one of their parents must also have the genetic disease. A child of two parents, one with an autosomal dominant disease (genotype **A**a, where the bold A is the affected allele) and one without (genotype aa), has a 50% chance of inheriting the disease (genotype **A**a) and a 50% chance of being disease free (genotype aa) (Figure 3.2a). Examples of autosomal dominant diseases are hypertrophic cardiomyopathy, polycystic kidney disease and myotonic dystrophy.
- **Autosomal recessive.** In an autosomal recessive disease, the phenotype is only seen when both

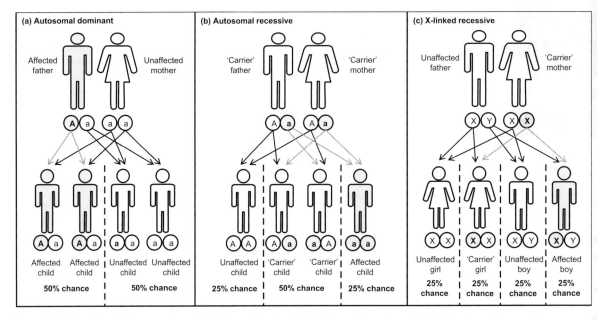

Figure 3.2 Mendelian inheritance patterns: (a) autosomal dominant; (b) autosomal recessive and (c) X-linked recessive.

alleles are recessive; that is, genotype aa (referred to as homozygous). The parents of a child with an autosomal recessive disease usually do not have the disease themselves: they are carriers (or heterozygotes) with the genotype Aa. A child of two heterozygous parents (genotype Aa) has a 50% chance of having genotype Aa (a carrier), a 25% chance of genotype AA (being disease free) and a 25% chance of having genotype aa (i.e. homozygous, having the autosomal recessive disease) (Figure 3.2b). Examples of autosomal recessive diseases are sickle cell disease, Wilson's disease and cystic fibrosis. Recessive diseases typically present at younger ages (often from birth) when compared to dominant conditions, which often present in young adulthood.

- **X-linked recessive**. These diseases are carried on the X chromosome. They usually only affect males (XY), because females (XX) are protected by a normal allele on the other X chromosome. Of the offspring of female carriers (XX), 25% are female carriers (XX), 25% are disease-free females (XX), 25% are disease-free males (XY) and 25% are males with the disease (XY) (Figure 3.2c). Examples of X-linked recessive diseases are haemophilia A, Duchenne muscular dystrophy and red–green colour blindness.

Mendelian inheritance refers to the inheritance of the genotype. However, genetic inheritance does not always result in phenotypic expression. This is known as 'penetrance'. For example, hypertrophic cardiomyopathy has a penetrance of ~70%, meaning that approximately 70 out of 100 patients who inherit the genetic mutation will actually get the disease. This is incomplete penetrance. Complete penetrance is when penetrance is 100%; an example would be neurofibromatosis. Incomplete penetrance usually refers to autosomal dominant conditions, but occasionally relates to autosomal recessive conditions.

Most inherited characteristics do not obey the simple monogenetic Mendelian rules. For example, diseases such as diabetes and ischaemic heart disease may certainly run in families, but their heritability is much more complex, often being polygenetic, age related and involving environmental as well as genetic factors.

Further reading

P. C. Turner, A. G. McLennan, A. D. Bates, M. R. H. White. *Instant Notes in Molecular Biology, 4th edition*. Oxford, Taylor and Francis, 2013.

A. Gardner, T. Davies. *Human Genetics, 2nd edition*. Banbury, Scion Publishing Ltd, 2009.

R. Landau, L. A. Bollag, J. C. Kraft. Pharmacogenetics and anaesthesia: the value of genetic profiling. *Anaesthesia* 2012; **67**(2): 165–79.

Chapter

4

The Cell Membrane

The cell membrane is the lipid bilayer structure that separates the intracellular contents from the extracellular environment. It controls the passage of substances into and out of the cell. This allows the cell to regulate, amongst other parameters, intracellular ion and solute concentrations, water balance and pH. The integrity of the cell membrane is of crucial importance to cell function and survival.

What is the structure of the cell membrane?

The cell membrane is composed of two layers of phospholipid, sandwiched together to form a phospholipid bilayer (Figure 4.1). Important features of this structure are:

- The phospholipid is composed of a polar hydrophilic phosphate head to which water is attracted and a non-polar hydrophobic fatty acid tail from which water is repelled.
- The phospholipid bilayer is arranged so that the polar groups face outwards and the non-polar groups are interiorised within the bilayer structure.

- The outer surface of the phospholipid bilayer is in contact with the extracellular fluid (ECF) and the inner surface of the bilayer is in contact with the intracellular fluid (ICF).
- The non-polar groups form a hydrophobic core, preventing free passage of water across the cell membrane. This is extremely important as it enables different concentrations of solutes to exist inside and outside the cell.
- The phospholipid bilayer is a two-dimensional liquid rather than a solid structure; the individual phospholipids are free to move around within their own half of the bilayer. The fluidity of the cell membrane allows cells to change their shape; for example, red blood cells may flex to squeeze through the small capillaries of the pulmonary circulation.

Which other structures are found within the cell membrane?

A number of important structures are found in and around the cell membrane:

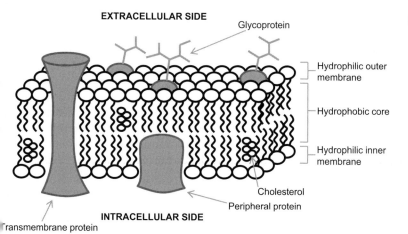

EXTRACELLULAR SIDE

Glycoprotein

Hydrophilic outer membrane

Hydrophobic core

Hydrophilic inner membrane

Cholesterol

Peripheral protein

INTRACELLULAR SIDE

Transmembrane protein

Figure 4.1 The phospholipid bilayer.

- **Transmembrane proteins**. As suggested by the name, these proteins span the membrane phospholipid bilayer. Importantly, the fluidity of the cell membrane allows these transmembrane proteins to float around, rather like icebergs on a sea of lipid.
- **Peripheral proteins**. These proteins are mounted on the surface of the cell membrane, commonly the inner surface, but do not span the cell membrane. Cell adhesion molecules, which anchor cells together, are examples of outer membrane peripheral proteins. Inner membrane peripheral proteins are often bound to the cytoskeleton by proteins such as ankyrin, maintaining the shape of the cell.
- **Glycoproteins and glycolipids**. The outer surface of the cell membrane is littered with short carbohydrate chains, attached to either protein (when they are referred to as glycoproteins) or lipid (when they are referred to as glycolipids). The carbohydrates act as labels, allowing the cell to be identified by other cells, including the cells of the immune system.
- **Cholesterol**. This helps strengthen the phospholipid bilayer and further decreases its permeability to water.

What are the functions of transmembrane proteins?

The hydrophobic core of the phospholipid bilayer prevents simple diffusion of hydrophilic substances. Instead, transmembrane proteins allow controlled transfer of large or charged solutes and water across the cell membrane.

The cell can therefore regulate intracellular solute concentrations by controlling the number, permeability and transport activity of its transmembrane proteins. There are many different types of transmembrane protein – the important classes are:

- **Ion channels**, water-filled pores in the cell membrane that allow specific ions to pass through the cell membrane along their concentration gradients.
- **Carriers**, which transport specific substances through the cell membrane via facilitated diffusion.
- **Pumps** (ATPases) use energy (from ATP hydrolysis) to transport ions across the cell membrane against their concentration gradients.
- **Receptors**, to which extracellular ligands bind, initiating an intracellular reaction either via a second messenger system (metabotropic) or an ion channel (ionotropic).
- **Enzymes**, which may catalyse intracellular or extracellular reactions.

By what means are substances transported across the cell membrane?

The behaviour of substances crossing the cell membrane is broadly divided into two categories:

- **Lipophilic substances** (e.g. O_2, CO_2 and steroid hormones) are not impeded by the hydrophobic core of the phospholipid bilayer and are able to cross the cell membrane by simple diffusion (Figure 4.2). Small lipophilic substances diffuse through the cell membrane in accordance with their concentration or partial pressure gradients: molecules diffuse from areas of high concentration (or partial pressure) to areas of low concentration (or partial pressure) (see Chapter 10).
- **Hydrophilic substances** (e.g. electrolytes and glucose) are prevented from passing through the hydrophobic core of the phospholipid bilayer. Instead, they traverse the cell membrane by passing through channels or by combining with carriers.

Hydrophilic substances can be transported across the cell membrane by passive or active means (Figure 4.2)

- **Passive transport**. Some transmembrane proteins act as water-filled channels through which hydrophilic molecules can diffuse along their concentration gradients. These protein channels are highly specific for a particular substance. There are two types of passive transport – ion channels and facilitated diffusion:
  - *Ion channels* are pores in the cell membrane that are highly specific to a particular ion. For example, the pore component of a voltage-gated sodium channel is the right size and charge to allow Na^+ to pass through 100 times more frequently than K^+ ions.[1] Ion channels may be classified as:

---

[1] It is easy to understand why a larger ion may not fit through an ion channel designed for a smaller ion, but the reverse is also true: a smaller ion does not fit through a

EXTRACELLULAR FLUID

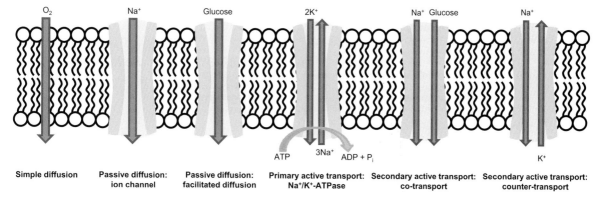

| Simple diffusion | Passive diffusion: ion channel | Passive diffusion: facilitated diffusion | Primary active transport: Na⁺/K⁺-ATPase | Secondary active transport: co-transport | Secondary active transport: counter-transport |

Figure 4.2 Means of transport across the cell membrane.

INTRACELLULAR FLUID

- Leak channels, which are always open, allowing continuous movement of the specific ion along its concentration gradient.
- Voltage-gated channels, which open by changing shape in response to an electrical stimulus, typically a depolarisation of the cell membrane (see Chapter 52).[2] When the ion channel is open, the specific ion diffuses through the cell membrane along its concentration gradient, but when the channel is closed or inactivated the membrane becomes impermeable.
- Ligand-gated channels, where the binding of a small molecule (ligand) causes the ion channel to open or close. For example, acetylcholine (ACh) binds to the nicotinic ACh receptor (a ligand-gated cation channel) of the neuromuscular junction, thereby opening its integral cation channel (see Chapter 53).

- Mechanically gated channels, which have pores that respond to mechanical stimuli, such as stretch. For example, mechanically gated Ca^{2+} channels open following distension of arteriolar smooth muscle – this is the basis of the myogenic response (see Chapters 34 and 56).

  - *Facilitated diffusion.* A carrier protein binds a specific substrate before undergoing a number of conformation changes to move the substrate from one side of the cell membrane to the other. Once the substrate has passed through the cell membrane, it is released from the carrier protein. The substance passes down its concentration gradient, facilitated by the carrier protein (Figure 4.3). Facilitated diffusion is much faster than simple diffusion, but is limited by the amount of carrier protein in the cell membrane. The most important example of facilitated diffusion is glucose transport into the cell through the glucose transporter (GLUT). An example of passive counter-transport is the Cl^-/bicarbonate (HCO_3^-)-antiporter in the renal tubule, where Cl^- and HCO_3^- are simultaneously transported in opposite directions down their respective concentration gradients.

- **Active transport.** Energy from ATP hydrolysis is used to move substances across the cell

---

channel designed for a larger ion. The reason for this is related to the number of water molecules that surround the ion (the hydration sphere): a smaller ion has a larger hydration sphere, which cannot pass through the wrong-sized ion channel.

[2] In contrast, the inward rectifying K^+ channels of the cardiac action potential open when the cell membrane *repolarises* (see Chapter 57).

EXTRACELLULAR FLUID

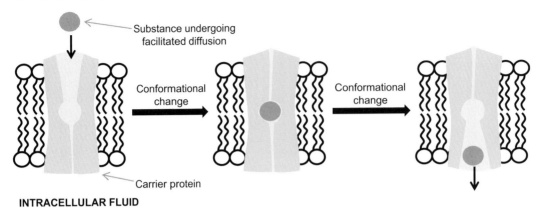

Figure 4.3 Facilitated diffusion.

membrane. Active transport is further subclassified as:

– *Primary active transport.* Here, ATP is hydrolysed by the carrier protein itself as it moves ions from one side of the cell membrane to the other. An example of primary active transport is the plasma membrane Ca^{2+}-ATPase, which pumps Ca^{2+} out of the cell, keeping the intracellular Ca^{2+} concentration very low. An important example of a more complicated system of primary active transport is the Na^+/K^+-ATPase pump, which uses one molecule of ATP to transport three Na^+ ions from the ICF to the ECF, whilst simultaneously transporting two K^+ ions from the ECF to the ICF. Unlike passive transport, whose direction of diffusion depends on the relative concentrations of the substance on either side of the cell membrane, active transport is usually unidirectional. The Na^+/K^+-ATPase can only move Na^+ intracellularly and can only move K^+ extracellularly.

– *Secondary active transport*, a combination of primary active transport and facilitated diffusion. Substances are transported alongside Na^+, driven by the low intracellular concentration of Na^+, which in turn is generated by the Na^+/K^+-ATPase pump. So whilst the transporter is not directly involved in hydrolysing ATP, it relies on primary active transport, which consumes ATP. Secondary active transport may be:

- Co-transport (or 'symport'), where both ions move in the same direction, such as the absorption of glucose with Na^+ in the renal tubules through the sodium–glucose-linked transporter (SGLT-2).[3]
- Counter-transport (or 'antiport'), where each ion is transported in opposite directions, such as the Na^+/K^+-antiporter in the principal cells of the renal collecting ducts.

Are there any other means by which substances are transported across the cell membrane?

An alternative method of transporting substances across the cell membrane is through vesicular transport:

- **Endocytosis.** This is an energy-consuming process whereby large extracellular substances are enveloped within a short section of cell membrane, forming a vesicle. The vesicle carries the substances, together with a small quantity of ECF, into the cytoplasm (Figure 4.4). Endocytosis is subclassified, depending on the type of substance transported:

---

[3] SGLT-2 transports glucose, along with Na^+, across the apical membrane of the proximal convoluted tubule by secondary active transport, which consumes ATP. Glucose then diffuses along its concentration gradient across the basolateral membrane of the tubular cell by facilitated diffusion (through GLUT-2), which does not require ATP.

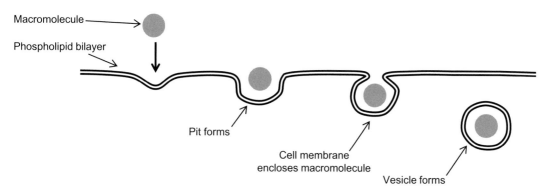

Macromolecule

Phospholipid bilayer

Pit forms

Cell membrane
encloses macromolecule

Vesicle forms

Figure 4.4 Mechanism of endocytosis.

- *Phagocytosis* is the intracellular transport of particulate matter by endocytosis – microbes (bacteria, viruses), cells and other debris. Phagocytosis is shown by neutrophils and macrophages; these cells engulf and kill microbes (see Chapter 75).
- *Pinocytosis* is the intracellular transport of macromolecules by endocytosis. An important example of pinocytosis is the transport of breast milk immunoglobulin A macromolecules through the cell membrane of the neonate's gut.
- *Receptor-mediated endocytosis*, in which the substance binds to a receptor located on the extracellular side of the cell membrane. The receptor–substance complex then undergoes endocytosis, transporting the substance across the cell membrane. Examples of substances transported by receptor-mediated endocytosis include iron and cholesterol.

- **Exocytosis**, the reverse process of endocytosis. Exocytosis is an energy-consuming process in which substances are transported across the cell membrane from the ICF to the ECF within a vesicle. Once the vesicle has reached the extracellular side of the cell membrane, it merges with the phospholipid bilayer via protein interactions (known as SNAREs), releasing its contents into the ECF. Exocytosis is an important mechanism by which neurotransmitters and hormones are released.
- **Transcytosis**, in which a substance undergoes endocytosis on one side of the cell is transported across the cell interior and is released on the far side of the cell through exocytosis.

Further reading

M. Luckey. *Membrane Structural Biology: With Biochemical and Biophysical Foundations, 2nd edition.* Cambridge, Cambridge University Press, 2014.

Chapter

5

Enzymes

Enzymes are biological catalysts whose function is to increase the rate of metabolic reactions.

What is a catalyst?

A catalyst is a substance that increases the rate of a chemical reaction without being itself chemically altered. As the catalyst is not consumed in the reaction, it can be involved in repeated chemical reactions – only relatively small numbers of catalyst molecules are required.

What are the main features of an enzyme?

Enzymes are complex, three-dimensional proteins that have three important features:

- **Catalysis.** Enzymes act as catalysts for biological reactions.
- **Specificity.** Their complex, three-dimensional structure results in a highly specific binding site – the active site – for the reacting molecules or substrates. The active site can even distinguish between different stereoisomers of the same molecule.
- **Regulation.** Many of the reactions in biochemical pathways (e.g. the glycolytic pathway) are very slow in the absence of enzymes. Therefore, the rate of a biochemical pathway can be controlled by regulating the activity of the enzymes along its path, particularly the enzyme controlling the rate-limiting step, which in the case of glycolysis is phosphofructokinase.

How does an enzyme work?

Enzymes work by binding substrates in a particular orientation, bringing them into the optimal position to react together. This lowers the activation energy for the chemical reaction, which dramatically increases the rate of reaction. The three-dimensional shape of the active site is of crucial importance. If the shape of the active site is altered (e.g. by increased temperature or pH), the function of the enzyme may be impaired and the chemical reaction slowed.

As an example, the reaction between CO_2 and water giving carbonic acid (H_2CO_3) is very slow:

$$CO_2 + H_2O \rightarrow H_2CO_3$$

However, addition of the enzyme carbonic anhydrase (CA), which contains a zinc atom at its active site, to the mixture of CO_2 and water increases the speed of the reaction considerably. First, water binds to the zinc atom, then a neighbouring histidine residue removes an H^+ ion from the water, leaving the highly active OH^- ion attached to zinc (Figure 5.1). Finally, there is a pocket within the active site that fits the CO_2 molecule perfectly: with CO_2 and OH^- in close proximity, the chemical reaction takes place quickly. Once CO_2 and water have reacted, the resulting H_2CO_3 diffuses out of the enzyme, leaving it unchanged chemically; that is, the enzyme acts as a catalyst.

The same enzyme can also catalyse the reverse reaction. This is indeed the case for CA, which catalyses

$$H_2CO_3 \rightarrow H_2O + CO_2$$

Carbonated drinks degas quite slowly when their container is opened, but degas very quickly on contact with saliva, which contains CA. This gives the sensation of carbonated drinks being 'fizzy' on the tongue.

The overall direction of the reaction obeys Le Chatelier's principle: if a chemical equilibrium experiences a change in concentration or partial pressure, the equilibrium shifts to counteract this change and a new equilibrium is reached. Enzymes increase the rate at which equilibrium is achieved.

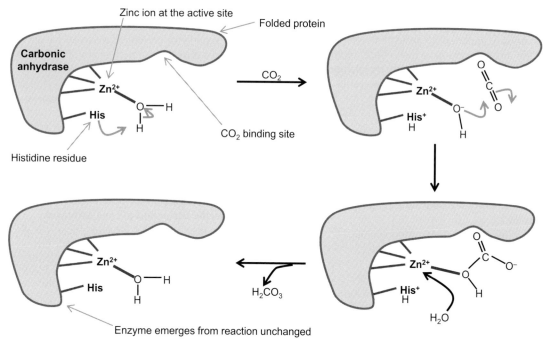

Figure 5.1 Catalysis of a reaction between water and CO_2 by carbonic anhydrase.

What types of enzyme are there?

Enzymes are classified by the type of biological reaction they catalyse:

- **Oxidoreductases**, which catalyse oxidation and reduction (redox) reactions.
- **Transferases**, which transfer functional groups (e.g. a kinase transfers a phosphate group) from one molecule to another.
- **Hydrolases**, which catalyse hydrolysis reactions.
- **Lyases**, which cleave bonds by means other than hydrolysis and oxidation.
- **Isomerases**, which allow a molecule to interconvert between its isomers.
- **Ligases**, which use energy (derived from ATP hydrolysis) to join two molecules together with covalent bonds.

What is meant by the terms 'cofactor' and 'coenzyme'?

Some enzymes consist purely of protein and catalyse biological reactions by themselves. Other enzymes require non-protein molecules (called cofactors) to aid their enzymatic activity. Cofactors can be:

- **Inorganic.** Many enzymes contain metal ions at their active site. For example:

  - CA contains Zn^{2+}, as discussed above.
  - The cytochrome P450 group of enzymes all contain Fe^{2+}.
  - Vitamin B_{12} contains Co^{2+}.
  - Superoxide dismutase contains Cu^{2+}.
  - Hexokinase contains Mg^{2+}.

- **Organic.** When the cofactor is organic, it is called a 'coenzyme'. Examples are:

  - Coenzyme A (CoA), a coenzyme used to transfer acyl groups by a variety of enzymes (e.g. acetyl-CoA carboxylase).
  - Nicotinamide adenine dinucleotide (NAD^+), a coenzyme that accepts a hydride (H^-) ion. NAD^+ is utilised, for example, in conjunction with the enzyme alcohol dehydrogenase.

Clinical relevance: enzymes and the anaesthetist

Enzymes are very important in anaesthetic practice. Many of the drugs we use have their effects terminated by enzymatic activity; others work by inhibiting enzymes directly. Some diseases are the result of reduced enzymatic activity. Examples include the following.

- **Cytochrome P450**. This superfamily of enzymes is responsible for the metabolism of most anaesthetic drugs. Notable exceptions include atracurium and cisatracurium (which degrade mainly by Hofmann elimination), catecholamines, suxamethonium, mivacurium and remifentanil (see below).
- **Monoamine oxidase** (MAO). Monoamine catecholamines (adrenaline, dopamine, noradrenaline) are metabolised by this mitochondrial enzyme. MAO inhibitors are antidepressants, with significant implications for the anaesthetist: indirect-acting sympathomimetics may precipitate a potentially fatal hypertensive crisis. Where necessary, direct-acting sympathomimetics can be used at a reduced dose, as they are also metabolised by another enzyme, catechol-O-methyl transferase (COMT). MAO inhibitors are also involved in the breakdown of serotonin. When used with other serotoninergic medications, such as pethidine, serotonin syndrome may be precipitated.
- **Pseudocholinesterase** (also known as plasma cholinesterase and butyrylcholinesterase). This is a plasma enzyme that metabolises suxamethonium and mivacurium. Patients who lack this enzyme or who have reduced enzyme activity experience prolonged muscular paralysis following a dose of suxamethonium or mivacurium – a condition known as 'suxamethonium apnoea'.
- **Acetylcholinesterase** (AChE). This is an enzyme found in the synaptic cleft of the neuromuscular junction. It hydrolyses the neurotransmitter ACh, terminating neurotransmission. Neostigmine, a reversible AChE inhibitor, is used to increase the concentration of ACh in the synaptic cleft. Increased ACh competitively displaces non-depolarising muscle relaxants from their receptors.
- **Non-specific tissue and plasma esterases**. These are responsible for the rapid hydrolysis of remifentanil, an ultra-short-acting opioid. This means that accumulation does not occur, and the context-sensitive half-time remains at 4 min, even after prolonged infusion. Esmolol, a 'cardioselective' β_1 receptor antagonist used to treat tachyarrhythmias during anaesthesia and for the control of heart rate and blood pressure during cardiac surgery, is rapidly degraded by red cell esterases. This results in rapid termination of effect following withdrawal.

Further reading

T. D. H. Bugg. *Introduction to Enzyme and Coenzyme Chemistry*, 3rd edition. London, John Wiley, 2012.

T. Palmer, P. L. Bonner. *Enzymes: Biochemistry, Biotechnology, Clinical Chemistry*, 2nd edition. London, Woodhead Publishing, 2007.

The Upper Airways

What are the components and functions of the upper respiratory tract?

The upper respiratory tract refers to the air passages that lie above the larynx, outside the thorax, and include:

- **Nose, nasal cavity and paranasal sinuses;**
- **Mouth;**
- **Pharynx,** which consists of the nasopharynx, oropharynx and laryngopharynx.

The main purpose of the upper respiratory tract is to conduct air from the atmosphere to the lower respiratory tract. However, the upper airways serve a number of additional functions:

- Nasal hairs filter any large inhaled particles.
- The superior, middle and inferior nasal turbinates (conchae) within the nasal cavity direct the inspired air over the warm, moist mucosa, promoting humidification. The epithelium of the posterior nasal cavity is covered in a thin mucous layer, which traps finer inhaled particles. Cilia then propel this mucus to the pharynx to be swallowed.
- The function of the four air-filled paranasal sinuses is of debate. They decrease the weight of the skull and protect the intracranial contents by acting as a 'crumple zone'. They may also have a role in air humidification, immunological defence and speech resonance.
- Olfactory receptors are located in the posterior nasal cavity. The proximal location of the olfactory receptors means that potentially harmful gases can be sensed by rapid, short inspiration (i.e. sniffing) before being inhaled into the lungs. They also play a major role in taste.
- The pharynx is a complex organ whose functions include the conduction of air, phonation and swallowing. The muscles of the upper airway are arranged to facilitate its multiple functions:
  - *Pharyngeal constrictors:* inferior, middle and superior constrictor muscles. During

swallowing, these muscles contract to propel food into the oesophagus.
  - *Pharyngeal dilators:* these muscles contract to maintain patency of the pharynx, so that air can flow to the lungs.

How does the upper airway remain patent during breathing?

During normal breathing, contraction of the diaphragm increases intrathoracic volume, which results in a negative airway pressure (see Chapter 7). Within the large airways, collapse is prevented by cartilaginous support. In contrast, the pharynx is largely unsupported and is therefore liable to collapse during inspiration. There are three groups of muscles responsible for maintaining upper airway patency:

- **Genioglossus,** the main dilator muscle of the pharynx, which causes the tongue to protrude forward and away from the pharyngeal wall.
- **Palatal muscles** control the stiffness and position of the palate, tongue and pharynx, as well as the shape of the uvula.
- **Muscles influencing the position of the hyoid,** such as geniohyoid, exhibit phasic activity. This means that their activity is increased during inspiration, thus stiffening and dilating the upper airway, counteracting the influence of negative airway pressure. When conscious, the airway will remain patent, even in the presence of intrathoracic pressures as low as -60 cmH$_2$O.

What happens to the upper airway during sleep?

During wakefulness, the activity of the pharyngeal dilator muscles is tightly controlled to maintain upper airway patency. Once an individual is asleep, the tone of the pharyngeal dilator muscles decreases significantly, leading to a reduced pharyngeal diameter. The greatest loss of pharyngeal muscle tone is associated with stage 3 non-rapid eye movement (NREM) sleep, the stage of sleep that is the most physically restorative.

In the majority of the population, upper airway patency is maintained during sleep. Susceptible individuals may experience pharyngeal obstruction:

- **Partial obstruction of the pharynx** results in turbulent airflow during breathing, resulting in the characteristic noise of snoring, an affliction that affects approximately 30% of the population (and their bed-partners!).
- **Complete obstruction of the pharynx**, as may occur in obstructive sleep apnoea (OSA).

What is OSA?

OSA is a sleep disorder characterised by recurrent episodes of complete upper airway obstruction during deep sleep. The pharyngeal collapse results in cessation of airflow despite the presence of diaphragmatic breathing effort. Each apnoeic period typically lasts 20–40 seconds, during which time hypoxia and hypercapnoea develop. The resulting chemoreceptor activation (see Chapter 22) rouses the individual from sleep sufficiently to restore pharyngeal muscle tone and therefore airway patency. A short period of hyperventilation occurs, until sleep deepens and airway obstruction recurs. This repeated cycle of sleep interruption (loss of stage 3 NREM *and* rapid eye movement sleep) and hypoxaemia is associated with the following problems:

- **Neuropsychiatric**: daytime sleepiness, poor concentration, irritability, anxiety, depression.
- **Endocrinological**: impaired glucose tolerance, dyslipidaemia, increased adrenocorticotropic hormone and cortisol levels.
- **Cardiovascular**: hypertension, atrial fibrillation, myocardial infarction, stroke.

OSA affects approximately 5–10% of the general population, but the prevalence is thought to be much higher in the surgical population. Risk factors for the development of OSA include:

- **Anatomical factors**: craniofacial abnormalities (such as Pierre Robin and Down's syndromes) and tonsillar and adenoidal hypertrophy (the major cause of OSA in children).
- **Obesity**, probably as a result of fat deposition around the pharynx. Abdominal obesity also decreases functional residual capacity (FRC), which exacerbates the hypoxaemia experienced during apnoeas.

- **Male gender**, possibly as a result of a relatively increased amount of fat deposition around the pharynx.

The effective treatment options are lifestyle modification (smoking cessation, alcohol reduction and weight loss), mouth devices and nasal continuous positive airway pressure (nCPAP). Overnight nCPAP set at between +5 and +20 cmH_2O probably works by acting as a pneumatic splint to maintain upper airway patency and has the effect of reducing daytime sleepiness and atrial fibrillation. It also improves mood, cognitive function and blood pressure control.

Clinical relevance: OSA and anaesthesia

Patients with OSA have a higher risk of perioperative complications, of which the most serious is airway obstruction due to the use of anaesthetic, sedative or opioid drugs.

Patients may present for surgery with a diagnosis of OSA or may be undiagnosed. A priority at preoperative assessment is to identify patients with undiagnosed OSA, as they benefit from a period of treatment with nCPAP prior to surgery. Screening is most commonly carried out using the STOP-BANG questionnaire, in which points are given for the presence of loud snoring, daytime sleepiness, observed apnoeas, hypertension, raised body mass index, age >50 years, neck circumference >40 cm and male gender.

With the exception of ketamine, all anaesthetic and sedative agents reduce central respiratory drive and pharyngeal muscle tone, leading to upper airway obstruction. Sedative premedication should therefore be avoided and regional or local anaesthetic techniques used where possible. Where general anaesthesia is required:

- Adequate preoxygenation prior to induction is key. This should involve oxygenating in the sitting position (to maximise functional residual capacity) and using CPAP (e.g. using a Water's circuit or high-flow nasal oxygen (HFNO)).
- An endotracheal tube is preferred over a laryngeal mask airway due to greater airway security and reduced risk of aspiration (gastroesophageal reflux is common in this patient group due to raised intra-abdominal pressure from obesity). However, both OSA and morbid obesity are associated with difficult laryngoscopy, and preparations should be made accordingly.
- At extubation, the patient should have any residual neuromuscular blockade fully reversed, be positioned to maximise FRC

(i.e. semi-upright or lateral) and should be fully awake.

- Post-operative CPAP, preferably with the patient's own machine, should be commenced.
- Multi-modal analgesia and regional anaesthetic techniques should be used to minimise post-operative opioid consumption and the associated central respiratory depressant effects.

Clinical relevance: HFNO therapy

Conventional O_2 delivery devices deliver cold, dry O_2 at a maximum flow rate of 15 L/min and have a number of disadvantages:

- **Masks are often poorly fitting**, which may result in damage to skin or entrainment of air. The maximum inspired O_2 concentration of a non-rebreathing mask is between 60% and 80% as a result of air entrainment.
- **The peak inspiratory flow** of a tachypnoeic patient may exceed the O_2 flow rate entering the mask, resulting in further air entrainment.
- **Delivery of dry oxygen** may result in thick, tenacious secretions and impaired mucociliary function.
- **Low flows**: conventional nasal cannulae improve patient compliance with O_2 therapy, as they allow the patient to eat, drink and communicate more effectively. But O_2 flows >4 L/min are poorly tolerated: the capacity of the nasal cavity to warm and humidify inspired gas is overwhelmed.

HFNO provides a method of delivering warmed, humidified O_2 to patients at flows of up to 60 L/min, with inspired O_2 concentrations of up to 100%. Because the inspired gas is warmed to 37°C and humidified to its saturation point, much higher gas flows can be tolerated – warming and humidification is no longer dependent on the nasal mucosa. HFNO offers a number of benefits:

- **Positive end-expiratory pressure** is generated at values between +3 and +7 cmH_2O depending on whether the patient's mouth is open or closed. This has the effect of recruiting alveoli and reducing upper airway collapse.
- **Pharyngeal dead space washout**: the high flow of O_2 washes expired CO_2 from the upper airway, reducing the effective anatomical dead space. A higher fraction of minute ventilation is therefore able to participate in gas exchange.
- **Reduced metabolic cost of breathing**. No longer having to warm and humidify inspired gases may provide a significant metabolic saving for a tachypnoeic patient.

HFNO is increasingly being used in ward and critical care settings as part of the management of patients with acute hypoxaemic respiratory failure and has an expanding role in the perioperative setting:

- **Preoxygenation** with HFNO allows denitrogenation of the lungs and provides an oxygen reservoir within the upper airway during laryngoscopy. The combination of a high fraction of inspired O_2 and positive end-expiratory pressure is especially useful in the preoxygenation of patients with reduced FRC, such as obese and obstetric patients and in the acute abdomen.
- **Intraoperative oxygenation**, to facilitate sedation techniques or tubeless airway surgery.
- **Extubation**, to re-recruit collapsed alveoli and to prevent post-operative upper airway collapse.

Further reading

A. B. Lumb. Functional anatomy of the respiratory tract. In: A. B. Lumb. *Nunn's Applied Respiratory Physiology*, 8th edition. London, Churchill Livingstone, 2016; 1–16.

T. Renda, A. Corrado, G. Iskandar, et al. High-flow nasal oxygen therapy in intensive care and anaesthesia. *Br J Anaesth* 2018; **120**(1): 18–27.

I. M. Gustafsson, Å. Lodenius, J. Tunelli, et al. Apnoeic oxygenation in adults under general anaesthesia using transnasal humidified rapid-insufflation ventilatory exchange (THRIVE) – a physiological study. *Br J Anaesth* 2017; **118**(4): 610–17.

F. Mir, A. Patel, R. Iqbal, et al. A randomised controlled trial comparing transnasal humidified rapid insufflation ventilatory exchange (THRIVE) pre-oxygenation with facemask pre-oxygenation in patients undergoing rapid sequence induction of anaesthesia. *Anaesthesia* 2017; **72**(4): 439–43.

G. Martinez, P. Faber. Obstructive sleep apnoea. *Continuing Educ Anaesth Crit Care Pain* 2011; **11**(1): 5–8.

R. B. Fogel, A. Malhotra, D. P. White. Sleep. 2: Pathophysiology of obstructive sleep apnoea/hypopnoea syndrome. *Thorax* 2004; **59**(2): 159–63.

I. Ayappa, D. M. Rapoport. The upper airway in sleep: physiology of the pharynx. *Sleep Med Rev* 2003; **7**(1): 9–33.

D. R. Hillman, P. R. Platt, P. R. Eastwood. The upper airway during anaesthesia. *Br J Anaesth* 2003; **91**(1): 31–9.

Chapter

7

The Lower Airways

What are the functions of the lung?

The lung has both respiratory and non-respiratory functions:

- **Respiratory functions** are those that facilitate gas exchange:
  - *Movement of gases* between the atmosphere and the alveoli;
  - *Passage of O_2* from the alveoli to the pulmonary capillaries;
  - *Passage of CO_2* from the pulmonary capillaries to the alveoli;
  - *Synthesis of surfactant.*
- **Non-respiratory functions** are:
  - *Acid–base balance;*
  - *Immunological and lung defence;*
  - *Vascular;*
  - *Metabolic and endocrine.*

Describe the functional anatomy of the lower airways

The lower airways can be divided into the larynx and tracheobronchial tree, which is subdivided into the conducting and respiratory zones. Important aspects of the anatomy are:

- **Larynx:**
  - During inhalation, the vocal cords are in an abducted position to reduce resistance to inward gas flow.
  - During exhalation, the cords adduct slightly, increasing the resistance to gas flow, which results in a positive end-expiratory pressure (PEEP) of 3–4 cmH$_2$O. This 'physiological' PEEP is important for vocalisation and coughing. It also maintains positive pressure in the small airways and alveoli during expiration, thus preventing alveolar collapse and maintaining functional residual capacity (FRC).

Clinical relevance: PEEP

When a patient is intubated, the vocal cords are no longer able to adduct during exhalation, leading to a loss of physiological PEEP. This can result in atelectasis and ventilation–perfusion ($\dot{V}/\dot{Q}$) mismatch. It is common practice to apply extrinsic PEEP (PEEP$_e$) at physiological levels (3–5 cmH$_2$O) to maintain FRC and prevent atelectasis following intubation.

However, PEEP increases intrathoracic pressure, which increases extravascular pressure on veins, causing collapse and reducing venous return. There are a small number of situations where not applying PEEP$_e$ may be advantageous – situations where raised venous pressure may have clinical consequences. For example:

- **Raised intracranial pressure** (ICP) – increased intrathoracic pressure may hinder venous drainage from the cerebral venous sinuses, leading to an increase in ICP.
- **Tonsillectomy** – raised venous pressure may increase bleeding at the tonsillar bed, obstructing the surgeon's view of the operative field.

Clinical relevance: humidification

Endotracheal and tracheostomy tubes bypass the upper airway, so the normal warming and humidification of inspired air cannot occur. Inhaling cold, dry gases results in increased mucus viscosity, which impairs the mucociliary escalator. This causes:

- Accumulation of mucus in lower airways;
- An increased risk of pulmonary infection;
- Microatelectasis.

Artificial humidification and warming of inspired gases are commonly achieved using a heat and moisture exchanger for surgical procedures or a hot water bath humidifier in the intensive care unit.

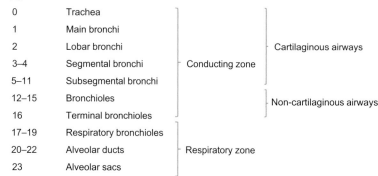

Airway generation

0	Trachea
1	Main bronchi
2	Lobar bronchi
3–4	Segmental bronchi
5–11	Subsegmental bronchi
12–15	Bronchioles
16	Terminal bronchioles
17–19	Respiratory bronchioles
20–22	Alveolar ducts
23	Alveolar sacs

Cartilaginous airways — Conducting zone

Non-cartilaginous airways

Respiratory zone

Figure 7.1 Generations of the tracheobronchial tree.

- **Tracheobronchial tree:**
  - The tracheobronchial tree consists of a series of airways that divide, becoming progressively narrower with each division. In total, there are 23 divisions[1] or generations between the trachea and the alveoli (Figure 7.1). As the generations progress, the total cross-sectional area increases exponentially (Figure 7.2).
  - The tracheobronchial tree is subdivided into the conducting zone (airway generations 0–16) and the respiratory zone (generations 17–23). As the names suggest, the conducting airways are responsible for conducting air from the larynx to the respiratory zone, whilst the respiratory zone is responsible for gas exchange.
  - In a 70-kg man, the volume of the conducting airways, known as the anatomical dead space, is approximately 150 mL. The volume of the respiratory zone at rest is approximately 3000 mL.

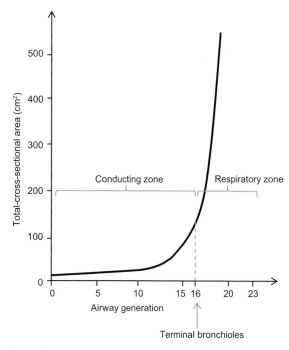

Figure 7.2 Increasing cross-sectional area with airway generation.

- **Conducting zone:**
  - The first generations of airways are lined by ciliated, pseudostratified columnar epithelium with scattered goblet cells. The goblet cells secrete a mucus layer that covers the epithelial cells and traps inhaled foreign bodies or microorganisms. The cilia beat in time, propelling mucus towards the oropharynx where it is either swallowed or expectorated. This system is known as the mucociliary escalator; its function is to protect the lungs from microorganisms and particulate matter and to prevent mucus accumulation in the lower airways.
  - The trachea starts at the lower border of the cricoid cartilage (C6 vertebral level) and

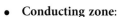

[1] Some studies claim that there are up to 28 airway generations in humans, but 23 generations are most commonly quoted.

25

bifurcates at the carina (T4/5 level).
The anterior and lateral walls of the trachea are reinforced with 'C'-shaped cartilaginous rings. The posterior gap of the cartilaginous rings is bridged by the trachealis muscle. At times of extreme inspiratory effort with associated high negative airway pressure, these cartilaginous rings prevent tracheal collapse.

- The trachea divides into the right and left main bronchi. The right main bronchus is shorter, wider and more vertical than the left. Inhaled foreign bodies and endotracheal tubes (ETTs) are therefore more likely to enter the right main bronchus than the left.

- The right lung has three lobes (upper, middle and lower) and the left has two lobes (upper and lower). The lingula (Latin for 'little tongue') is a part of the left upper lobe and is considered to be a remnant of the left middle lobe, which has been lost through evolution. There are 10 bronchopulmonary segments on the right (three upper lobe, two middle lobe, five lower lobe) and nine bronchopulmonary segments on the left (five upper lobe, four lower lobe).

Clinical relevance: double-lumen ETTs

The right upper lobe bronchus originates from the right main bronchus only 2 cm distal to the carina. In contrast, the left main bronchus bifurcates 5 cm from the carina.

Left-sided double-lumen ETTs (DLETTs) are often favoured over right-sided tubes for one-lung ventilation, even for some right-sided thoracic surgeries. This is because incorrect positioning of a right-sided DLETT risks occlusion of the right upper lobe bronchus by the ETT cuff. Right-sided DLETTs are available and have a hole positioned for ventilation of the right upper lobe. However, there are anatomical variations in the position of the right upper lobe bronchus; the position of the DLETT and the right upper lobe bronchus should therefore be checked using fibre-optic bronchoscopy.

- In segmental and subsegmental bronchi, the epithelium is surrounded by a layer of smooth muscle. Irregularly shaped cartilaginous plates prevent airway collapse.

- The bronchioles constitute the first airway generation that does not contain cartilage. They have a layer of smooth muscle that contracts (bronchoconstriction) and relaxes (bronchodilatation) to modulate gas flow:

  - Bronchodilatation results from sympathetic nervous system activity, such as during exercise: this reduces resistance to gas flow, allowing greater ventilation during periods of O_2 demand. Drugs that induce bronchodilatation include β_2-agonists and anticholinergics.

  - Bronchoconstriction is precipitated by the parasympathetic nervous system, histamine, cold air, noxious chemicals and other factors. At rest, the reduction in gas flow velocity causes particulate material to settle in the mucus, which is then transported away from the respiratory zone by the cilia.

- The terminal bronchioles are the last (16th) airway generation of the conducting zone.

- **Respiratory zone:**

  - Respiratory bronchioles are predominantly conducting, with interspersed alveoli that participate in gas exchange. These further divide into alveolar ducts, alveolar sacs and alveoli.

  - The alveoli form the final airway generation of the tracheobronchial tree. The human lungs contain approximately 300 million alveoli, resulting in an enormous surface area for gas exchange of 70 m^2. Each alveolus is surrounded by a capillary network derived from the pulmonary circulation.

Which cell types are found in the alveolus?

The wall of the alveolus is extremely thin, comprising three main cell types:

- **Type I pneumocytes.** These are specialised epithelial cells that are extremely thin, allowing efficient gas exchange. They account for around 90% of the alveolar surface area.

- **Type II pneumocytes.** These cover the remaining 10% of the alveolar surface. They are specialised secretory cells that coat the alveolar surface with pulmonary surfactant.

- **Alveolar macrophages**. Derived from monocytes, alveolar macrophages are found within the alveolar septa and the lung interstitium. They phagocytose any particles that escape the conducting zone's mucociliary escalator.

What is the alveolar–capillary barrier?

The barrier between the alveolus and the pulmonary capillary is extremely thin, which facilitates efficient gas exchange (see Chapter 10); in some places, it is as thin as 200 nm. There are three layers:

- Type I pneumocytes of the alveolar wall;
- Extracellular matrix;
- Pulmonary capillary endothelium.

Despite being very thin, the alveolar–capillary barrier is very strong owing to type IV collagen within the extracellular matrix. The barrier is permeable to small gas molecules such as O_2, CO_2, carbon monoxide, nitrous oxide (N_2O) and volatile anaesthetics.

The functions of the alveolar–capillary barrier are:

- To allow efficient gas exchange;
- To prevent gas bubbles entering the circulation;
- To prevent blood from entering the alveolus;
- To limit the transudation of water.

How does the lung inflate and deflate during tidal breathing?

The principal muscles involved in ventilation are the diaphragm and the intercostal muscles:

- **Inspiration**. The diaphragm is the main respiratory muscle during normal, quiet breathing (eupnoea); the external intercostal muscles assist during deep inspiration.
- **Expiration**. During eupnoea, the elastic recoil of the lungs produces passive expiration. The internal intercostal muscles are active during forced expiration.

Accessory muscle groups are used when additional inspiratory (sternocleidomastoid and scalene muscles) or expiratory (abdominal muscles) effort is required.

The forces acting on the lung at rest are:[2]

---

[2] Note: this account is simplified. The more complicated account includes transpulmonary pressure – the difference in pressure between the inside (i.e. alveolar) and the outside (i.e. intrapleural) of the lungs.

- **Intrapleural pressure** P_{pl}. There are two layers of pleura that encase the lungs: visceral and parietal. The inner visceral pleura coats each of the lungs, whilst the outer parietal pleura is attached to the chest wall. The space between the visceral and parietal pleurae (the intrapleural space) contains a few millilitres of pleural fluid whose role is to minimise friction between the pleurae. The pressure in the intrapleural space is normally negative (around -5 cmH$_2$O at rest) due to the chest wall's tendency to spring outwards.
- **Inward elastic recoil** P_{el}. The stretched elastic fibres of the lung parenchyma exert an inward force, tending to collapse the lung inwards.

At rest, the lung is at FRC: P_{pl} and P_{el} are equal and opposite (Figure 7.3a). The pressure in the alveoli equals atmospheric pressure and airflow ceases.

- **During tidal inspiration** (Figure 7.3b):
  - Diaphragmatic contraction increases the vertical dimension of the lungs. The diaphragm descends 1–2 cm during quiet tidal breathing, but can descend as much as 10 cm during maximal inspiration.
  - Contraction of the external intercostal muscles increases the anterior–posterior diameter of the thoracic cage; this is the so-called 'bucket handle' mechanism.

Arguably the most important aspect of lung mechanics is the airtight nature of the thoracic cage:

  - When inspiratory muscle contraction increases the volume of the thoracic cavity, P_{pl} falls from the resting value of -5 cmH$_2$O to -8 cmH$_2$O (as is typically generated during tidal breathing).
  - P_{pl} exceeds the inward elastic recoil of the lung and the lung expands.
  - As the alveolar volume increases:
    - The alveoli pressure P_A becomes subatmospheric, resulting in air entry.
    - The elastic fibres of the lung are stretched. P_{el} increases until end-inspiration, where P_{el} is again equal to P_{pl}. P_A is now equal to atmospheric pressure again and gas flow ceases (Figure 7.3c).

Transpulmonary pressure determines whether the lung has a tendency to inflate or deflate.

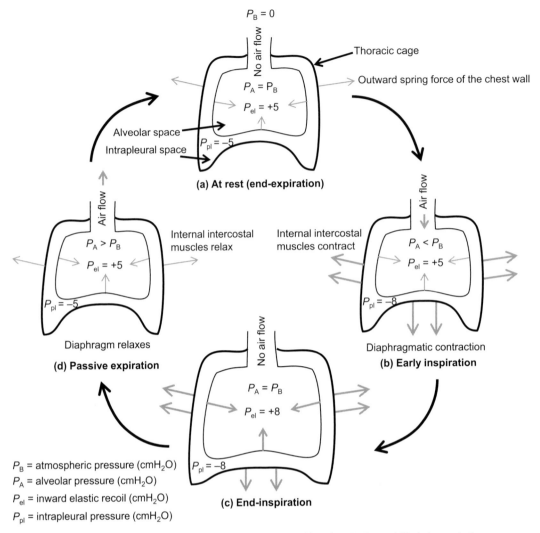

Figure 7.3 Forces acting on the lung: (a) at rest; (b) early inspiration; (c) end-inspiration and (d) during expiration.

- The volume of air inspired per breath depends on the lung compliance (volume per unit pressure change; see Chapter 20). For example, a decrease in intrapleural pressure of 3 cmH$_2$O may generate a 500-mL tidal volume (V_T) in normal lungs, but much less in a patient with acute respiratory distress syndrome.

- **During tidal expiration** (Figure 7.3d):

  - The inspiratory muscles relax.
  - The ribcage and the diaphragm passively return to their resting positions and the volume of the thoracic cavity decreases.

Because the thoracic cage is airtight:

- Decreasing thoracic cage volume causes P_{pl} to fall back to –5 cmH$_2$O.
- The stretched lung elastic fibres passively return lung volume to FRC.
- As lung volume decreases, the alveolar volume falls, resulting in an increase in alveolar pressure. P_A exceeds P_B and air is expelled from the lungs.
- Air continues to flow out of the lungs until P_A again equals P_B at end-expiration.

What are the non-respiratory functions of the lung?

The non-respiratory functions of the lung are:

- **Immunological and lung defence.** The lung has an enormous 70 m^2 of alveolar surface area to defend against microorganisms. This compares with a skin surface area of 2 m^2 and an intestinal surface area of 300 m^2. Lung defence mechanisms include:

  - Filtering inspired air;
  - The mucociliary escalator;
  - Alveolar macrophages;
  - Secretion of immunoglobulin A.

  The upper airway reflexes of coughing and sneezing also play key roles in lung defence.

- **Vascular.** The pulmonary circulation is discussed in greater detail in Chapter 23.

- **Metabolic and endocrine.** As nearly the entire cardiac output passes through the lungs, they are ideally suited for metabolic and endocrine processes, most notably:

  - Inactivation of noradrenaline, serotonin, prostaglandins, bradykinin (see below) and acetylcholine. Adrenaline, antidiuretic hormone and angiotensin II pass through the lungs unaltered.

  - Conversion of angiotensin I to angiotensin II by angiotensin-converting enzyme (ACE). ACE is also one of three enzymes responsible for the metabolism of bradykinin. Inhibition of ACE with ACE inhibitors leads to excess bradykinin, which can cause an intractable cough and has been implicated in ACE inhibitor-induced angioedema.

  - Synthesis of surfactant, nitric oxide and heparins.

  - Synthesis, storage and release of pro-inflammatory mediators: histamine, eicosanoids, endothelin, platelet-aggregating factor and adenosine.

A number of anaesthetic drugs undergo significant uptake and first-pass metabolism in the lungs, including lignocaine (lidocaine), fentanyl and noradrenaline.

Further reading

A. B. Lumb. Elastic forces and lung volumes. In: A. B. Lumb. *Nunn's Applied Respiratory Physiology, 8th edition*. London, Churchill Livingstone, 2016; 13–32.

A. B. Lumb. Nonrespiratory functions in the lung. In: A. B. Lumb. *Nunn's Applied Respiratory Physiology, 8th edition*. London, Churchill Livingstone, 2016; 203–16.

V. Ashok, J. Francis. A practical approach to adult one-lung ventilation. *BJA Education* 2018; **18**(3): 69–74.

J. Spaeth, M. Ott, W. Karzai, et al. Double-lumen tubes and auto-PEEP during one-lung ventilation. *Br J Anaesth* 2016; **116**(1): 122–30.

A. R. Wilkes. Heat and moisture exchangers and breathing system filters: their use in anaesthesia and intensive care. Part 1 – history, principles and efficiency. *Anaesthesia* 2011; **66**(1): 31–9.

W. Mitzner. Airway smooth muscle: the appendix of the lung. *Am J Respir Crit Care Med* 2004; **169**(7): 787–90.

Chapter

8

Oxygen Transport

How is oxygen transported in the blood?

O_2 is carried within the circulation from the lungs to the tissues in two forms:

- **Bound to haemoglobin** (Hb), accounting for 98% of O_2 carried by the blood. Each gram of fully saturated Hb can bind 1.34 mL of O_2 (this is called Hüfner's constant).
- **Dissolved in plasma**, accounting for 2% of O_2 carried by the blood. The volume of O_2 dissolved in blood is proportional to the partial pressure of O_2 (this is Henry's law).

The total volume of O_2 carried by the blood is the sum of the two:

Key equation: oxygen content equation

O_2 content per 100 mL of blood = $(1.34 \times$ [Hb] $\times S_aO_2/100\%) + 0.023 \times PO_2$, where 1.34 mL/g is Hüfner's constant at 37°C for typical adult blood, [Hb] is the Hb concentration (g/dL), S_aO_2 is the percentage Hb O_2 saturation, 0.023 is the solubility coefficient for O_2 in water ($mLO_2.dL^{-1}.kPa^{-1}$) and PO_2 is the blood O_2 tension (kPa).

For typical arterial blood ([Hb] = 15 g/dL, S_aO_2 = 97% and PO_2 = 13.0 kPa):

O_2 content per 100 mL arterial blood (C_aO_2) = $(1.34 \times 15 \times 0.97) + 0.023 \times 13 = 19.50 + 0.30 = 19.8$ mL

whereas venous blood (Hb O_2 saturation of 75%, PO_2 = 5.3 kPa) contains

O_2 content per 100 mL venous blood (C_vO_2) = $(1.34 \times 15 \times 0.75) + 0.023 \times 5.3 = 15.08 + 0.12 = 15.2$ mL

The above worked example demonstrates that Hb is a much more efficient means of O_2 carriage than O_2 dissolved in plasma. However, it would be wrong to think that dissolved O_2 is unimportant. The O_2 tension of blood is determined from the amount of O_2 dissolved in plasma – the PO_2 within a red blood cell

(RBC) is low because all the O_2 is bound to Hb. Fick's law of diffusion states that diffusion occurs along a pressure gradient, so O_2 diffuses to the tissues from the dissolved portion in the plasma, not from Hb itself. O_2 then dissociates from Hb as plasma PO_2 falls, replenishing the O_2 dissolved in the plasma.

How do the body's oxygen stores compare with its consumption of oxygen?

Very little O_2 is stored in the body, which means that periods of apnoea can rapidly lead to hypoxia. In addition to O_2 in the lungs (within the functional residual capacity), O_2 is stored in the blood (dissolved in plasma and bound to Hb) and in the muscles (bound to myoglobin).

As described above, approximately 20 mL of O_2 is carried in each 100 mL of arterial blood and 15 mL of O_2 per 100 mL of venous blood. At sea level, a 70-kg man has approximately:

- 5 L of blood, containing approximately 850 mL of O_2;
- A further 250 mL of O_2 bound to myoglobin;
- 450 mL of O_2 in the lungs when breathing air.

This gives a total of 1550 mL of O_2.

An adult's resting O_2 consumption is approximately 250 mL/min, which means that apnoea need only occur for a few minutes before the onset of significant cellular hypoxia. Hypoxic damage occurs even more quickly when there is reduced O_2-carrying capacity (e.g. anaemia or carbon monoxide poisoning) or an increased rate of O_2 consumption (e.g. in children).

Clinical relevance: minimal-flow anaesthesia

Low-flow and minimal-flow anaesthesia are anaesthetic re-breathing techniques used to reduce the

---

cost and environmental impact of general anaesthesia. Fresh gas flow rates are set below alveolar ventilation, and the exhaled gases are reused once CO_2 has been removed. Either low (<1000 mL/min) or minimal (<500 mL/min) fresh gas flow rates are used. The other requirements for this technique are a closed (or semi-closed) anaesthetic circuit (usually a circle system), a CO_2 absorber, an out-of-circle vaporiser and a gas analyser.

When using low fresh gas flows, the anaesthetist must ensure that the gases absorbed by the patient (i.e. O_2 and volatile anaesthetic agents) are replaced. The resting adult O_2 consumption is 250 mL/min; therefore, the minimum required O_2 delivery rate is 250 mL/min. However, most anaesthetists would deliver a slightly greater rate of O_2 than this (300–500 mL/min) to ensure that the patient never becomes hypoxaemic.

Describe the structure of RBCs

RBCs are small, flexible, biconcave discs (diameter 6–8 μm) that are able to deform to squeeze through the smallest of capillaries (around 3 μm in diameter). The cell membrane exterior has a number of antigens that are important in blood transfusion medicine: the ABO blood group system is composed of cell surface carbohydrate-based antigens, while the rhesus blood group system is formed by transmembrane proteins (see Chapter 73).

RBCs are unique as they have no nucleus and their cytoplasm has no mitochondria – effectively, RBCs can be considered to be 'bags of Hb'. By the time blast cells have become reticulocytes – the final cell stage of erythropoiesis – their nuclear DNA has been lost. Reticulocytes instead have a network of ribosomal RNA (hence the name: reticular, meaning net-like). Reticulocytes normally make up 1% of circulating RBCs, but this proportion may be increased if erythropoiesis in the bone marrow is highly active, such as in haemolytic anaemia or following haemorrhage.

As the RBC cytoplasm does not contain mitochondria, aerobic metabolism is not possible. RBCs are unique, as they constitute the only cell type that is entirely dependent on glucose and the glycolytic pathway (see Chapter 77) to provide energy for metabolic processes – even the brain can adapt to use ketone bodies in times of starvation.

What is Hb?

Hb is a large iron-containing protein contained within RBCs. The most common form of adult Hb is HbA, accounting for over 95% of the circulating Hb in the adult. It has a quaternary structure comprising four polypeptide globin subunits (two α-chains and two β-chains) in an approximately tetrahedral arrangement. The four globin chains are held together with weak electrostatic forces. Each globin chain has its own haem group, an iron-containing porphyrin ring with iron in the ferrous state (Fe^{2+}). O_2 molecules are reversibly bound to each haem group through a weak coordinate bond to the Fe^{2+} ion. In total, four O_2 molecules can be bound to each Hb molecule, one for each haem group (Figure 8.1).

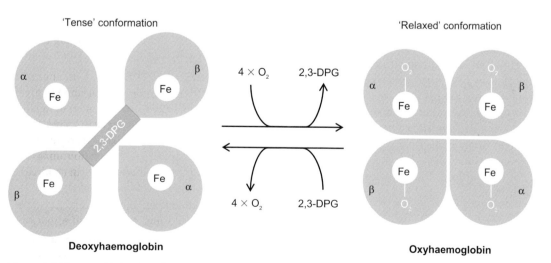

Figure 8.1 The reversible binding of O_2 to Hb (2,3-DPG = 2,3-diphosphoglycerate).

What is cooperative binding?

Hb is essentially either fully saturated with O_2 (oxy-haemoglobin) or fully desaturated (deoxyhaemoglobin) due to cooperativity.

Cooperative binding is the increase in O_2 affinity of Hb with each successive O_2 binding:

- The first O_2 molecule binds with relative difficulty – strong electrostatic charges must be overcome to achieve the required conformational changes in the Hb molecule. This conformation is referred to as the 'tense' conformation, where the β-chains are far apart.
- Once the first O_2 molecule has bound, the conformation of Hb changes and the β-chains come closer together.[1] This new conformation results in a second O_2 molecule having a higher binding affinity, thus requiring less energy to bind.
- Once the second O_2 molecule has bound, the third is easier to bind, and so on. In fact, the fourth O_2 molecule binds 300 times more easily than the first.
- Once the fourth O_2 molecule has bound, Hb is said to be in the 'relaxed' conformation.

What is the oxyhaemoglobin dissociation curve?

The oxyhaemoglobin dissociation curve describes the relationship between S_aO_2 and blood O_2 tension (Figure 8.2). As discussed above, the cooperative binding of Hb is responsible for the curve's sigmoid shape, which has important clinical consequences:

- The upper portion of the curve is flat. At this point, even if P_aO_2 falls a little, S_aO_2 hardly changes. However, when a patient's P_aO_2 is pathologically low (e.g. in patients with respiratory disease), the patient is at a much steeper part of the curve; here, a small decrease in P_aO_2 results in a large desaturation.
- The steep part of the curve is very important in the peripheral tissues, where PO_2 is low: a large quantity of O_2 is offloaded for only a small decrease in PO_2.

---

[1] The actual molecular mechanism of cooperative binding is still a subject of debate. It has been suggested that binding O_2 to Fe^{2+} simultaneously displaces a histidine residue, resulting in a conformation change.

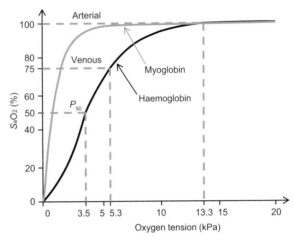

Figure 8.2 The oxyhaemoglobin and oxymyoglobin dissociation curves.

The position of the oxyhaemoglobin dissociation curve is described by the P_{50} value – the PO_2 at which 50% of Hb is bound to O_2. When the position of the curve moves to the right, the affinity of O_2 for Hb is reduced – O_2 is more easily offloaded (i.e. for a given PO_2, S_aO_2 is lower). Rightward shift is caused by (Figure 8.3):

- Increased PCO_2;
- Acidosis;
- Increased 2,3-diphosphoglycerate (DPG) concentration;
- Exercise;
- Increased temperature;
- The presence of sickle haemoglobin (HbS) in sickle cell disease.

(Mnemonic: CADETS – CO_2, acidosis, DPG, exercise, temperature, sickle cell disease)

This rightward shift of the curve is an important physiological mechanism:

- **The Bohr effect.** Metabolically active tissues produce CO_2, heat and H^+ ions. When blood arrives at these capillaries, the oxyhaemoglobin dissociation curve is shifted to the right, offloading O_2 where it is most needed.
- **Anaerobic metabolism.** When cellular PO_2 falls below a threshold value, anaerobic metabolism predominates. Energy is produced through the breakdown of glucose to pyruvate (in a process called glycolysis – see Chapter 77), which is then

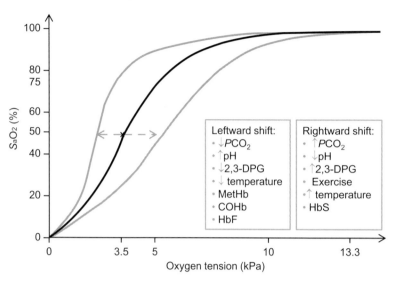

Figure 8.3 Displacement of the P_{50} of the oxyhaemoglobin dissociation curve (2,3-DPG = 2,3-diphosphoglycerate; COHb = carboxyhaemoglobin; MetHb = methaemoglobin; HbF = foetal haemoglobin; HbS = sickle haemoglobin).

converted to lactate. One of the intermediates of the glycolytic pathway is converted to 2,3-DPG in a side pathway.[2] The greater the extent of anaerobic metabolism, the greater the 2,3-DPG concentration. 2,3-DPG binds specifically to the β-chains of deoxyhaemoglobin, stabilising this configuration (Figure 8.1), thus reducing the O_2-binding affinity of Hb. This mechanism means that additional O_2 is offloaded to cells undergoing anaerobic metabolism.

- **O_2 loading in the lungs**. When blood reaches the lungs, CO_2 is excreted and the pH normalises. The P_{50} of the oxyhaemoglobin dissociation curve then returns to its central position. The binding affinity of O_2 therefore increases: dissolved O_2 binds to Hb, which in turn lowers the blood O_2 tension, facilitating O_2 diffusion across the alveolar–capillary barrier.

The oxyhaemoglobin dissociation curve is shifted to the left by the following (Figure 8.3):

- The reverse of the above – that is, low PCO_2, alkalosis, reduced 2,3-DPG levels, hypothermia;
- Carboxyhaemoglobin (COHb);
- Methaemoglobin (MetHb);
- Foetal Hb (HbF).

Leftward shift of the oxyhaemoglobin dissociation curve results in an increase in O_2-binding affinity. This is an important physiological mechanism in foetal life. HbF must be able to extract O_2 from maternal oxyhaemoglobin – HbF must therefore have a higher O_2-binding affinity than maternal Hb. This is achieved by two mechanisms:

- HbF causes a leftward shift in the oxyhaemoglobin dissociation curve, increasing O_2-binding affinity.
- While 2,3-DPG is present in foetal RBCs, it cannot bind to HbF: 2,3-DPG is only bound by β-globin chains, not the foetal γ-chain. This mechanism further increases the binding affinity of HbF for O_2.

Clinical relevance: blood transfusion

Erythrocyte 2,3-DPG concentration rapidly decreases in stored blood and is effectively zero after 1–2 weeks' storage. Low 2,3-DPG concentration shifts the oxyhaemoglobin dissociation curve to the left, increasing O_2 binding. When stored blood is transfused, it takes up to 24 h for erythrocyte 2,3-DPG concentration to return to normal.

The increased O_2-binding affinity means that transfused blood is not as effective at offloading O_2 as native blood. In contrast, cell-salvaged blood maintains almost all of its 2,3-DPG; O_2-binding affinity and O_2 offloading are unaffected.

---

[2] This is thought to be controlled by an O_2-sensitive enzyme in the glycolytic pathway, likely phosphofructokinase.

What other forms of Hb are there?

Types of Hb may be classified as physiological or pathological.

- **Physiological**:

  - *HbA*, which, as discussed above, is the most common form, has two α- and two β-globin subunits ($\alpha_2\beta_2$).

  - *HbA$_2$*, the other normal adult variant of Hb, accounts for around 2–3% of total Hb. It has two α- and two δ-globin subunits ($\alpha_2\delta_2$).

  - *HbF* is the normal variant during foetal life and is composed of two α- and two γ-globin subunits ($\alpha_2\gamma_2$). HbF has a higher affinity for O_2 than HbA and may therefore displace O_2 across the placenta from maternal blood (see Chapter 83). HbF is produced up to 3 months of age, when γ-globin synthesis switches to the adult β-globin; by 6 months of age, all HbF should have been replaced by normal adult variants. However, HbF can persist in conditions where β-globin synthesis is impaired, such as β-thalassaemia.

- **Pathological**:

  - *HbS*. Found in people with sickle cell disease, HbS has an abnormal β-globin subunit: a point mutation where glutamate has been replaced by valine at the sixth position.

  - *MetHb*. Methaemoglobinaemia is where the ferrous iron (Fe^{2+}) within the Hb molecule is oxidised to ferric iron (Fe^{3+}). Fe^{3+} cannot bind O_2, so MetHb cannot participate in O_2 transport.

  - *COHb*. This is formed when Hb binds inhaled carbon monoxide molecules.

  - *CyanoHb*. Cyanohaemoglobin is formed when Hb is exposed to cyanide ions.

How does the single point mutation cause clinical disease in sickle cell disease?

Sickle cell disease is a genetic disease inherited in an autosomal recessive pattern. Symptomatic sickle cell disease is only seen in homozygous patients; that is, where both β-globin chains have amino acid point mutations. Heterozygotic patients are said to have a sickle cell trait and are normally asymptomatic; the trait confers disease resistance to malaria.

Substitution of a single amino acid has a significant impact on how the Hb molecule behaves: under hypoxic conditions, Hb molecules aggregate, distorting the RBC into a sickle shape. Unfortunately, the O_2 tension of normal venous blood can be sufficiently low to cause sickling, especially within the sluggish flow of the spleen. As the RBCs move from arterial to venous O_2 tensions and back to arterial, repeated aggregation and de-aggregation results in reduced RBC membrane elasticity. Clinical disease occurs through two main mechanisms:

- **Vascular occlusion**. The reduced elasticity of the sickled cells means that they are less able to deform as they pass through narrow capillaries, resulting in increased blood viscosity, venous thrombosis and ischaemia. Capillary and venous occlusions threaten whole-organ infarction, resulting in ischaemic pain and organ dysfunction. In childhood, vascular occlusion commonly causes splenic infarction – patients are subsequently susceptible to encapsulated bacterial infection, such as meningococcal septicaemia and salmonella osteomyelitis. Vaso-occlusive crises are managed by hydration, analgesia and blood exchange transfusion.

- **Reduced red cell survival**. Normally, RBCs survive in the circulation for 100–120 days. In contrast, RBCs in sickle cell disease survive for a mere 10–20 days due to chronic haemolysis, resulting in an Hb concentration of 7–11 g/dL with a reticulocytosis. Sickle cell patients are susceptible to aplastic crises; for example, parvovirus B19 infection briefly stops erythropoiesis by destroying RBC precursors, preventing RBC production for 2–3 days. In normal patients, this is clinically unimportant, but the short RBC lifespan in sickle cell disease means that the brief cessation of bone marrow production can lead to profound anaemia.

Clinical relevance: anaesthesia for patients with sickle cell disease

The principles of management are:

- **Identifying undiagnosed sickle cell disease**. Sickle cell status may not be known by the patient: all patients of at-risk ethnic backgrounds should be tested. Formal screening test is by Hb electrophoresis, but in an emergency the rapid 'sickledex test' can be used (but it cannot distinguish sickle cell trait from sickle cell disease).

- **Preoperative optimisation**:
  - Identification and optimisation of end-organ dysfunction, Abnormal physiology for example, hypoxia, acidosis, hypothermia or hypotension should be addressed.
  - Exchange transfusion is sometimes undertaken before major elective surgery, but there is rarely sufficient time before emergency surgery.

- **Intraoperative management**:
  - Avoidance of known sickling precipitants: hypoxia, acidosis, hypothermia and hypotension.
  - Tourniquets are traditionally avoided, but are occasionally used if the benefits outweigh the risk of precipitating sickling.
  - Regional anaesthesia has many advantages over general anaesthesia, but neuraxial blockade risks hypotension.

- **Post-operative management**:
  - Patients should be managed in a high-dependency unit, given supplemental O_2 and kept warm and well hydrated.
  - Analgesia can be challenging, as sickle cell patients are rarely opiate naïve.

What is the clinical significance of MetHb?

Normally, MetHb makes up less than 1% of the total Hb concentration. The low level of MetHb is maintained by two mechanisms:

- **Glutathione/nicotinamide adenine dinucleotide phosphate (NADPH) system**. Oxidising agents within the RBC are reduced by glutathione before they are able to oxidise the haem Fe^{2+} to Fe^{3+}. The pentose phosphate pathway (PPP) (see Chapter 77) is integral to this process, as it supplies NADPH to return glutathione back to its reduced form.
- **MetHb reductase/nicotinamide adenine dinucleotide (NADH) system**. Any MetHb formed has its Fe^{3+} ion reduced back to Fe^{2+} by a protective reduction system involving the enzyme MetHb reductase and NADH.

Methaemoglobinaemia occurs as a result of:

- **Oxidising agents overwhelming the glutathione system**. Implicated drugs include sulphonamide antibiotics, nitric oxide and the amide local anaesthetic prilocaine (used in Bier's block or as a constituent of the topical local anaesthetic EMLA™).
- **Failure of the protective reduction system**; for example, as a result of glucose-6-phosphate dehydrogenase (G6PD) deficiency, in which a genetic defect of the PPP leads to a deficiency of reduced glutathione.

The clinical problems arising from methaemoglobinaemia are twofold:

- **MetHb cannot bind O_2**. This results in a reduced total blood O_2 concentration; that is, a 'functional anaemia'.
- **Altered O_2-binding affinity**. The presence of MetHb changes the O_2-binding affinity of the remaining normal Hb molecules. The oxyhaemoglobin dissociation curve shifts to the left, resulting in less O_2 being offloaded to the tissues.

Of further clinical significance: pulse oximeters 'misread' MetHb, displaying values of 85% irrespective of the MetHb concentration. Accurate MetHb concentrations can be measured using a CO-oximeter. Treatment of methaemoglobinaemia is with supplemental O_2 for mild cases and with methylene blue for severe cases.

How does carbon monoxide poisoning affect oxygen carriage?

Carbon monoxide is a very similar molecule to O_2 and can therefore reversibly bind to the Hb Fe^{2+} ion in a similar way to O_2. However, the Hb-binding affinity of carbon monoxide is 250 times greater than that of O_2. In the presence of carbon monoxide, Hb preferentially forms COHb rather than oxyhaemoglobin, resulting in a reduced O_2-carrying capacity. Like methaemoglobinaemia, tissue hypoxia is exacerbated by a leftward shift of the oxyhaemoglobin dissociation curve, reducing the offloading of O_2 to the tissues.

Normally, the proportion of COHb in the blood is $<2\%$. Owing to the high binding affinity of carbon monoxide, a patient exposed to low levels of carbon monoxide can still have a significant plasma COHb concentration – in heavy smokers, COHb can be as high as 9%. Even higher COHb concentrations may occur due to faulty gas appliances, house fires and following suicidal inhalation of car fumes.

Unsurprisingly, higher COHb concentrations result in more significant clinical features:

- A COHb concentration of 15–20% causes mild symptoms – headache and confusion.
- At higher concentrations – weakness, dizziness, nausea and vomiting.
- At COHb >60% – convulsions, coma and death.

Despite their reduced O_2-carrying capacity, patients with high COHb concentrations do not appear cyanosed. Cyanosis is only clinically evident when there is at least 5 g/dL of deoxyhaemoglobin, and any Hb that has not bound to carbon monoxide is usually fully saturated with O_2. Rarely, patients have a cherry-red discoloration of the skin and mucous membranes. Treatment involves competitively removing the reversibly bound carbon monoxide from Hb by providing a high P_aO_2, which may be achieved either by high F_iO_2 or by use of a hyperbaric chamber.

What are the mechanisms of cyanide toxicity?

The toxicity of cyanide is the result of two mechanisms:

- **Reduced O_2-carrying capacity.** In contrast to carbon monoxide, cyanide binds irreversibly to the O_2-binding site of the Hb Fe^{2+} ion, resulting in a functional anaemia that cannot be treated with O_2.
- **Inhibition of the electron transport chain.** The main toxic effect of cyanide is inhibition of cytochrome c oxidase (Complex IV) of the mitochondrial electron transport chain (see Chapter 77).

Thus, in cyanide poisoning, not only is there a reduced O_2-carrying capacity, but also the mitochondria are unable to make use of the O_2 that reaches them. One of the clinical signs of cyanide poisoning is the bright red colour of venous blood, where the blood has passed through the tissue capillary network without offloading O_2. In other words, mixed venous Hb O_2 saturation is raised, with a lactic acidosis resulting from anaerobic metabolism.

Clinical relevance: cyanide poisoning

Although cyanide poisoning is a popular mode of death in fiction books (in part due to the lethal dose

---

being only 1 mg/kg), cyanide toxicity is relatively rare. Cyanide toxicity occasionally occurs in the industrial setting and following administration of sodium nitroprusside, but most commonly occurs following inhalation of smoke from burning nylon materials in house fires.

The management of cyanide poisoning has recently changed. In addition to the usual supportive measures, hydroxocobalamin (vitamin B_{12a}) is given in high doses. The cobalt cation of hydroxocobalamin binds cyanide ions, forming cyanocobalamin (vitamin B_{12}), which is non-toxic and renally excreted. Crucially, hydroxocobalamin can enter the mitochondria, where it irreversibly binds cyanide ions, thus restoring oxidative metabolism.

What about myoglobin? What is its structure and oxygen-binding profile?

Like Hb, myoglobin is a large, O_2-binding, iron-containing protein, but it contains only one globin chain and one haem group. The role of myoglobin is O_2 storage; it is therefore located in skeletal muscle, where O_2 demand is high. Myoglobin Fe^{2+} pigments are responsible for the red colour of red meats.

Owing to its single globin chain, myoglobin is unable to exhibit the cooperative binding of Hb. The oxymyoglobin dissociation curve is a hyperbolic shape, positioned well to the left of the oxyhaemoglobin dissociation curve (Figure 8.2). The P_{50} value of myoglobin is much lower than Hb to allow transfer of O_2 from oxyhaemoglobin to myoglobin.

Further reading

A. B. Lumb. Oxygen. In: A. B. Lumb. *Nunn's Applied Respiratory Physiology, 8th edition*. London, Churchill Livingstone, 2016; 169–202.

L. Herbert, P. Magee. Circle systems and low-flow anaesthesia. *BJA Education* 2017; **17**(9): 301–5.

J.-O. C. Dunn, M. G. Mythen, M. P. Grocott. Physiology of oxygen transport. *BJA Education* 2016; **16**(10): 341–8.

P. Gill, R. V. Martin. Smoke inhalation injury. *BJA Education* 2015; **15**(3): 143–8.

M. Wilson, P. Forsyth, J. Whiteside. Haemoglobinopathy and sickle cell disease. *Continuing Educ Anaesth Crit Care Pain* 2010; **10**(1): 24–8.

A. D. Pitkin, N. J. H. Davies. Hyperbaric oxygen therapy. *Contin Educ Anaesth Crit Care Pain* 2001; **1**(5): 150–6.

Carbon Dioxide Transport

How does carbon dioxide production and storage compare with that of oxygen?

CO_2 is produced in the tissues as a by-product of aerobic metabolism. One of the important roles of the circulation is to transport CO_2 from the tissues to the lungs, where it is eliminated.

A typical adult produces CO_2 at a basal rate of 200 mL/min (at standard temperature and pressure), a slightly lower rate than the basal O_2 consumption (250 mL/min). During vigorous exercise, CO_2 production can rise as high as 4000 mL/min.

As discussed in Chapter 8, the body contains only 1.5 L of O_2. In contrast, an estimated 120 L of CO_2 is stored throughout the body in various forms.

How is carbon dioxide transported in the circulation?

CO_2 is transported in the circulation in three forms:

- **Dissolved in plasma.** Like O_2, the volume of CO_2 dissolved in the plasma is proportional to the partial pressure of CO_2 above it (according to Henry's law). Dissolved CO_2 makes a much greater overall contribution to total CO_2 carriage than dissolved O_2 does to O_2 carriage, because the solubility coefficient of CO_2 is 20 times greater than that of O_2.

- **Bound to Hb and other proteins as carbamino compounds.** Not to be confused with COHb (carbon monoxide bound to Hb), carbaminohaemoglobin is a compound formed when CO_2 reacts with a terminal amine group within the Hb molecule. The amine groups involved are the side chains of arginine and lysine within the globin chains: $CO_2 + HbNH_2 \rightarrow HbNHCOOH$ – this is carbaminohaemoglobin. Deoxyhaemoglobin forms carbamino compounds more readily than does oxyhaemoglobin (see Haldane effect below).

- **As bicarbonate.** The enzyme carbonic anhydrase (CA) catalyses the reaction between CO_2 and water to form H_2CO_3. The cytoplasm of red blood cells (RBCs) contains ample CA, whereas CA is absent in plasma. The reaction between CO_2 and water can therefore only occur within the RBC. Almost all the H_2CO_3 then dissociates into HCO_3^- and protons (H^+):

$$CO_2 + H_2O \rightleftharpoons H_2CO_3 \rightleftharpoons H^+ + HCO_3^-$$

  CO_2 and water are able to directly diffuse through the RBC membrane, whilst H^+ and HCO_3^- cannot. As the CA reaction between CO_2 and water is an equilibrium reaction, it would cease if the H^+ or HCO_3^- formed were allowed to build up within the RBC. This is prevented by two processes:

  - *Chloride shift (or Hamburger effect).* HCO_3^- is transported across the RBC membrane down its electrochemical gradient by a specific transmembrane Cl^-/HCO_3^- exchanger. Therefore, while the HCO_3^- ions leave the RBC, joining the blood bicarbonate buffer system, chloride ions enter the RBC (Figure 9.1) to maintain electrical neutrality.

  - *Binding of H^+ to histidine residues.* As H^+ cannot cross the cell membrane of the RBC, it instead binds to histidine side chains of the Hb molecule, thereby reducing the intracellular concentration of H^+ and facilitating the Bohr shift. Deoxyhaemoglobin is able to bind H^+ ions better than is oxyhaemoglobin (see the Haldane effect below).

By keeping the levels of HCO_3^- and H^+ in the RBC low, the reaction between CO_2 and water proceeds and there is a continual conversion of CO_2 to HCO_3^-. The net effect of both processes is that a molecule of CO_2 produced by the tissues results in the addition of a Cl^- ion to the RBC, whereas the H^+ is bound and HCO_3^- is removed to the extracellular fluid. CO_2 is not osmotically active

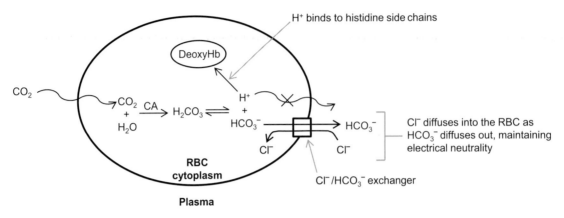

Figure 9.1 Chloride shift.

but Cl^- is; following the chloride shift, there is a small entry of water into the RBC. This is why venous RBCs have a 3% higher volume than arterial RBCs.

What is the Haldane effect? How is it related to the Bohr effect?

The Haldane effect is the observation that deoxyhaemoglobin is a more effective net carrier of CO_2 than is oxyhaemoglobin. As discussed above, this is for two reasons:

- Deoxyhaemoglobin more readily forms carbamino compounds.
- Deoxyhaemoglobin is a stronger base than oxyhaemoglobin, and hence more readily accepts H^+ than oxyhaemoglobin, allowing increased HCO_3^- formation.

The Bohr effect describes the finding that increased CO_2 tension or reduced pH shifts the P_{50} of Hb to higher PO_2 values (i.e. shifts the oxyhaemoglobin dissociation curve to the right), thereby resulting in Hb having an apparently lower O_2-binding affinity (see Chapter 8). The Haldane and Bohr effects are important physiological mechanisms in both the peripheral tissues and in the lungs with regard to gas exchange and acid–base balance:

- Metabolically active tissues produce H^+ and CO_2. Through the Bohr effect and its effect on P_{50}, additional O_2 is offloaded to the most metabolically active tissues. According to the Haldane effect, the newly formed deoxyhaemoglobin is better at binding H^+ and carrying CO_2 than is oxyhaemoglobin. The metabolic waste products are therefore efficiently transported away from the tissues to the lungs.

- In the lungs, PO_2 is high. As O_2 molecules bind to deoxyhaemoglobin, its ability to bind H^+ and CO_2 decreases, in a reversal of the Haldane effect. In consequence:
  - There is a release of H^+. The H^+ ions combine with HCO_3^- to form H_2CO_3. Catalysis by CA results in the liberation of CO_2.
  - There is a release of CO_2 directly from carbaminohaemoglobin.

As the liberated CO_2 diffuses into the alveoli and away from the blood, the Hb O_2-binding affinity increases, facilitating the loading of O_2 onto Hb, in a reversal of the Bohr effect.

What proportion of carbon dioxide is in each transported form?

In both arterial and venous blood, CO_2 is primarily transported as HCO_3^-.

- Dissolved CO_2 forms the smallest proportion of the three CO_2 transport forms.
- Venous blood has a higher CO_2 content than arterial blood, and also has a higher concentration of deoxyhaemoglobin. As discussed above, deoxyhaemoglobin more readily forms carbamino compounds than does oxyhaemoglobin, by the Haldane effect. The additional CO_2 carried in venous blood has a six times higher concentration of carbaminohaemoglobin than does arterial blood (Table 9.1).

The proportions of the different transport forms of CO_2 can be represented graphically in the CO_2 dissociation curve (Figure 9.2).

What are the principal features of the carbon dioxide dissociation curve?

The CO_2 dissociation curve describes the relationship between the partial pressure of CO_2 (PCO_2) and the blood CO_2 content (note the difference from the oxyhaemoglobin dissociation curve, which relates PO_2 and S_aO_2).

The CO_2 dissociation curve is often drawn as two curves: arterial and venous (Figure 9.2a). The typical PCO_2 in arterial blood is 5.3 kPa (resulting in a CO_2 content of 48 mL/100 mL blood), whilst in mixed venous blood it is 6.1 kPa (CO_2 content of 52 mL/100 mL blood). The two CO_2 dissociation curves are, of course, diagrammatic representations of the Haldane effect: deoxygenated blood (the upper curve) carries more CO_2 than oxygenated blood (the lower curve).

Important features of the CO_2 dissociation curve are:

- At physiological PCO_2, the CO_2 dissociation curve is essentially linear.
- As PCO_2 increases, CO_2 content continues to increase due to an increase in the fraction of CO_2 dissolved in the plasma.

Table 9.1 Approximate proportions of CO_2 transport forms.

	Dissolved	Carbamino compounds	Bicarbonate
Arterial blood	5%	5%	90%
Additional CO_2 in venous blood	10%	30%	60%

Clinical relevance: blood gas changes in apnoea

In total, the circulation and lungs contain approximately 2.5 L of immediately available CO_2 and 1550 mL of O_2 (see Chapter 8). If a healthy patient stops breathing (e.g. on induction of general anaesthesia), basal processes will continue: 250 mL/min of O_2 will be consumed and 200 mL/min of CO_2 will be produced. Therefore:

- PCO_2 will increase by 0.4–0.8 kPa/min.
- PO_2 will fall. The rate of fall is complicated, involving factors such as Hb concentration and total blood volume. Typically, S_aO_2 falls to 70% (PO_2 5.0 kPa) after 2 min.

However, if the patient breathes O_2 for sufficient time to completely de-nitrogenate their functional residual capacity prior to the period of apnoea, the quantity of stored O_2 increases to over 3 L – even after 5 min of apnoea, S_aO_2 will remain at 100%. Basal metabolic processes will continue, and after 5 min the P_aCO_2 will approach 10 kPa.

Further reading

A. B. Lumb. Carbon dioxide. In: A. B. Lumb. *Nunn's Applied Respiratory Physiology, 8th edition*. London, Churchill Livingstone, 2016; 151–68.

I. Caulder, A. Pearce. Physiology of apnoea and hypoxia. In: *Core Topics in Airway Management, 2nd edition*. Cambridge, Cambridge University Press, 2011; 9–18.

G. J. Arthurs, M. Sudhakar. Carbon dioxide transport. *Continuing Educ Anaesth Crit Care Pain* 2005; 5(6): 207–10.

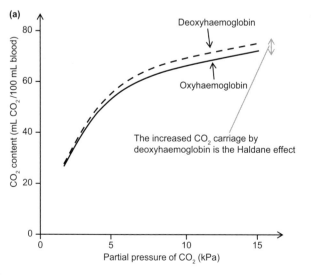

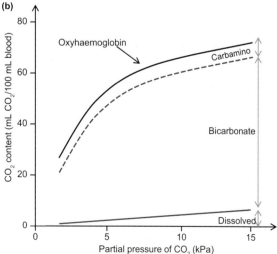

Figure 9.2 (a) The CO_2 dissociation curve and (b) proportions of CO_2 transport forms (arterial blood shown).

Chapter

10

Alveolar Diffusion

Which factors affect the rate of diffusion across a biological membrane?

The diffusion of molecules across a biological membrane is governed by five factors:

- **Fick's law.** The rate of diffusion of a substance across a membrane is directly proportional to the concentration gradient (or partial pressure gradient for gases).
- **Graham's law.** The rate of diffusion of a substance across a membrane is inversely proportional to the square root of its molecular weight (MW).
- **Surface area.** The rate of diffusion is directly proportional to the surface area of the membrane.
- **Membrane thickness.** The rate of diffusion is inversely proportional to the thickness of the membrane.
- **Solubility.** The rate of diffusion of a substance is directly proportional to its solubility.

Combining all these factors:

Key equation: rate of alveolar diffusion

$$\text{Rate of diffusion} \, \alpha \, \frac{\text{surface area} \times \text{concentration gradient} \times \text{solubility}}{\text{thickness} \times \sqrt{\text{MW}}}$$

Of the five factors:

- **Two factors relate to the diffusion barrier:** surface area and thickness.
- **Two factors are inherent properties of the substance diffusing:** solubility and MW.

So, for a given clinical situation, the only factor that can be altered is the concentration gradient; for example, by increasing the inspired fraction F_iO_2 in the case of O_2.

How is the lung alveolus designed for efficient gas diffusion?

Two aspects of lung anatomy are responsible for efficient gas exchange:

- A large surface area for diffusion. The lungs contain around 300 million alveoli, which provide a massive 70 m² surface area for gas exchange.
- A thin alveolar–capillary barrier, as little as 200 nm in some places.

It takes an average of 0.75 s for a red blood cell (RBC) to pass through a pulmonary capillary at rest, so the time available for diffusion is limited. However, gaseous diffusion within the lung is so efficient that O_2 diffusion is usually complete within 0.25 s: at rest, there is normally a threefold safety factor for diffusion. The high degree of safety for O_2 diffusion means that hypoxaemia is rarely due to a diffusion defect when compared with other factors such as $\dot{V}/\dot{Q}$ mismatch.

How do diffusion of oxygen and carbon dioxide compare in the lungs?

As discussed above, the rate of diffusion is affected by two factors specific to the substance diffusing: MW and solubility. Despite O_2 and CO_2 having similar MWs (32 Da and 44 Da, respectively), the rate of diffusion of CO_2 is 20 times higher than that of O_2 owing to the much higher solubility coefficient of CO_2. Therefore, in clinical situations where there is a diffusion defect (e.g. in pulmonary fibrosis), O_2 diffusion is more likely to be limited than CO_2 diffusion, resulting in type 1 respiratory failure. Thus, clinically significant hypercapnoea is never caused by impaired diffusion.

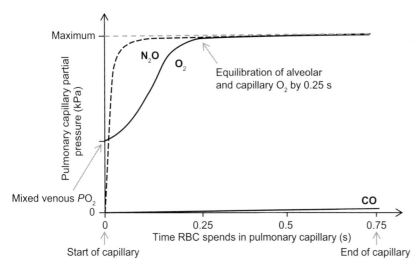

Figure 10.1 Diffusion of O_2, N_2O and carbon monoxide across the alveolar–capillary barrier at rest.

How does the diffusion of oxygen compare with the diffusion of other gases?

Comparing the diffusion of O_2 with other gases is complicated. As O_2 diffuses into the blood, most is bound to Hb, but some is dissolved in the plasma (see Chapter 8). It is the O_2 dissolved in the plasma that determines its partial pressure PO_2. At rest, an RBC takes 0.75 s to traverse a pulmonary capillary. As the RBC transits through the pulmonary capillary, diffusion of O_2 into the plasma increases its PO_2, which in turn reduces the pressure gradient across the alveolar–capillary barrier. An equilibrium is reached between the alveolar and plasma PO_2 after 0.25 s, after which net diffusion ceases (Figure 10.1).

The inspired gases relevant to anaesthesia are N_2O, volatile anaesthetics and carbon monoxide. These are all small molecules with low MWs. Carbon monoxide and N_2O are both considerably more water soluble than O_2.

Carbon monoxide binds to Hb with an affinity 250 times greater than that of O_2. Because carbon monoxide binds so strongly to Hb, virtually no carbon monoxide is dissolved in the plasma – consequently, the plasma partial pressure of carbon monoxide (P_{CO}) is very low. Even when the RBC has transited the entire length of the pulmonary capillary, there is still a substantial partial pressure difference across the alveolar–capillary barrier: an equilibrium is

never reached between alveolar and plasma P_{CO}. The transfer of carbon monoxide is thus said to be 'diffusion limited' because transfer of carbon monoxide is limited by the rate of diffusion rather than the amount of blood available (Figure 10.1). For this reason, carbon monoxide is used for testing diffusing capacity (see later).

The transfer of N_2O and the volatile anaesthetics across the alveolar–capillary barrier is different. Unlike O_2 and carbon monoxide, N_2O and the volatile anaesthetics do not bind to Hb. Because these gases are relatively insoluble and can only be carried in plasma in a dissolved form, an equilibrium is rapidly reached between the alveolus and the plasma, well before the RBC has traversed the pulmonary capillary (Figure 10.1). N_2O reaches equilibrium the most rapidly, within 0.075 s. N_2O is therefore said to be *perfusion limited* because more N_2O would diffuse from the alveolus if there were additional blood available. The volatile anaesthetics behave in a similar manner, but equilibrium is reached slightly later than for N_2O.

Is the transfer of oxygen perfusion or diffusion limited?

Under normal conditions (as exist in Figure 10.1), the transfer of O_2 across the alveolar–capillary barrier is perfusion limited. Like N_2O, an equilibrium is reached between the alveolar and capillary PO_2 before the RBC has traversed the pulmonary capillary.

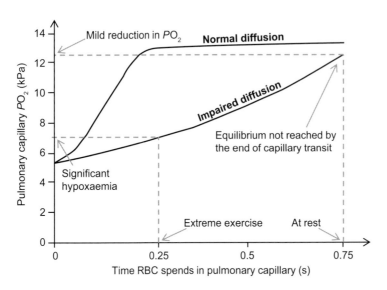

Figure 10.2 The effect of a thickened alveolar–capillary barrier and exercise on O_2 diffusion.

However, there are a number of circumstances where the transfer of O_2 may become diffusion limited:

- **Thickened alveolar–capillary barrier** (e.g. pulmonary fibrosis), which decreases the rate of diffusion. Equilibrium between alveolar and capillary PO_2 is not achieved by the time the RBC reaches the end of the pulmonary capillary, resulting in hypoxaemia (Figure 10.2).
- **Exercise.** Cardiac output increases during exercise, which reduces the length of time that an RBC spends in the pulmonary capillary. Extreme exercise can reduce RBC transit time to as little as 0.25 s. In patients with a normal alveolar–capillary barrier, alveolar and plasma PO_2 only just reach equilibrium during the available pulmonary capillary transit time (Figure 10.2). In patients with disease of the alveolar–capillary barrier, any exercise-induced reduction in RBC transit time results in hypoxaemia.
- **Altitude.** At high altitude, the lower barometric pressure P_B causes a reduction in alveolar PO_2 (see Chapters 18 and 87). This results in the transfer of O_2 becoming diffusion limited at a lower threshold (Figure 10.3). The patient with mild lung disease in Figure 10.2, where alveolar and plasma PO_2 just reach equilibrium at rest at sea level, will develop impaired O_2 diffusion at altitude. Even with normal lungs, intense exercise

can result in diffusion limitation and hypoxaemia.

What is meant by 'lung diffusion capacity'?

The diffusion capacity of the lung for carbon monoxide (abbreviated DLCO, or alternatively called 'transfer factor' or 'TLCO') is a measurement of the lungs' ability to transfer gases. It is one of the measurements taken during pulmonary function testing.

As discussed above, carbon monoxide is a diffusion-limited gas. The test involves a single vital capacity breath of 0.3% carbon monoxide, which is held for 10 s and then exhaled. The inspired and expired P_{CO} are measured – the difference is the amount of carbon monoxide that has diffused across the alveolar–capillary barrier and bound to Hb. The diffusion capacity is usually corrected for the patient's Hb concentration, but is also affected by altitude, age and sex.

The diffusion capacity is used to diagnose disease of the alveolar–capillary barrier. Diffusion capacity is reduced as a result of:

- **Thickened alveolar–capillary barrier.** For example, pulmonary fibrosis and other interstitial lung diseases (chronic), or pulmonary oedema (acutely).

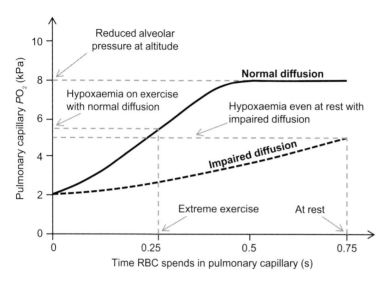

Figure 10.3 The effect of altitude on O_2 diffusion.

- **Reduced surface area for gas exchange.** For example, emphysema, pulmonary embolus and following pneumonectomy or lobectomy.

In patients who have previously undergone a pneumonectomy or lobectomy, a correction (called the transfer coefficient K_{CO}) is made to account for the loss of alveolar volume so that the diffusion capacity of the remaining alveoli can be assessed.

An increased diffusion capacity is less common, but can be found with:

- **Exercise,** following recruitment and distension of pulmonary capillaries;
- **Pulmonary haemorrhage;**
- **Asthma,** but DLCO may also be normal;
- **Obesity.**

Clinical relevance: lung resection

Pneumonectomy is associated with mortality rates of up to 8% (lobectomy mortality is around 2%). As part of the preoperative assessment, it is important to be able to predict a patient's post-operative lung function. Patients being considered for lung resection routinely undergo pulmonary function tests.

Post-operative pulmonary function is estimated using a calculation based on the measured preoperative forced expiratory volume in 1 s (FEV_1) and DLCO, and then comparing these with predicted values. By considering both the mechanical abilities of the lung and chest wall (FEV_1) and a gross measure of the alveolar/capillary function (DLCO), patients can be categorised as being at low or high risk of death and post-operative pulmonary complications.

Clinical relevance: management of a patient with diffusion impairment

As discussed above, the consequence of impaired alveolar diffusion is hypoxaemia. When managing a patient with a diffusion defect, the prevention and management of hypoxaemia is the anaesthetist's main concern.

Of the five factors that govern the rate of diffusion, solubility and MW of O_2 are fixed, but the anaesthetist has a degree of control over the other three factors:

- **Pressure gradient.** The reduction in the rate of diffusion due to a thickened alveolar–capillary barrier can be offset by increasing F_iO_2, thus increasing the O_2 pressure gradient. For example, portable supplemental O_2 is used to overcome exercise-induced hypoxaemia in patients with pulmonary fibrosis.
- **Surface area/thickness of alveolar–capillary membrane.** In the specific case of acute pulmonary oedema, raised pulmonary venous pressure results in fluid extravasation into the alveoli and pulmonary interstitium. The alveolar–capillary barrier is thickened and the area available for gas exchange is reduced, both of which reduce the rate of diffusion. In addition to increasing the F_iO_2, positive end-expiratory pressure can be applied, which:

  - Recruits collapsed alveoli, thus increasing the surface area for diffusion.
  - Increases alveolar pressure to redistribute alveolar oedema, thus reducing the thickness of the alveolar–capillary barrier.

Further reading

A. B. Lumb. Diffusion of respiratory gases. In: A. B. Lumb. *Nunn's Applied Respiratory Physiology, 8th edition*. London, Churchill Livingstone, 2016; 137–50.

J.-O. C. Dunn, M. G. Mythen, M. P. Grocott. Physiology of oxygen transport. *BJA Education* 2016; **16** (10): 341–8.

G. Gould, A. Pearce. Assessment of suitability for lung resection. *Continuing Educ Anaesth Crit Care Pain* 2006; **6**(3): 97–100.

P. Agostoni, M. Bussotti, G. Cattadori, et al. Gas diffusion and alveolar–capillary unit in chronic heart failure. *Eur Heart J* 2006; **27**(21): 2538–43.

Ventilation and Dead Space

In the lungs, what is meant by the term 'dead space'?

The air inspired during a normal breath V_T is divided into:

- **Alveolar volume** V_A, the volume of air which reaches perfused alveoli.
- **Dead space** V_D, the volume of inspired air that plays no part in gas exchange; that is, the air remaining in either the conducting airways or non-perfused alveoli.

Mathematically:

$$V_T = V_A + V_D$$

What are the different types of dead space?

Dead space is classified as 'anatomical', 'alveolar' or 'physiological':

- **Anatomical dead space** V_D^{Anat} is the volume of the upper airways and first 16 generations of the tracheobronchial tree, which form the conducting airways (see Chapters 6 and 7).
- **Alveolar dead space** V_D^{Alv} is the total volume of the ventilated alveoli that are unable to take part in gas exchange due to insufficient perfusion (i.e. due to $\dot{V}/\dot{Q}$ mismatch; see Chapter 15).
- **Physiological dead space** V_D^{Phys} is the total dead space; that is, the sum of anatomical and alveolar dead space:

$$V_D^{Phys} = V_D^{Anat} + V_D^{Alv}$$

What factors affect anatomical dead space? How is anatomical dead space measured?

V_D^{Anat} is measured using Fowler's method (see p. 47). Typical V_D^{Anat} is 150 mL for a 70-kg man; that is,

approximately 2 mL/kg, or around a third of the normal V_T (7 mL/kg). V_D^{Anat} may be altered by a number of factors:

- **Size of patient**: V_D^{Anat} increases as the size of the lungs increases.
- **Lung volume**: at high lung volumes, radial traction on the airway walls increases airway diameter, thus increasing V_D^{Anat}.
- **Posture**: lung volume decreases in the supine position, which reduces airway diameter and therefore reduces V_D^{Anat}.
- **Bronchoconstriction** reduces airway diameter: V_D^{Anat} therefore decreases.
- **Bronchodilatation** increases airway diameter: V_D^{Anat} therefore increases.

How is alveolar dead space measured and what factors affect it?

Alveolar dead space cannot be measured directly. As $V_D^{Phys} = V_D^{Anat} + V_D^{Alv}$, the alveolar dead space can be calculated if V_D^{Phys} and V_D^{Anat} are known. V_D^{Phys} is measured using the Bohr equation (see p. **48**) and V_D^{Anat} is measured using Fowler's method. In normal lungs, V_D^{Alv} is negligible as alveolar ventilation and perfusion are well matched. However, V_D^{Alv} may increase as a result of:

- **Upright posture**. Owing to the effect of gravity, blood only just perfuses the lung apices (i.e. West zone 2 – see Chapter 16). The apical alveoli are well ventilated but not adequately perfused, which increases V_D^{Alv}.
- **Low pulmonary artery pressure**; for example, as a result of reduced right ventricular output. Like upright posture, this leads to insufficient perfusion of the lung apices, a high $\dot{V}/\dot{Q}$ ratio and thus an increase in V_D^{Alv}.
- **Positive end-expiratory pressure** and positive pressure ventilation both increase alveolar

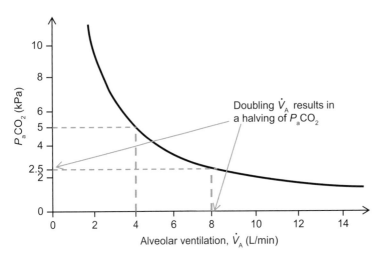

Figure 11.1 Inverse relationship between V_A and P_aCO_2.

pressure. In the lung apices, the increase in alveolar pressure causes compression of the pulmonary capillaries, reducing alveolar perfusion. This is West zone 1 (see Chapter 16). In addition, the increase in intrathoracic pressure reduces venous return to the right ventricle, which in turn reduces pulmonary artery pressure. Both effects increase V_D^{Alv}.

- **Pulmonary artery obstruction** by an embolus (arising from thrombus, gas, fat or amniotic fluid) results in the downstream alveoli being ventilated but not perfused, thus increasing V_D^{Alv}.
- **Chronic obstructive pulmonary disease.** The associated destruction of alveolar septa results in enlarged air spaces. The surface area available for gas exchange is therefore reduced. Much of the air entering the enlarged airspaces cannot participate in gas exchange, which results in an increase in V_D^{Alv}.

What is dead-space ventilation? How does it differ from minute ventilation?

Ventilation is the movement of air in and out of the lungs. There are many key definitions and formulae related to ventilation:

- **Minute ventilation** $\dot{V}_E$ is the volume of air inspired per minute,[1] written mathematically as:

---
[1] Note: V represents volume in millilitres, whilst $\dot{V}$ represents volume per unit time.

$$\dot{V}_E = V_T \times RR$$

where RR is the respiratory rate (breaths per minute).

- **Alveolar ventilation** $\dot{V}_A$ is the proportion of $\dot{V}_E$ that takes part in gas exchange, written mathematically as:

$$\dot{V}_A = V_A \times RR$$
$$= (V_T - V_D) \times RR$$

- **Dead-space ventilation** $\dot{V}_D$ is the proportion of $\dot{V}_E$ that cannot take part in gas exchange. It can be written mathematically as:

$$\dot{V}_D = V_D \times RR$$
$$= (V_T - V_A) \times RR$$

- **Overall:** $\dot{V}_E = \dot{V}_A + \dot{V}_D$

How are alveolar ventilation and arterial carbon dioxide tension related?

As $\dot{V}_A$ increases, there is an increased exchange of alveolar gas with atmospheric air. Therefore:

- As atmospheric air contains negligible CO_2, alveolar CO_2 tension (P_ACO_2) falls.
- The lower P_ACO_2 facilitates diffusion of CO_2 across the alveolar–capillary barrier, leading to a fall in arterial CO_2 tension (P_aCO_2).

In consequence, there is an inverse mathematical relationship between P_aCO_2 and $\dot{V}_A$ (Figure 11.1).

Key equation: P_aCO_2 equation

$$P_aCO_2 = K \frac{\dot{V}_{CO_2}}{\dot{V}_A}$$

where $\dot{V}_{CO_2}$ is the rate of CO_2 production through metabolism; K is a correction factor for the dissimilar units of $\dot{V}_{CO_2}$ (mL/min), $\dot{V}_A$ (L/min) and P_aCO_2. If P_aCO_2 is measured in kilopascals, $K = 0.015$.

The P_aCO_2 equation indicates three important principles:

- For a given metabolic rate, doubling $\dot{V}_A$ will halve P_aCO_2.
- If metabolic rate increases without a compensatory increase in $\dot{V}_A$, hypercapnoea will result. This is exemplified by the increasing end-tidal CO_2 concentration observed in ventilated patients with malignant hyperpyrexia.
- *Alveolar* ventilation is the key factor that determines P_aCO_2. $\dot{V}_E$ does not take into account dead-space ventilation.

Clinical relevance: hyperventilation

Consider two different patients with normal lungs:

- Patient 1: breathing with V_T of 500 mL and RR of 15 breaths per minute, resulting in $\dot{V}_E$ of 7500 mL.
- Patient 2: breathing with V_T of 250 mL and RR of 30 breaths per minute, resulting in $\dot{V}_E$ of 7500 mL.

Would you expect both patients to have equal P_aCO_2?

The answer is 'no'. Assuming both patients have a V_D^{Anat} of approximately 150 mL:

- For patient 1, $V_A = 500$ mL $-$ 150 mL $= 350$ mL

$$\Rightarrow \dot{V}_A = 350\,\text{mL} \times 15 \text{ breaths per minute}$$
$$= 5250\,\text{mL}.$$

- For patient 2, $V_A = 250$ mL $-$ 150 mL $= 100$ mL

$$\Rightarrow \dot{V}_A = 100\,\text{mL} \times 30 \text{ breaths per minute}$$
$$= 3000\,\text{mL}.$$

As patient 1 has a higher $\dot{V}_A$ than patient 2, patient 1's P_aCO_2 will be lower.

Clinical relevance: anaesthesia and dead space

In addition to alveolar and anatomical dead space, there is a third type of dead space associated with anaesthesia: that of the equipment. Mechanical dead space is the part of the anaesthetic breathing system that contains exhaled gases at the end of expiration. Whether it is a Bain circuit, a circle system or merely a

Hudson mask, all airway devices inevitably increase a patient's mechanical dead space.

Imagine a person breathing through a snorkel. When the individual exhales:

- The first gas exhaled is the anatomical dead space, which has not undergone gas exchange.
- Next, alveolar gas is exhaled. As this gas has undergone gas exchange, it contains CO_2 and water vapour and has a lower PO_2.
- At end-expiration, the entire volume of the snorkel contains alveolar gas.

When the individual comes to take their next breath, the alveolar gas within the snorkel is inspired before any fresh gas from the atmosphere – this is known as re-breathing. The problem with re-breathing is that the used alveolar gas has a lower PO_2 and a higher PCO_2 than atmospheric air, risking hypoxaemia and hypercapnoea. The higher the mechanical dead space (i.e. the volume of the snorkel), the greater the re-breathing that occurs. If the mechanical dead space exceeds V_T, the individual will solely inspire 'used' gases and become progressively more hypoxaemic.

As mechanical dead space is inevitable, anaesthetic circuits have various designs to prevent re-breathing. For example:

- The Bain circuit (Mapleson D) requires a high fresh gas flow for spontaneous ventilation – used gases are flushed along the tubing during the expiratory pause.
- The circle system is designed to allow re-breathing of gases – CO_2 is absorbed (e.g. by soda lime) and O_2 is replenished.

Some re-breathing is inevitable as a result of the volume of airway devices and tubing between the patient and the anaesthetic circuit. Because of the additional $\dot{V}_D$, $\dot{V}_E$ must increase if $\dot{V}_A$ is to stay the same. This is particularly important in paediatric anaesthesia, where mechanical dead space may represent a significant proportion of V_D^{Phys}. For this reason, mechanical dead space should be minimised; for example, by cutting endotracheal tubes, by reducing the length of catheter mounts and by minimising the use of angle pieces.

What is Fowler's method for the measurement of anatomical dead space?

Fowler's method is a single-breath nitrogen (N_2) washout used to calculate V_D^{Anat} and closing capacity (CC; see Chapter 12):

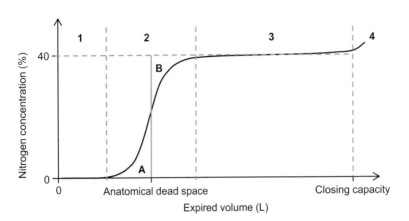

Figure 11.2 Fowler's method for measuring anatomical dead space and closing capacity.

- The patient starts by breathing tidal volumes of room air.
- At the end of a normal tidal expiration (i.e. functional residual capacity), the patient takes a vital capacity breath of 100% O_2.
- The patient then expires slowly into a mouthpiece to maximal expiration (i.e. residual volume).
- The mouthpiece is attached to a spirometer, which measures the volume of expired air. Also attached to the mouthpiece is a rapid N_2 analyser, which measures the concentration of expired N_2.

The result is a plot of expired N_2 against volume of expired gas. This graph has four phases (Figure 11.2):

- *Phase 1*: gas from the anatomical dead space is expired – it contains only O_2; no N_2 is present.
- *Phase 2*: a mixture of dead-space gas and alveolar gas is expired. The midpoint of this curve (where area A equals area B) is taken as being V_D^{Anat}.
- *Phase 3*: expired N_2 concentration reaches a plateau. All the gas expired is now alveolar gas. Note that the plateau has a slight upwards slope.
- *Phase 4*: there is a sharp increase in N_2 concentration at the CC, the lung volume at which the smallest airways in the dependent parts of the lung begin to collapse during expiration. The basal alveoli are more compliant than the apical alveoli: during inspiration, the basal alveolar volume increases more than the apical alveolar volume. Therefore, during the O_2 breath, most of the inspired O_2 enters the basal alveoli. At the start of expiration, the process reverses: the basal alveoli empty first. When the lower airways close,

the N_2-rich gas from apical alveoli is exhaled, resulting in the sudden increase in expired N_2 concentration.

What is the Bohr method for the measurement of physiological dead space?

The Bohr method is used to calculate V_D^{Phys}. The Bohr equation calculates the ratio of physiological dead space to tidal volume, V_D/V_T. The 'normal' value is 0.2–0.35 during tidal breathing.

Key equation: the Bohr equation

$$\frac{V_D}{V_T} = \frac{P_aCO_2 - P_{ET}CO_2}{P_aCO_2}$$

where P_aCO_2 is the arterial tension of CO_2 and $P_{ET}CO_2$ is the end-tidal tension of CO_2.[2]

So, to measure V_D/V_T, an arterial blood gas must be taken at the same time as end-tidal CO_2 is measured.

The Bohr equation can be derived using simple mathematics. It is based on the principle that all CO_2 comes from alveolar gas, and thus from alveoli that are both ventilated and perfused, and none comes from the dead space.

- We know that $V_T = V_A + V_D$.
- Rearranging: $V_A = V_T - V_D$.
- If we define

---

[2] Note: this is a usable, simplified version of the Bohr equation.

- – F_A as the fractional concentration of alveolar CO_2,
- – F_E as fractional concentration of expired CO_2,
- – F_D as the fractional concentration of dead-space CO_2,

then $V_T = V_A + V_D$ can be written as

$$V_T \times F_E = V_A \times F_A + V_D \times F_D,$$

which essentially states that all expired CO_2 comes from either the alveolus or the dead space.

- Dead-space CO_2 content should be zero; that is, $F_D = 0$.

$$\Rightarrow V_T \times F_E = V_A \times F_A$$

- Substituting in $V_A = V_T - V_D$:

$$V_T \times F_E = (V_T - V_D) \times F_A$$

- Multiplying out the brackets:

$$V_T \times F_E = V_T \times F_A - V_D \times F_A$$

- Rearranging:

$$V_D \times F_A = V_T(F_A - F_E)$$

- Rearranging:

$$\frac{V_D}{V_T} = \frac{F_A - F_E}{F_A}$$

- Because partial pressures are proportional to concentrations:

$$\frac{V_D}{V_T} = \frac{P_A CO_2 - P_E CO_2}{P_A CO_2}$$

This is the Bohr equation.

For ease of measurement, $P_A CO_2 \approx P_a CO_2$ and $P_E CO_2 \approx P_{ET} CO_2$, which gives the 'simplified' Bohr equation in the box above.

Further reading

S. Shaefi, M. Eikermann. Analysing tidal volumes early after a positive end-expiratory pressure increase: a new way to determine optimal PEEP in the operating theatre? *Br J Anaesth* 2018; **120**(4): 623–6.

G. Tusman, F. S. Sipmann, S. H. Bohm. Rationale of dead space measurement by volumetric capnography. *Anesth Analg* 2012; **114**(4): 866–74.

J. M. Raurich, M. Vilar, A. Colomar, et al. Prognostic value of the pulmonary dead-space fraction during the early and intermediate phases of acute respiratory distress syndrome. *Respir Care* 2010; **55**(3): 282–7.

Static Lung Volumes

What is the difference between a lung volume and a lung capacity?

A lung volume is measured directly, by a spirometer (Figure 12.1) or by a gas dilution technique (see p. 52). A lung capacity is the sum of two or more lung volumes; it is therefore a derived value. There are four lung volumes and four lung capacities (values given are typical for a 70-kg man when standing):

- **Four volumes:**
  - *Tidal volume* V_T = 500 mL. V_T is the volume of air inspired per breath during normal, quiet breathing.
  - *Inspiratory reserve volume* IRV = 2500 mL. IRV is the volume of additional air that can be inspired over and above V_T.

- *Expiratory reserve volume* ERV = 1500 mL. ERV is the volume of additional air that can be expired following normal tidal exhalation.
- *Residual volume* = 1500 mL. Residual volume is the volume of air that remains in the lungs following maximum expiration.

- **Four capacities:**
  - *Functional residual capacity* FRC = residual volume + ERV = 3000 mL.
  - *Vital capacity* VC = ERV + V_T + IRV = 4500 mL.
  - *Inspiratory capacity* IC = V_T + IRV = 3000 mL.
  - *Total lung capacity* TLC = residual volume + ERV + V_T + IRV = 6000 mL.

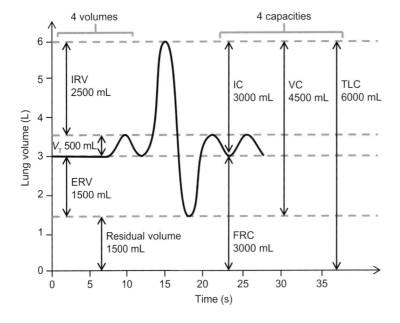

Figure 12.1 Spirometry trace with lung volumes and capacities.

Normal V_T is typically around 500 mL for a 70-kg adult, or 7 mL/kg. In mechanically ventilated patients, ventilator-associated lung injury can occur as a result of:

- **Volutrauma** – diffuse alveolar damage caused by overdistension of the lung. Traditionally, tidal volumes of 12 mL/kg were delivered to mechanically ventilated patients. This high-volume ventilation strategy is now thought to cause volutrauma and lung damage. Most intensive care units have adopted a low-V_T ventilation strategy (6 mL/kg), as it has been shown to reduce mortality in patients with acute respiratory distress syndrome (ARDS).
- **Barotrauma** – damage to the lung as a result of high airway pressure. Strategies to prevent barotrauma include maintenance of peak airway pressure P_{peak} below 35 cmH$_2$O or plateau airway pressure P_{plat} below 30 cmH$_2$O.

If a patient has particularly poor lung compliance (e.g. in ARDS), ventilation using lung-protective parameters (V_T = 6 mL/kg and $P_{plat} \leq$ 30 cmH$_2$O) may not achieve sufficient $\dot{V}_A$ to maintain normocapnoea. In this situation, it is preferable to practice 'permissive hypercapnoea' rather than increase V_T or inspiratory pressure, which may risk volutrauma or barotrauma, resulting in further lung damage. This is referred to as a lung-protective ventilation strategy.

What is the importance of the FRC?

FRC is the starting point of tidal breathing. At end-expiration, the inspiratory and expiratory muscles are relaxed – the inward elastic force of the lung parenchyma is exactly equal and opposite to the force with which the chest wall springs outwards (see Chapter 7, Figure 7.3).

FRC is physiologically important for three reasons:

- **O$_2$ buffer**. The air within the FRC acts as an O$_2$ buffer during normal breathing. O$_2$ continuously diffuses from the alveoli to the pulmonary capillaries. If FRC did not exist, there would be fewer aerated alveoli and therefore less O$_2$ in the lungs – alveolar partial pressure of O$_2$ (P_AO_2) would decrease during expiration. Pulmonary capillary blood would be intermittently oxygenated, only being fully oxygenated during inspiration.

- **Prevention of alveolar collapse**. If FRC did not exist (i.e. expiration to residual volume), alveoli would collapse. Atelectasis would result in $\dot{V}/\dot{Q}$ mismatch and hypoxaemia. Re-expansion of atelectatic alveoli with every tidal breath would significantly increase the work of breathing.
- **Optimal lung compliance**. Conveniently, lung compliance is at its highest at FRC. Pulmonary vascular resistance is also at its lowest (see Chapter 23).

FRC is of crucial importance to anaesthetists:

- **Apnoea**. FRC not only buffers swings in P_AO_2 during tidal breathing, but also crucially acts as an O$_2$ reservoir at times of apnoea, such as at induction of general anaesthesia.
- **Small airway closure**. If FRC falls below a certain volume (the closing capacity, CC), small airways close, resulting in $\dot{V}/\dot{Q}$ mismatch and hypoxaemia.

Which factors affect FRC?

FRC is not fixed; its volume is affected by surgical, anaesthetic and patient factors:

- **FRC is reduced by**:
  - *Position*. FRC falls by 1000 mL just by the patient lying supine.
  - *Raised intra-abdominal pressure*; for example, obesity, pregnancy, acute abdomen, laparoscopic surgery.
  - *Anaesthesia*, irrespective of whether ventilation is spontaneous or controlled. The cause is not known, but is thought to be related to decreased thoracic cage muscle tone and loss of physiological positive end-expiratory pressure (PEEP).
  - *Younger age*; that is, neonates, infants and young children.
  - *Lung disease*; for example, pulmonary fibrosis, pulmonary oedema, atelectasis, ARDS.

- **FRC is increased by**:
  - *PEEP*, which is commonly used to maintain FRC intraoperatively, especially in paediatric anaesthesia and following intubation (where physiological PEEP has been lost – see Chapter 7).
  - *Emphysema*. Lung elastic tissue is destroyed, resulting in reduced inward elastic recoil. The

balance between the forces of inward elastic recoil and outward springing of the thoracic cage is found at a higher volume, resulting in patients having a 'barrel chest'.

- *Increasing age.* The elderly have a reduced quantity of lung elastic tissue: FRC increases in a similar manner to emphysema.
- *Asthma*, caused by air trapping and high intrinsic PEEP.

Clinical relevance: pre-oxygenation for general anaesthesia

A normal adult lying supine (i.e. with an FRC of about 2000 mL) with a typical O_2 consumption (250 mL/min) will exhaust the O_2 within their lungs in just over 1 min. Critical hypoxaemia occurs even more rapidly in patients with reduced FRC or an increased rate of O_2 consumption.

Pre-oxygenation involves the patient breathing 100% O_2 for a period of time (traditionally 3 min) prior to induction of anaesthesia. Over time, N_2 molecules within the FRC are replaced by O_2 molecules. If the same supine patient as above had an FRC full of O_2, their lungs would contain 1800 mL of O_2 (slightly less than a full FRC of 2000 mL, as the alveoli also contain CO_2). The increased O_2 reservoir would allow the anaesthetist 8 min to secure the airway before onset of hypoxaemia.

For every five molecules of O_2 consumed, four molecules of CO_2 are produced, corresponding to the normal respiratory quotient of 0.8 (see Chapter 18). Therefore, during periods of apnoea, the total volume of the lungs decreases. If 100% O_2 is applied to a patent airway, some additional O_2 is drawn into the lungs as O_2 is consumed, further prolonging the time before onset of hypoxaemia. This is the principle behind passing O_2 into the lungs via a suction catheter as part of the 'apnoea test' during brainstem death testing.

Can all lung volumes and capacities be measured with a spirometer?

All lung volumes, with the exception of residual volume, can be measured with a spirometer. By definition, residual volume is the volume of gas that remains in the lungs at the end of maximal expiration; therefore, it cannot be directly measured. In consequence, any capacities that include residual volume also cannot be directly measured by spirometry; that is, TLC and FRC.

Instead, FRC can be calculated by one of the following three methods:

- *Gas dilution*;
- *Body plethysmography*;
- *Multiple-breath N_2 washout*.

How is FRC calculated using gas dilution?

The gas dilution method involves a patient breathing helium (He), an inert gas, through a spirometer. As He does not diffuse across the alveolar–capillary barrier, any drop in He concentration can be attributed to distribution in the lung rather than absorption into the body (Figure 12.2):

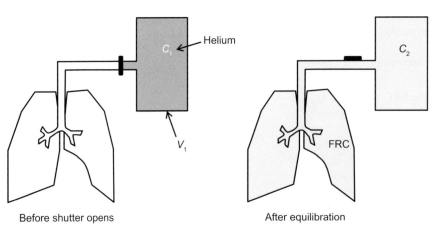

Before shutter opens   After equilibration

Figure 12.2 Gas dilution method for calculation of functional residual capacity (FRC).

- At the end of tidal expiration, a spirometer containing a known concentration of He is opened to the patient.
- The patient then breathes in and out through the spirometer for sufficient time to allow He to equilibrate between the lungs and the spirometer.
- The new concentration of He in the spirometer is then measured. From this, the FRC is calculated.

Mathematically:

- **Before equilibration**:
    - The initial amount of He is calculated from the equation:
      $$\text{Number of moles} = \text{Concentration (M)} \times \text{Volume (L)}$$
    - The volume of the spirometer is V_1 and the initial concentration in the spirometer is C_1, so the amount of He before connection to the patient is equal to C_1V_1.
- **After equilibration**:
    - The total volume is now the initial spirometer volume V_1 plus the volume in the lungs (FRC).
    - The concentration of He measured in the spirometer is lower (C_2).
    - He cannot diffuse across the alveolar–capillary barrier, so the amount of He before equilibration equals the amount of He after equilibration:

$$C_1 V_1 = C_2(V_1 + \text{FRC})$$
$$\Rightarrow \text{FRC} = V_1 \frac{C_1 - C_2}{C_2}$$

If the same spirometer is opened to the patient after a full inspiration (i.e. at TLC), the TLC can be calculated instead of FRC.

The gas dilution method may underestimate lung volumes. It is reliant on He equilibrating with all the air in the lungs, which it can only do if all airways are patent. For example, air-trapping can occur in chronic obstructive pulmonary disease (COPD): not all of the alveolar air is in direct communication with the mouth. Inspired He cannot access these closed-off alveoli, so these alveoli will not be included in the calculation of FRC.

How is FRC calculated using body plethysmography?

In contrast to the gas dilution method, body plethysmography takes into account all gas within the lung, including any gas trapped behind closed airways.

The body plethysmograph (the 'body box') is a large, airtight box in which the patient sits. The patient breathes in and out through a mouthpiece that has a shutter and a pressure transducer. There is also a pressure transducer in the wall of the box (Figure 12.3).

The physical principle behind this method is Boyle's law, which states that, 'at a constant temperature, the volume of a fixed mass of gas is inversely

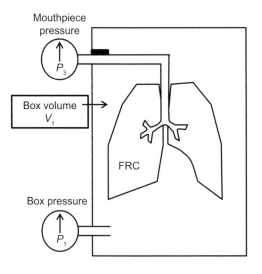

Before mouthpiece shutter closes

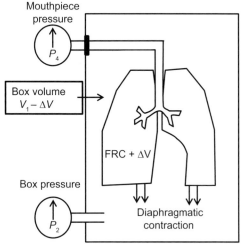

Mouthpiece shutter closes, patient tries to inspire

Figure 12.3 The body plethysmograph.

proportional to its absolute pressure'. Mathematically, Boyle's law states:

$$Pressure(P) \times Volume(V) = a \text{ constant}$$

The body plethysmograph calculates FRC as follows:

- At the end of normal expiration, the mouthpiece shutter closes.
- The patient tries to inhale against the closed mouthpiece. Respiratory effort increases the anterior–posterior diameter of the thoracic cage, increasing lung volume. The gas remaining in the lungs expands.
- As lung volume increases, the volume within the body plethysmograph decreases by an equal amount.
- The body box is airtight, so a decreased volume within the box must result in an increased pressure (according to Boyle's law, as PV = constant). This increase in pressure is measured by the pressure transducer in the wall of the box.
- First, the change in volume within the box is calculated:
  - Before closure of the mouthpiece shutter, the box pressure P_1 and the box volume V_1 are measured.
  - After inspiration against a closed mouthpiece, box pressure P_2 is measured.
  - ΔV is the change in volume in the box after inspiration:

    $P_1 V_1 = P_2(V_1 - \Delta V)$ according to Boyle's law.

  As P_1, P_2 and V_1 are measured, ΔV can be calculated.
- Then the lungs are considered:
  - Before closure of the mouthpiece shutter, the mouthpiece pressure P_3 is measured. The mouthpiece shutter closes at the end of tidal expiration, so the initial lung volume is the FRC.
  - After inspiration, the mouthpiece pressure P_4 is measured. The increase in lung volume is the same as the decrease in body box volume; that is, ΔV, which has already been calculated above.
  - Therefore, according to Boyle's law:

    $$P_3 \times FRC = P_4 \ (FRC + \Delta V)$$

All values except FRC are known, so FRC can be calculated:

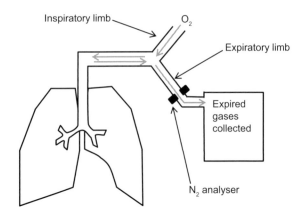

Figure 12.4 The multiple-breath N_2 washout method.

$$P_3 \times FRC = P_4 \times FRC + P_4 \Delta V$$
$$\Rightarrow FRC(P_3 - P_4) = P_4 \Delta V$$
$$\Rightarrow FRC = \frac{P_4 \Delta V}{P_3 - P_4}$$

In reality, all these calculations are made by computer.

How is FRC calculated using the multiple-breath nitrogen washout method?

Normally, N_2 makes up 79% of dry inspired air. The multiple-breath N_2 washout technique[1] involves a spirometer circuit with an N_2 analyser on the expiratory limb (Figure 12.4).

Like the gas dilution method, the N_2 washout method underestimates lung volume when there is gas-trapping. The procedure is carried out as follows:

- Initially, the patient breathes room air.
- At the end of tidal expiration (i.e. FRC), the inspired gas is switched from air to 100% O_2.
- From the next exhalation, all expired gases pass through the N_2 analyser and are collected.
- As the patient breathes in and out, N_2 in the lungs is replaced by O_2.
- The test finishes when the expired N_2 concentration is less than 1%, when all N_2 in the lungs has been exchanged for O_2.
- The total volume of expired N_2 is calculated from the total volume of expired gas multiplied by the concentration of N_2 within the collected gas.

---

[1] Note: this method is different from the single-breath N_2 washout known as Fowler's method, which is used to calculate anatomical dead space and CC (see Chapter 11).

- The FRC can then be calculated using the equation

$$\text{FRC} = \text{total expired gas volume} \times \frac{[\text{N}_2]_f}{[\text{N}_2]_i}$$

where $[\text{N}_2]_f$ is the final fractional N_2 concentration of expired gas and $[\text{N}_2]_i$ is the initial fractional N_2 concentration of expired gas.

What is the CC?

The lungs are affected by gravity. When the subject is upright, the lung parenchyma is more stretched at the apices and more compressed in the bases. One consequence of basal lung parenchymal compression is that the basal airways have a reduced radius; these airways are the first to be compressed during active expiration, resulting in a $\dot{V}/\dot{Q}$ mismatch. The lung volume at which this occurs is called the CC. Being a capacity, CC is the sum of two volumes: residual volume and closing volume.

In young, healthy adults, airway closure is not usually a problem because CC is well below FRC. If CC were to exceed FRC, airway closure would occur during normal tidal breathing, resulting in $\dot{V}/\dot{Q}$ mismatch and hypoxaemia. CC may exceed FRC because either:

- **FRC is lower than normal**, for one of the reasons discussed above. For example, CC exceeds FRC in neonates because of their reduced FRC.
- **CC is increased** – CC increases with age, encroaching on FRC at age 45 when supine and age 60 when standing.

Airway closure during tidal expiration also means that airways must be reopened during inspiration. This can increase the work of breathing significantly and is one of the factors that predisposes both the elderly and the very young to respiratory failure.

Clinical relevance: emergency anaesthesia, FRC and CC

Consider a 65-year-old patient with an acute abdomen lying supine, awaiting a rapid sequence induction (RSI) for an emergency laparotomy.

- **FRC is significantly reduced**: the patient is lying supine with an acute abdomen.
- **CC is increased**: CC ordinarily exceeds FRC at age 65.

Small-airway closure during tidal breathing results in $\dot{V}/\dot{Q}$ mismatch, even before any co-morbidities are taken into account (e.g. COPD or obesity).

Prior to RSI, the patient should have 100% O_2 administered for at least 3 min. Pre-oxygenation and induction of general anaesthesia could take place with the patient sitting at 45° to maximise FRC. Rapid and profound hypoxaemia can be expected if pre-oxygenation is insufficient. High-flow nasal oxygen therapy allows continued oxygenation during the apnoeic period and laryngoscopy attempts.

How is CC measured?

CC is measured using Fowler's method (single-breath N_2 washout method – see Chapter 11).

Further reading

K. Ray, A. Bodenham, E. Paramasivam. Pulmonary atelectasis in anaesthesia and critical care. *BJA Education* 2014; **14**(5): 236–45.

B. Kilpatrick, P. Slinger. Lung protective strategies in anaesthesia. *Br J Anaesth* 2010; **105**(Suppl. 1): i108–16.

C. R. O'Donnell, A. A. Bankier, L. Stiebellehner, et al. Comparison of plethysmograhic and helium dilution lung volumes: which is best for COPD? *Chest* 2010; **137**(5): 1108–15.

R. Sirian, J. Wills. Physiology of apnoea and the benefits of pre-oxygenation. *Continuing Educ Anaesth Crit Care Pain* 2009; **9**(4): 105–8.

The Acute Respiratory Distress Syndrome Network. Ventilation with lower tidal volumes as compared to traditional tidal volumes for acute lung injury and acute respiratory distress syndrome. *N Engl J Med* 2000; **342**(18): 1301–8.

C. J. L. Newth, P. Enright, R. L. Johnson. Multiple-breath nitrogen washout techniques: including measurements with patients on ventilators. *Eur Respir J* 1997; **10**(9): 2174–85.

Spirometry

What are the clinical uses of pulmonary function tests? What equipment is needed?

Pulmonary function tests (PFTs) are used to quantify an individual patient's respiratory physiology. A battery of tests and manoeuvres are performed to measure the performance of the different lung components:

- *Large and small airways*;
- *Alveoli*;
- *Pulmonary vasculature*;
- *Respiratory muscles*.

The clinical uses of PFTs are:

- Diagnosis of respiratory disease;
- Grading the severity of respiratory disease and guiding its pharmacological management;
- Estimation of surgical risk, in particular of thoracic surgery.

Spirometers are used for performing PFTs. There are many types of spirometer, classified as:

- **Volume-sensing**; for example, the vitalograph, based on a bellows mechanism;
- **Flow-sensing**; for example, the pneumotachograph, which is much more portable.

Which variables are measured using spirometry?

Spirometers are used to take many different lung measurements, broadly classified as:

- **Static lung volumes**. The patient breathes in and out of a spirometer, first with tidal volume breaths and then with vital capacity breaths. As discussed in Chapter 12, all static lung volumes and capacities can be measured, with the exception of

residual volume, functional residual capacity (FRC) and total lung capacity (TLC).

- **Dynamic spirometry**. Lung measurements that depend on the rate (i.e. volume per unit time) at which air flows in and out of the lungs are called 'dynamic'. Dynamic PFTs include:
  - *Forced expiratory volume in 1 second* (FEV_1);
  - *Forced vital capacity* (FVC);
  - *Peak expiratory flow rate* (PEFR);
  - *Expiratory flow–volume curve*;
  - *Flow–volume loops*.
- **Special tests** such as diffusion capacity (which gives a measure of alveolar diffusion – see Chapter 10), gas dilution and N_2 washout (used to calculate FRC – see Chapter 12).

How are FEV_1, FVC and PEFR measured?

Forced spirometry is a simple bedside test. From full inspiration, the patient breathes out as hard and as rapidly as possible into the spirometer, to full expiration, resulting in the expiratory volume–time graph (Figure 13.1).

Two parameters are measured: FEV_1 and FVC. These are compared with their 'predicted' values, based on normal patients matched for age, gender, height and ethnic origin. One parameter is calculated: FEV_1/FVC ratio – an FEV_1/FVC ratio less than 0.7 is considered abnormal. Use of this ratio identifies a relative difference between FEV_1 and FVC: a patient with low FVC will also have a low FEV_1 simply as there is less gas to be expelled, rather than necessarily being due to an obstructive pathology.

PEFR can also be calculated from the forced spirometry trace: flow is volume per unit time, so the gradient of the spirometry curve represents flow. The 'peak' flow is therefore the initial gradient of the forced volume–time curve (Figure 13.1). However,

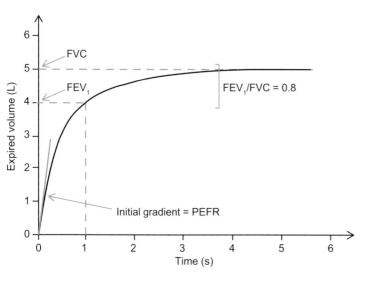

Figure 13.1 Normal forced expiratory volume–time graph.

PEFR is more commonly measured by a separate device: the peak flow meter.

Forced spirometry is particularly useful for the diagnosis of obstructive and restrictive lung diseases:

- **Obstructive airways diseases** (asthma and chronic obstructive pulmonary disease, COPD) can be diagnosed by comparing forced spirometry measurements with predicted values (Figure 13.2a). Diagnostic criteria are:

    - FEV_1 < 80% predicted;
    - FEV_1/FVC ratio < 0.7.

Severity of disease can be assessed using the FEV_1:

    - *Mild disease*, FEV_1 50–79% predicted;
    - *Moderate disease*, FEV_1 30–49% predicted;
    - *Severe disease*, FEV_1 < 30% predicted.

PEFR can also be used for the diagnosis of obstructive airways disease (a diurnal variation of >20% is suggestive of asthma), but is more commonly used to compare a patient's baseline respiratory function with that during an exacerbation.

Differentiation between asthma and COPD is based on the history and the reversibility of airway obstruction. Forced spirometry is performed before and 15 min after administration of a bronchodilator – an improvement in FEV_1 of 400 mL is said to correspond to significant airway reversibility, suggesting asthma. Some patients, usually over the age of 40 years, have chronic airways obstruction that is only partially reversible, as well as features suggestive of both asthma and COPD. This is referred to as 'asthma–COPD overlap syndrome' (ACOS). ACOS may represent an intermediary condition in the spectrum from asthma to COPD.

- **Restrictive lung diseases** (e.g. lung fibrosis, kyphoscoliosis, respiratory muscular weakness) are characterised by (Figure 13.2b):

    - FVC_1 < 80% predicted;
    - FVC < 80% predicted;
    - FEV_1/FVC ratio > 0.7; that is, 'normal' or even 'high', the latter due to increased FEV_1 from decreased pulmonary compliance.

Clinical relevance: Guillain–Barré syndrome

Guillain–Barré syndrome (GBS) refers to a collection of acute polyneuropathies characterised by motor, sensory and autonomic dysfunction. The most common variant of GBS is acute inflammatory demyelinating polyneuropathy, which is caused by autoimmune attack of the myelin-producing Schwann cells that surround the peripheral nerve axon. This variant has the classic presentation of ascending motor paralysis.

Around 25% of patients with GBS will require respiratory support due to respiratory muscle weakness or failure to clear secretions with a secondary pneumonia. Invasive ventilation is preferred over non-invasive ventilation as it enables secretions to be cleared.

It is important to be able to identify patients in need of respiratory support before respiratory failure occurs. Clinical features such as bulbar weakness and poor cough suggest a need for intubation. In addition, there are a number of well-recognised criteria for intubation, many based on spirometry.

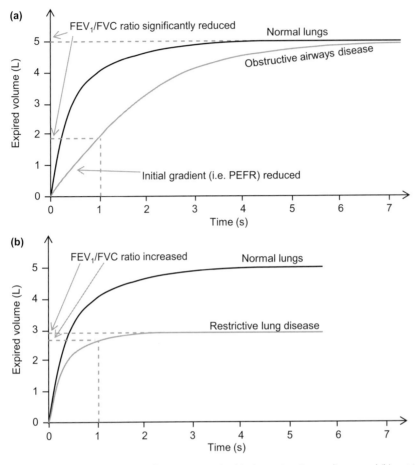

Figure 13.2 Forced expiratory volume–time graphs: (a) obstructive airways disease and (b) restrictive lung disease.

Most commonly, serial FVC is measured (at least every 6 h initially) and intubation considered if FVC falls below 20 mL/kg, or if FVC falls by >30% from baseline.

What is an expiratory flow–volume curve? What is it used for clinically?

Expiratory flow can be measured by forced spirometry. When plotted against expired volume, this results in an expiratory flow–volume curve (Figure 13.3).

The expiratory flow–volume curve can give additional diagnostic information:

- **Normal expiratory flow–volume curve** (Figure 13.3a). There is an initial rapid rise in expiratory flow, reaching a maximum at the PEFR. This part of the curve is effort dependent.

This is followed by a steady, uniform decline in flow rate until all air is expired – this part of the curve is effort independent, as it is limited by dynamic airway compression.

- **Obstructive airways disease** (Figure 13.3b). Small-airways obstruction increases the resistance to gas flow, reducing the expiratory flow rate:

  - In the effort-dependent part of the curve, PEFR is reduced.
  - The effort-independent part has a characteristic change from linear to concave, with the concavity related to the severity of disease (Figure 13.3c).

The other major difference in obstructive airways disease is the presence of air-trapping at full expiration, represented graphically by increased residual volume (Figure 13.3b). Air-trapping increases with disease severity (Figure 13.3c).

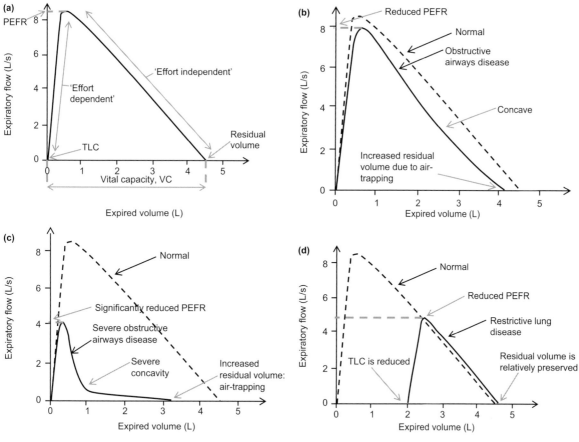

Figure 13.3 Expiratory flow–volume curve: (a) normal; (b) mild obstructive airways disease; (c) severe obstructive airways disease and (d) restrictive lung disease.

- **Restrictive lung disease** (Figure 13.3d):
  - The expiratory flow–volume curve has a characteristic reduction in TLC.
  - In the effort-dependent part of the curve, PEFR may be reduced: respiratory muscle weakness reduces the maximal expiratory effort that can be generated.
  - The effort-independent part of the curve remains linear.

Can you explain the shape of the forced expiratory flow–volume curve?

The shape of the forced expiratory flow–volume curve can be explained by considering the airway radius at different lung volumes (Figure 13.4):[1]

---

[1] This account is simplified – the more complete account is based on the 'equal pressure point hypothesis'.

- **At the start of forced expiration**, lung volume is high:
  - At high lung volume (Figure 13.4a), the lung parenchyma is generally more stretched and the radius of the airways is at its greatest. According to the Hagan–Poiseuille equation (see Chapter 21), airways of greater radius allow a much greater rate of gas flow.
  - On forced expiration, the expiratory muscles generate a high intrapleural pressure P_{pl}. This in turn generates a high alveolar pressure P_A (Figure 13.4b). Expiratory flow rate is initially 'effort dependent' – the greater the positive P_{pl} generated by the expiratory muscles, the greater the PEFR and FEV_1.

- **As forced expiration continues**, lung volume decreases:
  - The lung parenchyma becomes less stretched and the radius of the airways decreases.

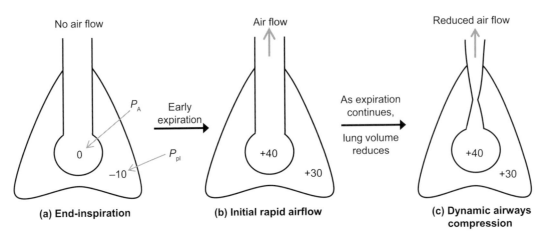

Figure 13.4 Schematic to illustrate the mechanism of dynamic airway compression.

- P_{pl} remains high.
- The smallest airways without any cartilaginous support become squashed by the high intrapleural pressure. This is called dynamic airway compression (Figure 13.4c).
- Resistance to gas flow increases, leading to a reduced expiratory flow.
- Expiratory flow is now said to be effort independent. Expiratory flow is instead dependent on lung volume, reducing linearly as lung volume approaches residual volume (Figure 13.3a).

What is the difference between a flow–volume curve and a flow–volume loop?

A flow–volume loop has an inspiratory flow–volume curve in addition to the expiratory flow–volume curve, thus completing a loop. The spirometry trace should be followed clockwise; that is, forced expiration from TLC to residual volume, followed by inspiration at maximal effort back to TLC (Figure 13.5a). The tidal volume flow–volume loop is also shown (Figure 13.5a). Note that the end-expiratory point of tidal breathing on the x-axis is FRC.

Clinically, flow–volume loops are especially useful when there is diagnostic uncertainty about the anatomical location of airway obstruction, as additional information can be gained from the inspiratory portion of the flow–volume loop. For example, a patient may present with wheeze and a history inconsistent with asthma or COPD.

- **Obstructive airways disease** (Figure 13.5b and c). As described above, the expiratory portion of the loop has a reduced PEFR, a concave rather than linear appearance of the effort-independent part of the curve and may have an increased residual volume due to air-trapping. Inspiration is relatively unaffected by small-airways obstruction.
- **Restrictive lung disease** (Figure 13.5d). As described above, the expiratory flow–volume curve has a reduced PEFR, a normal appearance of the effort-independent portion of the curve and a significantly reduced vital capacity. Depending on the severity of disease, the TLC is substantially lower whilst the residual volume is proportionally less reduced. This is shown graphically as a rightward-shifted loop with a substantially reduced FRC.
- **Fixed upper airway obstruction**; for example, tracheal stenosis or foreign body (Figure 13.6a). 'Fixed' refers to airway narrowing that is unchanged throughout the respiratory cycle. Lung volumes are unchanged, but there is a reduction in both peak expiratory and inspiratory flows, resulting in a characteristic flattening of both the inspiratory and expiratory flow–volume curves. Additional respiratory effort cannot overcome this obstruction – it is said to be effort independent.
- **Variable extrathoracic airway obstruction**; for example, vocal cord palsy (Figure 13.6b). 'Extrathoracic' refers to a level above the sixth tracheal ring and 'variable' refers to airway obstruction that is free to move with the changes

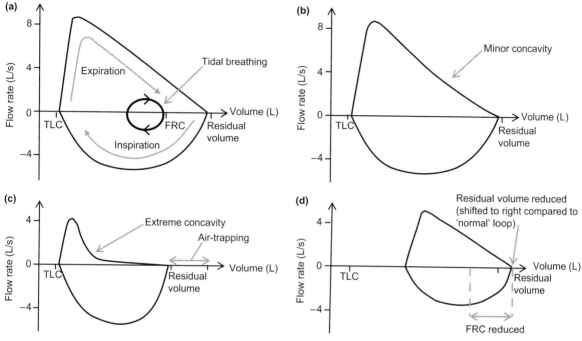

Figure 13.5 Flow–volume loops: (a) normal; (b) mild small-airways obstructive disease; (c) severe small-airways obstructive disease and (d) restrictive lung disease.

in airway pressure throughout the respiratory cycle. Again, lung volumes are unchanged. During inspiration, the subatmospheric airway pressure P_{aw} in the trachea 'pulls' the obstructing lesion inwards, reducing the inspiratory flow and thus leading to flattening of the inspiratory flow–volume curve. During expiration, positive P_{aw} 'pushes' the obstructing lesion outwards – the expiratory flow is therefore unaffected. This makes sense if you consider a patient with partial laryngospasm following extubation (i.e. a variable extrathoracic airway obstruction) – the patient has great difficulty with inspiration but not with expiration.

- **Variable intrathoracic airway obstruction;** for example, by a tumour (Figure 13.6c). 'Intrathoracic' refers to airway obstruction at or below the sixth tracheal ring. Once the airways enter the thoracic cage, they become subject to intrathoracic pressure. During inspiration, P_{pl} (and therefore intrathoracic pressure) is negative – radial traction pulls the airways apart. An obstructed airway is 'opened up', so that inspiratory flow is unaffected. However, in forced expiration, positive P_{pl} results in dynamic airway

compression, compounded by the obstructing lesion. Expiratory flow is limited and effort independent, resulting in a flattening of the expiratory flow–volume curve.

Clinical relevance: lung resection and spirometry

Spirometry is a key investigation in the preoperative workup for patients undergoing lung resection. Simple forced spirometry can predict patient suitability for lung resection:

- $FEV_1 > 2.0$ L indicates suitability for pneumonectomy.
- $FEV_1 > 1.5$ L indicates suitability for lobectomy.

When a patient's FEV_1 is less than these gross thresholds, further spirometric measurements are taken; for example:

- **Predicted postoperative FEV$_1$** (ppoFEV$_1$): a patient with a ppoFEV$_1$ < 30% of the predicted FEV_1 is more likely to require post-operative ventilation and has a higher mortality rate.
- **Predicted post-operative transfer factor** (ppoTLCO) estimates post-operative diffusion capacity. ppoTLCO < 40% of the predicted value is associated with increased morbidity and mortality.

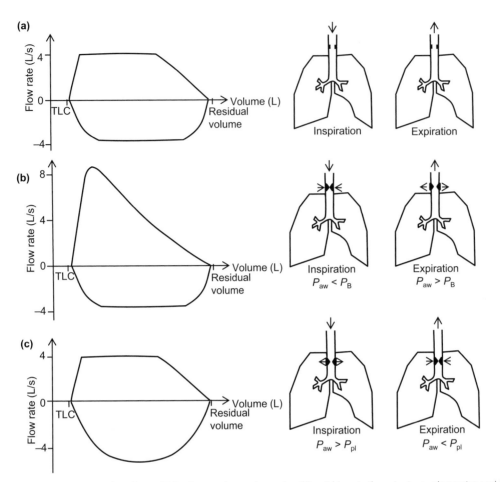

Figure 13.6 Flow–volume loops: (a) fixed upper airway obstruction; (b) variable extrathoracic airway obstruction and (c) variable intrathoracic airway obstruction (P_B = atmospheric pressure).

Clinical relevance: stridor

Stridor is an airway noise resulting from turbulent airflow during breathing. The consequence of turbulent airflow is an increase in the work of breathing. Stridor may be inspiratory, expiratory or biphasic:

- **Inspiratory stridor** usually results from a dynamic upper airway (extrathoracic trachea and above) obstruction: soft upper airway structures collapse inwards due to negative airway pressure on inspiration. Examples include croup, epiglottitis, tracheomalacia and partial laryngospasm.
- **Expiratory stridor** is due to dynamic lower airway (intrathoracic trachea and below) obstruction. Examples include tracheal or bronchial foreign bodies.

- **Biphasic stridor** is the result of fixed upper or lower airway obstruction (usually more pronounced in inspiration for upper airway lesions and in expiration for lower airway lesions). Examples include subglottic stenosis and tracheitis.

Further reading

D. Porch, B. McCormick. Pulmonary function tests and assessment for lung resection. *Update Anaesth* 2009; **25** (1): 13–21.

D. Hayes, S. S. Kraman. The physiologic basis of spirometry. *Respir Care* 2009; **54**(12): 1717–26.

K. J. C. Richards, A. T. Cohen. Guillain–Barré syndrome. *Continuing Educ Anaesth Crit Care Pain* 2003; **3**(2): 46–9.

14

Hypoxia and Shunts

What is meant by the term 'hypoxia'?

Hypoxia refers specifically to the situation in which tissues are unable to undergo aerobic metabolism. Hypoxaemia refers specifically to reduced P_aO_2. This can result from either a failure of O_2 delivery or a failure of O_2 utilisation. The following conditions must be fulfilled for cells to utilise O_2 for aerobic metabolism:

- **Adequate arterial O_2 tension** (P_aO_2) – blood leaving the lungs must be adequately oxygenated.
- **Adequate O_2-carrying capacity** – blood must have an adequate haemoglobin (Hb) concentration.
- **Adequate cardiac output (CO) and arterial flow** ensures that the O_2 carried by Hb reaches the tissues.
- **Adequate mitochondrial function** – the cells must be able to use O_2 effectively for aerobic metabolism.

Hypoxia is therefore classified in terms of failure of one or more of the processes above:

- **Hypoxaemic hypoxia** – caused by low P_aO_2. When P_aO_2 falls below 8 kPa, there is a steep fall in the saturation of Hb (see Chapter 8, Figure 8.2), which reduces O_2-carrying capacity.
- **Anaemic hypoxia** – P_aO_2 is normal but O_2-carrying capacity is reduced. This is exemplified by severe anaemia and carbon monoxide poisoning (see Chapter 8).
- **Stagnant hypoxia** – P_aO_2 and Hb concentration are normal, but circulatory failure means that tissue O_2 delivery is reduced. This is exemplified by cardiogenic shock and acute limb ischaemia following an arterial embolus.
- **Cytotoxic hypoxia** – P_aO_2, O_2-carrying capacity and O_2 delivery are normal, but the mitochondria fail to utilise O_2 effectively. This is exemplified by severe sepsis and cyanide poisoning.

What are the causes of hypoxaemic hypoxia?

Hypoxaemia can be classified according to aetiology:

- Hypoventilation;
- Diffusion limitation;
- Shunt;
- $\dot{V}/\dot{Q}$ mismatch.

How does hypoventilation cause hypoxaemia?

Hypoxaemia resulting from hypoventilation is described in detail in Chapter 18. In brief:

- $\dot{V}_A$ and P_aCO_2 are inversely related (see Chapter 11); hypoventilation therefore leads to high P_aCO_2.
- According to the alveolar gas equation (AGE; see Chapter 18), P_AO_2 decreases: the O_2 partial pressure gradient across the alveolar–capillary barrier is reduced, leading to low P_aO_2.

Is diffusion limitation an important cause of hypoxaemia?

Alveolar diffusion is discussed in detail in Chapter 10, but in summary:

- Diffusion limitation is rarely a cause of hypoxaemia.
- P_AO_2 and pulmonary capillary O_2 tension have normally reached equilibrium before the red blood cell has travelled a third of the way along the pulmonary capillary.
- Diffusion limitation can cause hypoxaemia when:
  - *The alveolar–capillary barrier is thickened*, as occurs in pulmonary fibrosis or severe pulmonary oedema.

- *Inspired O_2 tension is low*, as occurs at high altitude (altitude may also cause pulmonary oedema – see Chapter 87).
- *Exercising*, in the presence of mild disturbances of either of the above.

What is meant by the term 'shunt'?

Shunting is said to occur when blood passes from the right side to the left side of the heart without taking part in gas exchange. Deoxygenated venous blood consequently passes directly into the arterial system and mixes with arterial blood, decreasing P_aO_2.

A shunt can either be physiological or pathological:

- **Physiological shunt**, subclassified as either anatomical or functional:

  - *Anatomical shunt.* Deoxygenated blood enters the left side of the heart for anatomical reasons, such as:

    - Bronchial circulation. Most of the venous blood from the large airways drains directly into the pulmonary veins, returning to the left side of the heart.
    - Thebesian veins. A small amount of coronary venous blood drains directly into the four chambers of the heart via the Thebesian veins. The blood that drains into the left atrium and the left ventricle (LV) contributes to the anatomical shunt.

  - *Functional shunt.* A proportion of the pulmonary blood passes through poorly ventilated alveoli in the lung base. Blood leaving these alveolar capillaries will therefore not be fully oxygenated (i.e. there is a local $\dot{V}/\dot{Q}$ mismatch; see Chapter 15).

The normal physiological shunt fraction is 2–5%, approximately half of which is due to anatomical shunt and half due to functional shunt. Physiological shunt can be thought of as being analogous to physiological dead space: physiological dead space is the sum of anatomical dead space (analogous to anatomical shunt) and alveolar dead space (analogous to functional shunt).

- **Pathological shunt**, classified on the basis of its location:

  - *Intra-cardiac*; for example, as the result of a ventricular septal defect (VSD). Normally, the pressure in the LV is higher than that in the right ventricle. Accordingly, blood flows through a VSD in a left-to-right direction. However, if there were an increase in right ventricular pressure (such as in Eisenmenger's syndrome or when there is right ventricular outflow tract obstruction such as in tetralogy of Fallot), blood flow may change to a right-to-left direction, resulting in a pathological shunt.

  - *Through large communicating vessels*, exemplified by a direct communication between the pulmonary artery and either the pulmonary vein (pulmonary arteriovenous malformation, AVM) or the aorta (patent ductus arteriosus, PDA). Shunts may also be iatrogenically created, such as in the Blalock–Taussig shunt used to palliate tetralogy of Fallot. In common with a VSD, the direction of blood flow depends on the pressure in each vessel:

    - A pulmonary AVM has right-to-left blood flow and therefore results in a pathological shunt because pulmonary arterial pressure is greater than pulmonary venous pressure. Pulmonary AVMs are classified as congenital or acquired. The latter is exemplified by the multiple pulmonary AVMs that occur in hepatic cirrhosis, resulting in hepatopulmonary syndrome.
    - A PDA usually has left-to-right blood flow because aortic pressure is normally higher than pulmonary arterial pressure. However, the direction of blood flow may change if pulmonary arterial hypertension develops, as can occur with hypoxic pulmonary vasoconstriction in a neonate, resulting in pathological shunt.

  - *Intra-pulmonary shunts.* These constitute by far the commonest cause of pathological shunts. Shunting occurs when alveoli are perfused but are unable to participate in gas exchange. This may occur when alveoli are completely filled with fluid (e.g. as occurs in pulmonary oedema or pneumonia) or as a result of a proximal airway occlusion (e.g. with bronchial obstruction or one-lung ventilation).

What is the difference between shunt and ventilation–perfusion mismatch?

Ideally, ventilation and perfusion in the lung are matched. Ventilation ($\dot{V}$, L/min) in a particular area of the lung is then approximately the same as that area's perfusion ($\dot{Q}$, L/min), giving a $\dot{V}/\dot{Q}$ ratio of 1. $\dot{V}/\dot{Q}$ mismatch occurs when there is either:

- **Ventilation with relatively less perfusion**, giving a $\dot{V}/\dot{Q}$ ratio > 1. Pulmonary capillary blood transits through ventilated alveoli; gas exchange takes place, resulting in a normal P_aO_2. However, as there is a relative excess of ventilation, some of this ventilation is wasted (i.e. an increase in alveolar dead space). This results in increased work of breathing.
- **Perfusion with relatively less ventilation**, giving a $\dot{V}/\dot{Q}$ ratio < 1. Some of the pulmonary capillary blood transits through alveoli that are not being ventilated. Gas exchange cannot take place at these alveoli and therefore venous blood is allowed to enter the arterial circulation, causing a venous admixture. As a result, P_aO_2 decreases and the patient's arterial blood desaturates.

The important difference between shunt and $\dot{V}/\dot{Q}$ mismatch concerns the response to O_2 administration:

- Hypoxaemia due to a pathological shunt responds poorly to the administration of supplemental O_2. This is because, by definition, shunted blood bypasses aerated alveoli and so is never able to take part in gas exchange. P_aO_2 does improve a little with supplemental O_2 administration due to the small amount of additional dissolved O_2 in the blood.
- In contrast, hypoxaemia due to mild $\dot{V}/\dot{Q}$ mismatch does respond to O_2 administration. Increasing F_iO_2 increases P_AO_2, according to the AGE. In underventilated alveoli, this increases the concentration of O_2 available for diffusion, and P_aO_2 subsequently increases.
- Hypoxaemia due to a large $\dot{V}/\dot{Q}$ mismatch (where the $\dot{V}/\dot{Q}$ ratio approaches zero) responds poorly to O_2 administration, behaving more like a right-to-left shunt. Therefore, the difference between a severe $\dot{V}/\dot{Q}$ mismatch and a shunt is largely academic: clinically, neither responds to O_2 therapy.

What happens to arterial carbon dioxide tension in the presence of a shunt?

P_aCO_2 is related to:

- The rate of production of CO_2, which is determined by the metabolic rate.
- The rate of elimination of CO_2, which depends on $\dot{V}_A$.

In the presence of a shunt, blood bypasses the alveolar–capillary barrier. CO_2 cannot diffuse out of the shunted blood, so P_aCO_2 might be expected to increase. However, the respiratory centre responds to any increase in P_aCO_2 by increasing $\dot{V}_A$ (see Chapter 22). Therefore, in the presence of a shunt, P_aCO_2 usually remains in the normal range, but $\dot{V}_A$ increases.

What is the shunt equation?

The shunt equation is used to calculate the proportion of the CO that is shunted from the venous to the arterial system.

Key equation: the shunt equation

The shunt equation is in the form of a ratio, the shunt fraction:

$$\frac{\dot{Q}_S}{\dot{Q}_T} = \frac{C_cO_2 - C_aO_2}{C_cO_2 - C_vO_2}$$

where $\dot{Q}_S$ (L/min) is the flow of blood through the shunt, $\dot{Q}_T$ (L/min) is the total flow of blood (i.e. CO), C_cO_2 (mLO$_2$/100 mL blood) is the O_2 content of end-capillary blood, C_aO_2 (mLO$_2$/100 mL blood) is the O_2 content of arterial blood and C_vO_2 (mLO$_2$/100 mL blood) is the O_2 content of mixed venous blood.

The proportion of CO involved in a shunt can therefore be calculated if the O_2 contents of arterial, mixed venous and end-capillary blood are known (Figure 14.1).

Using the O_2 content equation (see Chapter 8):

- $C_aO_2 = [Hb] \times 1.34 \times S_aO_2 + (P_aO_2 \times 0.023)$. C_aO_2 can therefore be calculated from peripheral arterial blood gas analysis.
- $C_vO_2 = [Hb] \times 1.34 \times S_vO_2 + (P_vO_2 \times 0.023)$, where S_vO_2 is the Hb O_2 saturation of venous blood and P_vO_2 is the venous O_2 tension.

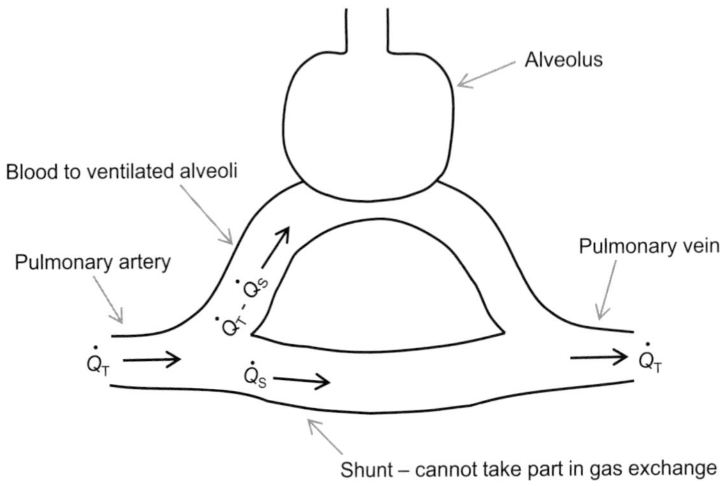

Figure 14.1 Schematic representing a shunt.

Alveolus

Blood to ventilated alveoli

Pulmonary vein

Pulmonary artery

$\dot{Q}_T - \dot{Q}_S$

$\dot{Q}_T$

$\dot{Q}_S$

$\dot{Q}_T$

Shunt – cannot take part in gas exchange

C_vO_2 can therefore be calculated by sampling blood from a central line (for *mixed* venous blood, this should strictly be from a pulmonary artery catheter).

- End-capillary blood cannot be measured directly. Instead, C_cO_2 can be estimated: as end-capillary blood has just left the alveolus, it is assumed to have an Hb O_2 saturation of 100%, with pulmonary capillary O_2 tension equal to P_AO_2. Therefore, $C_cO_2 = [Hb] \times 1.34 \times 100\% + (P_AO_2 \times 0.023)$. P_AO_2 can be calculated from the AGE using P_aCO_2 (see Chapter 18).

Overall, the shunt fraction can be calculated using arterial and central venous blood gas analysis, together with Hb concentration.

For example: normal [Hb] is 15 g/dL, P_aO_2 is 13.0 kPa with an S_aO_2 of 99%, P_vO_2 is 5.3 kPa with venous Hb saturation of 75% and P_aCO_2 is 5.3 kPa. Atmospheric pressure is 101 kPa, the saturated vapour pressure of water is 6.3 kPa and the respiratory quotient $R = 0.8$. Therefore:

$$C_aO_2 = 15 \times 1.34 \times 0.99 + 13.0 \times 0.023$$

$$= 20.2 \text{ mL}/100 \text{ mL blood}$$

$$C_vO_2 = 15 \times 1.34 \times 0.75 + 5.3 \times 0.023$$

$$= 15.2 \text{ mL}/100 \text{ mL blood}$$

Using the AGE:

$$P_AO_2 = F_iO_2(P_B - P_{SVP \text{ water}}) - \frac{P_aCO_2}{R}$$

$$P_AO_2 = 0.21 \times (101 - 6.3) - \frac{5.3}{0.8} = 13.3 \text{ kPa}$$

Therefore:

$$C_cO_2 = 15 \times 1.34 \times 100\% + 13.3 \times 0.023$$

$$= 20.4 \text{ mL}/100 \text{ mL blood}$$

Substituting these values into the shunt equation:

$$\frac{\dot{Q}_S}{\dot{Q}_T} = \frac{20.4 - 20.2}{20.4 - 15.2} \times 100 = 4\% \text{ shunt}$$

which is fairly typical for healthy lungs.

How is the shunt equation derived?

The shunt equation is not too difficult to derive.

- First, consider pulmonary blood flow:
  - According to Figure 14.1, the total pulmonary blood flow is $\dot{Q}_T$ and the blood flow to unventilated alveoli is $\dot{Q}_S$
  - Therefore, the blood flow to ventilated alveoli is $\dot{Q}_T - \dot{Q}_S$:
- Next, consider the volume of O_2:
  - The volume of O_2 in the pulmonary vein must equal the volume of O_2 in the ventilated capillaries plus the volume of O_2 in shunt capillaries.
  - The same statement written mathematically is:

$$\dot{Q}_T C_aO_2 = (\dot{Q}_T - \dot{Q}_S)C_cO_2 + \dot{Q}_S C_vO_2$$

- Multiplying out the brackets gives:

$$\dot{Q}_T C_aO_2 = \dot{Q}_T C_cO_2 - \dot{Q}_S C_cO_2 + \dot{Q}_S C_vO_2$$

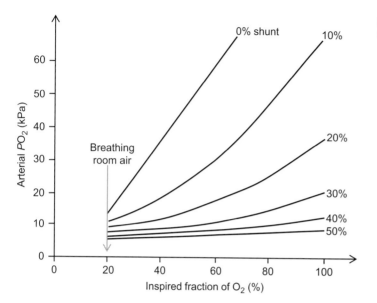

Figure 14.2 The effect of F_iO_2 on P_aO_2 at different shunt fractions.

- Rearranging gives:

$$\dot{Q}_S C_c O_2 - \dot{Q}_S C_v O_2 = \dot{Q}_T C_c O_2 - \dot{Q}_T C_a O_2$$

or:

$$\dot{Q}_S (C_c O_2 - C_v O_2) = \dot{Q}_T (C_c O_2 - C_a O_2)$$

- This leads to the shunt equation:

$$\frac{\dot{Q}_S}{\dot{Q}_T} = \frac{(C_c O_2 - C_a O_2)}{(C_c O_2 - C_v O_2)}$$

What is the effect of administering oxygen at different shunt fractions?

According to the AGE (see Chapter 18), O_2 administration (i.e. an increase in F_iO_2) leads to an increase in P_AO_2, which increases the O_2 pressure gradient across the alveolar–capillary barrier. In turn, the increased rate of O_2 diffusion leads to an increase in P_aO_2.

As discussed above, blood that bypasses the ventilated alveoli is not exposed to any extra O_2 administered to the patient. As the shunt fraction increases, more and more blood bypasses the ventilated alveoli – the higher F_iO_2 has less and less impact on P_aO_2 (Figure 14.2).

Further reading

A. B. Lumb. Distribution of pulmonary ventilation and perfusion. In: A. B. Lumb. *Nunn's Applied Respiratory Physiology, 8th edition.* London, Churchill Livingstone, 2016; 109–36.

J. R. Gossage, G. Kanj. Pulmonary arteriovenous malformations. A state of the art review. *Am J Respir Crit Care Med* 1998; **158**(2): 643–61.

Chapter

15

Ventilation–Perfusion Relationships

How does gravity affect blood flow to the lungs?

Lung perfusion[1] increases linearly from the top to the bottom of the lungs (Figure 15.1, lung perfusion line). The difference in perfusion at the top and bottom of the lung can be explained by the effect of gravity on the alveolar volume, which in turn determines the pulmonary capillary pressure. The difference in pulmonary capillary pressure between the lung apex and base is equivalent to the hydrostatic pressure exerted by a column of blood. The distance from apex to base is 30 cm, so the pressure difference is 30 cmH_2O (equivalent to 22 mmHg). The pulmonary circulation is a low-pressure system: mean pulmonary artery pressure (MPAP) is typically just 15 mmHg. A pressure difference of 22 mmHg between the top and the bottom of the lungs is therefore potentially significant (this is discussed further in Chapter 16).

The regional differences in lung perfusion are altered by:

- **Exercise.** When cardiac output (CO) increases, MPAP also increases. The difference in capillary hydrostatic pressure between the lung apex and base therefore becomes less significant; blood is distributed more evenly throughout the lung.
- **Body position.** When a patient is supine, the vertical difference between the apex and base is abolished. Instead, the anterior lung becomes vertically higher than the posterior lung. For the same reasons as above, perfusion of the posterior lung becomes greater than that of the anterior lung. Similarly, in the lateral position, the dependent lung (the lowermost) has a greater perfusion than the non-dependent lung (the uppermost).

What is the effect of gravity on alveolar ventilation?

The effect of gravity on alveolar ventilation $\dot{V}_A$ is discussed in detail in Chapter 20. In summary:

- The weight of the lung parenchyma results in intrapleural pressure being more negative at the apex than the base. At functional residual capacity (FRC), the apical alveoli are nearly fully inflated, whereas the basal alveoli are hardly inflated at all.
- At FRC, the basal alveoli have a greater compliance (i.e. a greater increase in volume per unit pressure applied) than the apical alveoli, as they are less distended by the weight of the lung parenchyma.
- During inspiration, intrapleural pressure becomes more negative, which causes the volume of the basal alveoli to increase more than the apical alveoli. $\dot{V}_A$ therefore increases from apex to base (Figure 15.1, alveolar ventilation line).

What is meant by the term 'ventilation–perfusion ratio'?

For ideal gas exchange, the ventilation and perfusion to each alveolus should be matched, giving exactly the right amount of $\dot{V}_A$ to fully oxygenate all the passing blood; that is, a ventilation–perfusion ratio $\dot{V}/\dot{Q} = 1$. Too little ventilation would lead to partial oxygenation of blood, whereas too much ventilation is unnecessarily wasteful of respiratory effort. However, normal lung perfusion is 5 L/min (i.e. normal CO) and $\dot{V}_A$ is 4 L/min.[2] The average $\dot{V}/\dot{Q}$ ratio is therefore 0.8.

Whilst the global $\dot{V}/\dot{Q}$ ratio in healthy lungs is 0.8, there is considerable regional variation. Owing to the

---

[1] Pulmonary blood flow is referred to as the 'perfusion', termed $\dot{Q}$.

[2] Note: $\dot{V}_E$ is around 5 L/min, but approximately a fifth is dead-space ventilation (see Chapter 11).

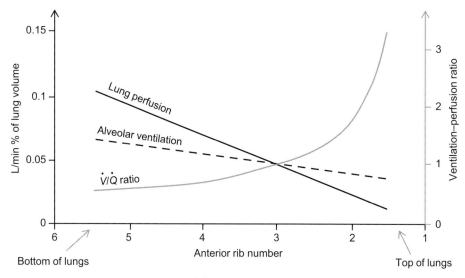

Figure 15.1 Perfusion, ventilation and the $\dot{V}/\dot{Q}$ relationship.

direct and indirect effects of gravity respectively, both ventilation and perfusion are increased in the lung bases compared with the apices. However, there is a greater effect on perfusion than on ventilation, as represented by the steeper gradient of the lung perfusion line in Figure 15.1. The $\dot{V}/\dot{Q}$ ratio therefore increases from the bottom to the top of the lungs:

- **In the bases**, the $\dot{V}/\dot{Q}$ ratio is approximately 0.6. As perfusion is greater than ventilation, blood may leave the pulmonary capillaries without being fully oxygenated, resulting in a right-to-left shunt. A greater amount of O_2 is extracted from the alveoli, resulting in a low alveolar O_2 tension (P_AO_2).

- **In the apices**, $\dot{V}/\dot{Q} > 3$. As ventilation is proportionally greater than perfusion, blood leaving the apical pulmonary capillaries is fully oxygenated. However, as only a small volume of blood passes by the apical alveoli, little gas exchange takes place: P_AO_2 is high and P_ACO_2 is low.

What are the causes of abnormal $\dot{V}/\dot{Q}$ ratio?

There are many pathological causes of $\dot{V}/\dot{Q}$ mismatch. These are broadly grouped into:

- **Problems with lung ventilation resulting in low $\dot{V}/\dot{Q}$ ratio.**
  This is the most common cause of hypoxaemia. Causes include:

- Upper airway obstruction;
- Foreign body aspiration;
- Pneumonia;
- Pneumothorax;
- Atelectasis;
- Acute respiratory distress syndrome;
- Emphysema;
- One-lung ventilation;
- Normal ageing;
- Increased closing capacity associated with obesity.

- **Problems with lung perfusion resulting in high $\dot{V}/\dot{Q}$ ratio.**
  Causes include:

- Pulmonary embolus (PE);
- Reduced right ventricular stroke volume due to hypovolaemia, right ventricular infarction or pericardial tamponade.

How might you manage hypoxaemia associated with $\dot{V}/\dot{Q}$ mismatch?

The commonest cause of hypoxaemia (defined as a $P_aO_2 < 8$ kPa) is $\dot{V}/\dot{Q}$ mismatch with a low $\dot{V}/\dot{Q}$ ratio. The mainstay of treatment is:

- **O_2 administration.** Hypoxaemia associated with low $\dot{V}/\dot{Q}$ ratio is responsive to O_2 therapy. As discussed earlier, poorly ventilated alveoli with normal perfusion have low P_AO_2. By

69

administering a higher F_iO_2, P_AO_2 is increased. The O_2 partial pressure gradient across the alveolar–capillary barrier is increased and blood leaving the pulmonary capillaries becomes better oxygenated.

- **Reversing the cause of the $\dot{V}/\dot{Q}$ mismatch.** For example, using antibiotics for pneumonia or positive end-expiratory pressure for atelectasis.

Clinical relevance: hypoxaemia with PE

Why do patients with PE become hypoxaemic? At first glance, this seems a facile question, but if you consider the $\dot{V}/\dot{Q}$ relationship associated with PE, it becomes intriguing.

PE results in obstruction (by a blood clot, gas, fat or amniotic fluid) of one or more major branches of the pulmonary arterial tree. Downstream of the arterial obstruction, the $\dot{V}/\dot{Q}$ ratio is high, as alveolar ventilation continues as normal whilst alveolar perfusion ceases. Since the affected alveoli are ventilated but no longer perfused, P_AO_2 increases and P_ACO_2 decreases. However, all the blood leaving the pulmonary capillaries should still be fully oxygenated. Therefore, one would expect a patient with PE to have an increased $\dot{V}_E$ (due to the increased alveolar dead space), but a normal P_aO_2.

Clinically, patients with PE become hypoxaemic. The mechanism for this has been a topic of some controversy for many years. The most accepted explanation is:

- Embolus settles in a branch of the pulmonary arterial tree, causing mechanical obstruction and stopping blood flow to the downstream pulmonary capillaries. This causes a high $\dot{V}/\dot{Q}$ ratio and increased alveolar dead space, as discussed above.
- J-receptors in the alveolar walls are activated by pulmonary emboli, causing a feeling of breathlessness and stimulating an increase in $\dot{V}_E$. This explains the low P_aCO_2 found in patients with PE.
- In addition to mechanical obstruction, the embolus causes local release of inflammatory mediators, causing:
  - bronchoconstriction of small airways;
  - alveolar–capillary barrier damage, leading to pulmonary oedema;
  - reduced pulmonary surfactant production, leading to atelectasis.

All three factors lead to a low $\dot{V}/\dot{Q}$ ratio, resulting in hypoxaemia.

Is gravity the only factor influencing $\dot{V}/\dot{Q}$ matching?

The gravitational model of lung ventilation and perfusion described above has been used to explain whole-lung $\dot{V}/\dot{Q}$ matching for nearly 50 years. However, the model cannot explain certain differences in $\dot{V}/\dot{Q}$ matching discovered more recently. For example, it has been shown that different areas of the lung at the same vertical height can have a different $\dot{V}/\dot{Q}$ ratio. In addition, even under zero gravity, the lung has been shown to have a non-uniform $\dot{V}/\dot{Q}$ relationship.

During embryonic development, the airways and blood vessels develop together. The branching of the vessels and airways is quite asymmetric, but because the airways and blood vessels branch at the same points, the diameters of the vessels and airways are well matched. This leads to similarities in ventilation and perfusion at the alveolar level, which contributes to $\dot{V}/\dot{Q}$ matching.

In addition, the lung has a physiological mechanism – hypoxic pulmonary vasoconstriction – that directs blood away from poorly ventilated alveoli (see Chapter 23). In a region of the lung with relatively less ventilation, P_AO_2 is low. In response, pulmonary arteriolar vasoconstriction reduces perfusion to this region, thus normalising the $\dot{V}/\dot{Q}$ ratio. Blood is instead redirected to well-ventilated regions, which accommodate the increased volume through the recruitment and distension of pulmonary capillaries, which again normalises the $\dot{V}/\dot{Q}$ ratio.

Further reading

A. B. Lumb. Distribution of pulmonary ventilation and perfusion. In: A. B. Lumb. *Nunn's Applied Respiratory Physiology, 8th edition.* London, Churchill Livingstone, 2016, 109–36.

J. B. West. *Ventilation/Blood Flow and Gas Exchange, 6th edition.* Hoboken, Wiley-Blackwell, 1990.

I. Galvin, G. B. Drummond, M. Nirmalan. Distribution of blood flow and ventilation in the lung: gravity is not the only factor. *Br J Anaesth* 2007; **98**(4): 420–8.

R. P. Mahajan. Acute lung injury: options to improve oxygenation. *Continuing Educ Anaesth Crit Care Pain* 2005; **5**(2): 52–5.

G. Stratmann, G. A. Gregory. Neurogenic and humoral vasoconstriction in acute pulmonary thromboembolism. *Anesth Analg* 2003; **97**(2): 341–54.

16

Ventilation–Perfusion Zones in the Lung

What are the West zones of the lung?

In the upright position, ventilation and perfusion both increase from the top to the bottom of the lung. This was previously attributed to the effect of gravity (the so-called gravitational model), but it is now thought that structural similarities between the pulmonary arteries and bronchioles contribute (see Chapter 15).

J. B. West built on a gravitational model of ventilation and perfusion. This assumes that capillary blood flow to the alveolus is dependent on the pressure of the gas within the alveolus. This is particularly important in anaesthesia, as positive-pressure ventilation significantly alters alveolar pressure. West divided the upright lung into three vertical zones, numbered 1 (at the apex) to 3 (at the base). The arterial, venous and alveolar pressures differ in each zone, which has implications for the $\dot{V}/\dot{Q}$ ratio.

How do the changes in arterial, venous and alveolar pressures affect alveolar perfusion?

The variation in alveolar perfusion in the three West zones (Figure 16.1) is most easily explained by starting from West zone 3, at the base of the lung:

- **In West zone 3**, $P_a > P_v > P_A$ (a: arterial; v: venous; A: alveolar). Both arterial and venous pressures are greater than alveolar pressure. This is because of the effects of gravity on alveolar volume. The lungs are suspended superiorly in the chest from the large airways and therefore there is little weight acting upon the base of the lung. For this reason, the basal alveoli are not particularly distended and thus sit upon a more compliant part of the pressure–volume loop.

As the alveoli occupy a small volume, they exert minimal extramural pressure on the pulmonary vasculature. Capillary blood flows continuously throughout the cardiac cycle – flow is dependent on the arterial–venous pressure difference, which is generated by the right ventricle. West zone 3 is how normal, healthy lungs behave below the level of the hilum.

- **In West zone 2**, $P_a > P_A > P_v$. As the lung is ascended, there is an increasing effect of the weight of the lung. Alveoli are pulled open and become less compliant. P_A therefore increases and the lung exerts increased extramural pressure on the pulmonary vasculature: alveolar pressure thus exceeds venous pressure, causing compression of the venous end of the pulmonary capillary. Capillary blood flow is therefore dependent on the arterial–alveolar pressure difference. Systolic pulmonary arterial pressure is greater than alveolar pressure, but diastolic pulmonary arterial pressure is not – blood therefore only flows through the pulmonary capillary during systole. The intermittent nature of blood flow causes a mismatch between alveolar ventilation and perfusion. Thus, the $\dot{V}/\dot{Q}$ ratio is higher, with an increased alveolar dead space, than in West zone 3 with consequently wasted ventilation. West zone 2 is how normal lungs behave between the apex and the hilum.

- **In West zone 1**, $P_A > P_a > P_v$. Alveolar pressure exceeds systolic pulmonary arterial pressure as the alveoli are maximally distended by the weight of the whole lung. The pulmonary capillary is completely compressed by the alveolus, with alveolar perfusion ceasing. The apical alveoli are still ventilated – $\dot{V}/\dot{Q}$ ratio is therefore high, with a high alveolar dead space. West zone 1 does not exist in normal lungs.

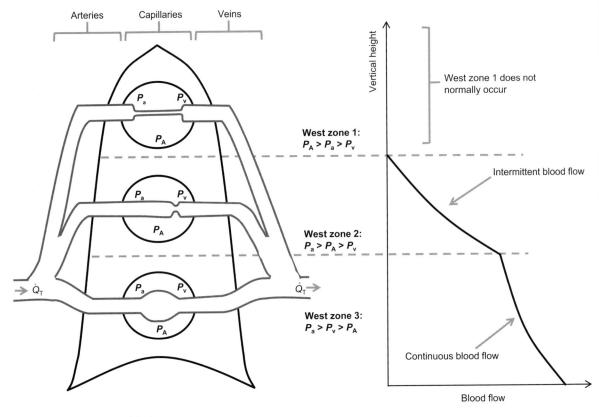

Figure 16.1 West zones of the lung.

When does West zone 1 become clinically significant?

In a healthy, non-anaesthetised person, alveolar pressure is approximately equal to atmospheric pressure, with small pressure variations due to inspiration and expiration (0 ± 2 cmH$_2$O). The situation of West zone 1, where alveolar pressure exceeds systolic pulmonary arterial pressure, therefore does not normally occur.

However, West zone 1 can occur when:

- **Pulmonary arterial pressure is abnormally low**, such as in haemorrhagic shock. Normal alveolar pressure may therefore exceed pulmonary arterial pressure.
- **Alveolar pressure is abnormally high**, such as during positive-pressure ventilation or high intrinsic positive end-expiratory pressure associated with acute severe asthma.

When West zone 1 does occur, the increase in alveolar dead space means that ventilation is wasted. In the case of acute severe asthma, the increased ventilatory effort required may precipitate respiratory failure.

Clinical relevance: pulmonary artery catheters (PACs)

One of the key measurements obtained from the PAC is the pulmonary capillary wedge pressure (PCWP). When inflated, the balloon-tipped end of the PAC is 'floated' through the right ventricle and into the pulmonary arterial tree until it wedges in a branch of the pulmonary artery.

For accurate measurement of PCWP, the PAC must wedge in a pulmonary artery within West zone 3. It is essential that the PAC is in communication with an uninterrupted static column of blood between the pulmonary artery and the left atrium. As discussed above, this can only occur in West zone 3 where capillary blood flow is continuous.

Because the majority of pulmonary blood flow is to West zone 3, the tip of the flow-directed PAC is likely to position itself correctly. A clinical method of

---

checking the position of the PAC is to increase positive end-expiratory pressure by 10 cmH$_2$O – if the PCWP increases by more than 25%, it is likely that the tip is not in West zone 3.

Further reading

J. B. West. *Ventilation/Blood Flow and Gas Exchange*, 6th edition. Hoboken, Wiley-Blackwell, 1990.

I. Galvin, G. B. Drummond, M. Nirmalan. Distribution of blood flow and ventilation in the lung: gravity is not the only factor. *Br J Anaesth* 2007; **98**(4): 420–8.

Oxygen Delivery and Demand

What is meant by the term 'global oxygen consumption'?

Global O_2 consumption $\dot{V}O_2$ (mL/min) is the volume of O_2 that is consumed by the body per minute.

During aerobic metabolism, $\dot{V}O_2$ is closely matched to the body's metabolic rate. Resting $\dot{V}O_2$ for a 70-kg man is typically 250 mL/min (at sea level and standard temperature). During exercise, $\dot{V}O_2$ increases as the body consumes additional O_2 to power muscle contraction. As exercise intensity increases, $\dot{V}O_2$ increases. There comes a point where $\dot{V}O_2$ is limited by the rate of O_2 delivery to the tissues, which is likely due to diffusion limitation being reached in the muscle microcirculation. When this happens, the muscles switch from aerobic metabolism, where O_2 is consumed, to anaerobic metabolism, where energy is obtained from glycolysis. The O_2 consumption at this transition point is termed $\dot{V}O_{2max}$ and is closely related to maximal exercise performance (see Chapter 43). Training increases the $\dot{V}O_{2max}$ and therefore performance.

Global $\dot{V}O_2$ can be calculated using the reverse Fick principle:

Key equation: reverse Fick principle

$$\dot{V}O_2 = CO \times (C_aO_2 - C_vO_2) \times 10$$

where CO (L/min) is the cardiac output, C_aO_2 is the O_2 content of arterial blood (mLO_2/100 mL of blood), C_vO_2 is the O_2 content of venous blood (mLO_2/100 mL of blood), 10 is a unit conversion factor and

$$C_aO_2 = (1.34 \times [Hb] \times S_aO_2/100\%) + 0.023 \times P_aO_2$$

(see Chapter 8), where [Hb] (g/dL) is the Hb concentration.

The equation above essentially states that the $\dot{V}O_2$ is the same as the O_2 'taken out of the arterial blood', as reflected in the difference in arterial and venous O_2 contents. CO and C_vO_2 can be measured with the aid of a pulmonary artery catheter (as C_vO_2 should really be measured using mixed venous blood) and C_aO_2 can be measured by peripheral arterial blood gas analysis.

What is meant by the term 'global oxygen delivery'?

Global O_2 delivery $\dot{D}O_2$ (mL/min) is the volume of O_2 delivered to the tissues from the lungs per minute. $\dot{D}O_2$ can be calculated using the O_2 flux equation:

Key equation: oxygen flux equation

$$\dot{D}O_2 = CO \times C_aO_2 \times 10$$

where 10 is a unit conversion factor.

What is a typical resting global oxygen delivery?

Using the O_2 flux equation with typical values for a resting patient breathing room air (CO = 5 L/min, [Hb] = 15 g/dL, S_aO_2 = 98%, P_aO_2 = 13 kPa), first the C_aO_2 is calculated:

$$C_aO_2 = (1.34 \times [Hb] \times S_aO_2/100\%) + 0.023 \times P_aO_2$$

Therefore:

$$\begin{aligned} C_aO_2 &= (1.34 \times 15 \times 98/100) + 0.023 \times 13 \\ &= 20.0 \text{ mL}O_2/100 \text{ mL blood} \end{aligned}$$

Then $\dot{D}O_2$ is calculated:

$$\dot{D}O_2 = CO \times C_aO_2 \times 10$$

Therefore:

$$\dot{D}O_2 = 5 \times 20.0 \times 10 = 1000 \text{ mL}O_2/\text{min}$$

Clinical relevance: anaemia

What happens to $\dot{D}O_2$ if a patient is anaemic? If the patient described above became anaemic, with an Hb concentration of, say, 8 g/dL:

$$C_aO_2 = (1.34 \times 8 \times 98/100) + 0.023 \times 13$$
$$= 10.8 \text{ mLO}_2/100 \text{ mL blood}$$
$$\Rightarrow \dot{D}O_2 = 5 \times 10.8 \times 10$$
$$= 540 \text{ mLO}_2/\text{min}$$

This corresponds to a fall in $\dot{D}O_2$ to nearly half the normal value.

However, there is a flaw in the calculation above. The CO of an anaemic patient is not the normal value of 5 L/min. Anaemia causes a compensatory increase in CO in order that $\dot{D}O_2$ is maintained. The increased CO is in part a result of the reduced viscosity of anaemic blood.

How are $\dot{D}O_2$ and $\dot{V}O_2$ related?

At rest in a normal patient, $\dot{D}O_2$ (typical value 1000 mL/min) is much higher than $\dot{V}O_2$ (typical value 250 mL/min). Thus, the tissues are said to have an O_2 extraction ratio (OER) of 25%.

Key equation: OER

$$OER = \frac{\dot{V}O_2}{\dot{D}O_2}$$

Normal OER is 0.2–0.3; that is, only 20–30% of delivered O_2 is consumed by the tissues, the rest being returned to the lungs in the venous blood.

An OER of 0.2–0.3 corresponds to a mixed venous Hb O_2 saturation of 70–80%.

As $\dot{D}O_2$ falls (e.g. as a result of hypotension) or $\dot{V}O_2$ rises (e.g. as a result of exercise or sepsis), the tissues must extract more O_2 from the passing blood if they are to continue to undergo aerobic metabolism. There is also a considerable difference in the normal OER between different organs. For example:

- The carotid bodies have high $\dot{D}O_2$ but low $\dot{V}O_2$, resulting in a low OER, reflecting their role in sensing changes in blood composition.
- The heart has a high OER (approximately 0.6), which makes it very susceptible to ischaemia following a reduction in coronary artery perfusion pressure.

Is there a point where oxygen delivery becomes inadequate?

At rest, the tissues will continue to extract O_2 for aerobic metabolism from the passing capillary blood at a rate of 250 mL/min, until a critical value of $\dot{D}O_2$ is reached (Figure 17.1a). This critical $\dot{D}O_2$ is referred to as the anaerobic threshold.

Before the anaerobic threshold is reached, $\dot{V}O_2$ is said to be supply independent. Once $\dot{D}O_2$ falls below this critical value, $\dot{V}O_2$ rapidly decreases and the tissues are forced to gain their energy by anaerobic means – $\dot{V}O_2$ is now said to be supply dependent.

Clinical relevance: critical illness and oxygen delivery

In the critically ill patient, O_2 supply and demand are more complicated.

Additional factors may significantly increase $\dot{V}O_2$:

- Inflammation, sepsis and pyrexia;
- Administration of adrenergic drugs;
- Weaning from the ventilator;
- Interventions such as physiotherapy;
- Conditions such as burns, trauma and seizures.

There is an altered relationship between $\dot{V}O_2$ and $\dot{D}O_2$ in patients with severe sepsis or acute respiratory distress syndrome. $\dot{V}O_2$ becomes supply dependent at a much higher $\dot{D}O_2$ (Figure 17.1b) – the normal biphasic relationship between $\dot{V}O_2$ and $\dot{D}O_2$ is no longer observed. It is not clear whether this effect is the result of critical $\dot{D}O_2$ being much higher than normal in critical illness or whether the tissues are less able to extract O_2 from the blood.

Early goal-directed therapy has traditionally involved the invasive monitoring and aggressive haemodynamic management of patients at risk of organ failure. However, patient outcomes of the more recent randomised trials have had contradictory outcomes (see Further reading).

Clinical relevance: anaesthesia, oxygen consumption and oxygen delivery

In the perioperative period, $\dot{V}O_2$ is frequently higher than the 'resting' value of 250 mLO$_2$/min. A number of factors are implicated:

- Surgery;
- Pain and anxiety;
- Inflammation, sepsis and pyrexia;
- Post-operative shivering;

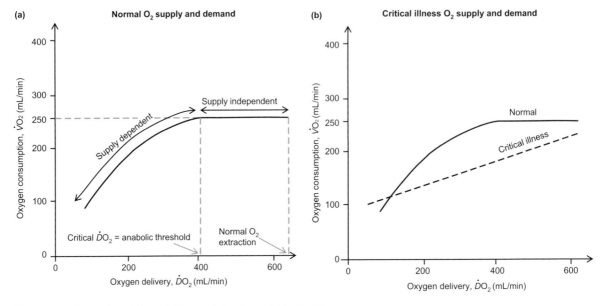

Figure 17.1 O_2 supply and demand: (a) normal situation and (b) critical illness.

Under general anaesthesia, some of this increase in $\dot{V}O_2$ is offset due to:

- **Sedatives/hypnotics**, which reduce cerebral metabolic rate, a major component of the resting $\dot{V}O_2$.
- **Mechanical ventilation and muscle paralysis**, which abolish the work of breathing.
- **Preoperative fasting**, which reduces O_2 consumption in the gut.

The inflammatory response following major surgery increases resting $\dot{V}O_2$ by 50% – this increase is then sustained over many days. It is important to know preoperatively that a patient has sufficient cardiopulmonary reserve to meet the required post-operative increase in $\dot{D}O_2$. A number of preoperative exercise tests are available, but cardiopulmonary exercise testing arguably offers the best assessment of cardiopulmonary reserve (see Chapter 43).

Further reading

L. Meng, P. M. Heerdt. Perioperative goal-directed haemodynamic therapy based on flow parameters: a concept in evolution. *Br J Anaesth* 2016; **117**(Suppl. 3): iii3–17.

J. G. Hopker, S.A. Jobson, J.J. Pandit. Controversies in the physiological basis of the 'anaerobic threshold' and their implications for clinical cardiopulmonary exercise testing. *Anaesthesia* 2011; **66**(2): 111–23.

C. M. Lilly. The PROCESS trial – a new era in sepsis management. *N Engl J Med* 2014; **370**(18): 1683–93.

N. Agnew. Preoperative cardiopulmonary exercise testing. *Continuing Educ Anaesth Crit Care Pain* 2010; **10**(2): 33–7.

E. Rivers, B. Nguyen, S. Havstad, et al. Early goal-directed therapy in the treatment of severe sepsis and septic shock. *N Engl J Med* 2001; **345**(19): 1368–77.

Chapter

18

Alveolar Gas Equation

Can you measure the partial pressure of oxygen in the alveolus?

The partial pressure gradient of O_2 between the alveolus and the pulmonary capillaries is one of the key factors that determine the rate of O_2 diffusion across the alveolar–capillary barrier (see Chapter 10). Unfortunately, it is not possible to directly measure the P_AO_2. Instead, P_AO_2 can be estimated using the alveolar gas equation (AGE).

What is the AGE?

The AGE[1] allows P_AO_2 to be estimated from variables that are easily measured.

Key equation: simplified AGE

$$P_AO_2 = F_iO_2(P_B - P_{SVP\ water}) - \frac{P_aCO_2}{R}$$

where F_iO_2 for dry air is 20.93%; P_B at sea level is 101.325 kPa. Inspired air becomes fully saturated with water vapour by the time it reaches the carina. $P_{SVP\ water}$ is the saturated vapour pressure of water, which at body temperature is 6.3 kPa. P_aCO_2 is measured in kilopascals. R is the respiratory quotient, usually taken as 0.8.

The AGE tells us that P_AO_2 is essentially dependent on three variables:

- **The inspired fraction of O_2.** According to the AGE, increasing F_iO_2 will result in a greater P_AO_2, thus increasing the pressure gradient across the alveolar–capillary barrier; the rate of O_2 diffusion will increase (Fick's law – see Chapter 10).

- **Barometric pressure.** P_B decreases exponentially with ascent to altitude (see Chapter 87). According to the AGE, as the elevation above sea level increases, the fall in P_B results in a lower P_AO_2 and thus a reduced rate of O_2 diffusion across the alveolar–capillary barrier.

- **Alveolar ventilation.** As P_aCO_2 is inversely proportional to $\dot{V}_A$ (see Chapter 11):

  - An increase in $\dot{V}_A$ (hyperventilation) results in a decrease in P_aCO_2. According to the AGE, P_AO_2 will increase, thus increasing the rate of O_2 diffusion across the alveolar–capillary barrier.

  - A decrease in $\dot{V}_A$ (hypoventilation) results in an increase in P_aCO_2. According to the AGE, P_AO_2 will decrease, thus reducing the rate of O_2 diffusion across the alveolar–capillary barrier.

What is the respiratory quotient? Why does it differ for different dietary substrates?

The respiratory quotient R is the ratio of CO_2 production and O_2 consumption:

$$R = \frac{\text{rate of } CO_2 \text{ produced}}{\text{rate of } O_2 \text{ consumed}}$$

R differs between the three dietary metabolic substrates: fat, protein and carbohydrate. R can be calculated for each substrate using the chemical formula of the overall aerobic metabolism reaction. For example, consider glucose:

$$C_6H_{12}O_6 + 6O_2 \rightarrow 6CO_2 + 6H_2O$$

Therefore, as six molecules of CO_2 are produced for every six molecules of O_2 consumed, $R = 1.0$ for a purely carbohydrate-based diet. Likewise:

- $R = 0.7$ for a purely fat-based diet.
- $R = 0.9$ for a purely protein-based diet.

---

[1] The derivation of the AGE is beyond the scope of this book; see Further reading for full details.

The respiratory quotient is usually taken as 0.8, the figure for a balanced Western diet.

Using the AGE, calculate the alveolar oxygen tension for a typical patient breathing room air at sea level

A typical patient has a P_aCO_2 of 5.3 kPa and a normal diet (i.e. $R = 0.8$). The values for F_iO_2, P_B and $P_{SVP\ water}$ are given above.

Substituting these values into the AGE:

$$P_AO_2 = F_iO_2(P_B - P_{SVP\ water}) - \frac{P_aCO_2}{R}$$

Therefore:

$$P_AO_2 = 20.93\% \times (101.325 - 6.3) - \frac{5.3}{0.8}$$
$$P_AO_2 = 13.3\ \text{kPa}$$

Clinical relevance: alveolar–arterial (A–a) gradient

The A–a gradient is the difference between the calculated alveolar P_AO_2 (using the AGE) and the measured arterial P_aO_2 (using arterial blood gas analysis).

In normal lungs, P_AO_2 and *pulmonary capillary* O_2 tension are approximately equal because there is sufficient time for the O_2 partial pressures on either side of the alveolar–capillary barrier to equilibrate before the red blood cells have traversed the capillary (see Chapter 10). But the *arterial* O_2 tension P_aO_2 is always lower than P_AO_2. Even in normal lungs with perfect $\dot{V}/\dot{Q}$ matching, there is always a small anatomical shunt as a result of the bronchial and Thebesian veins (see Chapter 14), resulting in a small A–a gradient:

- In a healthy, young adult, a normal A–a gradient is considered to be <1.5 kPa.
- A–a gradient increases with age due to a worsening of $\dot{V}/\dot{Q}$ matching in the ageing lung.

The A–a gradient is an index used clinically to diagnose the cause of hypoxaemia. Increased A–a gradient is seen in:

- **$\dot{V}/\dot{Q}$ mismatch**, by far the most common cause of an increased A–a gradient; for example, pneumonia, acute respiratory distress syndrome, atelectasis.
- **Right-to-left shunt**; for example, pulmonary arteriovenous malformation, intra-cardiac shunt.
- **Severe diffusion impairment**; for example, end-stage pulmonary fibrosis.

Normal A–a gradient is seen with:

- **Hypoxic mixtures**; for example, a faulty anaesthetic machine.
- **Alveolar hypoventilation**, as the AGE accounts for alveolar ventilation rate. Examples include airway obstruction, neuromuscular disease, drug-induced respiratory depression.

Clinical relevance: hypoventilation

A known intravenous drug user is admitted unconscious after an opioid overdose. His Hb saturations are only 91%, and arterial blood gas analysis shows a P_aCO_2 of 9 kPa – explain this.

Acute opiate overdose depresses the respiratory centre in the medulla, resulting in decreased $\dot{V}_A$, with a consequent rise in P_aCO_2. Using the AGE for a patient breathing room air with a P_aCO_2 of 9 kPa:

$$P_AO_2 = F_iO_2(P_B - P_{SVP\ water}) - \frac{P_aCO_2}{R}$$
$$P_AO_2 = 20.93\% \times (101.325 - 6.3) - \frac{9}{0.8}$$
$$P_AO_2 = 8.6\ \text{kPa, equivalent to an } S_aO_2$$
of approximately 91%.

How is the AGE relevant to the physiological adaptation to altitude?

At altitude, the proportion of O_2 in the air is the same as at sea level (i.e. F_iO_2 remains the same), but P_B is reduced. For example, P_B is 65 kPa at the Tibetan Plateau (one of the highest places to live in the world). Hyperventilation is an important physiological mechanism that increases P_AO_2. If a person did not hyperventilate at altitude (i.e. P_aCO_2 remained at 5.3 kPa), P_AO_2 would be calculated by the AGE as:

$$P_AO_2 = F_iO_2(P_B - P_{SVP\ water}) - \frac{P_aCO_2}{R}$$
$$P_AO_2 = 20.93\%(65 - 6.3) - \frac{5.3}{0.8}$$
$$P_AO_2 = 5.7\ \text{kPa}$$

Physiological shunt in the lungs would result in an even lower P_aO_2; that is, significant hypoxaemia. However, if a person were to hyperventilate and P_aCO_2 decreased to, say, 3.0 kPa, then:

$$P_AO_2 = 20.93\%(65 - 6.3) - \frac{3.0}{0.8}$$
$$P_AO_2 = 8.5\ \text{kPa}$$

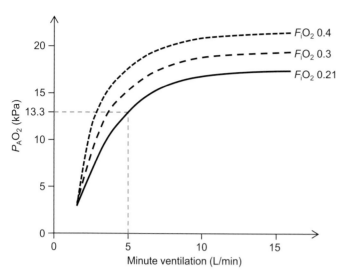

Figure 18.1 The relationship between P_AO_2 and minute ventilation.

Hyperventilation therefore increases P_AO_2 sufficiently to allow human existence at altitude, albeit with a chronic respiratory alkalosis.

However, there is a limit to the extent to which hyperventilation can increase P_AO_2 (Figure 18.1), The hyperbolic relationship between $\dot{V}_A$ and P_aCO_2 (see Chapter 11 and Figure 11.1) means that, beyond a modest increase in $\dot{V}_A$ (around 10 L/min), a large increase in $\dot{V}_A$ is required to achieve a small decrease in P_aCO_2. Therefore, as $\dot{V}_A$ increases, P_AO_2 reaches a plateau. As demonstrated in Figure 18.1, O_2 administration will increase P_AO_2 (and therefore P_aO_2) substantially more than hyperventilation.

Further reading

S. Cruickshank, N. Hirschauer. The alveolar gas equation. *Continuing Educ Anaesth Crit Care Pain* 2004; **4**(1): 24–7.

Oxygen Cascade

The O_2 cascade concept draws together areas of respiratory physiology covered in the previous few chapters. In an examination setting, it allows the examiner to assess your knowledge of more than one topic within a single question.

What is the oxygen cascade?

Aerobic metabolism is the body's most efficient method of energy production. O_2 tension (PO_2) is high in the atmosphere (21.2 kPa) and low in the mitochondria (<5 kPa). The O_2 cascade refers to the stepwise reduction in PO_2 as O_2 passes from the environment to the tissues (Figure 19.1).

Explain each of the steps in the oxygen cascade

The steps along the O_2 cascade are:

- **Atmosphere.** P_B at sea level is 101.325 kPa and F_iO_2 of dry air is 20.93%. Atmospheric PO_2 is calculated as follows:

$$PO_2 = P_B \times F_iO_2$$
$$\Rightarrow PO_2 = 101.325 \times 20.93\% = 21.2 \text{ kPa}$$

- **Trachea.** By the time inspired air reaches the carina, it has become fully saturated with water vapour. Water has a saturated vapour pressure $P_{SVP \text{ water}}$ of 6.3 kPa at 37°C. The PO_2 of humidified air at the carina is calculated as follows:

$$PO_2 = (P_B - P_{SVP \text{ water}}) \times F_iO_2$$
$$\Rightarrow PO_2 = (101.325 - 6.3) \times 20.93\% = 19.9 \text{ kPa}$$

- **Alveolus.** P_AO_2 is mainly dependent on F_iO_2, P_B and $\dot{V}_A$, as described by the AGE (see Chapter 18):

$$P_AO_2 = F_iO_2(P_B - P_{SVP \text{ water}}) - \frac{P_aCO_2}{R}$$

Figure 19.1 The O_2 cascade.

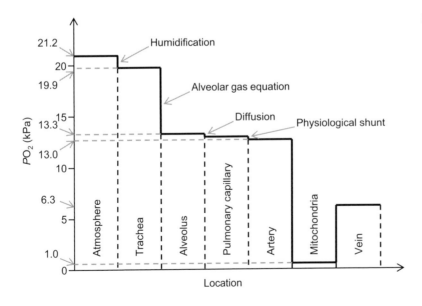

- P_AO_2 can be calculated using the typical values: $P_aCO_2 = 5.3$ kPa and R = 0.8:

$$P_AO_2 = 20.93\%(101.325-6.3)-\frac{5.3}{0.8}$$
$$\Rightarrow P_AO_2 = 13.3 \text{ kPa}$$

- **Arterial blood.** There is a 'step' reduction in PO_2 between the alveolus and the systemic arteries. This A–a gradient is the result of three factors:

  - *Diffusion across the alveolar–capillary barrier.* Normally, there is sufficient time for O_2 to diffuse across the alveolar–capillary barrier; that is, for P_AO_2 and pulmonary capillary PO_2 to equilibrate at 13.3 kPa. Transfer of O_2 is then said to be perfusion limited (see Chapter 10). However, in lungs with a thickened alveolar–capillary barrier or a decreased alveolar surface area, O_2 may become diffusion limited; pulmonary capillary PO_2 then becomes a step lower than P_AO_2.
  - *Shunts.* There is normally a small anatomical right-to-left shunt arising from the bronchial circulation and the Thebesian veins (see Chapter 14).
  - *$\dot{V}/\dot{Q}$ mismatch.* Any area of lung with relatively more perfusion than ventilation results in a functional right-to-left shunt, causing a further reduction in P_aO_2 (see Chapter 15). The normal physiological shunt fraction (the sum of anatomical and functional shunts) is 2–5%, which corresponds to a fall in P_aO_2 to 13.0 kPa.

- **Tissue capillaries.** As O_2 is taken up by the tissues, the PO_2 falls progressively from the arterial end to the venous end of the capillary. However, not all the arteriolar blood flows through the capillaries: pre-capillary sphincters control how much blood flows into each capillary network. The remaining blood bypasses the capillaries and flows directly into the venules via arteriovenous anastomoses, which in humans are likely to be dilated skeletal muscle capillary beds.

- **Mitochondria.** The mitochondrial PO_2 is very much lower than that of arterial blood and is related to the metabolic activity of the tissues. For example, in exercising skeletal muscle, O_2 utilisation is high and so the mitochondrial PO_2 is very low. Therefore, there is a large O_2 partial pressure gradient between the capillary blood and the mitochondria, increasing the rate of O_2 diffusion. In addition, metabolites (e.g. H^+ and CO_2) cause arteriolar vasodilatation, increasing local blood flow and hence O_2 delivery.

Clinical relevance: the Pasteur point and anaerobic metabolism

If the mitochondrial PO_2 falls below a critical point (between 0.15 and 0.3 kPa), there is insufficient O_2 tension for aerobic metabolism. Anaerobic metabolism then takes over as the dominant mechanism of ATP production. This critical threshold is called the Pasteur point.

For mitochondrial PO_2 to be adequate, capillary blood PO_2 must be high enough for O_2 to diffuse readily from the blood to the tissues. Well-oxygenated capillary blood is dependent on all the preceding steps of the O_2 cascade. Anaerobic metabolism can occur if any of the 'steps' of the cascade are disturbed. For example:

- High altitude reduces atmospheric PO_2, the starting point of the cascade. All subsequent steps will then have a lower PO_2 than at sea level.
- Hypoventilation increases P_aCO_2, which in turn reduces P_AO_2 (see Chapter 18).
- Pneumonia causes a $\dot{V}/\dot{Q}$ mismatch, resulting in a lower P_aO_2.

Further reading

C. C. W. Hsia, A. Schmidt, M. Lambertz, et al. Evolution of air breathing: oxygen homeostasis and the transitions from water to land and sky. *Compr Physiol* 2013; 3(2): 849–915.

20 Lung Compliance

What is lung compliance?

Compliance is defined as the change in lung volume produced by a unit change in transpulmonary pressure. Lung compliance is represented by the gradient of the pressure–volume curve:

$$\text{Compliance} = \frac{\Delta \text{Volume}}{\Delta \text{Transpulmonary pressure}}$$

Essentially, compliance is the property that determines the volume by which the lungs expand when pressure is applied to them: either negative pressure (as in spontaneous ventilation) or positive pressure (as in intermittent positive-pressure ventilation). For a spontaneously breathing patient:

- **When compliance is high**, the respiratory muscles only need to generate a small transpulmonary pressure to achieve inspiration to V_T. However, as less work is done in expansion, so too is less work stored as elastic potential energy. Therefore, exhalation becomes more difficult as there is less elastic recoil of the lungs.
- **When compliance is low**, a high transpulmonary pressure is required to expand the lung to the same V_T: the respiratory muscles must then work harder during inspiration and respiratory failure may ensue.

Normal tidal breathing starts from the functional residual capacity (FRC), the rest point where inward elastic recoil is equal and opposite to the force tending to spring the thoracic cage outwards. Conveniently, the lungs are at their most compliant at FRC, which means that the work of breathing at rest is minimal:

- For a typical patient at FRC, compliance is 200 mL/cmH$_2$O.
- Therefore, at FRC, a V_T of 500 mL is achieved with a transpulmonary pressure of just 2.5 cmH$_2$O.

What is respiratory compliance? How does it differ from lung compliance?

Respiratory compliance refers to the compliance of the whole lung–chest unit. It is made up of two components:

- Lung compliance;
- Thoracic cage compliance.

> **Key equation: respiratory compliance**
>
> Respiratory, lung and thoracic cage compliances are mathematically related:
>
> $$\frac{1}{RC} = \frac{1}{LC} + \frac{1}{TCC}$$
>
> where RC is respiratory compliance, LC is lung compliance and TCC is thoracic cage compliance. Typical values for both lung and thoracic cage compliance are 200 mL/cmH$_2$O. Therefore, a typical value for respiratory compliance is 100 mL/cmH$_2$O. Thus as compliances in series add as inverses, the overall compliance is always less than the sum of its parts.

Which factors affect lung and thoracic cage compliance?

Thoracic cage compliance is affected by:

- **Chest wall shape**, including the spine and rib cage;
- **Muscle tone**.

Lung compliance is broadly affected by two factors:

- **Elastic recoil** of the lung connective tissue;
- **Surface tension** at the air–fluid interface in the alveoli.

Outline some clinical situations in which respiratory compliance is increased or decreased.

Respiratory compliance may be affected by both physiological and pathological factors.

- **Causes of increased respiratory compliance include**:
  - *Emphysema*, in which there is destruction of lung elastic tissue.
  - *Advancing age*, in which there is degeneration of lung elastic tissue, similar to mild emphysema.
  - *Neuromuscular conditions*: decreased muscular tone results in an easier expansion of the thoracic cage, as occurs in motor neurone disease.

- **Causes of decreased respiratory compliance include**:
  - *Posture*: the lung is generally less compliant when supine.
  - *Pregnancy*: lung compliance is relatively unaffected, but thoracic cage compliance is reduced in late pregnancy.
  - *Fluid within the alveoli or lung interstitium*, exemplified by pneumonia and pulmonary oedema. Owing to the effects of surface tension, fluid-filled alveoli require a much higher transmural pressure to expand than aerated alveoli do. Consequently, compliance is significantly reduced.
  - *Atelectasis*: collapsed alveoli (i.e. alveoli with small radii) require a much higher transmural pressure than larger alveoli do to overcome surface tension forces (see Laplace's law below).
  - *Pulmonary hypertension*, in which the pulmonary capillaries are engorged with blood. This hinders alveolar enlargement, thus decreasing lung compliance.
  - *Pulmonary fibrosis*: the lung interstitium becomes stiff and less easily distensible.
  - *Extremes of lung volume*: at high lung volume, compliance is reduced because the elastic fibres are stretched to their limit. At low lung volume, lung compliance is reduced as a result of atelectasis.
  - *Obesity*: thoracic cage compliance is reduced due to the increased weight of the chest wall opposing thoracic expansion.
  - *Chest wall deformity/rigidity*: hinders the expansion of the thoracic cage, such as in kyphoscoliosis and ankylosing spondylitis.

How does surfactant increase lung compliance?

Surface tension is caused by forces of attraction between water molecules. These forces act to minimise the air–liquid interface by causing the water to form a spherical droplet. As the inner surface of the alveolus has a thin layer of fluid, an inward force – the surface tension – is created as the water tends to form a droplet. Opposing this inward force of surface tension is the alveolar transpulmonary pressure. As alveoli are approximately spherical, they obey Laplace's law.

Key equation: Laplace's law

For a sphere with only one surface,

$$P = \frac{2T}{r}$$

where, in this case, P is the transpulmonary pressure required to keep the alveolus open, T is the surface tension and r is the radius of the alveolus.

Surface tension poses a number of problems:

- **An alveolus has reduced compliance when its radius is low**. In expiration, the alveolus becomes smaller; that is, its radius decreases. According to Laplace's law, if surface tension is constant, a larger transmural pressure will be required to reinflate the alveolus.
- **Smaller alveoli empty into bigger alveoli**. When two connected alveoli are of different sizes, the alveolus with the smaller radius will require a higher transpulmonary pressure to remain inflated than the larger alveolus. As airway pressure is uniform throughout the lung, the smaller alveolus would collapse, emptying its air into the bigger alveolus.
- **Transudation of interstitial fluid**. The inward force of surface tension tends to suck fluid from

the interstitium into the alveolus via Starling filtration forces (see Chapter 36). This process is called 'transudation'.

These three problems are dealt with through the presence of pulmonary surfactant. Surfactant is produced by the type II pneumocytes in the alveolar wall. It is a mixture of phospholipids, of which dipalmitoylphosphatyldicholine (DPPC) is the most important, and proteins, particularly the surfactant apolipoproteins (SP-A, SP-B, SP-C).

Surfactant has three main roles through its action in reducing surface tension:

- **A general decrease in alveolar surface tension.** Surfactant increases global lung compliance, thus reducing the work required to expand the lung.
- **Stabilisation of small alveoli.** Surfactant is an especially elegant solution to the problem of surface tension. Reduction in surface tension is greater in small alveoli than large ones due to the way surfactant distributes itself. This offsets the mechanical disadvantage small alveoli have due to Laplace's law, resulting in a reduced tendency to collapse.
- **Prevention of fluid transudation.** As the surface tension forces are generally reduced by surfactant, less interstitial fluid is sucked into the alveolus.

What is the mechanism of this variation in surface tension?

The phospholipids within pulmonary surfactant are hydrophobic at one end and hydrophilic at the other. They therefore align over the surface of the liquid on the interior of the alveolus. The intermolecular repulsive forces between aligned DPPC molecules act to oppose the intermolecular attractive forces between water molecules and so surface tension is reduced. As the radius of the alveolus is reduced, the DPPC molecules are forced closer together, thus increasing the intermolecular repulsive forces and so further reducing surface tension.

Clinical relevance: infant respiratory distress syndrome

In utero, pulmonary surfactant is synthesised from about 24 weeks' gestation, stimulated by maternal corticosteroid release. However, full lung maturation is not complete until about 35 weeks' gestation. Infant respiratory distress syndrome (IRDS) is the condition that arises when premature neonates are born with lungs containing insufficient surfactant.

In the absence of surfactant, the lungs have low compliance, so alveoli become collapsed and fluid filled. Accordingly, IRDS is characterised by respiratory distress resulting from an increased work of breathing due to poorly compliant lungs, with areas of atelectasis and areas of pulmonary oedema. Treatment is either by administering steroids to the mother before birth to stimulate production of endogenous surfactant, if time allows, or by instilling artificial surfactant into the neonate's lungs.

A similar clinical picture is also seen in near-drowning: pulmonary surfactant is washed away, resulting in lungs of low compliance, with areas of atelectasis and areas of pulmonary oedema.

What is the difference between static and dynamic compliance?

As indicated above, lung compliance is represented by the gradient of the pressure–volume curve. However, the gradient of the pressure–volume curve depends on which technique is used for measuring pressure and volume. Static compliance and dynamic compliance refer to this dependence on how the pressure and volume are measured.

Static compliance is determined when pressure and volume measurements are taken at steady state; that is, when there is no gas flow:

- The patient inspires in 500-mL increments.
- In between increments there is a pause – gas flow stops and intrapleural pressure is measured using an oesophageal balloon catheter.
- The results are plotted on a pressure–volume graph (Figure 20.1). Note: the resultant sigmoid-shaped curve represents the combined thoracic cage and lung compliance.

The lung does not expand linearly with increasingly negative intrapleural pressure. Some key points to make about the static compliance curve are:

- *At low intrapleural pressure*, lung volume is low and the pressure–volume curve is flat, so lung compliance is low.
- *In the normal range of intrapleural pressure* (-5 to -10 cmH_2O), the pressure–volume curve is at its steepest; that is, a small change in transpulmonary pressure results in a large change in lung volume. The lung is therefore at its most

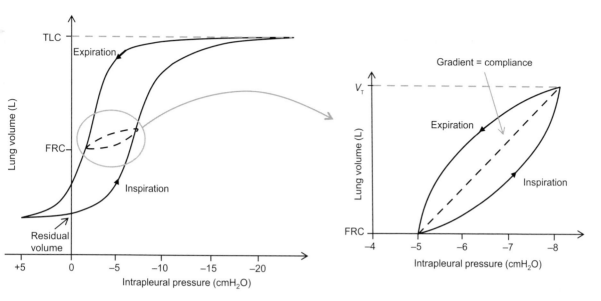

Figure 20.1 Static compliance curve (TLC = total lung capacity; V_T = tidal volume; FRC = functional residual capacity).

compliant at FRC during normal tidal breathing, resulting in low work during tidal inspiration.

- *At high intrapleural pressure*, the pressure–volume curve flattens out again. Alveoli are already well inflated and near to their elastic limit – a large decrease in intrapleural pressure is required for a small increase in lung volume; that is, compliance is low.

Dynamic compliance is calculated when continuous pressure and volume measurements are taken throughout the respiratory cycle; that is, there is no pause between measurements. There are two points in the respiratory cycle where gas flow ceases: end-inspiration and end-expiration. If these two points are plotted on a pressure–volume graph with a straight line joining them, the gradient (i.e. the dynamic compliance) is less than that of the static pressure–volume curve. The dynamic compliance is always lower than the static compliance. This reduction is due to airway resistance. In fact, the difference between static and dynamic compliance can be used as an indirect measure of the flow-resistive properties of the airways.

What is hysteresis?

Hysteresis is the phenomenon whereby a measurement differs depending on whether the value measured is rising or falling.

When lung volume is plotted against intrapleural pressure for both inspiration and expiration, the two curves follow different courses: a pressure–volume loop is formed. This loop effect is hysteresis – it is the result of viscous resistance to changes in lung volume. The area of the loop represents the amount of energy expended as heat in overcoming the resistive forces. The phenomenon of hysteresis occurs when both static and dynamic compliance are measured.

Dynamic hysteresis is illustrated in Figure 20.2a. The airway resistance increases when the velocity of gas flow is increased. The flow of air through the conducting airways is most rapid, and therefore most turbulent, at the beginning of inspiration and expiration. Consequently, airway resistance is at its greatest and compliance at its lowest (and accordingly the pressure–volume curve is at its flattest) at the beginning of inspiration and expiration. Similarly, if the respiratory rate increases but the V_T remains the same, inspiration must occur within a shorter time period. As the velocity of gas flow increases, airway resistance increases and dynamic compliance falls. Conditions that increase airway resistance (e.g. acute asthma) further decrease the dynamic compliance (Figure 20.2b).

Static hysteresis is illustrated in Figure 20.1. Unlike dynamic compliance, static compliance contains no airway resistance element because gas flow ceases during the pauses between measurements. Despite this, the inspiratory and expiratory curves still

(a) 10 breaths per minute

(b) Acute asthma, 30 breaths per minute

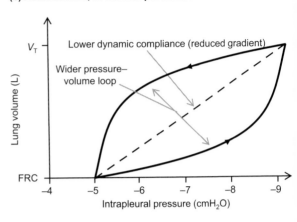

Figure 20.2 Dynamic hysteresis: (a) respiratory rate of 10 breaths per minute and (b) acute asthma with a respiratory rate of 30 breaths per minute.

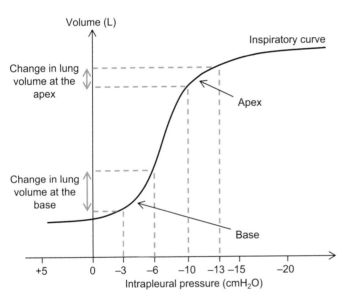

Figure 20.3 Effects of gravity and compliance on regional ventilation following a normal tidal inspiration (3-cmH₂O change in intrapleural pressure).

display hysteresis; that is, they follow different paths. Static hysteresis is attributed to the viscous resistance of the pulmonary surfactant and of the lung parenchyma itself.

How does the static compliance curve help to explain regional differences in lung ventilation?

The lung parenchyma is not uniformly distributed from top to bottom. Gravity acts on the lung parenchyma, resulting in intrapleural pressure being more negative at the apex (typically −10 cmH₂O) and less negative at the base (typically −3 cmH₂O). Consider the effect of this regional variation in intrapleural pressures on static lung compliance (Figure 20.3):

- **At the end of tidal expiration** (i.e. FRC), intrapleural pressure is −10 cmH₂O at the apex and −3 cmH₂O at the base. Therefore, at FRC, the apical alveoli are at near-maximum inflation, whereas the basal alveoli are barely inflated at all.

Thus, the lung apex is sometimes said to be 'more aerated' than the base.

- **During normal inspiration**. During tidal breathing, the inspiratory muscles decrease intrapleural pressure by 3 cmH$_2$O throughout the pleural cavity: apical intrapleural pressure decreases to –13 cmH$_2$O and basal intrapleural pressure decreases to –6 cmH$_2$O. The change in pressure results in a much greater volume change at the lung base than at the apex' that is, the lung base is more compliant (has a steeper pressure–volume curve gradient) than the apex. Because of the greater increase in volume of the basal alveoli, the lung base is said to be better ventilated than the apex.

Clinical relevance: optimum positive end-expiratory pressure

The static compliance curve (Figure 20.1) can be used in the intensive care unit to determine the optimum level of extrinsic positive end-expiratory pressure (PEEP):

- Tidal ventilation should take place on the most compliant (steepest) part of the pressure–volume curve. The point of end-expiration should therefore be above the lower inflection point.
- The point of end-inspiration should be below the upper inflection point to avoid lung hyperinflation.

In healthy lungs, the lower inflection point of the static compliance curve is at around 5 cmH$_2$O; that is, approximately the same as the physiological PEEP generated by the larynx (see Chapter 7). In contrast, diseases that significantly reduce lung compliance (e.g. acute respiratory distress syndrome, ARDS) have a significantly altered pressure–volume curve. If PEEP is applied to a pressure just above the lower inflection point, tidal breathing is shifted to a more compliant part of the pressure–volume curve.

In practice, this is difficult. Measuring static compliance in a patient with ARDS (i.e. increasing lung volume in 500-mL increments with pauses in between to allow gas flow to cease and intrapleural pressure to be measured) is likely to lead to life-threatening hypoxaemia. As discussed above, using dynamic compliance as a measure of the lower inflection point is not ideal. In practice, PEEP is increased using clinical judgement, with the intensivist aiming to identify a point where tidal volumes of 6 mL/kg can be achieved using 'safe' peak and plateau airway pressures.

Further reading

A. Aliverti, A. Pedotti. *Mechanics of Breathing: New Insights from New Technologies, 2nd edition*. Rome, Springer, 2014.

M. Wild, K. Alagesan. PEEP and CPAP. *Continuing Educ Anaesth Crit Care Pain* 2001; **1**(3): 89–92.

Chapter 21

Work of Breathing

What is meant by the term 'work of breathing'?

The work of breathing is the energy consumed by the respiratory muscles throughout the respiratory cycle.

Mathematically, for a single breath:

$$\text{Work(J)} = \text{Pressure(Pa)} \times \text{Volume(L)}$$

However, the work of breathing usually refers to the rate of work rather than the work for a single respiratory cycle. It should really be called the power of breathing and measured in watts (J/s).

Quiet tidal breathing is usually very efficient, requiring relatively little work. The energy required for tidal breathing is usually less than 2% of basal metabolic rate (BMR). Lung pathology can increase the work of breathing substantially, in some cases up to 30% of BMR, with the potential for respiratory muscle fatigue and respiratory failure.

What are the two main components that comprise the work of breathing?

The work of breathing is composed of elastic work and resistive work. In normal lungs, elastic work is responsible for most (approximately 65%) of the overall work of breathing:

- **Elastic work** is the work done on inspiration to overcome the elastic forces of the:

  - *Chest wall* (outward);
  - *Lung parenchyma* (inward);
  - *Alveolar surface tension* (inward).

  The work done against elastic forces is not all wasted. Some is stored as potential energy rather than being dissipated as heat. The stored potential energy is then used in expiration (see below). Elastic work is increased by diseases that affect the three factors above; for example:

  - *Obesity*, which opposes outward chest wall elastic recoil;
  - *Pulmonary fibrosis*, which reduces the compliance of the lung parenchyma;
  - *Infant respiratory distress syndrome*, in which there is insufficient pulmonary surfactant, leading to increased alveolar surface tension.

- **Resistive work** is the work done against friction – the energy used is 'wasted', as it is dissipated as heat (and sound). The resistive work of breathing is the work done to overcome:

  - *Tissue resistance*. As the tissues move against each other during lung inflation and deflation, frictional forces cause an increase in tissue resistance. Tissue resistance usually accounts for around 10% of the total resistive work. Tissue resistive work is increased by any condition that increases the amount of interstitial lung tissue, such as pulmonary fibrosis.
  - *Airway resistance*. Gas molecules are subject to frictional forces when they interact with each other and with the walls of the airways.

What factors affect airway resistance?

The resistance to gas flow is affected by two main factors: turbulence and the airway radius.

- **Turbulent gas flow** results in a much higher airway resistance than laminar gas flow does. During normal tidal breathing, gas flow is usually only turbulent in the trachea, but may become turbulent in the larger bronchi during peak inspiratory flow. If the velocity of gas flow increases (e.g. with increasing respiratory rate, RR), gas flow becomes turbulent in the larger bronchi for a greater portion of the respiratory cycle, increasing airway resistance. The point at which gas flow changes from laminar to turbulent is estimated using the Reynolds number.

Key equation: Reynolds number

$$\text{Reynolds number} = \frac{v\rho d}{\eta}$$

where v is velocity of gas flow, ρ is the density of gas, d is the airway diameter and η is the viscosity of gas. A Reynolds number of 2000 predicts an 80% chance of turbulent flow. A Reynolds number of 200 predicts an 80% chance of laminar flow.

- **Airway radius.** According to the Hagan–Poiseuille equation, resistance to gas flow is proportional to r^4 (r is the radius). Therefore, small reductions in airway radius can have a large impact on the resistance to flow.

Key equation: Hagen–Poiseuille equation for a tube

$$\Delta P = \frac{8\dot{Q}\eta l}{\pi r^4}$$

where ΔP is the pressure drop along the tube, $\dot{Q}$ is flow, η is the viscosity of the fluid, l is tube length and r is the radius.

Darcy's law[1] states:

$$\Delta P = \dot{Q}R$$

Therefore, if ΔP is pressure difference and $\dot{Q}$ is flow, then the resistance to flow $R = 8\eta l / \pi r^4$.

On the basis of the Hagan–Poiseuille equation in isolation, one would expect airway resistance to be highest in the terminal bronchioles, as these airways have the smallest radius. However, many terminal bronchioles are arranged in parallel, with a total cross-sectional area much larger than that of the more proximal airways. Overall, the main site of airway resistance is between the lobar bronchi and the sub-segmental bronchi.

Based on the discussion above, airway resistance is increased by:

- **Factors that result in turbulent flow.**
  - *High RR*: gas velocity increases, resulting in turbulent flow in the large bronchi.
  - *Increased airway diameter*: turbulent flow is more common in the larger upper airways such as the trachea. This is why bronchial breathing can be heard physiologically over these airways. Bronchodilatation by the sympathetic nervous system facilitates greater alveolar ventilation rates, but increases the amount of turbulent flow.
  - *Upper airway obstruction*, as exemplified by laryngeal oedema or the presence of a foreign body. The increased velocity of gas flow around the obstruction results in turbulent flow. Heliox, a mixture of helium (He) and O_2, is sometimes used in the management of upper airway obstruction: the lower density of heliox reduces Reynolds number, thereby reducing turbulent flow.
  - *Deep-sea diving*. The barometric pressure of air, and therefore its density, increases with increasing underwater depth. Because of the increased air density, Reynolds number predicts turbulent flow at lower gas velocity. As a result, gas flow becomes turbulent in the bronchi even during normal tidal breathing, increasing the airway resistance. Again, a mixture of He and O_2 is used by divers; the lower density promotes laminar gas flow, thereby reducing the work of breathing.

- **Factors that reduce airway radius.**
  - *Bronchoconstriction*, as occurs physiologically during parasympathetic nervous system activation or pathologically in asthma and chronic obstructive pulmonary disease (COPD). The radius of the small airways is reduced, which increases airway resistance.
  - *Low lung volume*. Airway radius increases during inspiration as a result of radial traction of the lung parenchyma. Likewise, airway radius decreases during expiration, which results in increased airway resistance. This partially explains why patients with asthma and COPD have more difficulty with expiration than inspiration.
  - *Dynamic airway compression*. During forced expiration, the respiratory muscles generate a

---

[1] Darcy's law of flow is analogous to Ohm's law of electricity: potential difference = current × resistance.

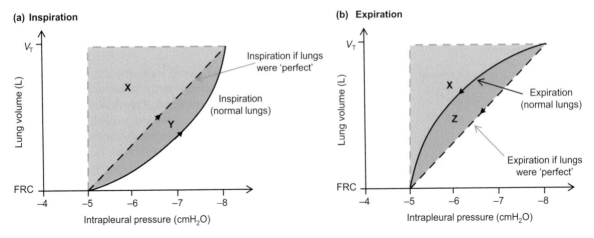

Figure 21.1 Pressure–volume curves: (a) normal tidal inspiration and (b) normal tidal expiration.

positive intrapleural pressure, which causes compression of airways that lack cartilaginous support, particularly the bronchioles, further reducing their airway radius and thus increasing airway resistance. In COPD, there is destruction of supportive elastic tissue with the lung parenchyma, which reduces radial traction on the airways, making these patients particularly susceptible to dynamic airway compression.

How can work of breathing be described graphically?

As mentioned above, work = pressure × volume. Therefore, the work of breathing can be represented as an area on the pressure–volume graph (Figure 21.1).

Pressure–volume loops exhibit hysteresis: the inspiratory and expiratory curves follow different paths (see Chapter 20). The area (i.e. pressure × volume) between the two curves represents the energy expended in overcoming the resistive forces; that is, the overall work done that is dissipated as heat:

- **During tidal inspiration** (Figure 21.1a).
  - The black dotted diagonal line represents inspiration for idealised lungs in which resistive forces are absent. In reality, this is not the case: the deviation of the black solid line from the black dotted line shows how much resistance there is to lung inflation.
  - The triangular area **X** is the elastic work done, which is stored as potential energy.

- The remaining area **Y** is the resistive work done, which is dissipated as heat.
- **During tidal expiration** (Figure 21.1b).
  - The black dotted diagonal line again represents expiration in the absence of resistive forces.
  - The triangular area **X** is the potential energy stored from inspiration that can now be used during expiration.
  - The area **Z** is the resistive work done during expiration.
  - So long as area **Z** is within area **X**, the stored potential energy is sufficient to overcome the resistive forces of expiration, resulting in passive expiration.
  - At the end of expiration, any potential energy not used for expiration is wasted, as it is dissipated as heat.

How does this graph change for patients with restrictive or obstructive lung disease?

In restrictive lung disease, lung compliance is reduced. A higher (more negative) intrapleural pressure is required to achieve a V_T of 500 mL. The work of inspiration is greater, as there is an increase in elastic work. Airway resistance is unchanged, so the resistive work is similar to normal lungs. Expiration remains passive, as the resistive work still lies within the area of potential energy (Figure 21.2a).

In obstructive lung disease, the problem is an increase in airway resistance. Both inspiratory and

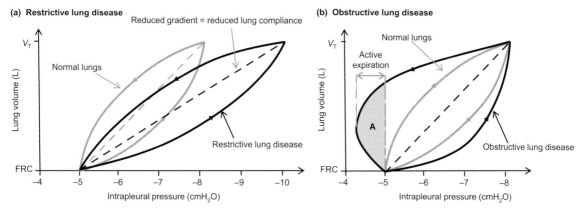

Figure 21.2 Pressure–volume loops: (a) restrictive lung disease and (b) obstructive lung disease.

expiratory work must increase to overcome the additional airway resistance. Graphically, this is represented by a wider pressure–volume loop. If the resistance to gas flow is severe enough, the expiratory work will exceed the stored potential energy, shown graphically as the expiratory curve bulging to the left. If compliance is also increased (as in COPD), expiration is no longer passive, requiring active effort by the expiratory muscles; the shaded area **A** is then the active expiratory work of breathing (Figure 21.2b).

Clinical relevance: anaesthesia and airway resistance

General anaesthesia inevitably results in increased resistance to gas flow:

- **Low lung volume**. Loss of respiratory muscle tone, the supine position and loss of physiological positive end-expiratory pressure (PEEP) result in low lung volume and thus increased airway resistance.
- **Pharyngeal resistance**. In some (unintubated) patients, relaxation of the pharyngeal muscles may result in partial or complete upper airway obstruction, increasing the resistance to airflow.
- **Airway devices**. To fit within the trachea, endotracheal tubes (ETTs) necessarily have a smaller radius. According to the Hagen–Poiseuille equation, reduced radius significantly increases airway resistance. ETT radius is especially important for small children, who are often not permitted to breathe spontaneously when intubated due to the substantially increased work of breathing. This is also why critically ill patients

should be intubated with as wide an ETT as possible, so that airway resistance is as low as possible for weaning.

- **Anaesthetic circuits**. These inevitably cause an increase in airway resistance, ranging from negligible to significant. Corrugated tubing, angle-pieces and high gas flow rates promote turbulent flow, whilst heat and moisture exchangers and adjustable pressure-limiting valves further increase resistance to gas flow.
- **Increased inspiratory gas flow**. Airway devices and anaesthetic circuits increase mechanical dead space. To maintain V_A, V_E must increase: inspiratory gas flow increases, resulting in an increase in turbulent flow.
- **Increased density and reduced viscosity**. Volatile anaesthetics, especially when used at high concentrations, significantly increase the density of the gas mixture, as well as causing a small decrease in viscosity. Both of these effects increase the amount of turbulence and therefore resistance.

Fortunately, airway resistance can be reduced by:

- **Bronchodilatation**. The volatile anaesthetics in current use are all potent bronchodilators. The radius of the small airways increases, thus offsetting some of the effects of general anaesthesia on lung volume and volatile anaesthetics on gas density. Halothane is especially potent due to its effects on vagal tone.
- **Application of extrinsic PEEP**, which increases lung volume: radial traction increases airway radius, thus reducing airway resistance.
- **Laryngeal mask airway** (LMA). In patients susceptible to pharyngeal collapse, the LMA

stents open pharyngeal tissues, thus reducing the resistance to gas flow.

If a patient is to breathe spontaneously under general anaesthesia, the airway resistance must be minimised as much as possible. LMAs are well designed for spontaneous ventilation: they have wide tubing to minimise resistance to gas flow.

Further reading

A. Carter, S. J. Fletcher, R. Tuffin. The effect of inner tube placement on resistance and work of breathing through tracheostomy tubes: a bench test. *Anaesthesia* 2013; **68**(3): 276–82.

S. Farrow, C. Farrow, N. Soni. Size matters: choosing the right tracheal tube. *Anaesthesia* 2012; **67**(8): 815–22.

S. H. Loring, M. Garcia-Jacques, A. Malhotra. Pulmonary characteristics in COPD and mechanics of increased work of breathing. *J Appl Physiol* 2009; **107**(1): 309–14.

V. G. Nyktari, A. A. Papaioannou, G. Prinianakis, et al. Effect of the physical properties of isoflurane, sevoflurane, and desflurane on pulmonary resistance in a laboratory lung model. *Anesthesiology* 2006; **104**(6): 1202–7.

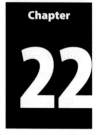

Control of Ventilation

Which anatomical sites are involved in the control of ventilation?

Ventilation is controlled by means of neuronal feedback loops. All feedback loops involve sensors, effectors and a control centre. For ventilation, these are:

- **Sensors** – the central and peripheral chemoreceptors, pulmonary stretch receptors, J-receptors, irritant receptors and joint proprioceptors.
- **Control centre** – the respiratory nuclei in the brainstem.
- **Effectors** – the muscles of respiration.

How does the respiratory centre control ventilation?

The respiratory centre has four main anatomical areas, each with a different function:

- **The dorsal respiratory group (DRG) of neurons** primarily controls the diaphragm and thus is responsible for normal tidal inspiration.
- **The ventral respiratory group (VRG) of neurons** controls the intercostal muscles; its function is to initiate forced expiration and to increase the force of inspiration. Additionally, the VRG contains the pre-Bötzinger complex, a cluster of neurons thought to be the respiratory pacemaker.[1]
- **The apneustic centre** modifies the activity of DRG neurons to prevent overexpansion of the lungs.
- **The pneumotaxic centre** modifies DRG impulses to reduce the depth of inspiration, acting to fine-tune the respiratory pattern. The pneumotaxic centre can also increase the respiratory rate (RR).

What are the inputs to the respiratory centre?

The major inputs to the respiratory centre are the peripheral chemoreceptors, central chemoreceptors, mechanoreceptors and bronchial irritant receptors.

- **Peripheral chemoreceptors.** These are located in the:

  - *Carotid bodies* at the bifurcation of the carotid artery. Their afferent nervous impulses are carried by the glossopharyngeal nerve. The carotid bodies are the most important peripheral chemoreceptors for respiratory responses.
  - *Aortic bodies* on the aortic arch. Their afferent nervous impulses are carried by the vagus nerve. They play a more important role in cardiovascular responses.

The peripheral chemoreceptors have a very high blood flow in relation to their weight. They are stimulated by:

  - *Low* P_aO_2. The aortic and carotid bodies are the only chemoreceptors in the body that respond to hypoxaemia. Note: the peripheral chemoreceptors are stimulated by low arterial O_2 *tension*, not low O_2 content – anaemia and carbon monoxide poisoning do not stimulate the chemoreceptors.
  - *High* P_aCO_2. The peripheral chemoreceptors are only responsible for 20% of the body's response to hypercapnoea, with the central chemoreceptors responsible for the remainder. However, the peripheral chemoreceptors respond the most rapidly, within the order of 1–3 s.
  - *Acidaemia* (pH < 7.35). Only the carotid bodies are stimulated by acidaemia.

---

[1] These neurons express hyperpolarisation-activated cyclic nucleotide-gated channels, the same channels as the pacemaker cells of the sinoatrial node.

- *Hypotension.* Reduced perfusion of the carotid and aortic bodies increases their neuronal output. This is why an increased RR is seen during the development of septic shock, even when there may not be any impairment of gas exchange.

- **Central chemoreceptors.** These are located on the ventral surface of the medulla close to, but separate from, the VRG neurons. In contrast to the peripheral chemoreceptors, central chemoreceptors are solely stimulated by a fall in cerebrospinal fluid (CSF) pH. However, because H^+ and HCO_3^- ions cannot cross the blood–brain barrier (BBB), changes in plasma pH do not directly affect ventilation. Instead, the course of events is as follows:

  - CO_2 freely diffuses from the blood into the CSF, and then from the CSF into the extracellular fluid (ECF) surrounding the central chemoreceptors.
  - The reaction between CO_2 and water results in the formation of H_2CO_3. H_2CO_3 then dissociates into H^+ and HCO_3^-.
  - H^+ diffuses into the chemoreceptor tissue, directly stimulating the chemoreceptors to activate the respiratory centre. The pH of the chemoreceptor ECF therefore provides an indirect measure of arterial P_aCO_2.
  - Therefore, as P_aCO_2 increases, the central chemoreceptors are stimulated and $\dot{V}_E$ increases.

There are a few important points to make about the central chemoreceptors:

  - The CSF protein concentration is much lower than that of plasma and thus minimal buffering of CO_2 occurs. This makes the CSF more sensitive to small changes in PCO_2 than plasma.
  - Respiratory acidosis stimulates the central chemoreceptors more than metabolic acidosis: CO_2 can diffuse across the BBB, whereas H^+ ions cannot. However, in profound metabolic acidosis, as exemplified by diabetic ketoacidosis, ventilation is stimulated via the carotid bodies, resulting in Kussmaul breathing.
  - The cerebral vasodilatation that accompanies hypercapnoea enhances the central

chemoreceptor mechanism by increasing the blood flow to the medulla.
- If hypercapnoea becomes chronic, as occurs in a subset of chronic obstructive pulmonary disease (COPD) patients, the increase in $\dot{V}_E$ cannot be sustained and returns to near normal. The underlying mechanism is as follows:

  - HCO_3^- ions are actively secreted into the CSF to buffer the change in pH.
  - CSF pH returns to normal and the central chemoreceptors are no longer stimulated: the activity of the respiratory centre is reduced.
  - The kidneys also reabsorb more HCO_3^-, which normalises arterial pH, thus reducing the stimulation of the respiratory centre by the carotid bodies.

These compensatory mechanisms result in a loss of sensitivity to CO_2, causing these patients to rely on hypoxaemic drive alone. Care must be taken when administering O_2 to COPD patients with chronic hypercapnoea as there is a theoretical risk that these patients will stop breathing.
- Unlike the peripheral chemoreceptors, the central chemoreceptors are not stimulated by hypoxaemia. In fact, in the absence of the peripheral chemoreceptors, hypoxaemia depresses the respiratory centre.

The inputs of the peripheral and central chemoreceptors are synergistic. For example, if hypoxaemia is sensed by the peripheral chemoreceptors and hypercapnoea by the central chemoreceptors, the resulting ventilatory response is greater than the sum of the two effects.

- **Mechanoreceptors.** The contribution that mechanoreceptors make to the stimulation of ventilation is controversial.[2] Mechanoreceptors that possibly affect the respiratory centre are:

  - *Lung stretch receptors,* located in bronchial smooth muscle. Overinflation of the lung stimulates these stretch receptors, whose

---

[2] It was thought that a number of mechanoreceptors contributed to the control of ventilation. This has been called into question, as denervated transplanted lungs have been shown to exhibit a normal ventilatory response.

impulses are conveyed to the apneustic centre by the vagus nerve, causing a reduction in the depth of inspiration. This is called the Hering–Breuer reflex. During normal physiological breathing, it is unlikely that sufficient stretch will occur to trigger the Hering–Breuer reflex. However, stretch responses may be important in neonates and ventilated patients.

- *Muscle spindles.* The ventilatory response to exercise is thought to be initiated by muscle spindle activity.

- **Other factors.** The respiratory centre also receives other inputs from the peripheral and central nervous systems:

  - *Juxtacapillary receptors* (J-receptors). These are non-myelinated C-fibres in the alveolar walls. Activation causes an increase in ventilation, a feeling of dyspnoea, bradycardia and hypotension. It is thought that J-receptors are stimulated by pulmonary oedema and pulmonary emboli.
  - *Irritant receptors.* Located in the airway epithelium, these cause bronchoconstriction and stimulate ventilation in the presence of noxious gases.
  - *Pain receptors.* Activation of pain receptors stimulates ventilation.
  - *Thalamus.* An increase in core body temperature stimulates ventilation.

- *Limbic system.* Extreme emotional states stimulate the respiratory centre, resulting in hyperventilation.
- *Cerebral cortex.* All of the other inputs to the respiratory centre can be transiently overridden by voluntary thought. However, one cannot breath-hold indefinitely; after a short period of apnoea, chemoreceptor stimulation by hypoxaemia or hypercapnoea overrides voluntary control, known as the 'break point'.

Summarise the ventilatory response to hypoxaemia

When P_aO_2 falls below 8 kPa, the peripheral chemoreceptors rapidly stimulate the respiratory centre, which significantly increases $\dot{V}_E$ (Figure 22.1a). This ventilatory response is further augmented in the presence of hypercapnoea. However, severe prolonged hypoxaemia has a depressive effect on the respiratory centre, causing apnoea.

Summarise the ventilatory response to hypercapnoea

The respiratory centre is stimulated by:

- **High P_aCO_2**, which activates both peripheral chemoreceptors;
- **Low arterial pH**, which activates the carotid bodies;

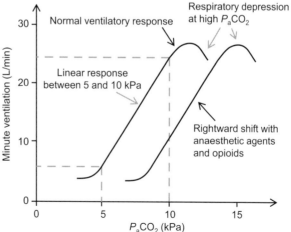

Figure 22.1 Ventilatory response to: (a) hypoxaemia and (b) hypercapnoea.

- **High CSF PCO_2**, leading to low central chemoreceptor ECF pH, which activates the central chemoreceptors.

The response of ventilation to CO_2 is linear within normal clinical limits (P_aCO_2 5–10 kPa), but experiments in animals have shown that $\dot{V}_E$ reduces with profound hypercapnoea (Figure 22.1b).

Clinical relevance: drugs and control of ventilation

All anaesthetic agents have a depressant effect on both the respiratory centre and the peripheral chemoreceptors, leading to reduced ventilatory response to both hypercapnoea and hypoxaemia. Graphically, anaesthetic agents shift the CO_2 response curve to the right (Figure 22.1b).

Opioids have no effect on the response of the peripheral or central chemoreceptors to hypoxaemia or hypercapnoea. In contrast, opioids have a significant depressant effect on the medullary respiratory centre. Thus, the ventilatory response to hypoxaemia and hypercapnoea is blunted, with the CO_2 response curve shifted to the right (Figure 22.1b).

The respiratory stimulant doxapram acts at the peripheral chemoreceptors, but the mechanism involved is unclear.

Further reading

A. B. Lumb. Control of breathing. In: A. B. Lumb. *Nunn's Applied Respiratory Physiology*, 8th edition. London, Churchill Livingstone, 2016; 51–72.

H. V. Forster, C. A. Smith. Contributions of central and peripheral chemoreceptors to the ventilatory response to CO_2/H^+. *J Appl Physiol* 2010; **108**(4): 989–94.

K. T. S. Pattinson. Opioids and the control of respiration. *Br J Anaesth* 2008; **100**(6): 747–58.

Pulmonary Circulation

What are the unique features of the pulmonary circulation?

The pulmonary circulation differs significantly in characteristics from the systemic circulation. The pulmonary circulation is a low-pressure, low-resistance, high-flow circulation: a blood flow of 5 L/min (i.e. 100% of cardiac output, CO) is achieved with a driving pressure (i.e. mean pulmonary artery pressure, MPAP) of only 15 mmHg. Important features of the anatomy of the pulmonary circulation are as follows:

- As may be expected, there are two pulmonary arteries: one for each lung. In contrast, there are at least four pulmonary veins: two arising from each lung.
- Initially, the arteries, veins and bronchi run in close proximity to each other, dividing at the same points. In the periphery of the lung, the vessels separate: the veins pass between lung lobules, whilst the arteries and bronchi travel together to the centre of the lobules.
- The pulmonary capillaries are fragile and very narrow (diameter 7–10 μm), just wide enough for red blood cells to squeeze through.
- The conducting airways of the lung also have their own blood supply, called the bronchial circulation. Some of the deoxygenated blood is carried away by the pulmonary veins, where it mixes with oxygenated blood and enters the systemic circulation. This is one of the causes of an anatomical shunt (see Chapter 14).

Clinical relevance: lung transplantation and the bronchial circulation

Historically during lung transplant surgery, despite the fact that the bronchial arteries normally receive 3–5% of CO, the donor bronchial artery was not re-anastomosed. Because most grafts survived despite the loss of the bronchial artery, the bronchial circulation had been considered to be unnecessary. However, a subset of lung transplant patients develop an ischaemic bronchiolitis obliterans, thought to be due to loss of the bronchial circulation. There is currently a trend towards direct bronchial artery revascularisation to overcome this problem.

Why can the pressure within the pulmonary circulation be low?

Unlike the systemic circulation, the pulmonary circulation does not need to direct blood flow from one region to another, with the exception of the property of hypoxic pulmonary vasoconstriction (see later). Therefore, pulmonary arterial pressure only needs to be high enough to propel blood to the lung apices.

The pulmonary capillaries are unique in being almost entirely surrounded by alveolar gas. They are also very fragile, with little connective tissue, and are therefore prone to distension or collapse. Transudation of fluid from the pulmonary capillary to the alveolus (i.e. pulmonary oedema) is dependent in part[1] on the transmural pressure, given by the difference in pressures between the capillary and the alveolus. As alveolar pressure is very low, having a low-pressure pulmonary capillary is essential if pulmonary oedema is to be avoided.

How do the pulmonary and systemic vascular resistances compare?

Key equation: Darcy's law

This is akin to Ohm's law in an electrical circuit:

---

[1] Pulmonary surfactant also contributes to the prevention of fluid transudation.

Potential difference = current × resistance, $V = IR$

Similarly, for the vascular system:

Pressure difference = total flow × vascular resistance

$$\Rightarrow vascular\ resistance = \frac{pressure\ difference}{total\ flow}$$

Therefore:

$$PVR = 80 \times \frac{MPAP-PCWP}{CO}$$

Similarly:

$$SVR \approx 80 \times \frac{MAP-mean\ right\ atrial\ pressure}{CO}$$

where MPAP (mmHg) is the mean pulmonary artery pressure, PCWP (mmHg) is the pulmonary capillary wedge pressure, MAP (mmHg) is the mean arterial pressure (MAP), SVR (dyn.s.cm^{-5}) is the systemic vascular resistance, PVR (dyn.s.cm^{-5}) is the pulmonary vascular resistance, CO (L/min) is the cardiac output and 80 is a constant related to unit conversion.

Calculating SVR using typical values (MAP = 100 mmHg, mean right atrial pressure is 2 mmHg and CO = 5 L/min):

$$SVR = 80 \times \frac{MAP-mean\ right\ atrial\ pressure}{CO}$$

$$\Rightarrow SVR = 80 \times \frac{100-2}{5} = 1568\ dyn\ s\ cm^{-5}$$

Likewise, calculating PVR with typical values (MPAP = 15 mmHg, PCWP = 5 mmHg, CO = 5 L/min):

$$PVR = 80 \times \frac{MPAP-PCWP}{CO}$$

$$\Rightarrow PVR = 80 \times \frac{15-5}{5} = 160\ dyn\ s\ cm^{-5}$$

PVR is approximately one-tenth of SVR. Note that all values required to calculate SVR and PVR (with the exception of MAP) can be measured with a pulmonary artery catheter (PAC).

Which factors affect PVR?

PVR is affected by three main factors:

- **Pulmonary artery pressure**. Increased MPAP results in a significant reduction in PVR (Figure 23.1a). This is the result of two mechanisms:

  - *Recruitment*, where collapsed pulmonary capillaries are reopened. This is the most important mechanism at low MPAP.
  - *Distension*, where open pulmonary capillaries are further distended. This is the most important mechanism at high MPAP.

During exercise, despite a large increase in CO, MPAP only rises moderately due to the recruitment and distension of pulmonary capillaries and the corresponding fall in PVR.

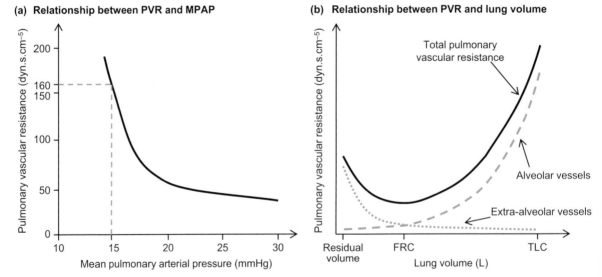

(a) Relationship between PVR and MPAP

(b) Relationship between PVR and lung volume

Figure 23.1 Relationship between (a) PVR and MPAP and (b) PVR and lung volume (FRC = functional residual capacity; TLC = total lung capacity).

However, there is a limit to recruitment and distension of the pulmonary capillaries. In racehorses, this limit is reached at moderate exercise – severe exercise can lead to very high MPAP and pulmonary haemorrhage can result. Fortunately, this is not common in humans.

- **Lung volumes.** Functionally, there are two types of pulmonary blood vessels:

    - *Alveolar capillaries*, which have little connective tissue and are compressed when subjected to raised alveolar pressure.
    - *Extra-alveolar vessels*, which are not exposed to alveolar pressure and can be pulled open by radial traction of the surrounding lung parenchyma.

    The changes in the shape of alveolar and extra-alveolar vessels account for the changes in PVR at different lung volumes (Figure 23.1b):

    - *At functional residual capacity* (FRC), PVR is at its lowest. This is a useful piece of design: tidal breathing takes place around FRC and PVR is therefore low for the majority of the time, reducing right ventricular workload.
    - *At high lung volume*, PVR increases primarily as a result of resistance to blood flow within the alveolar capillaries; these capillaries are stretched and distorted, which significantly increases their resistance to flow. The extra-alveolar vessels contribute little resistance to blood flow as lung volume increases; the radius of the vessels increases by radial traction, thereby reducing resistance to blood flow.
    - *At low lung volumes*, PVR is high primarily as a result of resistance to flow within the extra-alveolar vessels; these vessels are very narrow and offer high resistance to flow.

- **Hypoxic pulmonary vasoconstriction** (HPV). The response of the pulmonary circulation to hypoxia is unique. In the systemic circulation, tissue hypoxia causes vasodilatation of neighbouring blood vessels, so that local perfusion is matched to local metabolism. In contrast, the pulmonary vessels *vasoconstrict* in response to low alveolar O_2 tension ($P_AO_2 < 8$ kPa). This is a useful physiological mechanism: vasoconstriction of the pulmonary arterioles adjacent to hypoxic alveoli increases local vascular resistance, thus redirecting blood flow to better-ventilated areas of the lung. While the

pulmonary arterioles are the main site of vasoconstriction, venoconstriction of small pulmonary venules also contributes to HPV (albeit to a lesser degree). The response of HPV to low P_AO_2 is rapid, occurring within seconds; pulmonary lobar blood flow can halve within minutes. When alveolar hypoxia is prolonged, there is a second phase of slow, sustained pulmonary vasoconstriction.

- The exact mechanism for HPV is not fully established:

    - The main determinant of HPV is low *alveolar* PO_2, but low mixed venous PO_2 contributes around a fifth of the response.
    - HPV continues to operate in denervated lungs (i.e. following lung transplantation), so is not extrinsically (neurally) mediated.
    - The factors thought most likely to mediate HPV are:

        - *Nitric oxide* (NO), a potent pulmonary arteriolar vasodilator that is synthesised in the pulmonary endothelium when P_AO_2 is >9.3 kPa. Alveolar hypoxia decreases the amount of NO produced, resulting in arteriolar vasoconstriction.
        - *O_2-sensitive K^+ channels*, which are stimulated by alveolar hypoxia, leading to a depolarisation of the arteriolar membrane potential. Ca^{2+} channels are opened, resulting in arteriolar vasoconstriction.

Give some examples of HPV in clinical practice

HPV plays a key role in a number of physiological and pathological situations:

- **The foetal circulation.** *In utero*, the foetal lungs have yet to expand: P_AO_2 is zero, and HPV causes widespread pulmonary vasoconstriction. The resulting high PVR means that only 10% of the foetal CO passes through the foetal lungs, with blood instead being redirected through the ductus arteriosus. At the first breath, O_2 enters the alveoli; PVR decreases dramatically, resulting in an increase in pulmonary blood flow.
- **Infant respiratory distress syndrome.** Lack of surfactant results in increased surface tension, which leads to widespread atelectasis. The first breath is therefore extremely difficult, and PVR

remains high due to HPV. This results in poor alveolar perfusion and death of pneumocytes. Necrotic pneumocytes form a barrier (known as a hyaline membrane due to its histopathological appearance) that impairs diffusion and thus increases HPV, resulting in a vicious cycle.

- **Pneumonia**. HPV increases the PVR of the arterioles in the vicinity of hypoxic alveoli, which directs blood to better-ventilated alveoli, thereby reducing $\dot{V}/\dot{Q}$ mismatch.

- **High altitude**. Low P_B results in alveolar hypoxia throughout the lungs. The result is generalised pulmonary vasoconstriction and venoconstriction; pulmonary venoconstriction is implicated in the development of high-altitude pulmonary oedema (see Chapter 87).

- **Upper lobe diversion in cardiogenic pulmonary oedema**. In left ventricular failure, left ventricular end-diastolic pressure and pulmonary venous pressure are raised. Owing to the effect of West zones, pulmonary venous pressure is greater at the lung bases than the apices; the greater pressure results in transudation of fluid across the alveolar–capillary barrier (i.e. pulmonary oedema). The basal alveoli become hypoxic: HPV diverts blood to the better-ventilated apices.

Whilst HPV is primarily the result of *alveolar* hypoxia, some pulmonary vasoconstriction occurs in response to arterial hypoxaemia. Some patients with arterial hypoxaemia secondary to chronic lung disease (e.g. pulmonary fibrosis and chronic obstructive pulmonary disease, COPD) develop pulmonary arterial hypertension, which is thought to be due to widespread HPV. The resulting pulmonary hypertension can lead to right ventricular failure, known as cor pulmonale.

HPV is modified by various factors:

- HPV is enhanced by acidosis and hypercapnoea.
- HPV is reduced by alkalosis, hypocapnoea, vasodilators (nitrates, sodium nitroprusside, NO), bronchodilators and volatile anaesthetic agents.

Clinical relevance: HPV and the anaesthetist

By diverting blood away from hypoxic alveoli, HPV reduces $\dot{V}/\dot{Q}$ mismatch. Therefore, if HPV is inhibited, $\dot{V}/\dot{Q}$ mismatch and hypoxaemia may result.

HPV is inhibited by volatile anaesthetics. In a patient with pneumonia, intraoperative inhibition of HPV by volatile anaesthetic agents may cause a significant shunt, resulting in hypoxaemia. Fortunately, significant inhibition of HPV only occurs with the commonly used volatile anaesthetics above 1 MAC (minimum alveolar concentration). N_2O has little effect on HPV and intravenous agents have no effect.

HPV is important in one-lung anaesthesia. Without HPV, one-lung ventilation would result in a significant $\dot{V}/\dot{Q}$ mismatch. HPV redirects blood from the unventilated lung to the ventilated lung, minimising hypoxaemia.

Clinical relevance: positive end-expiratory pressure, PVR and one-lung ventilation

Positive end-expiratory pressure (PEEP) and positive-pressure ventilation both increase alveolar pressure, leading to compression of alveolar capillaries and therefore higher PVR. This can be an issue in one-lung ventilation:

- In the lateral position, the weight of the mediastinum and non-dependent (upper) lung tends to reduce the volume of the ventilated dependent (lower) lung. Atelectasis is more common at low lung volumes, leading to $\dot{V}/\dot{Q}$ mismatch and hypoxaemia.

- To counteract this, many anaesthetists apply PEEP to the dependent lung to prevent atelectasis. However, if too much PEEP is applied, the PVR of the dependent lung can increase – blood is diverted to the non-dependent lung, which increases $\dot{V}/\dot{Q}$ mismatch and worsens hypoxaemia.

- In this eventuality, continuous positive airways pressure can be applied to the non-dependent lung at the same pressure as PEEP is applied to the dependent lung (e.g. 5 cmH$_2$O). This increases the PVR of the non-dependent lung, diverting blood back to the dependent lung. The only problem with this strategy is that the volume of the non-dependent lung increases, which may hinder the surgeon (but arguably less than returning to two-lung ventilation!).

Bizarrely, patients with 'normal' lungs (i.e. good pre-operative spirometry) are more likely to develop hypoxaemia with one-lung ventilation than patients with poorer lung function (e.g. those with COPD). The reason for this paradox is not proven with any certainty, but it is likely that gas-trapping in patients with COPD causes intrinsic PEEP, which increases the volume of the dependent lung, reducing atelectasis and improving $\dot{V}/\dot{Q}$ matching.

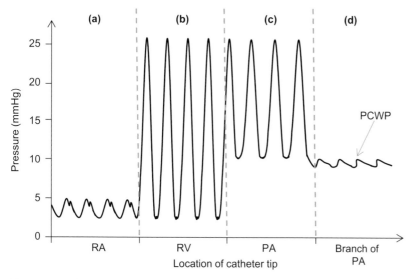

Figure 23.2 Characteristic pressure waveforms as a pulmonary artery catheter is advanced (RA = right atrium; RV = right ventricle; PA = pulmonary artery; PCWP = pulmonary capillary wedge pressure).

Describe the changes in pressure waveform seen when 'floating' a balloon-tipped PAC

The flow-directed, balloon-tipped PAC (also known as the Swan–Ganz catheter) has many uses:

- **Diagnostic**; for example, pulmonary hypertension and acute respiratory distress syndrome.
- **Measurement of haemodynamic parameters**; for example, CO and mixed venous O_2 saturation.
- **Therapeutic**; for example, aspiration of air emboli.

Despite its wide applicability in critical illness, the use of the Swan–Ganz catheter has declined in recent years: in the general adult intensive care population, using a PAC has not been shown to reduce mortality. In addition, the PAC is associated with several serious complications, such as line infection, pulmonary infarction and pulmonary artery rupture.

The PAC has a length of 150 cm and is usually inserted through a sheath in the right internal jugular vein. The pressure at the tip of the PAC is transduced and used to identify the tip's location (Figure 23.2). Once the PAC has been inserted as far as the right ventricle (Figure 23.2b) (about 20 cm), the balloon is inflated. The tip of the PAC is guided by the flow of blood through the pulmonary valve and into a pulmonary artery (Figure 23.2c), until it wedges in a branch of the pulmonary artery (Figure 23.2d), giving the PCWP.

Further reading

A. B. Lumb. The pulmonary circulation. In: A. B. Lumb. *Nunn's Applied Respiratory Physiology, 8th edition.* London, Churchill Livingstone, 2016; 89–108.

K. Nowak, M. Kamler, M. Bock, et al. Bronchial artery revascularisation affects graft recovery after lung transplantation. *Am J Respir Crit Care Med* 2002; **165**(2): 216–20.

J. Eastwood, R. Mahajan. One-lung anaesthesia. *Continuing Educ Anaesth Crit Care Pain* 2002; **2**(3): 83–7.

R. Naeije, S. Brimioulle. Physiology in medicine: importance of hypoxic pulmonary vasoconstriction in maintaining arterial oxygenation during acute respiratory failure. *Crit Care* 2001; **5**(2): 67–71.

Chapter

24

Oxygen Toxicity

What is oxygen toxicity?

Breathing O_2 at high partial pressure can have harmful effects on the body. Many organ systems can be affected by O_2 toxicity, but the most common are:

- **The central nervous system** (CNS), causing seizures and unconsciousness when breathing hyperbaric O_2, which is of obvious importance for divers. CNS toxicity is known as the Paul Bert effect.
- **The lungs**, causing bronchopulmonary dysplasia in premature neonates, whilst older children and adults develop absorption atelectasis and acute respiratory distress syndrome (ARDS). Lung toxicity is known as the Lorraine Smith effect.
- **The retina**, leading to retrolental fibroplasia in neonates, also known as the retinopathy of prematurity.

What is the mechanism of oxygen toxicity?

Toxicity is due to the unique structure of the O_2 molecule. The O_2 molecule is made up of two oxygen atoms, each with an unpaired electron in its outer shell. It is these unpaired electrons that give O_2 its property of paramagnetism. Molecules containing unpaired electrons – or free radicals – are usually highly reactive. Fortunately, the unpaired electrons of the O_2 molecule are fairly unreactive, requiring metal ions (such as those found in metalloproteins) to help the O_2 molecule accept electrons. This is of particular importance in the electron transport chain, where electrons are transferred to O_2 molecules, mediated by the copper-containing cytochrome c oxidase (Complex IV), to form water molecules.

The reduction of O_2 to $2H_2O$ requires four electrons: O_2 molecules accept one electron at a time, passing through a number of oxidation states along the way. Known intermediate molecules are the

superoxide anion ($O_2^{\bullet-}$), hydrogen peroxide (H_2O_2) and hydroxyl free radicals ($OH^{\bullet}$): these are collectively known as reactive oxygen species (ROS). ROS are also generated when cells are exposed to ionising radiation. O_2 toxicity is thought to be due to the harmful effects of ROS on nucleic acids, fatty acids, amino acids and sulphydryl-containing enzymes.

Is there a natural antioxidant system in the body?

Antioxidants can be either exogenous or endogenous. Exogenous antioxidants are obtained from the diet and include ascorbic acid (vitamin C). The body has many endogenous antioxidant systems to protect against oxidative stress. The most important are the glutathione, catalase and superoxide dismutase systems. However, at times of oxidative stress, these systems are overwhelmed by ROS, leading to cell damage.

Does the body make any use of ROS?

Despite their potential toxicity, ROS are also essential to the normal function of the body:

- Neutrophils and macrophages kill phagocytosed bacteria by synthesising and secreting ROS into the phagosome. The consumption of O_2 during this process is called the respiratory burst.
- Thyroid follicular cells synthesise H_2O_2, which is used to oxidise iodine anions (I^-) to iodine (I_2) (see Chapter 81).

How much oxygen is harmful?

Inspired O_2 below 50 kPa (an inspired fraction of O_2 F_iO_2 of 50% at atmospheric pressure) is considered to be safe. The risk of O_2 toxicity increases as the inspired partial pressure of O_2 increases and the duration of exposure increases.

Divers are particularly susceptible to CNS toxicity due to the breathing of gases at hyperbaric pressures and due to the consequences of losing consciousness underwater. To minimise the risk of O_2 toxicity, divers calculate their maximum O_2 exposure times based on the depth of the dive and the total time underwater.

Clinical relevance: intensive care and oxygenation

Studies have shown evidence of a reduction in pulmonary function in healthy volunteers following 24 h of exposure to 100% O_2. After 48 h of 100% O_2 exposure, subjects may develop early features of ARDS. However, there is significant variability in the length of exposure and F_iO_2 required to develop toxicity between patients.

Most intensive care guidelines recommend keeping the F_iO_2 below 50% where possible. If higher F_iO_2 is required, the time that the patient is exposed should be minimised. However, in the hypoxaemic patient, high inspired concentrations of O_2 should never be withheld for fear of O_2 toxicity.

What is the connection between bleomycin and oxygen toxicity?

Bleomycin is a chemotherapy drug used in the treatment of Hodgkin's lymphoma and testicular carcinoma. The most serious side effect of bleomycin is pulmonary fibrosis, which usually occurs within the first 6 months of treatment. Of concern to anaesthetists is that patients who have received bleomycin who subsequently require supplemental O_2 (e.g. owing to pneumonia or general anaesthesia) appear to be at increased risk of a rapidly developing life-threatening pulmonary fibrosis. Because of this, patients who have been treated with bleomycin carry an alert card – O_2 administration should be avoided if possible, and if O_2 is absolutely necessary, it should be titrated to an S_aO_2 of 88–92%.

The connection between bleomycin and O_2-induced lung injury is controversial, and the mechanism of bleomycin-induced lung toxicity is not completely resolved. However, it is known that bleomycin acts by chelating iron. The bleomycin–iron complex reacts with O_2, resulting in ROS (superoxide and hydroxide), which cleave DNA. It is certainly possible that administration of O_2 results in an excess of ROS, which overwhelm the body's protective mechanisms.

Further reading

A. B. Lumb. Oxygen toxicity and hyperoxia. In: A. B. Lumb. *Nunn's Applied Respiratory Physiology, 8th edition*. London, Churchill Livingstone, 2016; 341–56.

U. Nimmagadda, M. R. Salem, G. J. Crystal. Preoxygenation: physiologic basis, benefits, and potential risks. *Anesth Analg* 2017; **124**(2): 507–17.

N. Allan, C. Siller, A. Breen. Anaesthetic implications of chemotherapy. *Continuing Educ Anaesth Crit Care Pain* 2012; **12**(2): 52–6.

R. Taneja, R. S. Vaughan. Oxygen. *Continuing Educ Anaesth Crit Care Pain* 2001; **1**(4): 104–7.

I. Fridovich. Oxygen toxicity: a radical explanation. *J Exp Biol* 1998; **201**(8): 1203–9.

D. D. Mathes. Bleomycin and hyperoxia exposure in the operating room. *Anesth Analg* 1995; **81**(3): 624–9.

Chapter

25

Ventilatory Failure

What is meant by the term 'respiratory failure'?

Respiratory failure occurs when the respiratory system fails in one or both of its main functions; namely, the oxygenation of blood and the elimination of CO_2. Respiratory failure is categorised as 'type 1' or 'type 2' on the basis of blood gas analysis:

- **Type 1 respiratory failure** is defined as a P_aO_2 < 8.0 kPa with a normal or low P_aCO_2.
- **Type 2 respiratory failure** is defined as a P_aO_2 < 8.0 kPa with a raised P_aCO_2 > 6.0 kPa.

What is the difference between oxygenation and ventilation?

The respiratory system can be considered as two parts: a gas-exchange system and a 'bellows'.

- **The gas-exchange system** is made up of:
  - *Alveolar–capillary units*;
  - *Pulmonary circulation*.

  The gas-exchange system is responsible for oxygenation; deficiency leads to hypoxaemia and type 1 respiratory failure.
- **The bellows system** is made up of:
  - *Chest wall and pleura*;
  - *Respiratory muscles*;
  - *Airways*;
  - *Nerves*;
  - *Respiratory centre*.

  The bellows system is responsible for ventilation: moving air from the atmosphere to the alveoli on inspiration and from the alveoli to the atmosphere on expiration.

  Importantly, $\dot{V}_A$ facilitates the diffusion of CO_2 from the pulmonary capillaries to the alveoli: $\dot{V}_A$ (and not $\dot{V}_E$) is inversely proportional to P_aCO_2

(see Chapter 11). Failure of alveolar ventilation leads to increased P_aCO_2; that is, type 2 respiratory failure.

Which pathophysiological processes cause type 2 respiratory failure?

Normally, ventilation is controlled by a negative-feedback mechanism:

- A rise in P_aCO_2 stimulates the respiratory centre in the medulla oblongata via the peripheral and central chemoreceptors (see Chapter 22).
- The respiratory centre sends excitatory impulses to the respiratory muscles to increase the rate and depth of inspiration. $\dot{V}_E$ and $\dot{V}_A$ both increase.
- Owing to the inverse relationship between P_aCO_2 and $\dot{V}_A$, P_aCO_2 decreases.

In health, this system is very sensitive: P_aCO_2 is kept within tight limits. If P_aCO_2 rises above 6 kPa, $\dot{V}_A$ must be inadequate and one of the components of ventilation must be malfunctioning:

- **Failure of the respiratory centre** to respond appropriately. This may be due to:
  - *Respiratory centre depression* by opioids or general anaesthesia;
  - *Reflex desensitisation* of the respiratory centre to high P_aCO_2 in order to prevent respiratory muscle fatigue.
- **A problem with chest wall movement**. This could be:
  - *Mechanical*; for example, flail chest;
  - *Neuropathic*; for example, Guillain–Barré syndrome;
  - *Muscular*; for example, myopathies.
- **Respiratory muscle fatigue**. Fatigue occurs when the respiratory muscles cannot synthesise sufficient ATP to meet the demands of muscle contraction despite an intact respiratory drive and chest wall.

Describe how a patient with myasthenia gravis may develop respiratory failure

Myasthenia gravis is an autoimmune disease resulting in antagonism and destruction of postsynaptic nicotinic acetylcholine receptors at the neuromuscular junction (see Chapter 53). Clinically, this results in weakness of voluntary muscle with characteristic fatigability. The muscle groups most commonly affected are ocular, facial, bulbar and limb. Respiratory muscles are usually only mildly affected.

During a myasthenic crisis, the respiratory muscles may become profoundly weak. The inspiratory muscles become too weak to maintain normal V_T and breathing becomes shallow and rapid. Shallow breathing is particularly ineffective as dead space makes up a higher proportion of $\dot{V}_E$: $\dot{V}_A$ decreases, resulting in hypercapnoea (i.e. type 2 respiratory failure). In addition, the small inspiratory volumes cause microatelectasis, which decreases lung compliance and further increases the work of breathing. This situation can be worsened if there is an associated pneumonia or aspiration due to poor cough and secretion clearance, leading to a $\dot{V}/\dot{Q}$ mismatch.

Describe how patients with stable chronic obstructive pulmonary disease develop chronic hypercapnoea

Chronic obstructive pulmonary disease (COPD) is characterised by small-airways obstruction and destruction of lung elastic tissue, leading to chest hyperinflation. Hyperinflation has adverse consequences:

- **Diaphragmatic flattening**, which puts the diaphragm at a mechanical disadvantage. During inspiration, the diaphragm must contract with a greater force to generate the same negative intrapleural pressure as a normal patient.
- **Increased anterior–posterior diameter of the thoracic cage**, which results in an increased fibre length of the intercostal muscles. The sarcomere overlap is no longer ideal, so intercostal muscle contraction requires more energy to generate the same chest wall movement as a normal patient.

Patients with chronic, stable COPD therefore have increased inspiratory work of breathing compared with normal patients.

A subset of COPD patients develops chronic hypercapnoea. The mechanism behind this is not entirely clear. What is known is that:

- Most patients with chronic hypercapnoea can bring their P_aCO_2 back down to normal levels through voluntary hyperventilation.
- These patients start to develop respiratory muscle fatigue after a few minutes of voluntary hyperventilation.

It is likely, therefore, that these patients' respiratory centres have 'chosen' to hypoventilate rather than ventilating to achieve a normal P_aCO_2 and risking respiratory muscle fatigue. This is known as reflex desensitisation of the respiratory centre and highlights the concept of optimisation over homeostasis in physiology.

Clinical relevance: exacerbation of COPD

An exacerbation of COPD is defined as an acute change in a COPD patient's dyspnoea, cough and/or sputum that is beyond normal day-to-day variations. Exacerbations are commonly infective in origin, but also have a number of other causes, including atmospheric pollution.

During COPD exacerbations, there is a significant increase in the resistive and elastic work of breathing. During expiration, dynamic airway obstruction results in intrinsic positive end-expiratory pressure (PEEP), which must then be overcome on the next inspiration, causing further inspiratory work. Patients with COPD, especially those who have chronic hypercapnoea, are very susceptible to respiratory muscle fatigue. Owing to the high inspiratory work during exacerbations, the metabolic demand of the respiratory muscles cannot be met – $\dot{V}_A$ decreases and P_aCO_2 rises.

Decreased $\dot{V}_A$ and high inspiratory workload may be overcome by respiratory support – either invasive or non-invasive ventilation. Non-invasive ventilation acts in two ways:

- Extrinsic PEEP is applied to offset intrinsic PEEP and dynamic hyperinflation, thereby reducing the work of inspiration.
- Pressure support helps to overcome the increased inspiratory airway resistance, restoring V_T to normal.

The use of non-invasive ventilation in the management of COPD exacerbations has been shown to reduce the need for invasive ventilation. Intensive care complications are reduced, as are the lengths of intensive care and hospital stays.

Further reading

A. B. Lumb. Ventilatory failure. In: A. B. Lumb. *Nunn's Applied Respiratory Physiology, 8th edition*. London, Churchill Livingstone, 2016; 379–88.

S. Mehta. Neuromuscular disease causing acute respiratory failure. *Respir Care* 2006; **51**(9): 1016–23.

C. Roussos, A. Koutsoukou. Respiratory failure. *Eur Respir J* 2003; **22**(Suppl. 47): 3s–14s.

M. Thavasothy, N. Hirsch. Myasthenia gravis. *Contin Educ Anaesth Crit Care Pain* 2002; **2**(3): 88–90.

M. J. Garfield. Non-invasive ventilation. *Contin Educ Anaesth Crit Care Pain* 2001; **1**(5): 142–5.

Anaesthesia and the Lung

What effects do anaesthetic drugs have on the respiratory system?

Many of the drugs used by anaesthetists have effects on the medullary respiratory centre, the peripheral chemoreceptors and the airways. Their effects are most easily classified by drug class:

- **Volatile anaesthetic agents.** The inhalational agents have dose-dependent effects on the respiratory system:

  - *An increase in respiratory rate* (RR), but with reduced V_T.
  - *Blunted ventilatory response to hypercapnoea,* the extent of which varies between volatile agents: enflurane > desflurane > isoflurane > sevoflurane > halothane. The exceptions are N_2O (which has no effect) and ether (which may increase $\dot{V}_E$).

- **Intravenous anaesthetic agents.**

  - *Initial respiratory stimulation* following induction of general anaesthesia.
  - *Subsequent respiratory depression.* Respiratory stimulation is followed by abrupt respiratory centre depression. V_T falls and apnoea may occur, especially with the use of propofol.
  - *Specific to certain drugs*:

    - Propofol depresses laryngeal reflexes. This is used to the anaesthetist's advantage: depression of laryngeal reflexes allows the insertion of a laryngeal mask airway (LMA).
    - Propofol is thought to abolish the peripheral chemoreceptor response to hypoxaemia.
    - Ketamine differs from the other intravenous agents – in addition to its

cardiovascular stability, ketamine preserves airway reflexes and spontaneous ventilation.

Other drugs commonly used in anaesthesia with effects on the respiratory system are:

- **Opioids**, causing:

  - *Depression of the respiratory centre,* resulting in a reduced RR and blunting of the ventilatory response to hypercapnoea.
  - *Antitussive action,* depressing the cough reflex.
  - *Histamine release* (with morphine), which may precipitate bronchospasm in susceptible patients.
  - *Rarely, chest wall rigidity* (wooden chest syndrome) following the rapid intravenous injection of strong opioids, which can interfere with ventilation.

- **Benzodiazepines** cause depression of the respiratory centre, resulting in a decrease in RR and blunting of the ventilatory response to hypercapnoea.

- **Depolarising and non-depolarising muscle relaxants.** The most obvious effect of the muscle relaxants on the respiratory system is respiratory muscle paralysis necessitating mechanical ventilation. Adequate reversal of neuromuscular blockade is required to prevent post-operative respiratory failure. Other respiratory effects specific to particular agents are:

  - *Atracurium* may cause histamine release, resulting in bronchospasm.
  - *Suxamethonium and mivacurium* may cause prolonged respiratory muscle weakness in patients with reduced levels of plasma cholinesterase (suxamethonium apnoea).

- **Non-steroidal anti-inflammatory drugs** may precipitate bronchospasm in susceptible asthmatics.
- **Local anaesthetics** used in neuraxial blockade. During spinal anaesthesia, intrathecal local anaesthetic may rise high enough to cause weakness of the intercostal muscles. This occurs most commonly in obstetric anaesthesia, where sensory levels of T2 to T4 are typical. The diaphragm is unaffected (as it is supplied by nerve roots C3–5), unless the level of block is exceptionally high.

How are the lungs affected by general anaesthesia?

There are many physiological changes during the induction and maintenance of anaesthesia:

- **Airway devices.**
  - *Laryngospasm and bronchospasm.* Manipulation of the airway (by laryngoscopy, intubation or insertion of an LMA) can precipitate laryngospasm or bronchospasm. Bronchospasm is more common in patients who already have reactive airways (asthmatics, smokers), whilst laryngospasm is more common in children, particularly with inhalational inductions (as propofol is a useful depressant of laryngeal reflexes).
  - *Humidification.* Endotracheal tubes (ETTs) and LMAs both bypass the upper airway. The typical functions of the upper airway (humidification, filtration and warming of inspired gases) are usually performed instead by a heat and moisture exchanger. Inadequate warming and humidification may result in dry, tenacious secretions, leading to mucous plugging.
  - *Loss of physiological positive end-expiratory pressure* (PEEP). ETTs also bypass the larynx: the 3–5 cmH$_2$O of physiological PEEP is lost, predisposing the patient to atelectasis.
  - *Increased work of breathing.* The extent to which airway devices increase the resistance to gas flow depends on their internal radius, as determined by the Hagen–Poiseuille equation. The larger radius of the LMA makes it suitable for spontaneous ventilation. The narrower radius of the ETT increases the work of

breathing. This is of particular importance in small children (very small ETT radius) and when weaning intensive care patients.
  - *Increased dead space.* All airway devices increase mechanical dead space: $\dot{V}_E$ must increase (sometimes significantly) if $\dot{V}_A$ is to be maintained.

- **Lung volumes.** At induction of general anaesthesia, functional residual capacity (FRC; the essential store of O$_2$ during apnoea) is inevitably reduced due to:
  - *The supine position;*
  - *The relaxation of the chest wall muscles* associated with general anaesthesia;
  - *Co-morbidities,* such as acute abdomen, obesity;
  - *Patient population,* such as paediatric and obstetric patients.

Anaesthesia reduces FRC below closing capacity (CC) in otherwise-healthy middle-aged patients, leading to hypoxaemia.

To maximise FRC at induction of anaesthesia and therefore to maximise the volume of O$_2$ in the lungs, it may help if the patient is in a semi-recumbent position. Despite adequate pre-oxygenation, some patients are particularly prone to hypoxaemia on induction of anaesthesia, such as the obese. Intraoperative positioning (lithotomy and Trendelenburg) further reduce FRC by increasing the pressure of the abdominal contents on the diaphragm.

Low lung volumes also cause a reduction in airway radius (which increases resistance to gas flow, leading to an increased work of breathing) and an increase in pulmonary vascular resistance.

- **Atelectasis** has three causes: absorption of gases behind closed airways, alveolar compression and loss of pulmonary surfactant. The first two are common during general anaesthesia:
  - *Absorption atelectasis.* When breathing room air, very little N$_2$ diffuses across the alveolar–capillary barrier: N$_2$ remains in the alveoli, 'splinting' them open. During anaesthesia, the combination of diffusible gases (O$_2$ and N$_2$O) and small-airway closure (due to CC encroaching on the reduced FRC) means that all the alveolar contents may diffuse into the blood, leading to atelectasis.

- *Compression atelectasis.* Under general anaesthesia, a combination of reduced diaphragmatic tone and compression from the abdominal contents causes basal atelectasis. This is exacerbated by the loss of physiological PEEP and increased abdominal pressure (e.g. due to pneumoperitoneum).

- $\dot{V}/\dot{Q}$ **mismatch** as a result of:
  - *Low lung volume,* causing closure of small airways (due to CC encroaching on FRC).
  - *Increased tendency for atelectasis.*
  - *Positive pressure ventilation,* which alters intrathoracic pressure, reducing right ventricular preload and changing pulmonary capillary dynamics; West zone 1 occurs in the lung apex (see Chapter 16).
  - *Impairment of hypoxic pulmonary vasoconstriction* by volatile anaesthetic agents.

The hypoxaemia resulting from $\dot{V}/\dot{Q}$ mismatch can usually be managed simply by increasing F_iO_2 and adding extrinsic PEEP to reduce atelectasis and increase lung volume.

How does general anaesthesia affect post-operative respiratory function?

Post-operative pulmonary complications are common in the week following surgery, and include:

- *Atelectasis;*
- *Bronchospasm;*
- *Pneumonia;*
- *Pulmonary oedema;*
- *Ventilatory failure.*

Whilst underlying lung and cardiac disease may predispose patients to post-operative pulmonary complications, surgical and anaesthetic techniques also contribute:

- Upper abdominal and thoracic surgery carry the highest risk of post-operative pulmonary complications. Reduced FRC, basal atelectasis and $\dot{V}/\dot{Q}$ mismatch are inevitable and often persist for many days. $\dot{V}/\dot{Q}$ mismatch causes hypoxaemia, whilst atelectasis and reduced lung volume both contribute to an increased work of breathing.
- Inadequate analgesia following laparotomy, sternotomy and thoracotomy results in an inadequate cough and limited inspiration. This

exacerbates atelectasis and predisposes the patient to secretion retention and pneumonia.
- Post-operative shivering sometimes occurs at emergence from anaesthesia. Shivering increases metabolic demand at a time when the respiratory centre's response to hypercapnoea and hypoxaemia is blunted by the residual effects of anaesthetic agents and opioids. Respiratory failure (either type 1 or type 2) may then occur.
- Where neuromuscular blockade has been used, inadequate reversal may cause respiratory muscle weakness in the immediate post-operative period. Muscular weakness may be exacerbated by electrolyte disturbances (hypokalaemia or hypocalcaemia) resulting from fluid shift between body compartments and increased mineralocorticoid activity as part of the stress response.

One of the aims of anaesthetic management is to minimise the disturbance in post-operative lung function. The approach is multifactorial, taking into account many of the factors discussed above:

- **Preoperative assessment.** Risk stratification of patients based on type of surgery and presence of any underlying lung disease.
- **Regional versus general anaesthesia.** Depending on the type of surgery, the use of regional anaesthesia avoids many of the adverse effects of general anaesthesia on the lungs.
- **Laparoscopic surgery** reduces the prevalence of post-operative pulmonary complications.
- **Intraoperative ventilation strategy.** There is a significant reduction in postoperative pulmonary complications when patients are ventilated with low V_T (<8 mL/kg). The most effective level of intraoperative PEEP and the role of recruitment manoeuvres are yet to be determined.
- **Avoiding 100% O_2** to avoid absorption atelectasis. Even adding 20% nitrogen to the fresh gas flow is useful in splinting open alveoli.
- **Normothermia.** Intraoperative temperature management minimises the risk of post-operative shivering.
- **Neuromuscular monitoring and reversal of neuromuscular blockade.** Long-acting neuromuscular blocking agents (e.g. pancuronium) are more likely to lead to

post-operative respiratory failure than short- and intermediate-acting agents.

- **Adequate pain relief**. This is especially important in upper abdominal and thoracic surgery where a regional anaesthetic technique is commonly used; for example, a continuous infusion of local anaesthetic via a thoracic epidural or paravertebral catheter.

Further reading

A. B. Lumb. Ventilatory failure. In: A. B. Lumb. *Nunn's Applied Respiratory Physiology, 8th edition*. London, Churchill Livingstone, 2016; 379–88.

A. B. Lumb. Respiratory support and artificial ventilation. In: A. B. Lumb. *Nunn's Applied Respiratory Physiology, 8th edition*. London, Churchill Livingstone, 2016; 451–78.

E. Scarth, S. Smith. *Drugs in Anaesthesia and Intensive Care, 5th edition*. Oxford, Oxford University Press, 2016.

T. E. Peck. *Pharmacology for Anaesthesia and Intensive Care, 4th edition*. Cambridge, Cambridge University Press, 2014.

G. H. Mills. Respiratory complications of anaesthesia. *Anaesthesia* 2018; 73(Suppl. 1): 25–33.

A. Miskovic, A. B. Lumb. Postoperative pulmonary complications. *Br J Anaesth* 2017; **118**(3): 317–34.

V. A. Lawrence, J. E. Cornell, G. W. Smetana. Strategies to reduce postoperative pulmonary complications after noncardiothoracic surgery: systematic review for the American College of Physicians. *Ann Intern Med* 2006; **144**(8): 596–608.

G. Hedenstierna. Airway closure, atelectasis and gas exchange during anaesthesia. *Minerva Anestesiol* 2002; **68**(5): 332–6.

Chapter

27

Cardiac Anatomy and Function

What are the functions of the heart?

The mechanical function of the heart is to eject[1] blood into the vascular system:

- The right side of the heart generates *flow* around the pulmonary circulation, moving deoxygenated venous blood from the heart to the lungs.
- The left side of the heart generates *pressure* in the arterial circulation, moving oxygenated blood from the heart to the other organs of the body. Flow can then be regulated according to tissue demand.

The heart is also an endocrine organ with a role in the regulation of plasma volume. Stretch receptors in the cardiac atria and ventricles sense increases in plasma volume, secreting atrial natriuretic peptide (ANP) and brain natriuretic peptide (BNP) in response. Both ANP and BNP act on the kidney to produce a natriuresis, which restores plasma volume to normal.

Describe the structure of the heart

The heart is located in the thorax, enclosed within a fibrous sac called the pericardium. The pericardium forms attachments to surrounding structures that hold the heart in place.

The heart is made up of three tissue layers:

- **The epicardium**, the outer connective tissue layer. A small amount of pericardial fluid separates the epicardium from the pericardium, which helps reduce frictional forces as the heart moves.
- **The myocardium**, the middle layer, which is composed of cardiac muscle.
- **The endocardium**, a layer of epithelial cells that line the inner surface of the heart. The

endocardium is in contact with blood and is continuous with the endothelial layer of the blood vessels.

The heart can be divided into right and left sides, each consisting of an atrium and a ventricle. The two sides of the heart are separated by the interatrial and interventricular septae.

- **The right atrium** (RA) receives deoxygenated blood from the superior and inferior venae cavae. When the RA contracts, blood passes through the tricuspid valve (a trileaflet valve) and into the right ventricle (RV).
- **The RV** has a complex shape. Viewed in the transverse plane it is shaped as a crescent, whilst it is triangular in the longitudinal plane. Because of this complex shape, the structure of the RV is difficult to model mathematically. It is therefore difficult to estimate right ventricular volume by echocardiography. When the RV contracts, blood is driven through the pulmonary valve (a trileaflet valve) and into the pulmonary artery.
- **The left atrium** (LA). Oxygenated blood returns from the lungs through four (normal variation from three to five) pulmonary veins and enters the LA. When the LA contracts, blood passes into the left ventricle (LV) through the mitral valve (a bileaflet valve)
- **The LV** has a circular transverse section and a conical longitudinal section, amenable to accurate echocardiographic estimates of its volume. When the LV contracts, blood is forced through the aortic valve (a trileaflet valve) and into the aorta.

What is meant by the term 'functional syncytium'?

The myocardium is arranged in networks of striated cardiac muscle cells joined together by intercalated

---

[1] Technically, the heart does not operate as a true 'pump', as it does not suck from the venous system: negative pressure would cause these compliant vessels to collapse. However, the term 'pump' is commonly used.

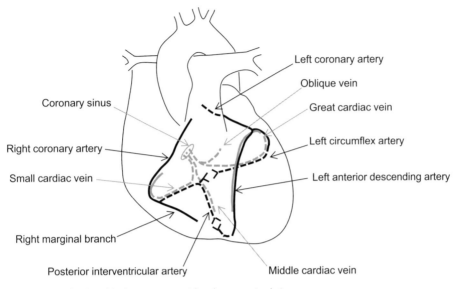

Figure 27.1 The (simplified) coronary arterial and venous circulations.

discs. Intercalated discs contain three different types of cell–cell interaction:

- **Gap junction complexes** permit the direct passage of intracellular ions and larger molecules from one cell to another. They form electrical synapses, allowing direct electrical spread of action potentials from cell to cell.
- **Fascia adherens** anchor the actin filaments within the sarcomere to the cell membrane.
- **Macular adherens** (also known as desmosomes) anchor cardiac cells to one another.

Cardiac muscle is therefore electrically, chemically and mechanically coupled together so that it behaves as a single coordinated unit, and it is often referred to as a functional syncytium.

Describe the coronary circulation

Whilst a large volume of blood passes through the cardiac chambers, the ventricular wall is too thick for effective diffusion of O_2 to occur; only the endocardium is nourished directly. The bulk of the cardiac muscle is perfused by the coronary circulation. Coronary arteries are end arteries: they represent the only source of blood for the downstream myocardium, with few native anastomoses. Consequently, acute obstruction of a coronary artery causes myocardial infarction.

The coronary circulation is divided into right and left sides, which both originate at the aortic root (Figure 27.1). The aortic root has three dilatations just above the aortic valve, known as the aortic sinuses (or sinuses of Valsalva). These sinuses produce eddy currents, which tend to keep the valve cusps away from the aortic walls and facilitate smooth valve closure. This is important, as the left and right coronary arteries originate from the left posterior and anterior coronary sinuses, respectively, and the eddy currents prevent their occlusion.

- **The left coronary artery** (left main stem) arises from the left posterior aortic sinus, just above the left cusp of the aortic valve. The left coronary artery travels a short distance in the left atrioventricular (AV) groove (less than 2.5 cm) before bifurcating into:

    - *The left anterior descending (LAD) artery* (left interventricular artery). This artery descends in the anterior interventricular groove, giving off septal and diagonal branches. The LAD supplies most of the LV, specifically:

        - The anterolateral myocardium;
        - The apex;
        - The interventricular septum.

    The LAD often forms an anastomosis with the posterior interventricular artery after passing over the apex.

– *The left circumflex artery.* This artery continues in the left AV groove, giving off one or more obtuse marginal branches. Normally, the terminal end of the left circumflex artery meets the right coronary artery in the AV groove, where the two arteries form an anastomosis. The left circumflex artery supplies:

  ▪ The posterolateral LV;
  ▪ The sinoatrial (SA) node in 40% of individuals.

● **The right coronary artery** originates from the anterior aortic sinus, just above the right cusp of the aortic valve. It travels along the right AV groove, before dividing into:

– *The SA branch*, which is present in 60% of individuals and supplies the SA node;
– *The right marginal artery*, which travels down the right margin of the heart towards the apex and supplies the RV; it is the right-sided equivalent of the left interventricular artery.

The right coronary artery continues in the AV groove until it reaches the posterior interventricular groove. In the majority of individuals, the right coronary artery then divides into:

– *The posterior interventricular artery* (posterior descending artery), which supplies the posterior part of the septum and the AV node. For this reason, occlusions of the right coronary artery predispose to bradycardia and AV block.

The right coronary artery continues in the AV groove, where it forms an anastomosis with the left circumflex artery.

The coronary circulation has a number of recognised variants, the most common of which is called 'left dominance'. In around 15% of the population, the posterior interventricular artery is not a branch of the right coronary artery, but is instead a branch of the left circumflex artery.

Describe the venous drainage of the heart

There are three different systems through which venous blood is drained from the myocardium:

● **The coronary sinus.** Venous blood from the LV (which accounts for around 85% of venous blood) is collected by the cardiac veins, which coalesce to form the coronary sinus. The sinus opens into the RA, between the inferior vena cava and the tricuspid valve. The cardiac veins lie in the grooves between atria and ventricles. Thus, they follow the same paths as the coronary arteries (Figure 27.1). They are:

– *The great cardiac vein*, which runs alongside the LAD in the anterior interventricular groove;
– *The middle cardiac vein*, which runs alongside the posterior interventricular artery in the posterior interventricular groove;
– *The small cardiac vein*, which runs alongside the right coronary artery in the posterior AV groove;
– *The oblique vein*, which traverses the back of the LA.

● **The anterior cardiac veins** are small veins that arise on the anterior surface of the RV and drain into the RA.
● **The Thebesian veins**, the smallest of the cardiac veins, drain directly into the four chambers of the heart. The Thebesian veins are predominantly found in the RA and RV. Note: the few Thebesian veins that drain into the left side of the heart pass deoxygenated blood directly into the stream of fully oxygenated blood returning from the lungs and thus contribute to anatomical shunt (see Chapter 14).

Clinical relevance: cardiac resynchronisation therapy

Cardiac resynchronisation therapy (CRT) is indicated in heart failure patients in sinus rhythm where ejection fraction is <35% and where there is a conduction defect (characterised by a widened QRS complex) resulting in asynchronous contraction of the left and right ventricles. A CRT device improves atrial and ventricular synchrony through the use of three pacemaker wires: atrial, right ventricular and left ventricular.

Like standard pacemakers, the CRT leads are usually inserted through the subclavian vein, which poses a question: how does the left ventricular wire reach the left ventricular myocardium?

- Atrial and right ventricular wires are passed through the subclavian vein and superior vena cava into the RA and RV.
- The left ventricular wire is also advanced into the RA, where it is passed into the coronary sinus and along the great cardiac vein until it reaches the left ventricular myocardium.

Is blood flow to the myocardium continuous or intermittent?

The heart is constantly beating, so has a high O_2 requirement even in an inactive subject:

- The resting heart receives 250 mL/min of blood, 5% of the cardiac output. Coronary blood flow may increase up to fivefold during strenuous exercise.
- Myocardial O_2 extraction is greater in the heart (around 70% at rest) than in any other organ; in contrast, resting skeletal muscle O_2 extraction is only 25%.

This requirement for high blood flow and efficient O_2 extraction makes the heart very susceptible to ischaemia.

The coronary arteries run along the epicardial surface, and their arterioles penetrate into the myocardium at an approximate right angle. During systole, the pressure within the contracting muscle of the LV exceeds coronary arterial pressure; the intramuscular arterioles are compressed, preventing blood flow to the myocardium. During diastole, the heart relaxes and its pressure falls; blood flow to the myocardium resumes (Figure 27.2). Blood flow to the LV is therefore intermittent. The pressure generated within the RV is much less than that of the LV; the right ventricular myocardium is therefore perfused throughout the cardiac cycle (Figure 27.2).

Which other factors influence coronary blood flow?

A number of factors are involved in the regulation of coronary blood flow:

- **O_2 demand.** As indicated above, the O_2 extraction ratio is higher in the heart than in any other organ. Any increase in O_2 demand requires a corresponding increase in coronary blood flow. Coronary blood flow is therefore tightly coupled to O_2 demand. One possible mechanism for this is:

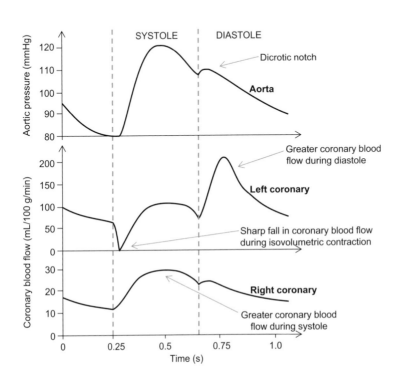

Figure 27.2 Coronary blood flow.

- An increase in cardiac work, as occurs in exercise, leads to a reduction in myocardial cytosolic ATP and an increase in AMP.
- Adenosine is released from the myocardial cells.
- In response, adenosine triggers vasodilatation of the coronary arterioles, thus increasing coronary blood flow.
- Other possible vasodilatory mediators are K^+, CO_2, H^+ and NO.

- **Autoregulation.** In common with blood flow to the brain and kidneys, coronary blood flow is autoregulated. The coronary arterioles vasoconstrict and vasodilate to maintain a constant coronary blood flow in the face of varying coronary perfusion pressure[2] between 60 and 180 mmHg. At a coronary perfusion pressure of 60 mmHg, the coronary arterioles are then maximally vasodilated and any further reduction in coronary perfusion pressure results in a fall in coronary blood flow.
- **Heart rate** (HR). An increase in HR encroaches on the diastolic time more than the systolic time, resulting in a decrease in left coronary blood flow. Right coronary blood flow is relatively unaffected.
- **Patency of coronary vessels:**

  - The presence of atheroma in the walls of the coronary arteries makes them unable to vasodilate in response to increased O_2 demand. Downstream myocardium then receives insufficient O_2 to meet its demand, resulting in myocardial ischaemia.
  - Acute obstruction of the coronary arteries by thrombosis, embolus or vasospasm can cause myocardial ischaemia even without an increase in O_2 demand.

  Chronic atheroma results in downstream ischaemic preconditioning in the tissues, allowing larger degrees of stenosis than acute occlusion. Collateral blood supplies derived from other coronary arteries may also form.
- **Autonomic control.** The autonomic nervous system has only a minor direct effect on coronary blood flow:

- *Parasympathetic activity* has a weak vasodilatory effect on the coronary arterioles.
- *Sympathetic activity* causes an increase in coronary blood flow. But this is mainly the result of increased O_2 demand secondary to an increase in inotropy and HR.

Clinical relevance: drugs and coronary blood flow

Drugs influence coronary blood flow through a number of mechanisms:

- **Nitrates** (e.g. glyceryl trinitrate) cause vasodilatation of the coronary arteries in common with their effects on other arterial beds. The consequent venodilatation and peripheral vasodilatation reduce cardiac preload and afterload, respectively. Myocardial O_2 demand falls and therefore overall coronary blood flow is reduced.
- **β-blockers** (e.g. bisoprolol) reduce HR, which prolongs the diastolic time. Coronary blood flow to the LV therefore increases. In addition, β-blockers inhibit catecholamine-induced increases in myocardial contractility, as occurs with exercise, which limits any increase in O_2 demand.
- **Ca^{2+} channel blockers** (e.g. nifedipine) cause coronary arteriolar vasodilatation, which increases coronary blood flow, and peripheral vasodilatation, which decreases afterload and therefore decreases myocardial O_2 demand.
- **K$^+$ channel openers** (e.g. nicorandil) increase K^+ efflux from arteriolar smooth muscle cells. This hyperpolarises the smooth muscle cells, reducing their cytosolic Ca^{2+} concentration, which causes smooth muscle relaxation. The resultant coronary arteriolar vasodilatation leads to an increase in coronary blood flow. Nicorandil dilates both normal and stenotic segments of coronary artery.
- **Ranolazine** inhibits the late Na^+ current during the cardiac action potential. This reduces intracellular Na^+ load, which facilitates Ca^{2+} efflux via the Na^+/Ca^{2+} exchanger. The resulting decrease in intracellular Ca^{2+} reduces the tension generated in the cardiac myocytes and aids cardiac relaxation, therefore reducing O_2 demand.
- **Antiplatelet agents** (e.g. aspirin and clopidogrel) prevent an occlusive thrombus forming within the coronary arteries.
- **Statins**. As well as reducing blood cholesterol levels, which are thought to be a driving factor in atheroma generation, statins also exert an

---

[2] Coronary perfusion pressure = aortic blood pressure – left ventricular end-diastolic pressure.

acute plaque stabilisation effect that improves coronary flow following a myocardial infarction. The mechanism is thought to be through both anti-inflammatory and anti-thrombotic effects.

Further reading

N. Herring, D. J. Paterson. Overview of the cardiovascular system. In: N. Herring, D. J. Paterson. *Levick's Introduction to Cardiovascular Physiology, 6th edition.* Boca Raton, CRC Press, 2018; 1–14.

N. Herring, D. J. Paterson. Specialisation in individual circulations. In: N. Herring, D. J. Paterson. *Levick's Introduction to Cardiovascular Physiology, 6th edition.* Boca Raton, CRC Press, 2018; 275–302.

R. H. Anderson, D. E. Spicer, A. M. Hlavacek, et al. *Wilcox's Surgical Anatomy of the Heart, 4th edition.* Cambridge, Cambridge University Press, 2013.

P. Barash, S. Akhtar. Coronary stents: factors contributing to perioperative major adverse cardiovascular events. *Br J Anaesth* 2010; **105**(Suppl. 1): u3–15.

B. M. Biccard, R. N. Rodseth. The pathophysiology of perioperative myocardial infarction. *Anaesthesia* 2010; **65**(7): 733–41.

T. Ramanathan, H. Skinner. Coronary blood flow. *Continuing Educ Anaesth Crit Care Pain* 2005; **5**(2): 61–4.

N. Herring, D. J. Paterson. ECG diagnosis of acute ischaemia and infarction: past, present and future. *Q J Med* 2006; **99**(4): 219–30.

Cardiac Cycle

What is the cardiac cycle?

The cardiac cycle refers to the complete sequence of physiological events that occur in the heart, from the beginning of one heartbeat to the beginning of the next.

The cardiac cycle consists of two phases:

- **The diastolic phase**, during which the ventricles are relaxed and are filling with blood. Diastole consists of four stages:
    - Isovolumetric relaxation;
    - Rapid ventricular filling;
    - Slow ventricular filling;
    - Atrial contraction.

- **The systolic phase**, during which the ventricles contract and eject blood into the aorta and pulmonary artery. Systole consists of two stages:
    - Isovolumetric contraction;
    - Ejection.

Describe the events making up the cardiac cycle

Traditionally, the cardiac cycle is described from late diastole, when the atria and ventricles are relaxed and the atrioventricular (AV) valves are open:

- **Slow ventricular filling.** The pressure within the atria is slightly higher than the intraventricular pressure. The AV valves are therefore open, allowing blood to flow slowly from atrium to ventricle.
- **Atrial contraction.**
    - The pacemaker cells of the sinoatrial (SA) node spontaneously depolarise, generating an action potential (see Chapter 57). The resulting electrical impulse is rapidly

conducted throughout the atria, triggering atrial contraction.
- As a result of atrial contraction, much of the remaining atrial blood is ejected through the AV valves into the ventricles. At rest, this atrial 'kick' accounts for only 10% of ventricular filling: 90% of the blood flows into the ventricle passively. However, during exercise, when diastole is shortened, atrial contraction contributes up to 40% of ventricular filling.
- The pressure generated during atrial contraction is transmitted along the venae cavae and pulmonary veins as they have no valves: atrial contraction is represented by the a-wave on the atrial pressure waveform (Figure 28.1).
- The volume of blood within the ventricle at the end of atrial contraction is the end-diastolic volume.

- **Isovolumetric contraction.** The action potential continues through the AV node and is conducted throughout the ventricles by the His–Purkinje system, represented on the electrocardiogram by the QRS complex. Initially, ventricular contraction causes a rapid rise in intraventricular pressure:

    - Once intraventricular pressure exceeds atrial pressure, the AV valves close, resulting in the first heart sound, S_1. The mitral valve normally closes slightly earlier than the tricuspid valve, resulting in a 'split' S_1.
    - There is a period of time between the closure of the AV valves and the opening of the aortic and pulmonary valves (semilunar valves) during which ventricular pressure rises without a change in ventricular volume – this is the phase of isovolumetric contraction.

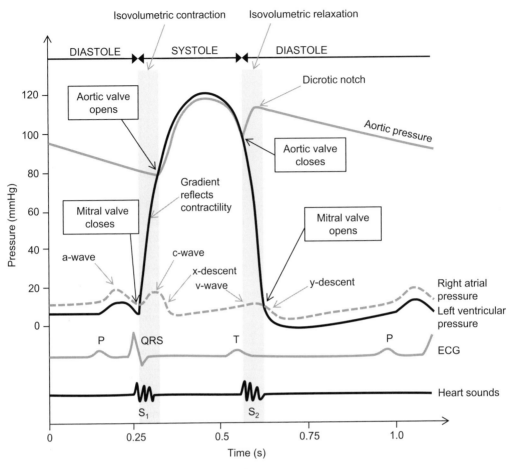

Figure 28.1 The cardiac cycle (ECG = electrocardiogram).

- During isovolumetric contraction, the increased right ventricular pressure causes the tricuspid valve to bulge into the right atrium. This corresponds to the c-wave on the atrial pressure waveform. Similarly, increased left ventricular pressure causes the mitral valve to bulge into the left atrium.

- **Ejection.** Once ventricular pressure exceeds the pressure in the aorta and pulmonary artery, the semilunar valves open and blood is ejected from the ventricles.

  - Right ventricular contraction pulls the tricuspid valve downwards. As the length of the right atrium increases, its pressure falls to zero and it is rapidly filled with blood. This is the origin of the x-descent on the atrial pressure waveform.

- Initially, the flow of blood through the semilunar valves is rapid, but as the ventricular myocytes start to repolarise, the force of contraction wanes.

- In the course of ventricular relaxation, the ventricular pressure falls below that of the aorta and pulmonary artery; the semilunar valves close, resulting in the second heart sound, S_2. The aortic valve usually closes slightly earlier than the pulmonary valve. Inspiration can accentuate this difference, particularly in young people, resulting in a 'physiological split' S_2.

- Aortic valve closure is represented on the aortic pressure curve (Figure 28.1) by the dicrotic notch, a positive deflection caused by the elastic recoil of the aortic valve and the aorta.

– The volume of blood within the ventricle following valve closure is the end-systolic volume.

- **Isovolumetric relaxation.** Following the closure of the semilunar valves, it takes a short time for the ventricles to further relax and their pressure to fall below that of the atria. Throughout late systole and isovolumetric relaxation, atrial pressure slowly rises due to venous return from the lungs and venae cavae. This corresponds to the v-wave of the atrial pressure waveform (Figure 28.1).
- **Rapid ventricular filling.** Once atrial pressure exceeds ventricular pressure, the AV valves open. Blood flows down its pressure gradient from the atria to the ventricles. During the early part of diastole, the ventricles are still undergoing relaxation and intraventricular pressure continues to decrease, and blood therefore flows rapidly into the ventricles. The fall in atrial pressure is represented by the y-descent of the atrial pressure waveform (Figure 28.1).

Ventricular filling is normally silent, but an increased volume of atrial blood (e.g. in mitral regurgitation) flowing into a poorly compliant left ventricle (LV; e.g. as occurs following a myocardial infarction or in dilated cardiomyopathy) results in reverberation of the ventricular wall and a third heart sound, S_3.

What is stroke volume?

The stroke volume (SV) is the volume of blood ejected from the LV per heartbeat. The volume of blood in the LV prior to contraction is the left ventricular end-diastolic volume (LVEDV) and the volume of blood remaining in the LV after contraction is the left ventricular end-systolic volume (LVESV). Therefore:

Key equation: SV

$$SV = LVEDV - LVESV$$

Typical values for a 70-kg man are:

- LVEDV of 120 mL
- LVESV of 50 mL

So, SV = 70 mL.

The 'normal range' for SV is 55–100 mL, though this depends on the size of the individual.

Ejection fraction (EF) is also commonly used. EF is the proportion of blood ejected from the LV per heartbeat:

Key equation: EF

$$EF = \frac{SV}{LVEDV}$$

As typical values are SV = 70 mL and LVEDV = 120 mL:

$$EF = \frac{70}{120} \times 100$$
$$= 58\%$$

The 'normal range' for EF is 55–70%.

Clinical relevance: cardiac output, ageing and tachycardia

Cardiac output, CO = HR × SV (see Chapter 29). Therefore, it seems logical that as HR increases, so does CO. However:

- At rest (HR = 75), a single cardiac cycle lasts for 0.8 s: the typical duration of systole is 0.3 s and diastole is 0.5 s. The LV fills during diastole, when its pressure is low and the mitral valve is open.
- A young athlete at maximal exercise may have an HR of 200; each cardiac cycle lasts just 0.3 s: systole lasts 0.15 s and diastole 0.15 s. Such a short diastolic time limits ventricular filling.

Therefore, the relationship between HR, SV and CO is more complex than it first seems:

- When HR is high, diastolic filling time decreases and thus SV decreases, leading to a fall in CO.
- Likewise, when HR falls below 40 beats per minute (bpm), CO still decreases, despite a moderate increase in SV (to 80–90 mL due to the increased diastolic filling time).
- A (sinus) HR between 50 and 150 bpm is optimal in most people.

The heart undergoes changes with age:

- Reduced compliance of the aorta results in an increase in afterload. In response, the LV undergoes hypertrophy, which reduces its compliance.
- LV relaxation is less efficient in diastole, again leading to a decrease in its compliance.
- Atrial fibrosis predisposes to atrial fibrillation (AF).

As a result of the changes in LV compliance, the rate of ventricular filling during the rapid filling stage is reduced. The maximum HR achieved during exercise therefore decreases with age:

$$HR_{max} = 208 - (0.7 \times age)$$

Therefore, HR_{max} is 194 at age 20, whilst HR_{max} falls to 152 at age 80.

Atrial contraction becomes ever more important to ventricular filling with advancing age, contributing up to 40% of LVEDV. The onset of AF, in which there is an absence of atrial contraction, may therefore lead to a significant fall in CO. This may decompensate an underlying heart failure that was previously well tolerated.

Clinical relevance: valvular heart disease and anaesthesia

The perioperative management of patients with valvular heart disease requires an understanding of the accompanying alterations in cardiovascular physiology and the consequences of anaesthetic drugs and positive-pressure ventilation. Broadly, patients with stenotic valvular heart disease cause the most concern due to their relatively fixed CO and consequent inability to compensate for changes in systemic vascular resistance (SVR). In addition to maintaining normovolaemia, the summarised haemodynamic goals are:

- **Aortic stenosis:**
  - *Maintain sinus rhythm*: AF severely impairs left ventricular filling and is poorly tolerated.
  - *Low/normal HR (50–70 bpm)* to allow time for systolic ejection across the stenotic valve.
  - *Avoid precipitous reductions in SVR* due to the relatively fixed CO. Hypotension may impair coronary perfusion – neuraxial blockade is contraindicated, and anaesthetic drugs must be carefully titrated.

- **Mitral stenosis:**
  - *Low/normal HR (50–70 bpm)* to allow time for left ventricular filling across the stenotic valve.
  - *Maintain sinus rhythm*: immediate cardioversion is indicated if intraoperative AF occurs.
  - *Avoid hypercarbia, acidosis and hypoxia*, which may exacerbate pulmonary hypertension.
  - *Maintain SVR* due to a relatively fixed CO.

- **Aortic regurgitation** ('full, fast and forward'):
  - *High/normal HR (90–110 bpm)*: a shorter diastolic time reduces the regurgitant fraction.
  - *Maintain cardiac contractility*.
  - *Low SVR*, which promotes forward flow and reduces regurgitant fraction.

- **Mitral regurgitation:**
  - *High/normal HR (90–110 bpm)*: a reduced diastolic time decreases the regurgitant fraction.
  - *Low SVR* maintains forward flow and reduces the regurgitant fraction.
  - *Avoid hypercarbia, acidosis and hypoxia*, which may exacerbate pulmonary hypertension.

Further reading

N. Herring, D. J. Paterson. The cardiac cycle. In: N. Herring, D. J. Paterson. *Levick's Introduction to Cardiovascular Physiology*, 6th edition. Boca Raton, CRC Press, 2018; 15–28.

K. Holmes, H. A. Vohra. Mitral valve and mitral valve disease. *BJA Education* 2017; **17**(1): 1–9.

J. Brown, N. J. Morgan-Hughes. Aortic stenosis and non-cardiac surgery. *Continuing Educ Anaesth Crit Care Pain* 2005; **5**(1): 1–4.

M. D. Cheitlin. Cardiovascular physiology – changes with aging. *Am J Geriatr Cardiol* 2003; **12**(1): 9–13.

Chapter

29

Cardiac Output and Its Measurement

Which factors affect the cardiac output?

The cardiac output (CO) is the volume of blood ejected by the left ventricle (LV) or right ventricle (RV) per minute.

CO is directly dependent on two factors: heart rate (HR) and stroke volume (SV).

Key equation: CO

$$CO = SV \times HR$$

At rest, the typical SV is 70 mL and HR is 75 bpm. Typical resting CO is therefore $70 \times 75 = 5.25$ L/min, but CO may increase fivefold during maximal exercise.[1]

In turn, SV is determined by three factors: preload, myocardial contractility and afterload.

- **Preload** is defined as the intraluminal pressure that stretches the RV or LV to its end-diastolic dimensions. Preload is therefore related to the diastolic length of the cardiac myocyte. According to Starling's law, the force of cardiac myocyte contraction depends on the resting diastolic length of the ventricular fibres (see Chapter 30): increased preload produces an increased SV.

  In practice, preload is very difficult to measure. It is impossible to measure sarcomere length *in vivo*, so surrogate measurements are used: left ventricular end-diastolic volume (LVEDV; measured by echocardiography) or, more commonly, left ventricular end-diastolic pressure.[2] Similarly:

  - *Central venous pressure* provides an indication of right ventricular preload, as it affects right ventricular end-diastolic volume (RVEDV).
  - *Pulmonary capillary wedge pressure* provides an indication of left ventricular preload, as it affects LVEDV.

- **Afterload** is the stress developed in the left ventricular wall during ejection, and it reflects the force opposing the shortening of cardiac myocytes. As afterload increases, both the rate and extent of sarcomere shortening decrease, resulting in a reduction in SV. Like preload, afterload is not easily measured *in vivo* and is assessed through surrogate markers:

  - *Mean arterial pressure (MAP) and systemic vascular resistance (SVR)* reflect left ventricular afterload.
  - *Pulmonary vascular resistance* reflects right ventricular afterload.

- **Myocardial contractility** is the intrinsic ability of cardiac myocytes to generate mechanical power at a given preload and afterload. Factors that increase myocardial contractility are said to exert a positive inotropic effect, whilst factors that decrease contractility exert a negative inotropic effect. Contractility is difficult to measure directly, but an index of myocardial contractility is provided by the rate of change of pressure (i.e. the gradient) during the isovolumetric contraction phase of the cardiac cycle (see Chapter 28 and Figure 28.1).

How does the body regulate CO?

CO is not static; it varies depending on the changing requirements of the body. For example:

---

[1] In elite athletes, peak CO may be as high as 40 L/min.
[2] Note: the relationship between end-diastolic volume and end-diastolic pressure depends on ventricular compliance, which may vary between patients.

- **Age**. Taking into account their proportionately greater body surface area (BSA, m^2), children have a greater CO than adults.
- **Exercise**. CO may increase up to fivefold in normal individuals.
- **Pregnancy** is associated with an increase in resting CO of up to 50% at term.
- **Eating** is associated with an increase in CO of around 25%.

As discussed above, the main factors that influence CO are HR, preload, myocardial contractility and afterload. The regulation of these four factors is complex, as changes in each rarely occur in isolation. However, HR may undergo a threefold increase (e.g. from 60 bpm to 180 bpm), whereas SV may only increase by around 50% (e.g. from 70 mL to 105 mL). Under normal circumstances, the major factor that influences CO is therefore HR.

- **HR** is set by sinoatrial (SA) node pacemaker activity, which is in turn modulated by the autonomic nervous system (ANS):

  - A denervated heart has a basal HR of around 100–120 bpm.
  - At rest, the parasympathetic nervous system (via the vagus nerve) is tonically active in the heart (note: this is an exception for the ANS; elsewhere, it is the sympathetic nervous system that is tonically active). Acetylcholine is continually released from parasympathetic nerve terminals, reducing the resting HR to 60–70 bpm through its effect at muscarinic M_2 receptors.
  - At the onset of exercise, parasympathetic tone is withdrawn, which increases HR. Noradrenaline is released from sympathetic nerve terminals and adrenaline is released from the adrenal medulla, both of which increase HR through activation of β_1-adrenoceptors.

CO decreases with bradycardia and increases with tachycardia. However, tachycardia is not always beneficial:

- Up to around 140 bpm, CO increases with increasing HR.
- Above 150 bpm, the diastolic cardiac filling time becomes very short (~0.15 s). As ventricular filling can only occur during diastole, SV falls with a consequent reduction in CO (see Chapter 28).
  - When HR is rapid, as may occur with ventricular tachycardia, the fall in CO may be sufficient to cause myocardial ischaemia, thus further reducing myocardial contractility; a vicious cycle ensues.

- **Preload**. Starling's law ensures that the cardiac outputs of the RV and LV are exactly matched. Therefore, the main determinant of both right and left ventricular preloads is the venous return to the RV; that is, RVEDV. Venous return depends on a number of factors, which are discussed in detail in Chapter 37.
- **Myocardial contractility** is affected by four factors:

  - *The sympathetic nervous system*. Release of noradrenaline from cardiac sympathetic neurons (and to a lesser extent circulating noradrenaline and adrenaline) increases myocardial contractility through its action on β_1-adrenoceptors.
  - *Tachycardia*. Intrinsic myocardial contractility is increased when the HR is high. This is known as the 'Bowditch effect'.
  - *Drugs* with positively inotropic effects include dobutamine, isoprenaline, glucagon, enoximone and digoxin. Drugs with negatively inotropic effects include β-blockers, Ca^{2+} channel blockers and anaesthetic agents.
  - *Disease states* may reduce myocardial contractility, such as sepsis, myocarditis, ischaemic heart disease, electrolyte and acid–base disturbance.

  Positive inotropy increases myocardial O_2 demand. As myocardial contractility increases, there may come a point where O_2 delivery becomes insufficient, resulting in myocardial ischaemia. This is especially so in patients with coronary artery disease, where atherosclerosis limits coronary blood flow. Ischaemic myocardium cannot contract as effectively, and this compromises SV.

- **Afterload**, which is governed by SVR. As discussed above, an increase in afterload results in a reduction in SV. As less blood is ejected from the heart per beat, there is a greater volume of blood remaining in the ventricle at end-systole and therefore (following the ventricular filling phase) a greater LVEDV. According to Starling's law, a greater LVEDV produces a greater SV. Overall, following a sudden increase in afterload, SV transiently decreases before gradually returning to normal.

In addition, an increase in afterload causes an intrinsic increase in inotropy. This 'Anrep effect' ensures that increases in afterload cause smaller reductions in SV than would be predicted from the Frank–Starling mechanism alone.

What is the Bowditch effect?

The Bowditch effect (also known as the 'Treppe effect' or the 'staircase effect') is an intrinsic autoregulatory phenomenon in which tachycardia leads to increased myocardial contractility. The mechanism for this is thought to be:

- As HR increases, the time period for each cardiac cycle falls, with the diastolic interval shortened more than the systolic interval.
- At high HR, there is increased systolic Ca^{2+} influx through the L-type Ca^{2+} channels.
- In addition, the diastolic Na^+ efflux due to the Na^+/K^+-ATPase cannot keep pace with the systolic influx of Na^+.
- The Na^+/Ca^{2+} exchanger is normally responsible for the low intracellular Ca^{2+} concentration. However, with tachycardia, the increase in cytosolic Ca^{2+} and Na^+ concentrations leads to an accumulation of intracellular Ca^{2+}, with a consequent positive inotropic effect. This is also seen with digoxin therapy, where the Na^+/K^+-ATPase is blocked.

What is the cardiac index?

The typical resting CO in a 70-kg adult is said to be 5–6 L/min, but varies with body size. Cardiac index (CI) is a means of standardising CO based on BSA.

Key equation: CI

$$CI = \frac{CO}{BSA}$$

Normal resting CI is 3.0–3.5 L min^{-1} m^{-2}.

Likewise, SV can be standardised based on BSA, resulting in the SV index (SVI):

Key equation: SVI

$$SVI = \frac{SV}{BSA}$$

Normal resting SVI is 33–47 mL m^{-2} beat^{-1}.

How is MAP related to CO?

MAP describes the average arterial pressure during a single cardiac cycle. Pressure and flow are related by Darcy's law:

Pressure = flow × resistance

In the case of MAP and CO:

Key equation: determinants of MAP

MAP ≈ CO × SVR

NB: This equation holds if right atrial pressure is assumed to be much smaller than MAP. The equation is an oversimplification – in formal terms, arterial and venous circulations should be considered separately, because pressure generation in each circulation occurs by different mechanisms.

In turn, SVR is dependent on the radius of the arterioles, and (to a much lesser extent) the blood viscosity.

Therefore, at a given CO:

- **MAP is increased by:**
  - *Vasoconstriction*, as might take place following catecholamine release.
  - *Increased blood viscosity*, as occurs in patients with paraproteinaemia or polycythaemia rubra vera, who are consequently often hypertensive.
- **MAP is decreased by:**
  - *Vasodilatation*, as occurs in septic shock or following general anaesthesia.
  - *Decreased blood viscosity*.

Clinical relevance: aortic stenosis

Aortic stenosis is a degenerative disease of the aortic valve. Lifetime incidence is estimated at 1%. The most common cause of aortic stenosis is repeated mechanical stress causing fibrosis and calcification of a previously normal trileaflet aortic valve, usually presenting over the age of 70. Patients with a congenital bicuspid aortic valve tend to develop aortic stenosis at a younger age.

The normal aortic valve area is 2.6–3.5 cm^2. As the area of the aortic valve decreases over time, there is an initial compensatory hypertrophy of the LV: systolic function is maintained, preserving SV and therefore CO. However, this pathological left ventricular hypertrophy has adverse effects:

- *A decrease in left ventricular compliance*, which impairs ventricular relaxation and diastolic filling. Atrial contraction becomes ever more important in left ventricular filling, contributing up to 40% of LVEDV. The development of AF may have devastating consequences in patients with aortic stenosis and occurs more frequently due to increased atrial stretch.
- *Increased myocardial O$_2$ demand*. As the aortic valve becomes increasingly stenotic, a greater left ventricular pressure is required to maintain SV. Therefore, left ventricular O$_2$ demand increases. At the same time, the increase in left ventricular mass and higher left ventricular pressure reduces coronary blood flow. The mismatch between myocardial O$_2$ delivery and demand is why patients with severe aortic stenosis develop angina, despite often having normal coronary arteries.

Patients with severe aortic stenosis (below 1.0 cm^2) effectively have a fixed CO. In consequence:

- *Exertional syncope*. Exercise causes a decrease in SVR, which is normally compensated for by an increase in CO, to maintain MAP. In severe aortic stenosis, the required increase in CO cannot be met; MAP falls, leading to a decrease in cerebral blood flow and thus syncope.
- *Central neuraxial blockade*. The decrease in SVR caused by sympathetic blockade cannot be met by an increase in CO, resulting in a devastating reduction in MAP.

Classify the methods of measuring CO

CO is a measure of overall cardiovascular blood flow and is therefore considered one of the most important cardiovascular parameters. In 1928, Adolf Jarisch wrote: 'It is a source of regret that measurement of flow is so much more difficult than measurement of pressure. This has led to an undue interest in the

blood pressure manometer. Most organs, however, require flow rather than pressure.' This statement remains equally true today.

Since 1928, many methods of CO measurement have been developed; all have limitations and sources of error. The invasive nature of most techniques usually limits their use to critical care and theatre areas. Methods of CO measurement in clinical use can be classified as:

- **Invasive**, involving a pulmonary artery catheter (PAC), central line or arterial line;
- **Minimally invasive**, utilising ultrasound techniques and the proximity of the oesophagus to the heart and great vessels;
- **Non-invasive**, encompassing a variety of techniques, including trans-thoracic Doppler echocardiography, trans-thoracic electrical bioimpedance and magnetic resonance imaging.

Describe the invasive methods of CO measurement

Invasive methods may be divided into methods based on the Fick principle and methods using pulse contour analysis.

Methods based on the Fick principle

The Fick principle states that the uptake or excretion of a substance by an organ is equal to the difference between the amount of substance entering the organ and the amount of substance leaving the organ.

Therefore:

Key equation: Fick principle

Blood flow to an organ

$$= \frac{\text{Rate of uptake or excretion of substance}}{\text{Arterio} - \text{venous concentration difference}}$$

or:

$$Q = \frac{M}{A - V}$$

where Q is the blood flow to the organ per minute, M is the number of moles of substance added or removed from the blood per minute, A is the arterial concentration of substance and V is the venous concentration of substance.

The Fick principle can be applied in a number of ways to determine CO:

• **Using O_2 as the substance**, as in the direct Fick method. As the entire CO passes through the lungs (i.e. pulmonary blood flow equals CO) and the lungs add O_2 to the blood, the Fick principle can be applied to determine the CO:

Key equation: Fick principle applied to O_2

$$CO(mL/2pt\ min) = \frac{\dot{V}O_2}{C_aO_2 - C_vO_2}$$

where $\dot{V}O_2$ (mL/min) is the rate of O_2 uptake, C_aO_2 (mLO_2/mL blood) is the arterial O_2 content and C_vO_2 (mLO_2/mL blood) is the mixed venous O_2 content.

- C_aO_2 can be determined by peripheral arterial blood gas analysis (see Chapter 8).
- C_vO_2 can be determined by analysing a mixed venous sample from a PAC.[3] Some PACs are modified with a fibre-optic bundle incorporated in the catheter to continuously measure mixed venous haemoglobin O_2 saturation S_vO_2.
- $\dot{V}O_2$ over 1 min can be determined by asking the patient to breathe from a spirometer containing a known volume of 100% O_2 and a CO_2 absorber. After a minute, the volume of O_2 remaining in the spirometer allows the calculation of the O_2 uptake into the lungs.

For example, using typical resting values ($C_aO_2 = 0.2$ mLO_2/mL blood, $C_vO_2 = 0.15$ mLO_2/mL blood and $\dot{V}O_2 = 250$ mL/min):

$$CO = \frac{\dot{V}O_2}{C_aO_2 - C_vO_2}$$

$$= \frac{250}{0.2 - 0.15} = 5000\ mL/min$$

Measurement of CO by this method is cumbersome and is clearly not practical in the clinical setting.

---

[3] Note: the 'true' mixed venous sample taken from the tip of a PAC includes blood from the superior and inferior venae cavae and the coronary sinus. Blood samples taken from the tip of a central line are often used as surrogates of the 'true' mixed venous blood sample, introducing a source of error: the blood sampled mainly originates from the upper body (via the superior vena cava) and may not accurately reflect venous blood from the lower body and heart.

For this reason, other methods based on the Fick principle were developed.

• **Dye dilution method**. A known amount of indicator dye is injected directly into the pulmonary artery (a PAC is therefore required) and its concentration is continuously sampled at a peripheral arterial line. Indocyanine green was traditionally used as the indicator dye, as it has low toxicity and a short half-life. An alternative indictor is lithium, which can be measured using a lithium-sensitive electrode incorporated into an arterial catheter. The change in indicator concentration over time is recorded as a graph (Figure 29.1a). CO can then be calculated from the integral of this curve (i.e. the area under the curve) and the amount of indicator substance using a modification of the Fick equation:

Key equation: the Stewart–Hamilton equation

$$CO = \frac{amount\ of\ indicator}{\int_0^\infty concentration\ of\ indicator\ dt}$$

or simplified as:

$$CO = \frac{amount\ of\ indicator}{area\ under\ concentration - time\ graph}$$

One of the main drawbacks of the dye dilution method is recirculation of the indicator dye. Indicator that passes through the circulation for a second time causes a second peak in the concentration–time graph (Figure 29.1a), which makes accurate measurement of the area under the graph difficult. This drawback is partially overcome by using a logarithmic transformation of concentration. Using this logarithmic transformation, the area under the first curve is easier to measure (Figure 29.1b).

• **Thermodilution method**. Following the introduction of a balloon-tipped, flow-directed PAC with a thermistor located near its tip by Swan and Ganz in 1970, the thermodilution method became the most frequently adopted method of determining CO. The technique is as follows:

- Inflating the balloon at the tip of the PAC allows it to be floated through the right atrium (RA) and RV to the pulmonary artery.

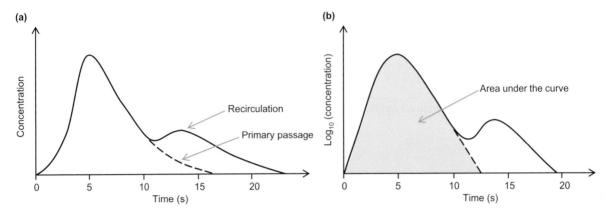

Figure 29.1 Indicator dye technique: (a) concentration–time graph and (b) logarithmic transformation.

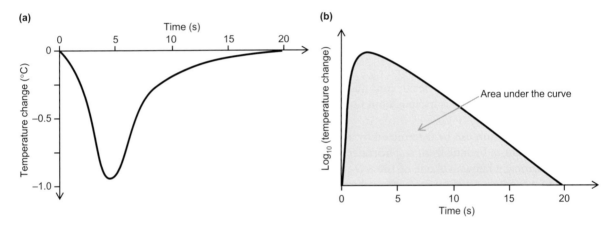

Figure 29.2 Thermodilution method: (a) temperature–time curve and (b) logarithmic transformation.

- 10–15 mL of cold saline is injected through the most proximal lumen of the PAC (located in the RA).
- The change in pulmonary arterial blood temperature is measured by the thermistor, resulting in a temperature–time graph (Figure 29.2a).
- CO is calculated using a modification of the Stewart–Hamilton equation:

Key equation: modified Stewart–Hamilton equation

$$CO = \frac{V(T_B - T_I)K_1 K_2}{\int_0^\infty T_B(t)\, dt}$$

where V is the volume of injectate, T_B is the initial blood temperature, T_I is the initial injectate temperature, K_1 is the density constant, K_2 is the computation constant and $\int_0^\infty T_B(t)\, dt$ is the area under the blood temperature–time curve.

The thermodilution method became the gold standard[4] against which other methods of CO assessment are compared. The thermodilution method became popular as:

- Blood sampling is not required.
- There is no second recirculation peak in the temperature–time graph, the main source of inaccuracies with the dye dilution method.
- It can be used accurately in the presence of intra-aortic balloon pumps and arrhythmias.
- Inaccuracies (such as variation in the speed of injection of the cold saline) can be reduced by performing three or four measurements and averaging the results.

---

[4] The direct Fick method described above is often considered the physiological 'gold standard' and was originally used to validate the thermodilution method, but it cannot be used practically in critical care patients.

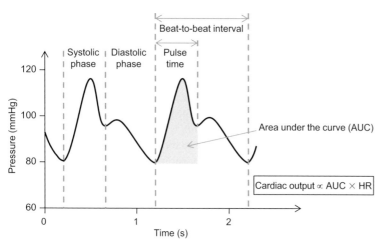

Figure 29.3 Pulse contour analysis.

However, the use of the PAC is associated with a number of serious complications: arrhythmias, infection, tricuspid and pulmonary valve damage and pulmonary artery rupture. In 2005, a study investigating the use of PACs in the management of intensive care patients (the PAC-Man study) found no clear evidence of benefit or harm. Since then, the worldwide use of the PACs has significantly reduced, as intensivists move towards other (arguably less accurate) methods of CO estimation or alternatively abandon CO monitoring entirely (see Further reading).

Methods based on pulse contour analysis

As discussed in Chapter 35, the morphology of the arterial pressure waveform is related to SV and SVR. A continuous estimate of CO is produced by means of a computer-based algorithm. The commercially available pulse contour analysis systems each use their own patented algorithm for estimating CO (Figure 29.3). In addition to CO, a number of other variables are measured or derived, including HR, SV, CI and SV variation (SVV).

SV varies throughout the respiratory cycle as a result of changes in venous return to the heart with changes in intrathoracic pressure. SVV is a measure of the difference between the maximum SV and the minimum SV within a respiratory cycle, and it is used as a measure of fluid responsiveness. The CO of a patient with an SVV $\geq$ 15% is likely to increase with fluid administration, whereas a patient with an SVV < 10% is unlikely to respond to additional fluid.

The commercially available pulse contour analysis systems can be classified as calibrated or non-calibrated. An overview is provided below.

- **Calibrated systems**: PiCCO and LiDCO.
  - *PiCCO (pulse contour CO)* uses a standard central line and a thermistor-tipped arterial line sited at the femoral, brachial or axillary artery. CO is estimated by analysis of the arterial pressure waveform. The PiCCO system is calibrated using a transpulmonary thermodilution method in which cold saline is injected into the central line and the resulting blood temperature change is detected at the arterial line. This introduces an element of error when compared with the thermodilution method using a PAC, as heat is dissipated as the cold injectate passes through the lungs.
  - *LiDCO (lithium dilution CO)* requires only a standard arterial line. The arterial pressure waveform is analysed in a similar way to PiCCO.[5] The LiDCO system is calibrated by a lithium dilution method whereby lithium chloride is injected into a peripheral or central vein and the fall in its arterial concentration is measured by a lithium electrode sampling the arterial line. Recalibration should be

---

5 There is a subtle difference in the analysis of the arterial pressure waveform using LiDCO – the algorithm is based on 'pulse power analysis' rather than 'pulse contour analysis'.

performed every 8 h, or whenever major haemodynamic changes occur. The use of lithium avoids the error introduced by heat dissipation when thermodilution is used for calibration. However, the LiDCO cannot be calibrated in patients who take therapeutic lithium (e.g. bipolar disorder), and frequent calibration (and therefore repeated doses of lithium) results in inaccuracies. In addition, muscle relaxants may cross-react with the lithium electrode.

- **Uncalibrated systems:** FloTrac/Vigileo and LiDCOrapid.

  - *FloTrac/Vigileo:* this system uses a specialised pressure sensor (FloTrac) attached to a standard arterial line. The pressure transducer is connected to a Vigileo monitor, where the arterial pressure waveform is analysed. The FloTrac/Vigileo algorithm is not externally calibrated; instead, it uses an estimate of aortic vascular compliance based on population demographics and the patient's age, height, gender and weight.

  - *LiDCOrapid:* this system is based on the same pulse power analysis algorithm as the LiDCO system. However, like the FloTrac/Vigileo system, LiDCOrapid is uncalibrated, using nomograms based on demographic data.

In general, pulse contour analysis shows good correlation with PAC thermodilution methods. However, a number of situations may make pulse contour analysis inaccurate:

- An over- or under-damped arterial line trace;
- Cardiac arrhythmias;
- Aortic regurgitation;
- An intra-aortic balloon pump.

Describe the minimally invasive methods of CO estimation

The proximity of the heart and great vessels to the oesophagus allows the use of ultrasound-based techniques to estimate CO. Two methods are commonly used in clinical practice:

- **Oesophageal Doppler** (CardioQ). A small ultrasound transducer mounted on the tip of a flexible probe is inserted through the nose or

mouth into the oesophagus. The tip of the probe is adjusted so that it lies immediately alongside the descending thoracic aorta. The ultrasound beam is orientated at an angle of 45° to the aortic blood flow, where it reflects off the passing red blood cells (RBCs). As the RBCs are in motion, the ultrasound beam is reflected at a different frequency – this is the Doppler principle. Using the Doppler equation, the velocity of blood flow within the descending thoracic aorta can be calculated:

Key equation: the Doppler equation

$$V = \frac{F_d c}{2F_0 \cos \theta}$$

where V is the velocity of blood in the descending thoracic aorta, F_0 is the transmitted ultrasound frequency, F_d is the change in frequency (Doppler shift) of the reflected ultrasound, θ is the angle between the ultrasound beam and the bloodstream (45°) and c is the velocity of ultrasound in tissue (1540 m/s).

Blood flow in the descending thoracic aorta is determined by multiplying the measured blood velocity by the cross-sectional area of the descending thoracic aorta, which is estimated from a nomogram (using the patient's height and weight) based on cadaveric studies.[6] CO is calculated from aortic blood flow on the basis that 70% of SV passes through the descending thoracic aorta, with the remainder flowing to the upper body.

In addition to SV, HR and CO, a number of other cardiovascular parameters are derived from the oesophageal Doppler waveform (Figure 29.4), including:

- *Stroke distance* (SD), the area under the velocity–time curve. SD is the distance in centimetres that a column of blood moves along the aorta with each heartbeat.
- *Peak velocity* (PV), the highest blood velocity recorded during systole. PV is an indicator of left ventricular contractility. The normal range of PV alters with age: 90–120 cm/s for a 20-year-old, decreasing to 50–80 cm/s for a 70-year-old.

---

[6] Newer machines use M-mode ultrasound to measure the diameter of the aorta.

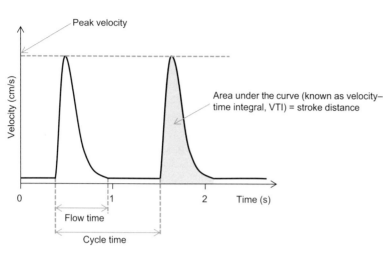

Figure 29.4 Oesophageal Doppler waveform.

- *Flow time corrected* (FTc), the duration of blood flow when corrected for HR, which reflects left ventricular preload. Normal FTc is 330–360 ms. A low FTc suggests hypovolaemia or increased afterload, whilst a high FTc suggests vasodilatation.

Oesophageal Doppler offers a number of advantages over other methods:

- There is no requirement for arterial or central lines (though these are often already present in a patient for whom CO monitoring is being considered).
- Oesophageal tone helps to keep the probe in position, though repositioning is intermittently required.
- No calibration is required.
- It provides continuous cardiovascular measurements.

However, there are a number of disadvantages:

- Oesophageal Doppler probes are poorly tolerated in awake patients.
- Movement of the probe may lead to a poor trace.
- Surgical diathermy interferes with the trace.
- The estimates of aorta cross-section and the division of SV may be inaccurate.
- The use of oesophageal Doppler probes is contraindicated in patients with pharyngoesophageal pathology, such as oesophageal varices.

- **Trans-oesophageal echocardiography** (TOE). The use of TOE is now standard practice in cardiothoracic anaesthesia and cardiac intensive care. Manipulation of a large, multiplane ultrasound transducer in the oesophagus of an anaesthetised patient allows detailed, two-dimensional views of the heart and great vessels.

CO may be calculated in two ways using TOE:

- *Calculation from estimated volumes.* The conical shape of the LV allows its EDV and ESV to be estimated with reasonable accuracy by measuring the longitudinal and transverse diameters in systole and diastole. The difference between EDV and ESV is SV, which, when multiplied by HR, gives CO.
- *Calculation using Doppler.* Blood flow is measured across the left ventricular outflow tract using the Doppler principle and the measured cross-sectional area.

In addition to CO, SV and HR, TOE gives useful information on the mechanical function of the heart, identifying valve dysfunction and regional wall motion abnormalities. However, the bulk and expense of the equipment and the extensive training required currently limit the widespread use TOE.

Further reading

N. Herring, D. J. Paterson. Control of stroke volume and cardiac output. In: N. Herring, D. J. Paterson. *Levick's Introduction to Cardiovascular Physiology*, 6th edition. Boca Raton, CRC Press, 2018; 87–112.

N. Herring, D. J. Paterson. Assessment of cardiac output and arterial pulse. In: N. Herring, D. J. Paterson. *Levick's Introduction to Cardiovascular Physiology, 6th edition.* Boca Raton, CRC Press, 2018; 113–20.

D. A. Reuter, S. Kalman. From 'goal-directed haemodynamic therapy' to 'individualised perioperative haemodynamic management'. *Br J Anaesth* 2018; **120**(4): 615–6.

F. Michard, M. T. Giglio, N. Brienza. Perioperative goal-directed therapy with uncalibrated pulse contour methods: impact on fluid management and postoperative outcome. *Br J Anaesth* 2017; **119**(1): 22–30.

B. Saugel, M. Cecconi, J. Y. Wagner, et al. Noninvasive continuous cardiac output monitoring in perioperative and intensive care medicine. *Br J Anaesth* 2015; **114**(4): 562–75.

S. Ghosh, B. Arthur, A. A. Klein. NICE guidance on CardioQ™ oesophageal Doppler monitoring. *Anaesthesia* 2011; **66**(12): 1081–7.

S. Jhanji, J. Dawson, R. M. Pearse. Cardiac output monitoring: basic science and clinical application. *Anaesthesia* 2008; **63**: 172–81.

Chapter

30

Starling's Law and Cardiac Dysfunction

What is Starling's law of the heart?

The Frank–Starling law (also known as Starling's law of the heart) states that the strength of ventricular contraction is dependent on the length of the resting fibres. In other words, when all other factors are kept constant, an increase in left ventricular preload causes stroke volume (SV) to increase, without the need for extrinsic neural or humoral regulatory mechanisms. As left ventricular preload (i.e. left ventricular end-diastolic volume, LVEDV) is difficult to measure, left ventricular end-diastolic pressure (LVEDP) is often used as its surrogate marker. The relationship between SV and LVEDP is nonlinear (Figure 30.1).

The mechanism of Starling's law remains incompletely understood. It has been traditionally attributed to the degree of overlap of the actin and myosin myofilaments in diastole, which in turn determines the extent of crossbridge formation on activation. This is known as the length–tension relationship:

- The maximal force of contraction occurs when the sarcomere is stretched to around 2.2 μm. This length corresponds to an optimal point where the number of actin and myosin crossbridges formed is high (Figure 30.2b) but there is no overlapping of the thin filaments. In a normal heart, this optimal sarcomere length corresponds to an LVEDP of approximately 10–12 mmHg.

- When the sarcomere is shorter than 2.2 μm (i.e. end-diastolic volume is decreased and the sarcomere is less stretched), overlapping of thin filaments reduces the tension that may be generated (Figure 30.2a):

  – Contractile energy is lost due to work against friction.

  – The sarcomere becomes distorted.

- When the sarcomere is stretched beyond 2.2 μm, fewer actin–myosin crossbridges are formed; the force of contraction is thus reduced (Figure 30.2c). This situation does not occur in the normal heart, but may occur in ventricular failure.

- At 3.6 μm, there is no overlap between actin and myosin myofilaments; the active tension developed is zero (Figure 30.2d).

Figure 30.1 The Frank–Starling curve.

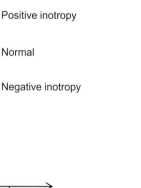

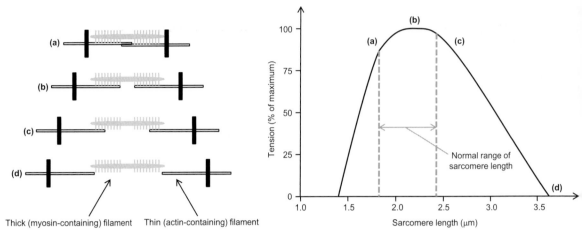

Figure 30.2 Tension developed at different cardiac sarcomere lengths.

The most important consequence of the Frank–Starling mechanism is the matching of SV between the right and left sides of the heart. An increase in venous return to the right ventricle (RV) increases its SV, resulting in a greater pulmonary blood flow, a greater LVEDV and hence a greater left ventricular SV. If the left ventricle (LV) ejected just 1 mL of blood less than the RV per cycle, after an hour the pulmonary circulation would contain over 3 L of additional blood.

What is cardiac failure?

Cardiac failure (or heart failure) is said to occur when the heart is unable to provide sufficient cardiac output (CO) to meet the demands of the tissues. Heart failure may either be:

- **High-output heart failure**: CO is normal, but the tissue O_2 demand is high, such as in thyrotoxicosis and pregnancy.
- **Low-output heart failure**: the tissue's O_2 demand is normal, but the CO is insufficient to meet it.

In low-output failure, either the RV or LV may be affected in isolation, resulting in right ventricular failure (RVF) or left ventricular failure, respectively. In addition, progressive pump failure of the LV may lead to RVF – this is known as congestive cardiac failure. Heart failure may be classified as follows:

- **Systolic heart failure**, in which the pump function of the heart is impaired; that is, ejection fraction is reduced to below 45% (Figure 30.3). At 20%, the annual mortality of patients with systolic heart failure is higher than many cancers; patients also suffer considerable morbidity. Systolic heart failure occurs when the strength of myocardial contraction is inadequate due to:

  - *Dysfunction of myocytes* as a result of ischaemia (coronary artery disease), inflammation (myocarditis), congenital disease (Duchenne muscle dystrophy) or following myocardial infarction and scar formation. The reduction in SV leads to an increased LVEDV, and in turn the size of the heart is increased; this pathological dilatation of the heart is known as cardiomegaly.

  - *Chronically raised afterload*; for example, systemic hypertension or aortic stenosis. Chronically increased afterload causes a compensatory left ventricular concentric hypertrophy. Over time, further increases in afterload exceed the heart's ability to compensate by hypertrophy. SV becomes reduced and LVEDV increased.

  Whatever the cause, the heart must then expend more energy to achieve a normal SV. This increases myocardial O_2 demand, thus reducing cardiac reserve. A vicious positive feedback ensues during periods of increased demand (e.g. during exercise), where increased myocardial O_2 demand in the face of low output exacerbates the failure.

- **Diastolic heart failure**, in which ventricular compliance is reduced, either as a result of impaired ventricular relaxation (e.g. in ischaemic heart disease, restrictive cardiomyopathy) or as a result of pathological ventricular hypertrophy (e.g.

in hypertension, hypertrophic obstructive cardiomyopathy, aortic stenosis). Reduced ventricular compliance leads to impaired ventricular filling and thus reduced SV. Because atrial contraction makes a significant contribution to ventricular filling in these patients, a fourth heart sound may be heard. The development of atrial fibrillation significantly reduces ventricular filling; a high heart rate results in reduced diastolic filling time, thus reducing LVEDV further. Rate control using β-blockers or Ca^{2+} channel antagonists helps prevent this.

Diastolic heart failure is being recognised increasingly commonly, and often coexists with systolic heart failure. Annual mortality in diastolic heart failure is 8% – less than that of systolic heart failure. Again, these patients suffer significant morbidity.

What is compensated heart failure?

Compensated heart failure refers to the situation in which ventricular function is impaired, but CO is still normal as a result of two compensatory mechanisms (Figure 30.4):

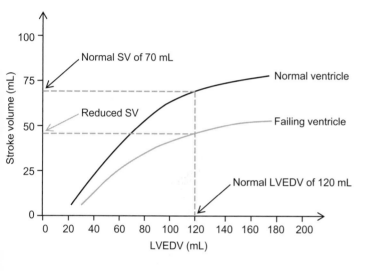

Figure 30.3 Reduced contractility in systolic heart failure.

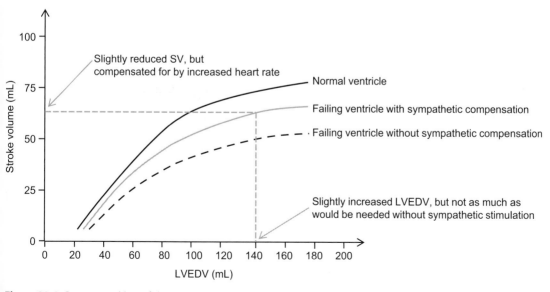

Figure 30.4 Compensated heart failure.

- **Sympathetic stimulation**. This causes both an increase in myocardial contractility and an increase in heart rate, thereby maintaining CO despite the reduced SV. Over time, the heart becomes less responsive to this sympathetic nervous system activity, as β-receptors are downregulated.
- **An expansion in blood volume**. A reduction in CO results in a fall in renal blood flow (RBF). The kidneys respond by increasing plasma volume through the renin–angiotensin–aldosterone (RAA) axis; the increase in blood volume results in an increase in left ventricular preload. An increase in LVEDV results in an increase in SV, according to Starling's law. This is offset to some extent through the production of atrial natriuretic peptide and brain natriuretic peptide by the heart, which causes a natriuresis.

As the disease progresses, the heart reaches a point where, despite compensatory mechanisms, it can no longer eject a normal SV. CO then falls, resulting in a situation termed 'decompensated heart failure'.

The cardiac sarcomeres are stretched beyond their optimal length and the tension generated during contraction is reduced (Figure 30.2). Beyond the optimum sarcomere length, increases in preload only serve to further decrease SV, represented by the Frank–Starling curve in Figure 30.5. Additionally, when the heart has a large ventricular radius, it is at a mechanical disadvantage due to Laplace's law (see Chapter 20). Therefore, for the same active tension generated in the ventricular wall, an LV of greater radius will produce a lower pressure than a ventricle of smaller radius. This again increases the myocardial work required to generate the same pressure.

What are the clinical consequences of decompensated heart failure?

Decompensated heart failure has many effects, classified into forward heart failure and backward heart failure:

- **Forward heart failure**. The heart is unable to pump sufficient blood to meet the metabolic demands of the body. Consequences of left ventricular forward heart failure include:
  - *Renal failure*. Reduced RBF causes kidney dysfunction and activation of the RAA axis. This has the effect of further expanding plasma volume, exacerbating backward heart failure.
  - *Exercise*. The LV cannot meet the increased O_2 demand associated with exercise, resulting in fatigue. As heart failure worsens, the onset of fatigue occurs after minimal exercise, and then at rest. This is reflected in the New York Heart Association classification of heart failure.
  - *Coronary circulation*. Acute left ventricular dysfunction may lead to cardiogenic shock: reduced CO causes a fall in coronary blood flow. In turn, myocardial ischaemia reduces myocardial contractility, reducing CO further and leading to a vicious cycle.
- **Backward heart failure**. The increase in LVEDV results in an abnormally high atrial pressure:
  - *Increased left atrial pressure* causes an increase in interstitial pressure in the pulmonary

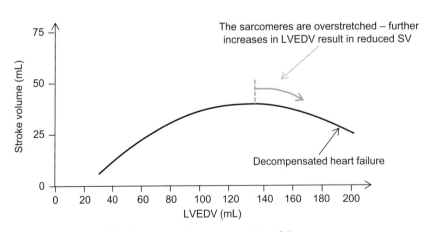

Figure 30.5 The Frank–Starling curve in decompensated heart failure.

circulation. As left atrial pressure increases, the balance of Starling filtration forces (see Chapter 36) favours fluid extravasation in the lung bases, resulting in pulmonary oedema and dyspnoea. Chronically increased pulmonary venous pressure increases right ventricular afterload, which may cause RVF.

When the patient is supine (e.g. overnight), redistribution of blood from the legs further increases the venous return to the heart. As the LV is unable to increase its output any further, the effect of this increase in blood volume is further pulmonary oedema. This leads to paroxysmal nocturnal dyspnoea.

- *Increased right atrial pressure* results in an increase in central venous pressure. The Starling filtration forces favour fluid extravasation, initially in the dependent areas, resulting in ankle and sacral oedema. More advanced RVF results in ascites and hepatomegaly, which may be associated with liver dysfunction (e.g. coagulopathy). Extravasation of fluid into the intestine results in gut wall oedema, which can reduce the absorption of nutrients (leading to the condition of cardiac cachexia) and drugs. Gut wall oedema may also facilitate the translocation of intestinal flora across the gut wall. Bacteria may produce vasodilatory cytokines, which can further decompensate heart failure.

Further reading

N. Herring, D. J. Paterson. Control of stroke volume and cardiac output. In: N. Herring, D. J. Paterson. *Levick's Introduction to Cardiovascular Physiology, 6th edition.* Boca Raton, CRC Press, 2018; 87–112.

H. Fukuta, W. C. Little. The cardiac cycle and the physiological basis of left ventricular contraction, ejection, relaxation and filling. *Heart Fail Clin* 2008; **4** (1): 1–11.

R. Pirracchio, B. Cholley, S. De Hert, et al. Diastolic heart failure in anaesthesia and critical care. *Br J Anaesth* 2007; **98**(6): 707–21.

L. Groban, J. Butterworth. Perioperative management of chronic heart failure. *Anesth Analg* 2006; **103**(3): 557–75.

L. Mandinov, F. R. Eberli, C. Seiler, et al. Diastolic heart failure. *Cardiovasc Res* 2000; **45**(4): 813–25.

Chapter

31

Cardiac Pressure–Volume Loops

Describe the left ventricular pressure–volume loop

The left ventricular pressure–volume loop provides a useful representation of left ventricular performance through the cardiac cycle (Figure 31.1; see also Chapter 28, Figure 28.1).

In a normal left ventricle (LV), the pressure–volume loop is approximately rectangular and can be divided into four phases:

- **Isovolumetric contraction**, a vertical line representing the increase in intraventricular pressure without a change in ventricular volume.

- **Ventricular ejection**, in which the stroke volume (SV) is ejected into the aorta.
- **Isovolumetric relaxation**, a vertical line representing the fall in intraventricular pressure without a change in ventricular volume.
- **Diastolic ventricular filling**, in which the ventricle fills with blood ready for the next contraction.

How does the pressure–volume loop change when preload is increased?

Preload can be thought of as the volume of blood within the ventricle prior to contraction (see

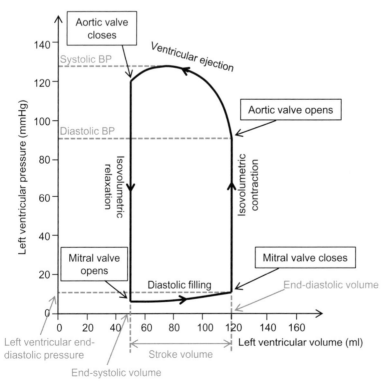

Figure 31.1 Pressure–volume loop of the normal left ventricle (BP = blood pressure).

Chapter 29). For the LV, it is the left ventricular end-diastolic volume (LVEDV). According to Starling's law, an increase in preload results in a greater diastolic stretch of the contractile myocardial fibres (see Chapter 30). The stretched sarcomeres contract more forcefully, thus increasing SV (Figure 31.2).

Figure 31.2 illustrates a number of important features:

- The width of the pressure–volume loop, which represents SV, is increased due to the increase in LVEDV. The left ventricular end-systolic volume (LVESV) increases slightly due to an increase in afterload (aortic pressure) caused by the greater cardiac output.
- The end-diastolic pressure–volume relationship (EDPVR) line reflects the passive diastolic compliance of the LV. Beyond a certain preload, left ventricular end-diastolic pressure (LVEDP) increases sharply, reflecting the nonlinear compliance of the left ventricular wall. This is due to the elastic proteins and connective tissue within the myocardium reaching their elastic limit.

How does the pressure–volume loop change when afterload is increased?

Afterload is the stress developed in the left ventricular wall during ejection, and it reflects the force opposing the shortening of cardiac myocytes. As afterload increases (e.g. due to an increase in diastolic aortic pressure), both the rate and extent of sarcomere shortening decrease, resulting in a reduction in SV:

- As a reduced volume of blood is ejected from the LV, the LVESV is increased.
- In turn, the addition of the venous return leads to an increase in LVEDV.
- According to Starling's law, an increase in LVEDV causes an increase in myocardial contractility. Thus, SV increases, returning LVEDV to near normal.

Overall, the increase in LVESV is greater than that of LVEDV. SV is slightly decreased, and the left ventricular pressure–volume loop looks taller and thinner (Figure 31.3a).

How does an increase in myocardial contractility alter the pressure–volume loop?

Myocardial contractility may be altered extrinsically by the autonomic nervous system, circulating hormones or positively inotropic drugs. It is therefore independent of preload and afterload. Graphically, increased contractility (positive inotropy) increases the gradient

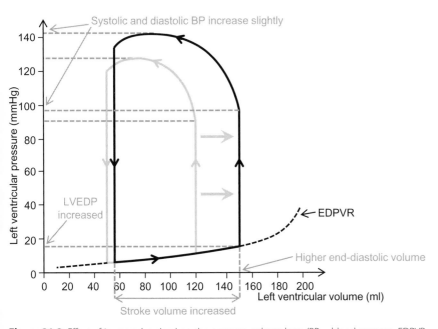

Figure 31.2 Effect of increased preload on the pressure–volume loop (BP = blood pressure; EDPVR = end-diastolic pressure–volume relationship; LVEDP = left ventricular end-diastolic pressure).

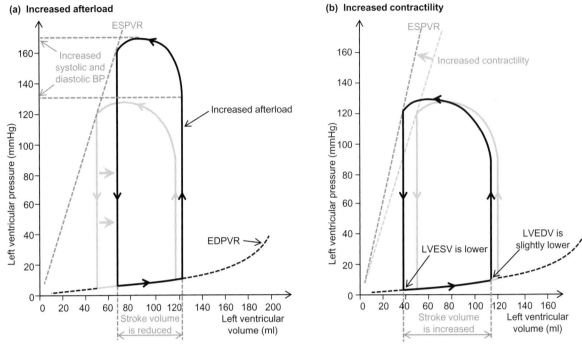

Figure 31.3 Effect of (a) increased afterload and (b) increased contractility on the pressure–volume loop (BP = blood pressure).

of the end-systolic pressure–volume relationship (ESPVR) line (Figure 31.3b).

The increased strength of myocardial contraction ejects additional blood, resulting in a lower LVESV. Following the addition of venous return, LVEDV is reduced. As positive inotropy decreases LVESV more than LVEDV, overall SV is increased.

How is the left ventricular pressure–volume loop related to cardiac work?

The mechanical work of the heart can be divided into:

- **External work** (or stroke work), the kinetic energy expended when blood is ejected under pressure from the ventricle. The area enclosed by the ventricular pressure–volume loop (i.e. pressure × volume) represents the external work done during a single cardiac cycle (Figure 31.4).
- **Internal work**, the energy expended during isovolumetric contraction. It is sometimes known as 'pressure work'. As myofilament shortening does not occur, the energy expended during isovolumetric contraction is converted to heat energy during diastole; that is, the energy

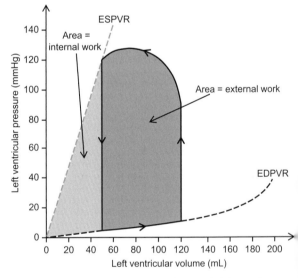

Figure 31.4 External and internal work expended during the cardiac cycle.

expended is potential energy. The area enclosed within the ESPVR, the EDPVR and the isovolumetric relaxation lines represents the internal work.

The total work done – that is, the sum of external and internal work – is known as the pressure–volume area (PVA). PVA correlates surprisingly well with the myocardial O_2 consumption for the heart. Note: whilst mechanical work accounts for most of the heart's energy expenditure, basal metabolism accounts for a small percentage, resulting in a small discrepancy between PVA and myocardial O_2 consumption.

Looking back at Figures 31.2 and 31.3, it can be seen that:

- Increased preload leads to increased external work (Figure 31.2); thus, myocardial O_2 demand is higher.

- Increased afterload may not increase external work significantly, but does increase internal work (Figure 31.3a); thus, myocardial O_2 demand increases.
- Increased myocardial contractility may not increase internal work, but does increase external work (Figure 31.3b). Overall, myocardial O_2 consumption is increased.

How does the pressure–volume loop of the right ventricle compare with that of the left?

The right ventricular pressure–volume loop has a characteristic triangular shape (Figure 31.5). Some important points regarding Figure 31.5 are:

- The pressure developed within the right ventricle (RV) is significantly lower than that of the LV; the RV must overcome a much lower afterload, as pulmonary vascular resistance and thus pulmonary artery pressure are low.
- Despite pumping the same volume of blood (i.e. the SV), the area enclosed by the right ventricular pressure–volume loop (i.e. the stroke work) is only 20–25% that of the left ventricular loop.
- Ejection of blood from the RV begins early in systole: right ventricular volume starts to fall shortly after right ventricular pressure increases.

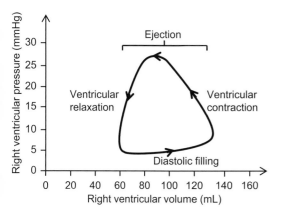

Figure 31.5 Right ventricular pressure–volume loop.

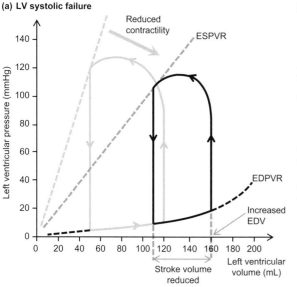

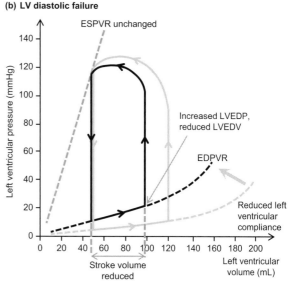

Figure 31.6 Left ventricular (a) systolic failure and (b) diastolic failure.

- In the RV, stroke work makes up a greater proportion of the total work than the LV does. The RV is therefore more susceptible to failure in the presence of pulmonary hypertension than the LV is in the presence of systemic hypertension.

How does the left ventricular pressure–volume loop change in heart failure?

As discussed in Chapter 30, left ventricular failure is classified as systolic, diastolic or mixed. Left ventricular systolic failure results in a reduction in myocardial contractility (reduced gradient of the ESPVR line) and an increase in LVEDV. A subnormal SV is ejected from the LV, resulting in a higher than normal LVESV (Figure 31.6a).

Left ventricular diastolic failure is due to reduced left ventricular compliance. The EDPVR line follows a different course, but the contractility of the LV (the ESPVR line) is unchanged. Overall, SV is reduced (Figure 31.6b).

Further reading

R. E. Klabunde. *Cardiovascular Physiology Concepts, 2nd edition*. Philadelphia, Lippincott Williams & Wilkins, 2011.

Chapter

32

Cardiac Ischaemia

How does the oxygen extraction ratio of the heart compare to other organs?

The oxygen extraction ratio (OER) is the ratio of oxygen consumption, $\dot{V}O_2$, to oxygen delivery, $\dot{D}O_2$ (see Chapter 17). At around 60%, the OER of the heart is near maximal. This is in contrast to the lower OERs of the liver (around 50%), the kidney (around 15%) and skeletal muscle (between 10% and 100% depending on activity).

During exercise, myocardial $\dot{V}O_2$ increases by up to fivefold. Normally, coronary blood flow increases to match the increase in $\dot{V}O_2$ through coronary vaso-dilatation (see Chapter 27). However, when the flow of blood is limited by coronary arterial stenosis, a mismatch between $\dot{V}O_2$ and $\dot{D}O_2$ occurs, resulting in myocardial ischaemia.

What is meant by the term 'acute coronary syndrome'?

Acute coronary syndrome encompasses a range of conditions that are due to an acute interruption of myocardial perfusion. It includes:

- ST-segment elevation myocardial infarction (STEMI);
- Non-ST-segment elevation myocardial infarction (NSTEMI);
- Myocardial ischaemia without evidence of myocyte necrosis (e.g. unstable or crescendo angina).

How is a myocardial infarction diagnosed?

The diagnosis of myocardial infarction (MI) requires evidence of myocardial necrosis in a clinical setting consistent with acute MI. In practice, this usually means a rise in measured serum cardiac troponin (either troponin T or troponin I isoform) above the upper reference range, with at least one of:

- Typical anginal symptoms;
- New significant ST-segment or T-wave changes on the electrocardiogram (ECG), which may be dynamic in nature, or new left bundle branch block (LBBB);
- Development of pathological Q-waves on the ECG in established infarct;
- New regional wall abnormality on echocardiography.

Describe the typical symptoms associated with MI

The most common symptom of myocardial ischaemia is severe central chest pain: tightness, pressure or squeezing. The pain may classically radiate to the left arm, neck or lower jaw, but also to the right arm, shoulder, back or upper abdomen. Other associated symptoms include autonomic features (sweating, nausea or vomiting), dyspnoea, syncope and fatigue. In a significant proportion of cases, patients experience no symptoms of MI – this is termed a 'silent MI'. Presentation in women is more likely to be atypical, which may delay presentation and diagnosis.

Anaesthetised patients cannot complain of chest pain. The anaesthetist must instead rely on clinical signs to detect myocardial ischaemia: ECG changes, cardiovascular instability, arrhythmias, hypoxia and increased airway pressures due to pulmonary oedema, as well as (if transoesophageal echo is being used) regional wall abnormalities.

What is the physiological mechanism for referred cardiac pain?

Visceral pain is often referred to (i.e. perceived as coming from) the surface of the body. In addition to efferent sympathetic and parasympathetic neurons (see Chapter 59), the heart is innervated by unmyelinated afferent sympathetic neurons. Myocyte ischaemia triggers these afferent neurons to transmit action potentials, through the cardiac plexus, to synapse in the dorsal horn of the spinal cord. It is thought that when the spinal cord is bombarded with sensory information from a viscus, the signal is instead interpreted as pain originating from a dermatome whose afferent sensory neurons also synapse in the same spinal cord segment.

Clinical relevance: silent MI

Up to half of all MIs occur either without any symptoms or with atypical symptoms, and as a result these patients often miss the opportunity for early treatment. Many of these patients develop pathological Q-waves on their ECG. Silent MI is as significant a clinical event as recognised MI, and both carry a similar mortality rate.

Two groups of patients at particular risk of silent MI are:

- **Diabetics**. As a result of autonomic neuropathy, there may be abnormal transmission of action potentials along the afferent sympathetic neurons.
- **Heart transplant recipients**. As the donor heart is completely denervated, there is no pathway for the afferent transmission of ischaemic pain signals. This is of real significance in heart transplant recipients, as the graft coronary arteries undergo accelerated atherosclerosis.

How is MI classified?

MI is classified into five types:

- Type 1 refers to a primary coronary event, such as atherosclerotic plaque rupture or coronary dissection.
- Type 2 is myocardial ischaemia due to either increased oxygen demand or decreased supply in the context of another acute illness.
- Type 3 is unexpected cardiac death with symptoms suggestive of MI.
- Type 4 is associated with percutaneous coronary intervention (PCI).
- Type 5 is associated with cardiac surgery.

The majority of cases of MI are due to spontaneous rupture of an atheromatous plaque. Thrombus rapidly forms around the damaged vascular lumen.

Complete occlusion of a coronary artery results in a full-thickness MI (with ST-segment elevation on the ECG), while partial occlusion of a coronary artery results in a partial thickness or subendocardial MI (with ST-segment depression and/or T-wave inversion on the ECG).

Clinical relevance: ECG changes with myocardial ischaemia

The ECG is a key investigation in the diagnosis of acute myocardial ischaemia and infarction. Both the depolarisation (Q-waves and bundle branch blocks) and repolarisation (ST-segment and T-wave) of ischaemic myocardium may be abnormal, resulting in characteristic changes to the ECG. These ECG changes are dependent on the extent and location of ischaemic myocardium. By correlating Einthoven's triangle (see Chapter 58) with the anatomical location of injured myocardium and its arteries, the angiographic appearance and certain complications may be predicted. As a rough guide:

- **Extent of myocardial ischaemia**:
  - *Subendocardial ischaemia/infarction* is associated with ST-segment depression.
  - *Subepicardial or transmural infarction* is associated with ST-segment elevation.

- **Location of ischaemia**:
  - *Inferior wall ischaemia* affects leads II, III and aVF. This inferior portion of the heart is supplied by the right coronary artery and the posterior interventricular artery. As the right coronary artery frequently supplies the sinoatrial (SA) and atrioventricular (AV) node, occlusion may result in hypotension and bradycardia. Complete heart block is a common presentation of inferior STEMI.
  - *Left main stem ischaemia* results in widespread ST-depression often affecting leads I, II and V4–6, with ST-elevation in aVR.
  - *Lateral wall ischaemia* affects leads I, aVL, V5 and V6. This area of the heart is supplied by the circumflex artery. Infarction results in left ventricular dysfunction.
  - *Septal ischaemia* affects leads V1 and V2, corresponding to occlusion of a septal branch of the left anterior descending artery. As the interventricular septum is the site of the bundle of His, infarction may cause LBBB.
  - *Apical ischaemia* affects leads V3 and V4, corresponding to occlusion of a terminal

portion of the left anterior descending artery or (in right-dominant circulations) the posterior interventricular artery. Apical involvement is associated with mural thrombus formation.

- *Anterior wall ischaemia* may affect up to eight leads: I, aVL, V1, V2, V3, V4, V5 and V6. This part of the myocardium is supplied by the left anterior descending artery: complete occlusion will result in ischaemia of a considerable portion of the left ventricle (LV) and is therefore associated with severe LV dysfunction, ventricular septal defects and aneurysm formation.
- *Posterior wall ischaemia* is difficult to diagnose. Posterior wall infarction causes ST-segment depression in leads V1, V2, V3 and V4 and results in LV dysfunction. The posterior wall is supplied by the circumflex artery and the posterior interventricular artery.

What is the treatment for a type 1 MI

A type 1 MI refers to an interruption in myocardial perfusion due to coronary artery pathology. The treatment pathway depends on the ECG changes:

- **STEMI or new-onset LBBB** is an emergency and requires an immediate primary PCI. Intracoronary thrombus is removed and blockages opened up using angioplasty and stents. Dual antiplatelet agents (aspirin plus an ADP/P2Y inhibitor such as ticagrelor) will be required to prevent reocclusion of the coronary artery. If PCI is not immediately available, pharmacological thrombolysis (e.g. recombinant tissue plasminogen activator) may be administered in the interlude.
- **NSTEMI** is typically managed with antiplatelet agents and low-molecular-weight heparin. An urgent coronary angiogram is used to assess the patient's coronary arteries for stenoses that may be amenable to stenting. The 'Thrombolysis in Myocardial Infarction' (TIMI) risk score can be used to guide the urgency of angioplasty.

What is the difference between type 2 MI and myocardial injury?

It was previously thought that cardiac troponin could only be released into the plasma through the necrosis

of cardiac myocytes. However, since the introduction of high-sensitivity cardiac troponin assays, it has been recognised that troponin may also be released when the myocardium is put under severe physiological stress. This myocardial injury may be due to aetiologies such as:

- Sepsis;
- Myocarditis;
- Catecholamine surge (e.g. following subarachnoid haemorrhage);
- Right ventricular strain (e.g. as a result of acute pulmonary embolus).

A type 2 MI is defined as a myocardial ischaemia due to an imbalance in oxygen demand and supply or in the context of another acute illness. There is considerable overlap between a type 2 MI and myocardial injury, and no clear definition separates the two. Therefore, in a patient who is critically ill with sepsis and has an increase in serum troponin, it may be difficult to determine whether the patient has had a type 2 MI or myocardial injury. Either way, the diagnosis is fairly academic: both carry a poor prognosis and, because an atheromatous plaque in a coronary artery is not the cause, neither is amenable to specific treatment (e.g. coronary angioplasty).

What is ischaemic reperfusion injury?

It is essential that the blood supply is restored to acutely ischaemic tissues to prevent necrosis; however, reperfusion is not without its own problems.

Tissue metabolic activity is reduced during periods of ischaemia, which has a relative protective effect against tissue damage. Normal cellular protective factors such as free radical scavengers may also be consumed. When the coronary blood supply is restored (e.g. by revascularisation aided by PCI and/or thrombolysis, ending the cardioplegic bypass or by stabilisation of mean arterial blood pressure), metabolic processes resume. This permits inflammation, cytosolic ionic homeostatic disturbance and the production of reactive oxygen species (ROS). Production of nitric oxide also becomes reduced, which promotes vasoconstriction. These processes result in microvascular endothelial damage with thrombosis and embolisation, as well as damage to the myocardial cells themselves directly and indirectly via apoptosis. This sequence of events is known as cardiac ischaemia reperfusion injury (IRI) and is most commonly associated with STEMI. Similar damage may also occur in other organs such as the brain following a stroke.

The complications of IRI are as follows:

- **Arrhythmias.** Reperfusion results in atrial and ventricular arrhythmias, likely secondary to disturbed ionic homeostasis and ROS. Accelerated idioventricular rhythm is commonly seen in the catheter laboratory following reperfusion and is usually well tolerated. Other ventricular arrhythmias, such as ventricular ectopy and ventricular tachycardia, may be seen in the following hours. This is why patients are usually monitored in a dedicated cardiac critical care unit following primary PCI. Reperfusion arrhythmias usually resolve spontaneously, although scar formation may result in an anatomical substrate for persistent rhythm disturbance.
- **Contractile dysfunction** (so-called myocardial stunning) occurs due to cytosolic Ca^{2+} overload. This can result in symptoms of heart failure, but these may resolve with good reperfusion and time. Immediate echocardiography is rarely useful for assessing long-term myocardial function.
- **Microvascular damage.** Inflammation, leukocyte debris, thrombosis, embolic events and myocardial oedema may prevent reperfusion of ischaemic tissue, even when blood flow has been restored to the blocked coronary artery. This is the 'no-reflow' complication that is associated with poor long-term outcomes.

Many therapeutic interventions have been suggested for IRI; however, none have a conclusive evidence basis. Approaches include ischaemic preconditioning, therapeutic hypothermia, therapeutic hyperoxaemia, anti-inflammatory drugs and free radial scavengers.

What is ischaemic preconditioning?

This is a largely experimental technique whereby controlled ischaemia is carried out with the intention of giving a protective effect to the myocardium against future ischaemic insults. Its mechanism remains incompletely understood but may result from:

- Genetic/energetic cellular changes;
- The production of ischaemic metabolites (e.g. adenosine);
- The production of paracrine factors (e.g. endogenous opiates).

In experimental studies, preconditioning reduces infarct size and complications. Strangely, preconditioning need not be via direct occlusion of the coronary arteries. Occluding the brachial artery appears to convey a similar benefit: this is known as remote preconditioning. Ischaemic preconditioning can be mimicked pharmacologically, such as through the use of isoflurane during coronary bypass surgery. This is known as anaesthetic preconditioning.

Further reading

J. C. Kaski, D. J. Hausenloy, B. J. Gersh, D. M. Yellon (Eds.). *Management of Myocardial Reperfusion Injury*. Berlin, Springer, 2012.

M. R. Pinski, A. Artigas, J. F. Dhainaut. *Coronary Circulation and Myocardial Ischemia*. New York, Springer-Verlag, 2002.

F. van Lier, F. H. I. M. Wesdorp, V. G. B. Liem, et al. Association between postoperative mean arterial blood pressure and myocardial injury after non-cardiac surgery. *Br J Anaesth* 2018; **120**(1): 77–83.

A. R. Chapman, P. D. Adamson, N. L. Mills. Assessment and classification of patients with myocardial injury and infarction in clinical practice. *Heart* 2017; **103**: 10–18.

S. Ekeloef, M. Alamili, P. J. Devereaux, et al. Troponin elevations after non-cardiac, non-vascular surgery are predictive of major adverse cardiac events and mortality: a systematic review and meta-analysis. *Br J Anaesth* 2016; **117**(5): 559–68.

Z.-M. Zhang, P. M. Rautaharju, R. J. Prineas, et al. Race and sex differences in the incidence and prognostic significance of silent myocardial infarction in the Atherosclerosis Risk In Communities (ARIC) study. *Circulation* 2016; **133**(22): 2141–8.

R. D. Foreman, K. M. Garrett, R. W. Blair. Mechanisms of cardiac pain. *Compr Physiol* 2015; **5**: 929–60.

R. Loveridge, F. Schroeder. Anaesthetic preconditioning. *Continuing Educ Anaesth Crit Care Pain* 2010; **10**(2): 38–42.

Systemic Circulation

The cardiovascular system distributes blood around the body. It is divided into the pulmonary circulation and the systemic circulation. The systemic circulation is a 'pressure-constant, flow-variable' system.

What are the functions of the circulation?

Functions include:

- Transport of O_2 from the lungs to the tissues;
- Transport of CO_2 from the tissues to the lungs;
- Transport of metabolic waste products from the tissues to the liver and kidneys for excretion;
- Distribution of nutrients from the sites of absorption (gut) or production (liver) to the tissues;
- Distribution of body water and electrolytes between intracellular, interstitial and intravascular body compartments;
- Transport of immunologically active substances (antibodies, leukocytes, complement);
- Transport of hormones from their site of production (e.g. the parathyroid gland) to their target site (e.g. the kidney);
- Production of hormones (e.g. atrial natriuretic peptide);
- Assisting in thermoregulation by redistributing blood flow between the core organs and the skin.

The transport and distributive properties of the circulation are utilised by anaesthetists to distribute a range of substances: drugs, fluids, nutrition and heat.

What are the constituent parts of the systemic circulation?

The systemic circulation is composed of:

- A 'pump' – the left ventricle (LV) – which drives blood through the vessels;

- The arterial system, consisting of arteries and arterioles;
- Capillaries;
- The venous system, consisting of venules and veins.

Only 15% of circulating blood volume is found within the arterial system. Most of the circulating blood (65%) is found within the venous system due to its greater compliance. The veins thus act as an important reservoir for blood, with venous tone responsible for maintaining venous return to the right atrium. The remainder of the circulating volume is found within the pulmonary circulation (10%), the cardiac chambers (5%) and the capillaries (5%).

What are the main differences between the systemic and pulmonary circulations?

The primary function of the pulmonary circulation is the transport of blood from the right ventricle (RV) to the lungs for participation in gas exchange (see Chapter 23). The RV therefore acts as a flow generator around a low-resistance pulmonary circulation. This is in contrast to the role of the systemic circulation, where the LV generates pressure in the arterial system. This pressure is then used as the energy gradient to perfuse tissues (create flow) according to the demand. The transport of blood from the LV to the rest of the body is thus determined by local tissue metabolism or by stereotyped responses (e.g. an increase in sympathetic outflow). The main differences between the two circulations stem from this pressure difference (Table 31.1).

What happens to blood velocity as blood passes through the systemic circulation?

There is an important relationship between blood velocity, flow and cross-sectional area:

Table 31.1 Differences between the systemic and pulmonary circulations (PVR = pulmonary vascular resistance; SVR = systemic vascular resistance).

	Systemic circulation	Pulmonary circulation
Arteries		
Typical pressure (systolic/diastolic)	140/80 mmHg	25/8 mmHg
Typical mean pressure	100 mmHg	15 mmHg
Vessel wall	Thick walled, elastic	Thin walled, distensible
Resting vasoconstrictor tone	Highly constricted at rest	No vasoconstrictor tone at rest
Arterioles		
Vessel wall	Thick walls, small lumen, muscular	Thin walls, large lumen
Vessel resistance	High resistance, typical SVR 1600 dyn.s. cm^{-5}	Low resistance, typical PVR 160 dyn.s. cm^{-5}
Response to hypoxia	Vasodilatation	Vasoconstriction
Capillaries		
Wall thickness	Thin, to allow exchange of O_2, CO_2 and nutrients	Extremely thin, to allow efficient gas exchange
Blood flow	Owing to high resistance in arterioles, flow is continuous	Low resistance in arteries and arterioles means blood flow is still pulsatile at the capillaries
Distensibility/compressibility	Little change in radius, as little change in external/internal pressures	Compressible with increased alveolar pressure; distensible with increased pulmonary venous pressure
Veins		
Typical mean pressure	2 mmHg	5 mmHg
Venous reservoir	High venous capacitance, holding >1000 mL, which can be released back into the circulation if required	Only holds around 500 mL of blood, which can be released back into the circulation if required

---

Key equations: blood velocity and flow

$$V = \frac{\dot{Q}}{A}$$

where V (cm/s) is the blood velocity (the distance travelled per unit time), $\dot{Q}$ (mL/s) is the blood flow (the volume of blood passing a point per unit time) and A (cm^2) is the cross-sectional area of the vessel.

For a typical adult, the aortic cross-sectional area is 4 cm^2, whilst the mean blood velocity in the aorta is 20 cm/s. Therefore, typical aortic blood flow is 80 cm^3/s (i.e. 80 mL/s). At a heart rate of 60 bpm, there is one cardiac cycle per second; that is, stroke volume is 80 mL.

As blood passes along the arterial system, large arteries branch into many small arteries, small arteries branch into many arterioles, and so on. The cross-section of each individual blood vessel decreases as its radius decreases. However, the overall cross-sectional area A summed over all of the vessels at a given level of bifurcation increases dramatically. The total blood flow $\dot{Q}$ remains the same (i.e. cardiac output of 80 mL/s); so, as $V = \dot{Q}/A$, if $\dot{Q}$ remains constant and A is significantly higher, then the velocity of blood flow must be significantly reduced (Figure 33.1).

The capillaries account for a combined cross-sectional area of around 4000 cm^2 (Figure 33.1). Total blood flow is the same, so the velocity of blood flow through the capillaries is:

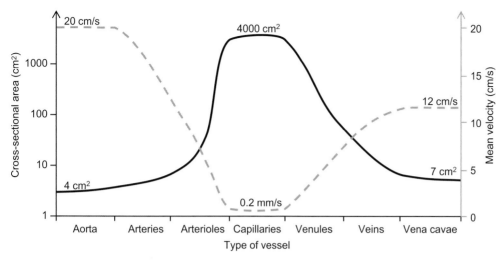

Figure 33.1 Changes in velocity (dotted grey line) and cross-sectional area (solid black line) across the systemic circulation.

$$V = \frac{\dot{Q}}{A} = \frac{80}{4000} = 0.2 \text{ mm/s}$$

that is, slow enough to allow capillary–tissue exchange.

As blood is moved from the capillaries to the venules and then to the veins, the cross-sectional area of each individual vessel increases, but the total cross-sectional area of the entire system decreases. Eventually, all veins in the lower half of the body combine to form the inferior vena cava, and those from the upper half of the body form the superior vena cava. The blood flow entering the right atrium is approximately equal to the cardiac output,

allowing for some fluid being filtered into the interstitial space and carried away by the lymphatics. The cross-sectional area of the venae cavae is 7 cm², so the velocity of blood flow rises to 12 cm/s (Figure 33.1).

Further reading

N. Herring, D. J. Paterson. Haemodynamics: flow, pressure and resistance. In: N. Herring, D. J. Paterson. *Levick's Introduction to Cardiovascular Physiology*, 6th edition. Boca Raton, CRC Press, 2018; 113–20.

L. Heller, D. Mohrman. The peripheral vascular system. In: L. Heller, D. Mohrman. *Cardiovascular Physiology*, 9th edition. New York, Lange McGraw-Hill, 2018; 104–27.

Chapter

34

Arterial System

The arterial system is the high-pressure component of the systemic circulation. The arterial system divides from the aorta into large arteries, smaller arteries and finally arterioles before joining the capillary networks. Arteries normally carry fully oxygenated blood to the capillaries. The two exceptions are the pulmonary arteries and the umbilical arteries in the foetus.

Describe the cross-section of an artery

A thick muscular wall surrounds the normally circular arterial lumen. The arterial wall is made up of three layers:

- **Tunica externa** (formerly known as the tunica adventitia), the outermost layer, made up of loose connective tissue, such as collagen fibres.
- **Tunica media**, a thick layer of circumferential smooth muscle and elastic tissue.
- **Tunica intima**, the innermost layer, comprising a single layer of endothelial cells. Some larger vessels also have a subendothelium, made up of connective tissue and basement membrane.

Larger arteries have their own blood supply: the vasa vasorum, a network of small blood vessels that supply the outer layers of the arterial wall.

Are there different types of artery?

Arteries are subclassified into two types:

- **Elastic arteries**: the more proximal, larger arteries; that is, the aorta and its immediate branches. Their role is the conduction of blood. The relatively large radius of these arteries results in their resistance to blood flow being low. Elastic arteries have more elastic tissue than muscular tissue in their tunica media, allowing them to accommodate the high pressure generated by the heart during systole. The arteries expand in systole, accommodating the blood ejected from the heart, and recoil in diastole, thereby

maintaining the diastolic pressure. The expansion and recoil of the elastic arteries acts to dampen the pulsatile arterial blood flow.
- **Muscular arteries**: medium-sized arteries, which follow on from the large elastic arteries and, in turn, divide into the smaller 'resistance' arterioles. Muscular arteries supply individual organs; examples include the renal and coronary arteries. Their tunica media are composed primarily of smooth muscle, whose diameter is tonically controlled by the sympathetic nervous system:
  - Increased sympathetic activity results in smooth muscle contraction (vasoconstriction), which narrows the vessel lumen and reduces blood flow.
  - Reduced sympathetic activity permits vasodilatation, which increases the lumen diameter and increases blood flow. The mechanism for vasodilatation in this context is an increase in sheer stress cause by higher intravascular pressure. This results in a rise in intracellular Ca^{2+}, leading to increased nitric oxide synthase activity in endothelial cells, and thus increased nitric oxide production. Nitric oxide acts as a potent vasodilator of vascular smooth muscle.

There is little or no parasympathetic innervation of the arterioles, although the walls do contain muscarinic acetylcholine (ACh) receptors, possibly mediating some local, paracrine effects.

What is the mathematical relationship between vessel radius and resistance to blood flow?

Laminar flow of an incompressible Newtonian fluid of constant viscosity in a rigid tube with a circular cross-section is normally governed by the Hagen–Poiseuille equation:

Key equation: Hagen–Poiseuille equation

$$\Delta P = \frac{8\dot{Q}\eta l}{\pi r^4}$$

where ΔP is the pressure drop along the tube, $\dot{Q}$ is flow, η is the viscosity, l is the tube length and r is the radius.

The equation can also be rearranged to give:

$$\dot{Q} = \frac{\Delta P \pi r^4}{8\eta l}$$

Darcy's law states: pressure = flow × resistance; so, if ΔP is pressure and $\dot{Q}$ is flow, then the resistance to flow is $8\eta l/\pi r^4$.

According to the Hagen–Poiseuille equation, the most important factor affecting flow is the tube radius, owing to its fourth power. For example, doubling the radius produces a 16-fold increased flow. However, the Hagen–Poiseuille equation provides only an approximation of *blood* flow, because:

- **The pressure drop along the vessel is not continuous** – it has a pulsatile component.
- **Blood does not behave like a Newtonian fluid.** Instead, its viscosity varies with:
  - *Flow rate.* At low blood flow, there is increased interaction between red blood cells (RBCs): they aggregate into rouleaux, thereby increasing blood viscosity, and thus resistance to flow is greater. At normal flow rates, aggregation is prevented by negatively charged sialic acid residues on the RBC surface repelling other RBCs.

  - *Haematocrit.* Interactions between RBCs mean that high haematocrit is associated with a greater overall blood viscosity. In anaemia, a reduced haematocrit increases blood flow; a haematocrit of around 0.3 is considered to be the optimal balance between blood flow and O_2-carrying capacity.
  - *Temperature.* Viscosity increases as temperature decreases. This has some relevance in intensive care: until recently, patients were cooled following cardiac arrest and therefore had an increased blood viscosity. Thus, blood flow was decreased at a time when flow may already be low due to coexisting cardiogenic shock.
  - *Fahraeus–Lindqvist effect.* At vessel diameters below 300 µm (i.e. arterioles), RBCs tend to stream towards the centre of the vessel, leaving the plasma at the vessel walls. As plasma has a lower viscosity than whole blood, the resistance to blood flow is reduced. This Fahraeus–Lindqvist effect opposes the tendency for resistance to increase as the vessel radius decreases, especially in arterioles and capillaries.

- **Vessels are not uniform rigid tubes**.
  - *Vessels are non-uniform.* They may have branches, turn corners or be narrowed due to atherosclerotic plaques or external compression. These factors increase the risk of turbulence.
  - *Vessels are distensible.* According to the Hagen–Poiseuille equation, a rigid tube has a constant resistance: flow is therefore proportional to pressure (Figure 34.1).

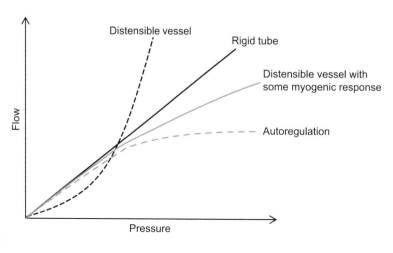

Figure 34.1 Comparison of distensible vessels, rigid tubes and myogenic response.

However, large vessels are distensible: an increase in pressure causes an increase in vessel radius, which reduces resistance and thus increases flow. In contrast, if the pressure falls near to zero (as may occur in veins), the vessel tends to collapse, resulting in no flow.

– *Myogenic autoregulation* is the intrinsic ability of an arteriole to maintain a constant blood flow despite changes in intraluminal pressure (see below) (Figure 34.1).

What are the functions of the arterioles?

The arterioles are the vessels with the smallest radii of the arterial tree and are therefore the main source of resistance to blood flow. Structurally, their tunica media is made up of one or two layers of circumferential smooth muscle. Vasoconstriction increases the vessel's resistance to blood flow; this is very sensitive owing to the fourth-power relationship of the radius in the Hagen–Poiseuille equation. Likewise, vasodilatation reduces the vessel's resistance to blood flow. Compared with arteries, the arterioles lack elastin in their tunica media. Pulsatile blood flow is damped, becoming continuous flow by the time the blood reaches the capillaries.

In addition to conducting blood from small arteries to the capillaries, the arterioles have three other roles:

- Control of the distribution of blood flow to different organs by altering organ vascular resistance;
- Control of total systemic vascular resistance (SVR);
- Alteration of capillary hydrostatic pressure, effectively controlling bulk flow of water between intravascular and interstitial body fluid compartments (see Chapter 36).

Which factors are involved in arteriolar vasoconstriction and vasodilatation?

The control of arteriolar smooth muscle is complex, influenced by local, humoral and neural factors.

- **Local factors**:
  - *Myogenic autoregulation*. This is an intrinsic property of the arteriolar smooth muscle in which the vessel vasoconstricts in response to increased intraluminal pressure. This occurs

because mechanically gated ion channels in the vascular wall are opened by stretch, leading to the opening of voltage-gated Ca^{2+} channels, Ca^{2+} influx and thus to contraction of arteriolar smooth muscle. Likewise, arterioles vasodilate in response to reduced intraluminal pressure via the sheer stress mechanism. The overall effect is the maintenance of a relatively constant blood flow over a range of intraluminal pressures. Autoregulation is an important feature of arterioles in the brain, heart and kidney, but does not occur in the skin.

- *Metabolites*. The tissues regulate blood flow in proportion to their metabolic rate. When an organ increases its metabolic activity, the local O_2 tension falls and the concentration of metabolites (CO_2, H^+ ions, lactate) increases. The arteriole vasodilates in response to increased metabolite concentration, increasing blood flow and therefore O_2 delivery to the tissues. This is thought to be the mechanism behind reactive hyperaemia: the large increase in blood flow following temporary cessation of organ perfusion (e.g. critical limb ischaemia) or following deflation of an arterial tourniquet in limb surgery.

- **Humoral factors**. A number of locally and systemically produced chemical substances affect arteriolar smooth muscle tone, including:

  - *Kinins* (e.g. bradykinin), which cause vasodilatation in the salivary glands, gut and skin.
  - *Histamine*, released from basophils and mast cells as part of the inflammatory response. The resulting arteriolar vasodilatation increases blood flow to the affected tissues. During allergic reactions, the systemic release of histamine is responsible for widespread arteriolar vasodilatation.
  - *Nitric oxide* (NO), previously known as endothelium-derived relaxing factor, released from the endothelium in response to shear stress. NO is a potent arteriolar vasodilator, increasing blood flow to the damaged area. NO also causes venodilatation; this is the mechanism underlying a technique familiar to all anaesthetists: tapping the skin overlying a peripheral vein prior to cannulation.

- *Serotonin and thromboxane A_2* are released from platelets when they are activated (e.g. when a blood vessel is cut). Both chemicals cause arteriolar vasoconstriction, which reduces the local blood flow, allowing the clot to form without it being washed away.
- *Adrenaline* activates both α_1-adrenoceptors, resulting in vasoconstriction, and β_2-adrenoceptors, resulting in vasodilatation. The response of arterioles to adrenaline differs between organs depending on their relative proportions of α_1- and β_2-adrenoceptors. In the gut and skin, there is a high concentration of arteriolar α_1-adrenoceptors: adrenaline causes vasoconstriction, resulting in reduced blood flow. In contrast, heart and skeletal muscles have high concentrations of β_2-adrenoceptors, the activation of which causes vasodilatation.
- *Anti-diuretic hormone* (ADH; or arginine vasopressin), which is synthesised in the hypothalamus and released from the posterior lobe of the pituitary gland in response to low plasma volume and high plasma osmolarity. In addition to its anti-diuretic effect on the collecting ducts, ADH is a potent arteriolar vasoconstrictor. This effect is unimportant in health, but it is an important mechanism for maintaining blood pressure in haemorrhage. Vasopressin is used clinically as an arteriolar vasoconstrictor in the intensive care unit: patients with septic shock have been shown to have relatively reduced ADH concentrations.
- *Other hormones.* Angiotensin II is a potent arteriolar vasoconstrictor, whilst atrial natriuretic peptide is an arteriolar vasodilator that also decreases the sensitivity of the arterioles to other vasoconstrictors. Together with ADH, these hormones are normally concerned with control of blood volume and total body water.
- **Neural factors**:
  - *Sympathetic nervous system.* The arterioles have a rich sympathetic nervous supply; the basal sympathetic outflow is responsible for setting the resting arteriolar smooth muscle tone. Activation of the sympathetic nervous system results in the release of noradrenaline from post-ganglionic neurons, which, like adrenaline, activates arteriolar α_1-adrenoceptors, resulting in vasoconstriction. In contrast to adrenaline, noradrenaline only weakly activates β_2-adrenoceptors, causing minimal arteriolar vasodilatation. Sympathetic nervous stimulation causes arteriolar vasoconstriction in the skin, kidneys and gut, where α_1-adrenoceptors are plentiful, but has minimal effect on the arterioles of the brain and heart, which have relatively few α_1-adrenoceptors. Sympathetic stimulation therefore preferentially directs blood flow to these vital organs.
  - *Parasympathetic nervous system.* Parasympathetic control of arteriolar smooth muscle tone is only found in the penis, where parasympathetic stimulation results in vasodilatation and erection.
  - *Skeletal muscle.* Skeletal muscle is unusual[1] in that it possesses a sympathetic cholinergic pathway, which is only activated following the onset or anticipation of exercise, fear, anger or pain. ACh is released at post-ganglionic nerve endings instead of noradrenaline, resulting in arteriolar vasodilatation and a substantial increase in skeletal muscle blood flow.

How can the combined resistance of all arterioles be calculated?

The combined resistance of all arterioles in the arterial system is the SVR. This can be calculated by using Darcy's law:

Key equation: SVR

Darcy's law states:

pressure difference = flow × resistance

When considering the systemic circulation as a single circuit:

- 'Pressure difference' refers to the difference in hydraulic pressure between the arterial and venous circulations.
- Flow is the cardiac output (CO; L/min).
- Resistance is the SVR (dyn.s.cm^{-5}).

---

[1] The eccrine sweat gland is also sympathetic cholinergic.

Therefore:

$$MAP - RAP = CO \times SVR$$

Rearranging:

$$SVR = 80 \times \frac{MAP - RAP}{CO}$$

where MAP (mmHg) is the mean arterial pressure, RAP (mmHg) is the right atrial pressure and 80 is a conversion factor between units. This equation is simplified to consider the circulation as a whole rather than its constituent arterial and venous parts.

Using typical values: MAP = 100 mmHg, RAP = 2 mmHg and CO = 5 L/min:

$$SVR = 80 \times \frac{MAP - RAP}{CO}$$

$$\Rightarrow SVR = 80 \times \frac{100 - 2}{5} = 1568 \text{ dyn.s.cm}^{-5}$$

How are systolic, diastolic and mean blood pressures measured?

For each cardiac cycle (Figure 34.2):

- The peak blood pressure is the systolic blood pressure (SBP).
- The lowest blood pressure is the diastolic blood pressure (DBP).
- MAP is somewhere in-between and is considered to be the most important of the three blood pressure measurements. Once arterial pulsations have been damped, the pressure within the arterioles (i.e. the pressure perfusing the organs) is the MAP. However, MAP is not simply the

average of the systolic and diastolic pressures. This is because the systolic portion of the cardiac cycle is shorter than the diastolic portion at rest. At resting heart rates (HRs), diastole is twice the length of systole; so:

$$MAP = \frac{2}{3}DBP + \frac{1}{3}SBP$$

or:

$$MAP = DBP + \frac{1}{3}PP$$

where PP is the pulse pressure, the difference between SBP and DBP; that is, PP = SBP – DBP.

The assumption that a third of the cardiac cycle is systole does not hold true in tachycardia; calculated values of MAP can therefore be inaccurate.

Whether SBP, DBP and MAP are directly measured or calculated depends on the method used:

- **Non-invasive blood pressure measurement**:
  - The *cuff and manometer* method. SBP is pressure measured at the onset of the first Korotkoff sound, whilst DBP is the pressure measured at the fifth Korotkoff sound. MAP is calculated using the equation above.
  - *Automated oscillometric method* (DINAMAP). SBP is the pressure measured when oscillations are first detected by the pressure transducer, whilst MAP is the pressure measured when oscillations are maximal. DBP is calculated using the formula above. As it is calculated and not measured, DBP may be inaccurate in tachycardia.
- **Invasive blood pressure measurement**: SBP is the peak and DBP is the trough of the arterial pressure

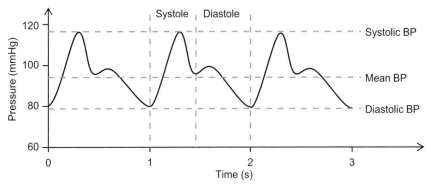

Figure 34.2 The arterial pressure waveform (BP = blood pressure).

waveform (Figure 34.2). MAP is calculated by integrating the area under the arterial pressure waveform and dividing it by the length of the cardiac cycle – this calculation is accurate at all HRs.

Which factors determine arterial blood pressure?

As discussed above:

$$MAP - RAP = CO \times SVR$$

As RAP is usually much smaller than MAP in a normal adult,[2] this can be approximated to

$$MAP \approx CO \times SVR$$

Therefore, the main determinants of MAP are:

- **SVR**, which depends on the degree of arteriolar smooth muscle contraction. As discussed above, arteriolar smooth muscle tone depends on complex interactions between local, humoral and neural factors.
- **CO**, which depends on stroke volume (SV) and HR (see Chapter 29):

$$CO = HR \times SV$$

In turn, SV depends on a complex interaction of:
- *Preload*;
- *Myocardial contractility*;
- *Afterload*.

HR results from the balance of cardioacceleratory sympathetic outflow and the cardioinhibitory parasympathetic outflow.

Clinical relevance: manipulation of blood pressure

In clinical practice, anaesthetists use a variety of pharmacological and non-pharmacological methods to increase or decrease MAP by manipulating the five factors described above: preload, myocardial contractility, afterload, HR and SVR. For example:

- **Neuraxial blockade** causes a decrease in sympathetic nervous activity below the level of the block. This causes arteriolar vasodilatation, which decreases SVR and therefore decreases MAP. Anaesthetists often use vasopressors to

counteract the decreased SVR, thereby increasing MAP, such as phenylephrine (α_1-agonist) or metaraminol (direct and indirect α_1-agonist with some β-effects).

- **Septic shock** causes hypotension through two mechanisms:
  - *Fluid leakage from the intravascular space to the interstitial space*, which reduces preload, thereby reducing SV and CO.
  - *Systemic release of vasodilatory inflammatory mediators*, which reduce SVR.

    Management of hypotension in septic shock is therefore by fluid resuscitation to restore intravascular volume and by vasopressors to counteract arteriolar vasodilatation. Two vasopressors commonly used in septic shock are noradrenaline (selective α_1-agonist) and vasopressin.

- **Cardiogenic shock.** When hypotension is due to left ventricular dysfunction, positively inotropic drugs may be used to increase myocardial contractility, thereby increasing MAP, such as dobutamine (β_1-agonist) or adrenaline (mainly a β_1- and β_2-agonist at low/moderate doses). An intra-aortic balloon pump is sometimes used to increase forward flow of blood whilst decreasing left ventricular afterload and improving coronary perfusion.

- **Hypotensive anaesthesia.** This is a (mainly historical) technique where controlled hypotension is induced in anaesthetised patients to establish a bloodless surgical field, being of particular interest in middle-ear surgery. Hypotension may be induced by:
  - *Patient position.* The reverse-Trendelenburg position reduces venous return, thereby reducing left ventricular preload.
  - *Drugs that cause arteriolar vasodilatation* and reduce SVR, such as volatile anaesthetics, glyceryl trinitrate and sodium nitroprusside.
  - *Drugs that reduce HR and myocardial contractility*, such as esmolol (β_1-antagonist) and labetalol (mixed α_1- and β-antagonist).

Further reading

N. Herring, D. J. Paterson. Haemodynamics: flow, pressure and resistance. In: N. Herring, D. J. Paterson. *Levick's Introduction to Cardiovascular Physiology*, 6th edition. Boca Raton, CRC Press, 2018; 113–20.

---

[2] RAP may become significant in right ventricular failure.

C. Vlachopoulos, M. O'Rourke, W. W. Nichols. *McDonald's Blood Flow in Arteries: Theoretical, Experimental and Clinical Principles, 6th edition.* Boca Raton, CRC Press, 2011.

K. Lakhal, S. Ehrmann, M. Martin, et al. Blood pressure monitoring during arrhythmia: agreement between automated brachial cuff and intra-arterial measurements. *Br J Anaesth* 2015; **115**(4): 540–9.

J. A. Russell, K. R. Walley, J. Singer, et al. Vasopressin versus norepinephrine infusion in patients with septic shock. *N Engl J Med* 2008; **358**(9): 877–87.

M. Ward, J. A. Langton. Blood pressure measurement. *Continuing Educ Anaesth Crit Care Pain* 2007; 7(4): 122–6.

Arterial Pressure Waveforms

The rate and character of the arterial pulse has been used for millennia for the diagnosis of a wide range of disorders. Perhaps more useful, however, is the direct cannulation of an artery, which allows quantitative information to be extracted.

What is the Windkessel effect?

During systole, the left ventricle (LV) ejects around 70 mL of blood into the aorta (the stroke volume, SV). The elastic aortic walls expand to accommodate the SV, moderating the consequent increase in intra-aortic pressure from a diastolic blood pressure (DBP) of 80 mmHg to a systolic blood pressure (SBP) of 120 mmHg. The ejected blood possesses kinetic energy, whilst there is storage of potential energy in the stretched aortic wall. In diastole, recoil of the aortic wall converts the stored potential energy back into kinetic energy. This maintains the onward flow of blood during diastole, thereby maintaining DBP; this is known as the 'Windkessel effect'. This effect, along with the cardiac valves, converts the sinusoidal pressure wave generated in the heart into a positive and constant pressure at the tissues, much like converting AC to DC electricity. With advancing age, there is degeneration of elastin in the wall of the aorta. The aortic wall becomes less compliant, and its ability to accommodate SV without a large increase in pressure reduces. This accounts for the development of systolic hypertension in the elderly.

What is the arterial pressure wave?

Ejection of blood into the aorta generates both an arterial pressure wave and a blood flow wave. The arterial pressure wave is caused by the distension of the elastic walls of the aorta during systole. The wave propagates down the arterial tree at a much faster rate (around 4 m/s) than the mean aortic blood velocity (20 cm/s). It is the arterial pressure wave that is felt as the radial pulse, not the blood flow wave.

Describe the arterial pressure waveform for the aorta

Starting from end-diastole (Figure 35.1), the pressure generated by the LV ejects the SV into the aorta. The intra-aortic pressure rises to a peak value (the SBP) and then falls to a trough (the DBP). The smooth descent of the curve is interrupted at the dicrotic notch, when the aortic valve closes.

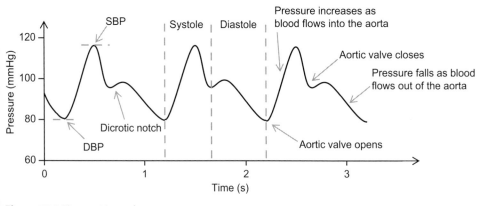

Figure 35.1 The arterial waveform.

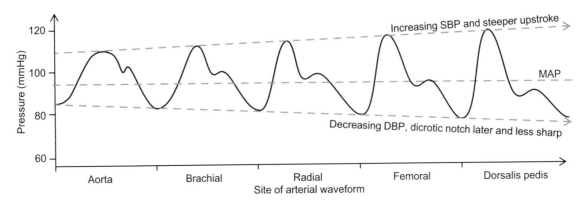

Figure 35.2 Arterial pressure waveform at different sites.

How does the arterial pressure waveform differ at peripheral arteries?

The morphology of the arterial pressure waveform differs depending on where it is measured (Figure 35.2). As the site of measurement moves more distally:

- The arterial upstroke is steeper and SBP is increased.
- DBP is decreased.
- Crucially, mean arterial pressure (MAP) is relatively constant wherever it is measured; this is another reason why MAP is the most important measure of blood pressure.
- The morphology of the dicrotic notch changes:
  - The dicrotic notch is positioned further down the pressure curve.
  - Rather than being a sharp interruption in the pressure descent, the dicrotic notch becomes more of a dicrotic wave.

The change in shape and position of the dicrotic wave is due to it being caused by reflections of the arterial pressure wave rather than aortic valve closure.

Can any other information be gathered from the arterial pressure waveform?

Although the arterial pressure waveform is often only used for measuring SBP, DBP, MAP and heart rate, it has many other clinical uses:

- **Myocardial contractility.** The slope of the waveform upstroke is a reflection of myocardial contractility: an increased upstroke gradient suggests a greater pressure generated per unit time. However, a reduced upstroke gradient is sometimes seen in aortic stenosis (Figure 35.3a). In contrast, aortic regurgitation is usually associated with normal myocardial contractility, but often has a pressure wave with a bisferiens appearance.
- **Systemic vascular resistance** (SVR). The downstroke of the arterial pressure waveform gives information about SVR: a steep downstroke with a low dicrotic notch indicates a low SVR – the arterial waveform looks thin and pointed (Figure 35.3a). Likewise, a high dicrotic notch implies a high SVR.
- **Hypovolaemia.** In positive pressure-ventilated patients, a respiratory swing in the arterial pressure waveform is an indicator of hypovolaemia. There is beat-to-beat variation in the systolic pressure of the waveform, caused by the variation in preload throughout the respiratory cycle (Figure 35.3b).
- **Arterial pulse contour analysis.** SV is proportional to the area under the systolic portion of the arterial pressure waveform; arterial pulse contour analysis allows calculation of the cardiac output (see Chapter 29). SV variation is calculated by dividing the minimum SV (Area 2) by the maximum SV (Area 1).

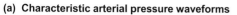

(a) Characteristic arterial pressure waveforms

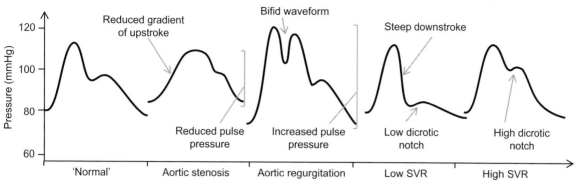

(b) Respiratory swing with hypovolaemia and positive-pressure ventilation

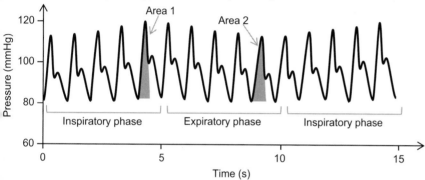

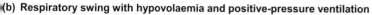

Figure 35.3 (a) Characteristic changes of the arterial waveform and (b) variation through the respiratory cycle with positive-pressure ventilation.

Further reading

N. Herring, D. J. Paterson. Haemodynamics: flow, pressure and resistance. In: N. Herring, D. J. Paterson. *Levick's Introduction to Cardiovascular Physiology, 6th edition.* Boca Raton, CRC Press, 2018; 113–20.

C. Vlachopoulos, M. O'Rourke, W. W. Nichols. Principles of recording and analysis of arterial waveforms. In: *McDonald's Blood Flow in Arteries: Theoretical, Experimental and Clinical Principles, 6th edition.* Boca Raton, CRC Press, 2011; 255–72.

S. J. Denardo, R. Nandyala, G. L. Freeman, et al. Pulse wave analysis of the aortic pressure waveform in severe left ventricular systolic dysfunction. *Circ Heart Fail* 2010; **3**(1): 149–56.

G. M. London, B. Pannier. Arterial functions: how to interpret the complex physiology. *Nephrol Dial Transplant* 2010; **25**(12): 3815–23.

B. Lamia, D. Chemla, C. Richard, et al. Interpretation of arterial pressure wave in shock states. *Crit Care* 2005; **9**(6): 601–6.

Capillaries and Endothelium

What are the roles of the capillaries?

The capillaries are tiny vessels (measuring 5–10 μm in diameter) arranged in an interweaving network called the capillary bed. Capillaries have two main roles:

- Delivery of nutrients to and removal of metabolites from the tissues;
- Distribution of body water between intravascular and interstitial fluid compartments.

In contrast to arteries and veins, the capillary wall is almost entirely composed of endothelium and is only one cell thick, supported by a basement membrane.

What are the different types of capillary?

There are three main capillary types:

- **Continuous capillaries,** the most common class of capillary, found in muscle, brain and connective tissue. Features include:
  - *A continuous basement membrane.*
  - *Neighbouring cells joined by tight junctions*; endothelial cells are closely associated.
  - *Blood–brain barrier.* In the brain, tight junctions hold the endothelial cells especially close and are surrounded by astrocyte foot processes (see Chapter 47). Only the smallest molecules such as water, O_2 and CO_2 can then freely diffuse from one side of the cell to the other. The diffusion of larger molecules (nutrients, metabolites and drugs) across the capillary is dependent on carrier-mediated transport mechanisms.
- **Fenestrated capillaries,** found in the renal glomeruli, intestinal mucosa and choroid plexus. Fenestrated capillaries have large pores within the endothelial cell called fenestrations, which makes them much more permeable than continuous capillaries. These fenestrations are large enough

(60–80 nm) to allow passage of all but the largest plasma proteins (i.e. albumin).

- **Sinusoidal capillaries,** a particular type of fenestrated capillary found in the bone marrow and lymph nodes. The fenestrations are large enough to allow white blood cells and red blood cells (RBCs) to pass through (up to 10 μm). In the liver and spleen, even greater movement of cells is required – in addition to large fenestrations, their sinusoidal capillaries also lack tight junctions. These vessels are called discontinuous sinusoidal capillaries.

How does capillary–tissue exchange occur?

Capillary exchange involves the matrix properties of the capillary basement membrane as well as the features of the endothelial layer itself. It takes place through three overall mechanisms:

- **Simple diffusion.**
  - Gases (e.g. O_2 and CO_2) and small lipophilic molecules (e.g. anaesthetic agents) are able to diffuse across the phospholipid bilayer of the endothelial cell.
  - Small water-soluble molecules traverse the capillary either through pores in the cell membrane or through gaps between endothelial cells.

    The rate of diffusion is affected by a number of factors; most importantly, the concentration (or partial pressure) gradient of the substance across the capillary wall (Fick's law – see Chapter 10).

- **Bulk flow.** Water is filtered through the fluid-filled pores within (fenestrations) or between (tight junctions) endothelial cells. Any dissolved solutes (e.g. electrolytes) can be dragged along with the water. This mechanism is particularly important in the fenestrated renal glomerular capillaries. Filtration and reabsorption of fluid across the capillary is governed by the balance of Starling filtration forces.

- **Pinocytosis**. This is an energy-consuming type of endocytosis where substances in the capillary lumen are enveloped by the endothelial cell membrane to form a vesicle. The vesicle is then transported across the endothelial cell and its contents released into the interstitium (see Chapter 4). Pinocytosis makes only a minor contribution to capillary exchange.

Capillary exchange is facilitated by a blood flow pattern known as bolus flow, which is another example of the non-Newtonian nature of blood. Capillaries have approximately the same diameter as the RBC at around 7 μm. For this reason, the RBC only just fits through the capillary, often having to deform its biconvex shape. Flow therefore takes place as intermittent RBC and plasma boluses. As previously discussed, turbulence increases resistance and therefore decreases flow; this is therefore usually avoided in the larger vessels. However, turbulence can be used advantageously in the capillary as a method of mixing the plasma and potentially facilitating exchange at the endothelium. Effective viscosity is only increased by approximately 30% in bolus flow, which is much less than would be expected from turbulent flow. Capillary bolus flow therefore allows controlled pockets of turbulence to occur for mixing whilst maintaining a relatively low resistance.

How do the Starling filtration forces determine transmembrane fluid flow?

The net fluid filtration across the capillary wall results from the balance of the four opposing Starling filtration forces (Figure 36.1):

- **Forces tending to move fluid out of the capillary**:
  - *Capillary hydrostatic pressure P_c*;
  - *Interstitial fluid oncotic pressure π_i*.
- **Forces tending to move fluid into the capillary**:
  - *Interstitial fluid hydrostatic pressure P_i*;
  - *Plasma oncotic pressure π_c*.

Key equation: the Starling filtration equation

Net fluid filtration pressure across capillary wall = K_f $[(P_c - P_i) - \sigma(\pi_c - \pi_i)]$, where K_f is the filtration coefficient, a constant related to the permeability of the capillary wall (high K_f indicates high water permeability, whilst low K_f indicates low water permeability); σ is the reflection coefficient, a constant that represents the permeability of the capillary to proteins ($\sigma = 1$ implies that the capillary wall is 100% impermeable).

As capillary walls are normally relatively impermeable to proteins, the Starling filtration equation can be simplified as:

Net fluid filtration pressure across capillary wall $\propto$ $[(P_c - P_i) - (\pi_c - \pi_i)]$

Note: Starling pressures are usually measured in mmHg.

Normally, three values are relatively constant:

- π_c is 24 mmHg.
- P_i and π_i are both low, being 2 mmHg and 3 mmHg, respectively.

P_c is therefore the main determinant of whether fluid is filtered or reabsorbed:

- **At the arterial end of the capillary**, $P_c = 36$ mmHg. Net filtration pressure = $(36 - 2) - (24 - 3) = 13$ mmHg. Therefore, there is bulk flow out of the capillary; that is, filtration.

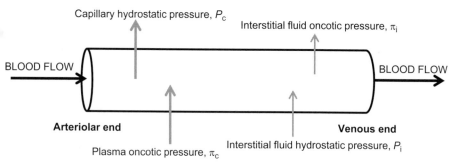

Figure 36.1 The balance of Starling filtration forces across a capillary.

- **At the venous end of the capillary**, $P_c = 10$ mmHg. Net filtration pressure $= (10 - 2) - (24 - 3) = -13$ mmHg. Therefore, there is bulk flow into the capillary; that is, absorption.

As the capillary hydrostatic pressure decreases from the arteriolar to the venous end of the capillary, the direction of bulk flow changes from net filtration to net absorption. The Starling filtration forces can be demonstrated graphically: Area 1 represents net filtration, whilst Area 2 represents net absorption (Figure 36.2a). Filtration and absorption are not exactly matched – overall, there is a daily net filtration of around 4 L of

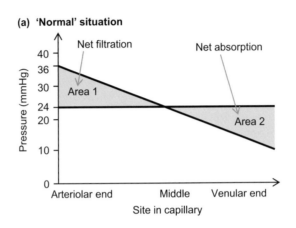

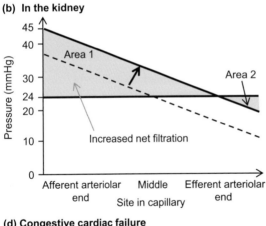

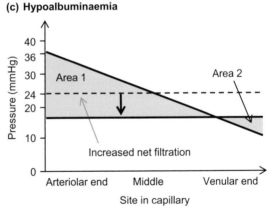

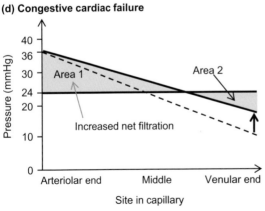

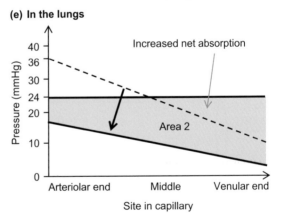

Figure 36.2 Graphical representation of Starling filtration forces.

fluid. This fluid is returned to the circulation via the lymphatic system at the thoracic duct.

The body controls the bulk flow of water through alterations in P_c. Arteriole and venule tone is controlled by the sympathetic nervous system:

- Arteriolar vasodilatation and venule venoconstriction both increase P_c, resulting in net filtration.
- Arteriolar vasoconstriction and venule venodilatation both reduce P_c, resulting in net absorption.

The Starling filtration forces can be used to explain a number of physiological and pathological situations.

- **In the kidney**: the system of afferent and efferent arterioles produces a high glomerular capillary hydrostatic pressure, which increases net filtration – this is how the kidney is able to filter a large volume (180 L) of plasma per day (Figure 36.2b). Additionally, glomerular disease may result in a decrease in the reflection coefficient σ. As a result, proteins such as albumin enter the filtrate, resulting in proteinuria.
- **In critical illness**: hypoalbuminaemia reduces plasma oncotic pressure, which increases net filtration. Clinically, this results in peripheral oedema (Figure 36.2c).
- **In congestive cardiac failure**: venous pressure is increased. This increases net filtration, again resulting in peripheral oedema (Figure 36.2d).
- **In the lungs**: the pulmonary circulation is a low-pressure system – mean capillary hydrostatic pressure is only 8 mmHg. The plasma constituents are unchanged, so plasma oncotic pressure remains the same (around 24 mmHg). Overall, there is net fluid absorption, which explains why alveoli are usually fluid free (Figure 36.2e). If pulmonary venous pressure were to increase, as occurs in left ventricular failure, capillary hydrostatic pressure would rise. Should pulmonary capillary pressure increase sufficiently, there would be net filtration of fluid into the alveolus, resulting in pulmonary oedema.

Clinical relevance: haemorrhage

Following haemorrhage, the sudden loss of intravascular blood volume risks organ hypoperfusion. The body responds to haemorrhage through a massive increase in sympathetic outflow, involving many reflexes and mechanisms (see Chapter 40). This sympathetic outflow causes arteriolar vasoconstriction, which has two effects:

- An increase in systemic vascular resistance to maintain mean arterial pressure and therefore organ perfusion pressure;
- A reduction in the hydrostatic pressure of downstream capillaries.

According to the Starling filtration equation, the reduced capillary hydrostatic pressure results in net absorption of fluid from the interstitial space. In an acute haemorrhage, around 500 mL of fluid can be mobilised within 30 min from the interstitial space to the intravascular space, known as autotransfusion. This constitutes an important compensatory mechanism for temporarily increasing the circulating volume.

Does blood always flow through all the capillary networks?

At rest, only around a quarter of capillaries are patent. Blood can entirely bypass the capillary networks, passing from arterioles to venules via short shunting vessels called metarterioles.

The flow of blood into each capillary network is controlled by small pre-capillary sphincters: one or two smooth muscle cells that form a cuff around the arteriolar end of the capillary. When the pre-capillary sphincter constricts, blood is prevented from entering the capillary network and is diverted elsewhere, either to other capillaries or along the metarterioles to the venules. Pre-capillary sphincter dilatation allows blood to flow through the capillary network, delivering O_2 and nutrients to the tissues. Like the arterioles (see Chapter 34), the tone of the pre-capillary sphincter is controlled by neural and local metabolic factors:

- At rest, the tissues are only minimally metabolically active. The demand for O_2 and nutrients is low and so most of the pre-capillary sphincters are closed.
- In metabolically active tissues, such as exercising muscle, a large proportion of the pre-capillary sphincters open in response to neural stimulation, low O_2 tension and high concentrations of metabolites (e.g. H^+ and CO_2). Blood is permitted to flow through the capillary networks, resupplying the tissues with O_2 and metabolic substrates.

What are the functions of the endothelium?

The endothelium is far from an inert blood vessel lining. In a typical adult, the endothelium comprises nearly 1 kg of cells. As described above, the endothelium acts as a semipermeable membrane, controlling the movement of gases, nutrients and metabolites across the capillary wall. In addition, the endothelium is involved in many other processes, including:

- **Synthesis of vasoactive substances**, the most important of which are nitric oxide (NO), prostacyclin (PGI$_2$) and endothelin (ET); NO and PGI$_2$ are vasodilators, whilst ET is a potent vasoconstrictor. These vasoactive substances are released in response to local metabolic and mechanical stimuli and play a major role in the control of vascular tone. NO is synthesised from L-arginine by nitric oxide synthase (NOS) and has a wide range of functions. It is of particular interest to anaesthetists:

  - *Inhaled NO* has been used in neonatal and adult pulmonary hypertension and in acute respiratory distress syndrome to reduce pulmonary vascular resistance through pulmonary arteriolar vasodilatation.
  - *NO is released* when a vein is traumatised (e.g. by tapping it), causing local venodilatation, which makes veins easier to cannulate.
  - *NO donors*, such as glyceryl trinitrate, are used as anti-anginal drugs. At therapeutic levels, NO dilates the capacitance veins, reducing venous return. The resulting decrease in preload leads to a reduction in myocardial O$_2$ demand, easing the pain of angina.

- **Haemostasis.** The endothelium normally has anticoagulant properties, but becomes procoagulant when injured (see Chapter 72):

  - *Anticoagulant properties.* The endothelial cell surface receptor thrombomodulin binds thrombin, effectively removing it from the circulation. The thrombomodulin–thrombin complex also activates protein C, a potent anticoagulant. NO and PGI$_2$ are both inhibitors of platelet aggregation.

Heparan sulphate is an endothelial cell membrane-bound molecule that activates the plasma protein antithrombin III, which in turn inactivates thrombin and factor Xa.

  - *Procoagulant properties.* Endothelial cells synthesise von Willebrand factor (vWF), which is released into the plasma where it binds to factor VIII. When blood vessels are damaged, vWF acts as an adhesion molecule, binding the exposed collagen (in the vessel basement membrane) to platelets, which leads to platelet activation.

- **Inflammatory system.** Inflammatory cytokines like interleukin 1 and tissue necrosis factor stimulate the endothelium to express adhesion molecules. These adhesion molecules attract neutrophils and lymphocytes, causing them to roll along the endothelial surface before migrating across the endothelial cell (see Chapter 75).

Further reading

N. Herring, D. J. Paterson. Endothelium. In: N. Herring, D. J. Paterson. *Levick's Introduction to Cardiovascular Physiology*, 6th edition. Boca Raton, CRC Press, 2018; 149–70.

N. Herring, D. J. Paterson. The circulation and solute exchange. In: N. Herring, D. J. Paterson. *Levick's Introduction to Cardiovascular Physiology*, 6th edition. Boca Raton, CRC Press, 2018; 171–90.

N. Herring, D. J. Paterson. Circulation of fluid between plasma, interstitium and lymph. In: N. Herring, D. J. Paterson. *Levick's Introduction to Cardiovascular Physiology*, 6th edition. Boca Raton, CRC Press, 2018; 191–220.

T. E. Woodcock. Plasma volume, tissue oedema, and the steady-state Starling principle. *BJA Education* 2017; **17**(2): 74–8.

J. R. Levick, C. C. Michel. Microvascular fluid exchange and the revised Starling principle. *Cardiovasc Res* 2010; **87**(2): 198–210.

H. F. Galley, N. R. Webster. Physiology of the endothelium. *Br J Anaesth* 2004; **93**(1): 105–13.

C. C. Michel. Fluid exchange in the microcirculation. *J Physiol* 2004; **557**(3): 701–2.

37

Venous System

What are the roles of the venous system?

The venous system has a number of roles:

- **Transport of deoxygenated blood** from the capillaries to the right side of the heart, which is the main role of the venous system. There are a few exceptions to this rule:

    - *The pulmonary veins* carry oxygenated blood from the pulmonary capillaries to the left side of the heart (see Chapter 23).

    - *The umbilical vein* carries oxygenated blood from the placenta to the foetus (see Chapter 83).

    - *A portal vein* is a vein that connects two capillary networks. For example:

        - The hepatic portal vein carries deoxygenated blood between two capillary beds: from the gut to the liver (see Chapter 65).

        - The long hypophyseal portal veins connect the capillary networks of the lower hypothalamus and the anterior lobe of the pituitary gland (see Chapter 80).

        - The short hypophyseal portal veins connect the capillary networks of the posterior and anterior lobes of the pituitary gland.

- **Storage of blood**. The venous system contains 65% of the circulating blood volume.

- **Venous return to the heart**. The rate at which blood returns to the right atrium determines the cardiac preload and is therefore a major factor determining the cardiac output (CO).

- **Thermoregulation**. Arteriovenous anastomoses are short channels that connect arterioles to venules, bypassing the capillary networks. Arteriovenous anastomoses are plentiful in the skin. They are opened when body temperature increases, allowing a large amount of blood to flow through the skin, dissipating heat to the environment.

How does the structure of a vein differ from an artery?

Arteries have three layers (see Chapter 34):

- The tunica externa;
- The tunica media;
- The tunica intima.

The tunica media is the thickest layer, with a much higher proportion of smooth muscle than elastin.

In contrast, veins:

- Have thinner walls and larger lumens than equivalent-sized arteries;
- Have much less smooth muscle and more elastin in their tunica media;
- Have as their thickest layer the tunica externa, containing elastin and collagen;
- Are much more distensible than arteries and are often collapsed;
- Have valves formed by folds of tunica intima that prevent backflow of blood. Note that there are no valves in the venae cavae, portal veins or cerebral veins.

What is compliance? How does this relate to the venous system?

Compliance is the change in volume caused by a unit change in distending pressure. The venous system is around 30 times more compliant than the arterial system. This means that the veins can accommodate large volumes of blood for only a small increase in intraluminal pressure. In fact, the venous system holds 65% of the circulating blood volume compared with only 15% within the arterial system, which is under considerably higher pressure.

The difference in compliance between arteries and veins is of critical importance to the systemic circulation. As previously discussed, the left ventricle acts as a pressure generator. It does this by moving a unit of blood (the stroke volume) from the highly compliant veins to the less compliant arteries. As compliance (C) is the change in volume per unit change in pressure, the pressure generated is: $\Delta P = \Delta V / C$. Therefore, as the veins have a high compliance, the same volume of blood gives a low pressure, whereas when it is moved to the low-compliance artery the pressure is much increased.

Which factors are involved in determining venous return to the heart?

When standing upright, the majority of the venous blood is situated vertically below the level of the heart. This blood must therefore return to the heart against the force of gravity. In addition to gravity, venous return is hindered by fluctuations in abdominal and thoracic pressures and disease states such as congestive cardiac failure. There are a number of mechanisms involved in venous return:

- **Valves.** One-way valves are positioned every few centimetres along the veins – an intact valvular system means that blood can only be propelled forwards.
- **Venous pressure** (or more correctly mean systemic filling pressure). As blood fills the venous capacitance vessels, the venous pressure increases, thus increasing venous return to the heart. Venous pressure is increased by filling the veins with a greater blood volume or by increasing venous tone through an increase in sympathetic nervous activity.[1] Similarly, loss of blood volume (e.g. haemorrhage) or loss of sympathetic tone (e.g. following central neuraxial blockade) results in a decrease in venous pressure and thus a fall in venous return.
- **The respiratory (or abdominothoracic) pump.** In the spontaneously breathing patient, negative

intrathoracic pressure pulls open the distensible venae cavae by radial traction, reducing their resistance to flow. At the same time, the increased intra-abdominal pressure propels blood towards the heart. The end result is increased venous return on inspiration. During exercise, an increase in respiratory rate produces a greater respiratory pump effect, increasing venous return.

- **The cardiac pump.** During ventricular contraction, the fibrous atrioventricular rings are pulled downwards, increasing the volume of the atria. Atrial pressure therefore decreases, sometimes to below zero, which aids the flow of blood from the venae cavae and pulmonary veins, but is limited by venous collapse.
- **The skeletal muscle pump.** Rhythmical contraction and relaxation of skeletal muscle, particularly the calf, propels blood through the deep veins. Blood is first drawn from the superficial to deep veins by skeletal muscle relaxation. Skeletal muscle contraction then compresses the deep veins, which propels blood forwards. Valves within the veins ensure unidirectional flow towards the heart. This mechanism increases venous return during exercise.
- **Body position.** Standing leads to venous pooling in the lower limbs. Venous pressure increases in the supine position, leading to an increase in venous return. The Trendelenburg position (head-down tilt) further increases venous return to the heart.

Clinical relevance: venous return and anaesthesia

Anaesthesia may be responsible for a fall in venous return:

- **Positive-pressure ventilation** increases intrathoracic pressure during inspiration, which reduces venous return, right ventricular preload and CO. Clinically, at induction of general anaesthesia, patients commonly become hypotensive; this is partly the result of propofol- or thiopentone-induced arteriolar vasodilatation, but also partly the result of positive-pressure ventilation.
- **Positive end-expiratory pressure** worsens this situation, increasing intrathoracic pressure and further reducing venous return.
- **Inferior vena cava (IVC) compression.** From mid-pregnancy, the gravid uterus compresses the IVC when lying supine, reducing venous return and thus resulting in hypotension (see

---

[1] Like arteries, venous smooth muscle is innervated by post-ganglionic sympathetic neurons, which act at α_1-adrenoceptors. Sympathetic stimulation results in venoconstriction, which reduces venous wall compliance. Owing to the relatively large radius of veins, venoconstriction causes only a small increase in the resistance to blood flow.

Chapter 82). When awake, pregnant women generally prefer any position other than being supine. When anaesthetised, patients obviously cannot alter their own position. It is then essential to perform a lateral tilt or position the pregnant patient in the full lateral position to relieve pressure on the IVC. Lateral tilt is especially important during cardiopulmonary resuscitation of a pregnant patient. Large intra-abdominal masses, such as tumours, may have a similar effect.

How does the venous pressure affect resistance to blood flow?

As discussed in Chapter 34, laminar blood flow is described by the Hagen–Poiseuille equation. According to this equation:

$$\text{Resistance to flow} = \frac{8\eta l}{\pi r^4}$$

Compared with vessels in the arterial system, veins and venules have a relatively large radius. As resistance is inversely proportional to the fourth power of the radius, resistance to blood flow in the venous system should therefore be markedly lower. However, veins do not necessarily have a circular lumen. In fact, the shape of the lumen alters with intraluminal pressure, and this has an effect on the resistance to blood flow:

- **Above 12 mmHg**, the vein lumen is circular; resistance to blood flow is relatively low.

- **At 4 mmHg**, the vein lumen is elliptical; resistance to blood flow is increased.
- **At 1 mmHg**, the vein lumen is often collapsed; the resistance to blood flow increases markedly.

Intraluminal pressure decreases along the venous system – typical pressures are:

- Venules 10–15 mmHg;
- Veins 4–8 mmHg;
- IVC 0–2 mmHg.

Venules, therefore, have a circular lumen, providing minimal resistance to blood flow. In contrast, a collapsed IVC can significantly increase flow resistance. During exercise, the increased sympathetic outflow increases the venomotor tone, increasing the intraluminal pressure. This makes the lumen more circular and reduces the venous resistance to blood flow. As the heart provides a negligible pressure to the venous system and the intravascular resistance is low, strangely the greatest contribution to venous resistance is the local pressure gradients generated by the skeletal muscle and respiratory pumps. In other words, the action of these mechanisms is to reduce the effective resistance to venous return during exercise.

Further reading

N. Herring, D. J. Paterson. Haemodynamics: flow, pressure and resistance. In: N. Herring, D. J. Paterson. *Levick's Introduction to Cardiovascular Physiology, 6th edition.* Boca Raton, CRC Press, 2018; 113–20.

K. Cooke, R. Sharvill, S. Sondergaard, et al. Volume responsiveness assessed by passive leg raising and a fluid challenge: a critical review focused on mean systemic filling pressure. *Anaesthesia* 2018; **73**(3): 313–22.

Venous Pressure Waveforms

Describe the key features of the central venous pressure waveform

The central venous pressure (CVP) waveform is measured using a central venous catheter positioned just above the right atrium (RA), within the superior vena cava. Starting from mid-diastole, key features of the normal CVP waveform are (Figure 38.1):

- **The a-wave** corresponds to the increase in pressure when the RA contracts, occurring just after the P-wave on the electrocardiogram.
- **The c-wave** occurs in time with the carotid pulsation. In early systole, right ventricular contraction causes the tricuspid valve to bulge into the RA, leading to a small increase in CVP.
- **The x-descent** corresponds to atrial relaxation and the downward movement of the RA during right ventricular contraction. The resultant low CVP leads to rapid right atrial filling.
- **The v-wave** corresponds to the continued venous return to the RA during ventricular systole; that is, right atrial filling with a closed tricuspid valve.

- **The y-descent** corresponds to the decrease in CVP after the tricuspid valve opens, when blood flows from the RA into the right ventricle (RV).

How can the shape of the CVP waveform help the diagnosis of arrhythmias?

A number of cardiac conditions impact on the CVP waveform:

- **Atrial fibrillation**. The loss of coordinated atrial contraction leads to the absence of a-waves.
- **Third-degree heart block**. Electrical impulses cannot pass through the atrioventricular node. As a result, atrial and ventricular contraction occur independently. There will be times when the atria contract at the same time as the ventricles (i.e. when the tricuspid valve is closed), resulting in the occasional larger a-wave on the CVP waveform; this is called a 'cannon a-wave'.
- **Tricuspid regurgitation**. During ventricular systole, blood is ejected from the RV into the RA, increasing the CVP. The CVP waveform has a 'giant v-wave', a large positive deflection that replaces the c-wave, the x-descent and the v-wave.

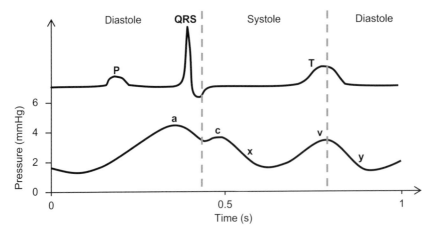

Figure 38.1 The CVP waveform.

What constitutes a normal CVP?

The normal mean CVP is said to be 2–8 mmHg when measured at the level of the RA. However, isolated CVP readings should be interpreted with care. CVP is not purely related to central venous blood volume. It is also affected by venous compliance, the compliance of the RA and RV and the intrathoracic pressure.

Common causes of raised CVP (>8 mmHg) are:

- Transducer below the level of the RA;
- Positive-pressure ventilation/positive end-expiratory pressure;
- Congestive cardiac failure;
- Isolated right ventricular failure; for example, following right ventricular infarction, cor pulmonale;
- Hypervolaemia;
- Pulmonary embolus;
- Constrictive pericarditis.

Common causes of low CVP (<2 mmHg) are:

- Transducer above the level of the RA;
- Acute hypovolaemia; for example, anaphylaxis, acute haemorrhage.

How can CVP be used to guide fluid management?

Because of its ease of measurement, CVP has historically been used to guide fluid management. The physiology underlying this is as follows:

- CVP provides a good approximation of right atrial pressure (RAP).
- RAP approximately correlates with right ventricular end-diastolic pressure (RVEDP) and right ventricular end-diastolic volume; that is, right ventricular preload.
- RVEDP approximately correlates with left ventricular end-diastolic pressure and left ventricular end-diastolic volume (LVEDV); that is, left ventricular preload.

- One of the determinants of cardiac output (CO) is left ventricular preload.
- CVP therefore reflects left ventricular preload and can be used to optimise CO.

Even in healthy patients, there are just too many assumptions and approximations for CVP to provide a precise guide to fluid management. LVEDV corresponds poorly with CVP, and individual CVP readings are of little use. However, trends of CVP readings can be used to assess the response to a fluid bolus:

- **A transient rise in CVP** implies that the RV is on the ascending part of the Starling curve; further fluid administration may be needed to optimise preload.
- **A sustained rise in CVP** implies that the RV is on the plateau of the Starling curve and at maximal preload. When operating at this part of the Starling curve, the RV is already at a mechanical disadvantage; any further increase in preload is likely to precipitate RVF. A further increase in CO can only be achieved by increasing myocardial contractility, increasing heart rate or reducing afterload.
- **A clinical deterioration and marked rise in CVP** implies that the RV is on the descending part of the Starling curve, with excessive preload overstretching the myocardial fibres, causing RVF.

CVP is still used in clinical practice to assess adequate venous filling, with a target CVP of 8–12 mmHg (12–15 mmHg in mechanically ventilated patients) commonly quoted. However, the Surviving Sepsis Guidelines (2016) have decreased the importance of using CVP over other methods of assessing volume status, reflecting the weakness of using CVP in this context.

Further reading

M. Singer, C. S. Deutschman, C. W. Seymour, et al. The third international consensus definitions for sepsis and septic shock (Sepsis-3). *JAMA* 2016; 315(8): 801–10.

Chapter

39

Lymphatics

Describe the anatomy of the lymphatic system

The lymphatic system is part of the systemic circulation. Its two main components are the conducting system and lymphoid tissue.

Key aspects of the conducting system are:

- Small lymphatic capillaries drain lymph into larger lymphatic vessels, which converge on the right lymphatic duct and the thoracic duct.
- The right lymphatic duct is quite short (around 1.5 cm). It drains lymph into the right subclavian vein.
- The thoracic duct (also known as the left lymphatic duct) is much larger, and drains into the left brachiocephalic vein. It collects lymph from the majority of the body (everywhere except the right arm, right chest and right side of the head and neck) and returns it to the systemic circulation.
- Lymphatic vessels are pulled opened as a result of radial traction by the surrounding connective tissue. This permits fluid, proteins and even cells to enter. Like veins, lymph flow is promoted by skeletal muscle activity and deep inspiration. The larger lymph vessels have valves to ensure unidirectional flow.

The lymphoid tissue consists of:

- **Primary lymphoid organs** – thymus and bone marrow. These organs are involved in the production of lymphocytes from progenitor cells.
- **Secondary lymphoid organs** – these include lymph nodes and lymphoid follicles within the tonsils, spleen, Peyer's patches and other mucosa-associated lymphoid tissue. This lymphoid tissue contains mature lymphocytes and is the site where foreign antigens activate the adaptive immune response (see Chapter 75).

Clinical relevance: central venous cannulation

Internal jugular and subclavian vein cannulation is a commonly performed procedure in major surgical and critical care patients. There is a long list of potential complications, including infection, air embolus, pneumothorax and arterial puncture.

Left-sided central venous cannulation also risks damage to the thoracic duct, which is in close proximity to the junction of the internal jugular and subclavian veins. Puncture of the thoracic duct can lead to a chylothorax. Damage to the thoracic duct can be prevented by using the right-sided internal jugular and subclavian veins, using a high-neck approach to the internal jugular vein and most importantly by cannulating under ultrasound guidance.

What are the functions of the lymphatic system?

The lymphatic system has three main functions:

- **Fluid balance.** As blood passes through the capillaries, most of the fluid filtered into the interstitium is then reabsorbed back into the capillary (see Chapter 36). Overall, there is slight excess of filtration. Each day approximately 4 L of interstitial fluid must consequently be returned to the circulation by the lymphatic system – this fluid is called lymph.
- **Immune.** In addition to fluid, the lymph capillaries are the only means by which filtered proteins, lymphocytes and other debris (including cells) can leave the interstitial space. Lymph passes through lymph nodes before passing back into the systemic circulation. The lymph nodes are packed full of lymphocytes, which detect foreign bodies and pathogens, triggering an immune response. Distribution by the lymphatic system is the most

common pathway through which carcinomas may metastasise.

- **Digestion**. Dietary triglycerides are esterified and combined with cholesterol esters, phospholipids and apolipoprotein B-48 to form chylomicrons (see Chapter 64). These chylomicrons pass into lacteals – the lymphatic capillaries of the intestine – and combine with lymph to form a fluid called chyle. Chyle is then conducted through the lymphatic vessels until it enters the systemic circulation via the thoracic duct.

Clinical relevance: subcutaneous and intramuscular drug administration

Protein-based drugs are frequently delivered by the subcutaneous route as they have a poor bioavailability when administered orally (e.g. insulin and low-molecular-weight heparins). Large, negatively charged proteins are unable to cross the capillary membrane and therefore remain in the subcutaneous extracellular space. Instead, they are absorbed by the lymphatic system and enter the systemic circulation via the thoracic duct.

Clinical relevance: lymphoedema

Lymphoedema is the accumulation of excess lymphatic fluid in the interstitium:

- Acute lymphoedema may occur during transplant procedures, as the transplanted organ or tissue has lost its lymphatic supply, or during thoracic surgery, due to excision or disruption of thoracic and mediastinal lymphatics.
- Chronic lymphoedema usually occurs following surgery for cancer, especially breast cancer, where lymph nodes have been resected.

Initially, the excess fluid gives a pitting oedema; however, with time, inflammation results in the tissue becoming firm and the oedema becomes non-pitting. This is often painful and cosmetically displeasing for the patient.

Non-pitting oedema may preclude non-invasive blood pressure monitoring. Cannulation of the affected limb should be avoided, as fluid administration can precipitate or worsen lymphoedema (although clearly in an emergency this might be required).

Further reading

N. Herring, D. J. Paterson. Circulation of fluid between plasma, interstitium and lymph. In: N. Herring, D. J. Paterson. *Levick's Introduction to Cardiovascular Physiology*, 6th edition. Boca Raton, CRC Press, 2018; 191–220.

A. Pikwer, J. Akeson, S. Lindgren. Complications associated with peripheral or central routes for central venous cannulation. *Anaesthesia* 2012; **67**(1): 65–71.

Cardiovascular Reflexes

Why is it important to minimise fluctuations in blood pressure?

The organs require a fairly constant mean arterial pressure (MAP) to ensure adequate perfusion. Some organs (most notably the brain, heart and kidneys), despite fluctuations in MAP, intrinsically maintain their blood flow through autoregulation (see Chapter 34), but are still unable to compensate if MAP is significantly reduced or increased.

How is MAP kept constant?

Normal activities (including changes in body position, exercise and digestion) can potentially result in major changes in MAP, as they can cause both vasodilatation or vasoconstriction of vascular beds and can increase or decrease venous return to the heart. The cardiovascular system rapidly responds to fluctuations in MAP through a series of neural reflexes. These cardiovascular reflexes may be classified as:

- **Reflexes originating from stimuli within the cardiovascular system**:
  - *The arterial baroreceptor reflex.* Changes in MAP are detected by mechanoreceptors in the aortic arch and carotid sinus. In response, sympathetic outflow from the central nervous system (CNS) is rapidly altered, which in turn modifies heart rate (HR) and systemic vascular resistance (SVR), returning MAP to its set point. This is the major cardiovascular reflex involved in short-term control of MAP.
  - *The Bainbridge reflex*, in which an increase in central venous pressure (CVP) results in an isolated tachycardia.
  - *The chemoreceptor reflex*, in which activation of the peripheral chemoreceptors triggers an increase in sympathetic nervous activity, thus increasing HR and MAP under conditions of extreme hypotension and cardiovascular

collapse. This reflex is only usually relevant during profound hypotension, such as during haemorrhage or sepsis.
  - *The CNS ischaemic response*, in which CNS ischaemia triggers an increase in sympathetic nervous activity, thus increasing HR and MAP.
- **Reflexes triggered by stimuli external to the cardiovascular system**: for example, pain, emotion or temperature.

Describe the arterial baroreceptor reflex

The arterial baroreceptor reflex is an extremely important mechanism for minimising fluctuations in MAP. The arterial baroreceptors are mechanoreceptors that sense the degree of distension of the walls of the carotid sinus, a dilatation at the bifurcation of the carotid artery and the aortic arch (of lesser importance):

- **An increase in MAP** distends the wall of the carotid sinus/aortic arch, which increases the frequency of action potentials generated by the baroreceptor afferent fibres.
- **A decrease in MAP** reduces carotid sinus/aortic arch wall distension, which decreases the frequency of action potential generation.

The baroreceptors transmit their action potentials to the vasomotor centre, located in the medulla oblongata, through the glossopharyngeal nerve (carotid sinus baroreceptors) and the vagus nerve (aortic arch baroreceptors). The vasomotor centre is divided into two functional areas:

- **The vasoconstrictor (pressor/defence) area.** This area triggers tachycardia, increased myocardial contractility and vaso- and venoconstriction and promotes adrenaline release from the adrenal medulla through sympathetic efferent neurons.

- **The vasodilator (depressor) area**. This area acts on the vasoconstrictor centre, decreasing its sympathetic outflow.

Overall:

- **An increase in MAP** increases the frequency of action potentials produced by the baroreceptors. In response, the vasodilator area inhibits sympathetic outflow, causing peripheral vasodilatation and a decrease in both HR and myocardial contractility, thus returning MAP to normal.
- **A decrease in MAP** reduces the frequency of action potentials produced by the baroreceptors. In response, the vasoconstrictor area increases sympathetic outflow, causing peripheral vasoconstriction and an increase in both HR and myocardial contractility, thus returning MAP to normal.

Some important points to note about this system are:

- In addition to short-term changes in HR, myocardial contractility and SVR, the baroreceptor reflex also influences plasma volume. Following a fall in MAP, the increased sympathetic outflow triggers renin secretion by the kidney, thus increasing plasma volume through the action of the renin–angiotensin–aldosterone (RAA) axis. Likewise, an increase in MAP decreases sympathetic outflow, which decreases renin secretion and thus plasma volume. In clinical practice, this can be observed in patients with pre-eclampsia, where persistently raised MAP results in a relative hypovolaemia.
- There are two types of neurons involved in the baroreceptor reflex. Large myelinated A fibres are activated at lower pressure, whilst small unmyelinated C fibres are activated at higher pressure. In combination, these neurons provide a system that is sensitive over a wide range of MAP, from 80 to 150 mmHg.
- In patients with chronic hypertension, the baroreceptors reset their working range and sensitivity.
- The compliance of the arterial tree is reduced with ageing and atherosclerosis. In turn, this affects the sensitivity and rapidity of the baroreceptor reflex; postural hypotension (i.e. a failure of the baroreceptor reflex to compensate for the postural changes in MAP) is common in the elderly.

What is the Bainbridge reflex?

Low-pressure mechanoreceptors are located within the great veins and the walls of the right atrium (RA) at its junction with the superior and inferior venae cavae and are activated by increased wall distension. An increase in CVP therefore stimulates these low-pressure mechanoreceptors, increasing their frequency of action potential generation – these action potentials are then relayed to the CNS via the vagus nerve. In response, the vasomotor centre increases sympathetic outflow to the sinoatrial node (but not to the cardiac ventricles or peripheral vasculature), resulting in an isolated tachycardia.

Physiological manifestations of the Bainbridge reflex are:

- **Respiratory sinus arrhythmia**. This occurs in children and young adults. During inspiration, negative intrathoracic pressure leads to a transient increase in venous return to the RA, which activates low-pressure mechanoreceptors. As a result, HR increases during inspiration and decreases during expiration.
- **Uterine autotransfusion**. Following delivery, sustained uterine contraction returns around 500 mL of uteroplacental blood to the maternal circulation. The resulting increase in CVP stretches the right atrial wall, resulting in a tachycardia.

What are the cardiovascular consequences of chemoreceptor activation?

The peripheral chemoreceptors (the carotid and aortic bodies) are activated by low arterial O_2 tension P_aO_2, high P_aCO_2 and, in the case of the carotid bodies, low arterial pH (see Chapter 22). In addition, the peripheral chemoreceptors are activated by severe hypotension (MAP < 60 mmHg). The action potentials generated by the peripheral chemoreceptors are relayed to the respiratory centre in the medulla and pons. The medullary respiratory centre is located in close proximity to the vasomotor centre, to which it is neurally connected; activation of the peripheral chemoreceptors therefore has a minor effect on blood pressure regulation. Hypoxia, hypercapnoea and acidosis therefore trigger an increase in sympathetic outflow from the vasomotor centre.

Outline the physiological changes that occur following haemorrhage

The fall in circulating volume that accompanies haemorrhage causes a reduction in mean systemic filling pressure and thus venous return to the heart falls. The consequent fall in cardiac output results in decreased MAP. Organ perfusion pressure falls, leading to organ dysfunction. The cardiovascular, nervous and endocrine systems act to redistribute blood flow to the vital organs, namely the brain, the heart and, to a lesser extent, the kidneys.

The physiological response to haemorrhage can be classified as immediate, early and late:

- **The immediate response** involves the cardiovascular reflexes, which act within seconds of the haemorrhage to restore MAP, maintaining the perfusion pressure of the vital organs. Haemorrhage is detected by low-pressure mechanoreceptors in the RA and arterial baroreceptors of the carotid sinus and aortic arch. In response, the vasomotor centre increases sympathetic outflow,[1] resulting in:

  - *Tachycardia and increased myocardial contractility.* HR increases in proportion to the degree of blood loss.

  - *Generalised arteriolar vasoconstriction.* Blood flow to the kidney, brain and heart initially falls, but quickly recovers to near normal due to autoregulation. Blood flow to the skin, gut and skeletal muscle dramatically falls; anaerobic metabolism results in lactic acid production. The resulting fall in arterial pH stimulates the respiratory centre (through the carotid bodies), leading to tachypnoea.

  - *Venoconstriction* of the capacitance veins. The compliance of the capacitance veins is reduced, thereby tending to restore venous return to the heart despite the reduction in total blood volume.

- **The early response.** In the minutes and hours following blood loss, the body attempts to restore circulating volume through a number of mechanisms:

  - *Transcapillary refill/autotransfusion.* Capillary hydrostatic pressure depends on arteriolar and venous pressures (see Chapter 36). Following the increase in sympathetic outflow, arteriolar vasoconstriction decreases capillary hydrostatic pressure. The balance of Starling filtration forces is altered – interstitial fluid is reabsorbed into the capillaries. 500 mL of interstitial fluid can be reabsorbed within 30 min by this mechanism.

  - *Increased plasma glucose concentration* through sympathetic nervous system-mediated glycogenolysis and gluconeogenesis in the liver. The raised glucose concentration causes plasma to have a greater osmotic pressure, which acts to draw water from the extracellular space. This mechanism approximately matches (or may even exceed) the volume of autotransfusion generated by alterations in hydrostatic pressure.

  - *Renal conservation of sodium and water.* Renal blood flow (RBF) decreases as a result of arterial hypotension, which in turn decreases glomerular filtration rate. Thus, a reduced volume of urine is produced. There are a number of additional mechanisms that further reduce fluid loss from the kidney:

    - The RAA axis is activated by the increase in sympathetic activity, the reduction in RBF and the reduction in Na^+ delivery to the macula densa. The RAA axis acts to reabsorb Na^+ and therefore water,

---

[1] Note: in severe haemorrhage, a massive sympathetic outflow is triggered by brainstem ischaemia, when cerebral perfusion pressure falls below the lower limit of autoregulation (50 mmHg).

predominately through actions on the distal convoluted tubule (DCT).

- Decreased venous return to the heart results in decreased stretch of the atrial and ventricular walls. As a result, atrial natriuretic peptide and brain natriuretic peptide secretion is decreased, which ordinarily promotes Na^+ and water excretion.

- Antidiuretic hormone (ADH) is released from the hypothalamus in response to plasma osmolarity and (to some extent) volume changes. ADH has three effects in severe haemorrhage: it acts as a vasopressor, augmenting noradrenaline-mediated arteriolar vasoconstriction, and it also acts at the renal collecting ducts, where it increases water reabsorption. Finally, ADH acts at the hypothalamus to stimulate thirst.

- Additional cortisol is released from the adrenal gland in response to major haemorrhage. Cortisol has a minor mineralocorticoid role, increasing the reabsorption of Na^+ and water at the DCT and collecting ducts. Cortisol also promotes gluconeogenesis.

- **The late response.** In the longer term, plasma volume is restored over the next 2 days by oral intake of water and renal reabsorption of electrolytes. However, because only water and electrolytes are returned to normal, blood has a reduced haematocrit and plasma protein concentration. The liver rapidly synthesises albumin, restoring plasma albumin concentration to normal within 4–6 days. Haemoglobin concentration usually returns to normal within 8 weeks if sufficient iron is available.

- **Decompensated shock.** If blood loss is extensive (>30%) and rapid, compensatory mechanisms may be unable to restore MAP. This level of blood loss reflects the change from stressed (contributes to stretching the vessel wall) to unstressed blood volume (simply fills the vessel lumen). Decompensated shock is characterised by a paradoxical vasodilatation and decrease in tachycardia, possibly as a result of endogenous opioid signalling. This results in myocardial ischaemia and thus cardiac depression, resulting in a rapid fall in MAP.

Clinical relevance: classes of haemorrhagic shock

The physiological response to haemorrhagic shock is proportional to the degree of haemorrhage (Table 40.1).

Table 40.1 Haemorrhagic shock divided into four classes (HR = heart rate; SBP = systolic blood pressure; DBP = diastolic blood pressure; RR = respiratory rate).

	Class 1	Class 2	Class 3	Class 4
Blood loss (%)	<15	15–30	30–40	>40
Blood loss (mL, 70-kg adult)	<750	750–1500	1500–2000	>2000
HR (bpm)	<100	>100	>120	>140
SBP (mmHg)	Normal	Normal	Reduced	Very low
DBP (mmHg)	Normal	Raised	Reduced	Very low
RR (breaths/min)	<20	20–30	30–40	>35
Urine output (mL/h)	>30	20–30	5–15	Negligible
Mental status	Normal	Anxious	Confused	Drowsy or unconscious

Class 1 and 2 haemorrhagic shock are referred to as compensated shock, as blood pressure is maintained, whilst Class 3 and 4 haemorrhagic shock are decompensated, as hypotension has occurred. Decompensated shock is associated with >50% mortality.

Note: 'pure' haemorrhagic shock is unusual. Haemorrhage usually occurs in conjunction with trauma. Following trauma, tissue damage triggers a cascade of inflammatory mediators, resulting in the systemic inflammatory response syndrome and organ dysfunction, further increasing mortality.

Further reading

N. Herring, D. J. Paterson. Cardiovascular receptors, reflexes and central control. In: N. Herring, D. J. Paterson. *Levick's Introduction to Cardiovascular Physiology*, 6th edition. Boca Raton, CRC Press, 2018; 303–24.

N. Herring, D. J. Paterson. Co-ordinated cardiovascular responses. In: N. Herring, D. J. Paterson. *Levick's*

Introduction to Cardiovascular Physiology, 6th edition. Boca Raton, CRC Press, 2018: 325–42.

N. Herring, D. J. Paterson. Cardiovascular responses in pathological situations. In: N. Herring, D. J. Paterson. *Levick's Introduction to Cardiovascular Physiology, 6th edition.* Boca Raton, CRC Press, 2018; 343–68.

G. Gutierrez, H. D. Reines, M. E. Wulf-Gutierrez. Clinical review: haemorrhagic shock. *Crit Care* 2004; **8**(4): 373–81.

R. P. Dutton. Haemostatic resuscitation. *Br J Anaesth* 2012; **109**(Suppl. 1): i39–46.

B. Boeuf, V. Poirier, F. Gauvin, et al. Naloxone for shock. *Cochrane Database Syst Rev* 2003; (4): CD004443.

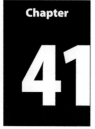

Chapter

41

Valsalva Manoeuvre

What is the Valsalva manoeuvre? What was it originally used for?

The Valsalva manoeuvre is performed by forced expiration against a closed glottis. It is attributed to Antonio Valsalva (1666–1723), who described it as a test of Eustachian tube patency and as a method of expelling pus from the middle ear.

How might a patient perform a Valsalva manoeuvre?

The Valsalva manoeuvre involves increasing intrathoracic pressure to ~40 cmH$_2$O and holding it for 10 s. The methods of achieving this depend on whether the patient is awake or anaesthetised:

- **Awake**. The patient attempts to forcibly exhale whilst keeping their mouth and nose closed. This can be difficult to explain to a patient – the same effect can be gained by asking a patient to try to blow the plunger out of a syringe.
- **Anaesthetised**. The adjustable pressure-limiting valve of the anaesthetic circuit is closed and the airway pressure is increased to 40 cmH$_2$O and held for 10 s. This is really only possible for intubated patients; laryngeal mask airways are prone to leak above pressures of 20 cmH$_2$O.

What are the cardiovascular changes that occur during the Valsalva manoeuvre?

A sudden generation of a high intrathoracic pressure, such as that occurring during the Valsalva manoeuvre, results in dramatic changes to mean arterial pressure (MAP), cardiac output and heart rate (HR). The Valsalva manoeuvre is divided into four phases (Figure 41.1):

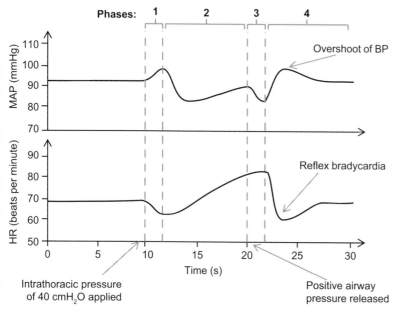

Figure 41.1 The Valsalva manoeuvre (BP = blood pressure).

- **Phase 1**. At the start of the Valsalva manoeuvre, the increase in intrathoracic pressure compresses the pulmonary vessels, squeezing blood into the left side of the heart. This transiently increases the stroke volume (SV), resulting in a transient increase in MAP. The baroreceptor reflex responds to the rise in MAP by transiently reducing HR.
- **Phase 2**. Next, the high intrathoracic pressure prevents venous return to the heart. SV is reduced, which leads to a steady fall in MAP. Again, the baroreceptor reflex is triggered: HR increases, which returns MAP to near normal.
- **Phase 3**. After 10 s, the high intrathoracic pressure is released. Venous return fills the empty intrathoracic vessels. SV decreases, resulting in a further fall in MAP and a further reflex rise in HR.
- **Phase 4**. As left ventricular preload is restored, the MAP increases. However, because the HR is still high, there is an overshoot in MAP. The baroreceptor reflex rapidly corrects this, causing a reflex bradycardia through vagal stimulation. Both MAP and HR then return to normal.

What are the uses of the Valsalva manoeuvre today?

Obviously, the Valsalva manoeuvre is no longer the primary method used to expel pus from the ear.

Instead, it has found a number of other uses, both clinical and non-clinical, including:

- **Termination of a supraventricular tachycardia.** The intense vagal stimulation of Phase 4 slows conduction through the atrioventricular node.
- **An aid to diagnosis of a murmur.** A Valsalva manoeuvre increases the intensity of the murmur of hypertrophic obstructive cardiomyopathy whilst decreasing the intensity of most other murmurs, including aortic stenosis, the main differential diagnosis of an ejection systolic murmur.
- **Diving.** During descent, a Valsalva manoeuvre helps the diver to open their Eustachian tubes and equalise middle-ear pressure with ambient pressure. However, it is not advisable to do this during ascent – there is a risk of opening a patent foramen ovale (PFO). A PFO in combination with decompression illness arising from dissolved N_2 coming out of solution, producing gas bubbles in the venous circulation, may result in an arterial gas embolus.
- **Temporary increase in venous pressure.** The Valsalva manoeuvre is often used intraoperatively to increase venous pressure to check for adequate haemostasis following, for example, a radical neck dissection.

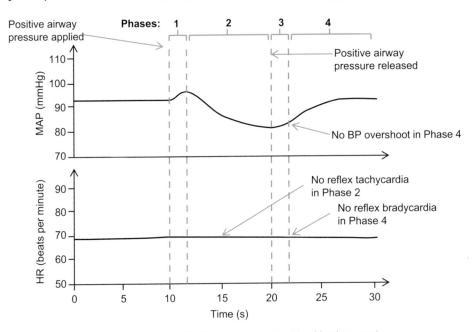

Figure 41.2 Autonomic dysfunction and the Valsalva manoeuvre (BP = blood pressure).

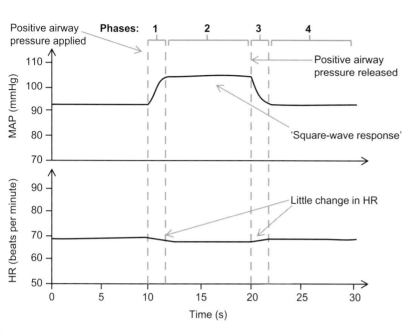

Figure 41.3 Square-wave response to the Valsalva manoeuvre.

How is the Valsalva manoeuvre used to test autonomic function?

The integrity of the autonomic nervous system (ANS) can be tested by demonstrating a normal cardiovascular response to the Valsalva manoeuvre. The baroreceptor reflex is often abnormal in conditions affecting the ANS, such as diabetic autonomic neuropathy and spinal cord injury (Figure 41.2):

- In Phase 2, there is no compensatory reflex tachycardia – MAP continues to fall until the intrathoracic pressure is released.
- In Phase 4, there is no overshoot of MAP and no compensatory bradycardia.

What other abnormal responses are there to the Valsalva manoeuvre?

A 'square-wave response' to the Valsalva manoeuvre is seen in conditions characterised by high venous pressure, such as congestive cardiac failure and constrictive pericarditis (Figure 41.3). These patients survive with the left ventricle operating on the plateau of the Starling curve, with a chronically raised sympathetic outflow resulting in near-maximal vaso- and veno-constriction. Performing the Valsalva manoeuvre leads to an elevation of MAP throughout the duration of raised intrathoracic pressure, with little change in HR and no MAP overshoot in Phase 4.

Further reading

N. Herring, D. J. Paterson. Co-ordinated cardiovascular responses. In: N. Herring, D. J. Paterson. *Levick's Introduction to Cardiovascular Physiology*, 6th edition. Boca Raton, CRC Press, 2018; 325–42.

G. Smith. Management of supraventricular tachycardia using the Valsalva manoeuvre: a historical review and summary of published evidence. *Eur J Emerg Med* 2012; **19**(6): 346–52.

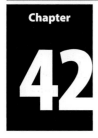

Exercise Physiology

Exercise is a major physiological challenge to the body, affecting all the main body systems. An accompanying increase in muscle metabolic rate results in an increase in O_2 demand and a requirement for an increased rate of removal of CO_2 and other metabolites, including lactic acid and ketone bodies. Exercise thus requires substantial increases in muscle blood flow with maintenance of mean arterial pressure (MAP). In addition, despite the increased rate of energy metabolism, normoglycaemia must be preserved. Finally, exercising muscle generates a large amount of heat, yet core temperature must be controlled.

What is the difference between dynamic and static exercise?

Exercise involves the activation of skeletal muscle. It may be classified as:
- **Dynamic** (or isotonic), where muscles rhythmically contract and relax, moving joints (e.g. running);
- **Static** (or isometric), where muscles contract against a resistance but do not lengthen or shorten (e.g. weight lifting).

Both types of exercise may involve the same muscles, but they differ in their effects on muscle blood flow and metabolism:
- **During dynamic exercise**, there is marked muscle capillary bed vasodilatation in response to aerobic metabolic activity. Accordingly, systemic vascular resistance (SVR) falls. The baroreceptors initiate a tachycardia in response to the consequent reduction in diastolic blood pressure (DBP).
- **During static exercise**, the muscle capillaries are externally compressed by sustained muscle contraction, with a resultant increase in anaerobic metabolism. Vessel compression results in an increase in SVR, which causes an increase in DBP. In addition, sympathetic nervous activity increases

heart rate (HR), but to a lesser extent than dynamic exercise.

What types of skeletal muscle fibres are there?

There are two main types of skeletal muscle fibre:
- **Type I (slow-twitch or fatigue-resistant) fibres**. This type of muscle fibre derives its metabolic energy from the oxidative metabolism of triglycerides and is therefore rich in myoglobin (hence its red appearance), mitochondria and capillaries. Type I fibres are found in groups of muscles where sustained contraction is required, such as the postural muscles. Type I fibres contract more slowly but are resistant to fatigue.
- **Type II (fast-twitch) fibres**. There are two types:
  - *Type IIa (fast-twitch oxidative) fibres*;
  - *Type IIb (fast-twitch glycolytic) fibres*.

  Type IIb fibres are more reliant on anaerobic metabolism (glycolysis) for ATP generation and thus have larger glycogen stores; their lack of myoglobin leads to a white appearance. These fibres occur in muscles that require short, rapid, powerful movements for activities such as sprinting. Because of the limited capacity of anaerobic metabolism to generate ATP, type IIb muscle fibres are more prone to fatigue. Type IIa fibres are functionally intermediate between type IIb and type I fibres. They utilise both aerobic and anaerobic metabolism using large glycogen stores and contract more slowly, but are more resistant to fatigue than type IIb fibres.

Individual muscles contain varying mixtures of type I, IIa and IIb fibres, with the proportions of each fibre type depending on the muscle's function. The percentage of each fibre type also differs widely between individuals. Individuals genetically equipped with a greater proportion of type IIb fibres will be better sprinters than those who have a higher proportion of type I fibres, who make better endurance athletes.

Which substrates are used by skeletal muscle to generate energy for contraction?

In common with other cells, skeletal muscle uses ATP as the direct energy source to power contractions. However, only a small amount of ATP is stored in the muscles, enough for 1–2 s of muscle contraction. It is therefore essential that ATP can be rapidly regenerated. There are a number of means by which the muscles do this:

- **Breakdown of phosphocreatine**. This is a high-energy molecule that is used to rapidly re-synthesise ATP from adenosine diphosphate (ADP). Despite muscles only having sufficient phosphocreatine stores for around 7 s of intense exercise, it acts as an important energy buffer that allows time for the more definitive energy-generating processes to occur.
- **Glycolysis** utilises either glucose or the muscle glycogen store to generate ATP without the need for O_2. Considering the number of steps involved (see Chapter 77), glycolysis results in a rapid but relatively inefficient increase in ATP synthesis:
  - The maximum glycolysis rate is achieved within a few seconds of the onset of exercise.
  - The glycolytic breakdown of glucose generates two ATP molecules, whilst that of glycogen generates three ATP molecules.

  Lactic acid is produced as a by-product of glycolysis. In strenuous exercise, lactic acid is not cleared from the circulation as quickly as it is produced, as the blood supply to the liver is reduced.
- **Oxidative phosphorylation**. This is the most efficient mechanism of generating ATP. Complete breakdown of glucose (through glycolysis, the citric acid cycle and oxidative phosphorylation by the electron transport chain) generates 36 ATP molecules.
- **Fat metabolism**. Metabolism of fats through β-oxidation (see Chapter 77) generates a greater number of ATP molecules than an equivalent weight of carbohydrate. However, such fat mobilisation takes place over a longer time course than the corresponding carbohydrate metabolism

and therefore contributes little in the early phases of exercise. Fat metabolism becomes more important during sustained exercise, when muscle and liver glycogen stores become depleted. In marathon running, the sudden fatigue associated with glycogen store depletion is called 'hitting the wall'.

What is muscle fatigue?

Muscle contraction cannot be sustained indefinitely; muscle fatigue is defined as the decline in the ability of a muscle to generate a force. Peak muscle tension and the velocity of contraction may be reduced.

Muscle fatigue is a protective mechanism; it stops the muscle from contracting to the point where it runs out of ATP, which would result in rigor mortis or even cell apoptosis. The exact mechanism underlying muscle fatigue is unknown, with a number of factors thought to be involved:

- **Increased ADP and phosphate** as a result of ATP breakdown, which has been variously suggested to reduce Ca^{2+} reuptake into the sarcoplasmic reticulum (see Chapter 54) or to trigger the opening of ATP-sensitive K^+ channels, which reduces muscle membrane excitability.
- **Increased extracellular K^+**. In severe exercise, arterial K^+ concentration can rise as high as 8 mmol/L (the exercising heart seems to be protected from the effects of hyperkalaemia). The muscle interstitial K^+ concentration rises even higher, up to 12 mmol/L. Hyperkalaemia is thought to contribute to muscle fatigue.
- **Accumulation of lactate within the muscle**. Intense exercise may inhibit enzymes involved in aerobic metabolism.
- **Exhaustion of muscle glycogen stores** following prolonged exercise.

What physiological changes occur in anticipation of exercise?

Some physiological changes occur before the onset of exercise. Merely anticipating exercise results in greater sympathetic outflow and parasympathetic nervous system inhibition, causing:

- **In the venous system**: venoconstriction, which causes an increase in the venous return to the heart.

- **In the heart**: an increase in HR and myocardial contractility, which, in conjunction with the increased venous return, leads to an increase in cardiac output (CO).
- **In skeletal muscle**: vasodilatation of capillary beds through activation of sympathetic cholinergic fibres. This is an important mechanism that prevents large increases in blood pressure following the anticipatory increase in CO.
- **In the peripheries**: vasoconstriction in the gut and skin.

The cardiovascular effects vary depending on the anticipated duration and intensity of the exercise. For example, anticipation of a short sprint results in a greater increase in HR than anticipation of an endurance run. This is because it would be impossible to increase HR to near-maximal levels over the short duration of a sprint distance, whereas in a marathon there is ample time to instigate the cardiovascular response. This is an example of feedforward control.

What are the physiological effects of exercise on each body system?

Considering each system in turn:

- **Skeletal muscle**. Exercising muscle requires a substantial increase in blood flow to increase the delivery of O_2 and metabolic substrates and to remove CO_2 and other waste products.
  - Resting skeletal muscle blood flow is around 2–4 mL/100 g of muscle/min. At rest, pre-capillary sphincters are closed and blood is diverted from the muscle capillary beds into large vessels.
  - In fit, healthy adults undergoing strenuous exercise, muscle blood flow increases up to 50–100 mL/100 g of muscle/min, depending on the type of muscle.
  - This marked increase in blood flow to muscle is caused by the local action of vasodilatory metabolites (e.g. H^+, AMP, K^+, phosphate). These metabolites are produced in proportion to O_2 consumption; they open pre-capillary sphincters, allowing blood to flow through the muscle capillary bed.
- **Cardiovascular system**. The cardiovascular system undergoes significant changes with exercise (Figure 42.1a):

  - *A large increase in CO.* Resting skeletal muscle blood flow accounts for around 20% of CO (1000 mL/min). In normal individuals, CO may increase fivefold with strenuous exercise, from 5 L/min to 25 L/min, to match the metabolic demands of exercising muscles. At maximum exercise intensity, skeletal muscle blood flow accounts for 80% of CO. The increase in CO is mediated by the sympathetic nervous system:

    - *Preload is increased* as a result of venoconstriction, the skeletal muscle pump and the respiratory pump (see Chapter 37).
    - *Afterload is reduced*: SVR falls due to the release of vasodilatory metabolites from the muscle.
    - *HR increases* in proportion to exercise intensity due to a reduction in parasympathetic nervous activity and an increase in sympathetic nervous activity in the heart. However, there is a limit to the value of tachycardia: above a certain rate, the diastolic filling time is so short that venous return is compromised and CO falls (see Chapter 29).
    - *Myocardial contractility increases* due to both sympathetic nervous system stimulation of the cardiac myocytes and the Bowditch effect, where tachycardia induces an increase in myocardial contractility (see Chapter 29).

  - *Changes in blood pressure.* Little change in blood pressure occurs in anticipation of and during early phases of dynamic exercise as the increased CO is mitigated by sympathetic cholinergic arteriolar vasodilatation in the skeletal muscle. Systolic blood pressure (SBP) increases as cardiac contractility increases.

    - *In dynamic exercise*, DBP remains similar or may even decrease due to a reduction in the SVR caused by skeletal muscle arteriolar vasodilatation. As the SBP increases more than the DBP falls, MAP may slowly increase with increased exercise intensity or duration.
    - *In static exercise*, the DBP increases as the muscle capillary beds are occluded. Therefore, MAP increases rapidly.

(a) Cardiovascular changes with dynamic exercise

(b) Respiratory changes with exercise

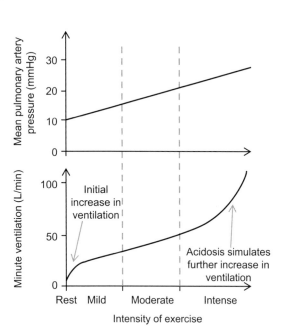

Figure 42.1 (a) Cardiovascular changes with dynamic exercise and (b) respiratory changes with exercise.

– *Changes in regional blood flow.* Whilst the greatest increase in blood flow is to the skeletal muscle, the blood flow to other organs is also altered during exercise:

- Coronary blood flow increases fivefold to meet the increased O_2 demand of the cardiac myocytes, from a resting value of 250 mL/min to 1250 mL/min.
- Blood flow to the skin substantially increases to aid heat dissipation.
- Splanchnic blood flow falls substantially during exercise.
- Renal blood flow falls, but to a lesser extent than splanchnic blood flow, due to a stronger autoregulatory mechanism.
- Cerebral blood flow does not alter at any exercise intensity.

- **Respiratory system.**
  – *A substantial increase in minute ventilation,* $\dot{V}_E$. In strenuous exercise, O_2 consumption may increase from a typical basal value of 250 mL/min to 5000 mL/min; CO_2 production increases proportionately. In healthy lungs, the respiratory system has a remarkable capacity: $\dot{V}_E$ increases in proportion to exercise intensity up to 20-fold, from a basal level of 5 L/min up to 100 L/min. This compares with a fivefold increase in CO by the cardiovascular system. The respiratory system is thus not usually the limiting factor in exercise performance. The control of ventilation is discussed in detail in Chapter 22. In brief:

    - At the onset of exercise, there is a rapid increase in $\dot{V}_E$: both respiratory rate and tidal volume, V_T, increase (Figure 42.1b). The respiratory centre is stimulated by two factors: increased activity of the motor cortex and afferent signals from limb joint proprioceptors.

▪ As CO_2 is a by-product of skeletal muscle metabolism, $\dot{V}_E$ increases in proportion to the intensity of exercise.

▪ With extremely intense exercise, $\dot{V}_E$ increases disproportionately (Figure 42.1b). There comes a point where O_2 delivery to the exercising muscle is unable to match O_2 consumption (the anaerobic threshold) and anaerobic metabolism commences. Lactic acid is produced as a consequence, which causes a fall in arterial pH. The lower arterial pH is sensed by the carotid bodies, resulting in further stimulation of the respiratory centre.

– *Increased pulmonary blood flow*. As discussed above, exercise results in a substantial increase in CO; pulmonary blood flow therefore increases to the same degree. If it were not for the pulmonary vasculature responding by recruitment and distension (see Chapter 23), mean pulmonary artery pressure (MPAP) would increase substantially. The mild increase in MPAP that actually occurs (Figure 42.1b) is physiologically important, as it diminishes the effect of gravity within the lung: the regional $\dot{V}/\dot{Q}$ ratio trends towards 1.0 (0.8 is typical in the resting lung). Gas exchange therefore becomes more efficient with exercise and physiological shunt is reduced.

– P_aO_2. Despite the high O_2 consumption of exercising muscle, P_aO_2 remains normal, even during intense exercise. As discussed in Chapter 10, transfer of O_2 across the alveolar–capillary barrier is not diffusion limited in normal lungs at sea level. S_aO_2 is therefore unchanged. However, the position of the oxyhaemoglobin dissociation curve changes: acidosis and raised temperature shift the P_{50} to the right (see Chapter 8), which aids O_2 offloading to the metabolically active tissues.

● **Thermoregulation**. Skeletal muscle activity is relatively inefficient: only 20–25% of the chemical energy within the metabolic substrates is converted to mechanical energy, with the rest dissipated as heat energy. As discussed in Chapter 89, thermoregulation is controlled through a complex negative-feedback loop involving peripheral and central sensors, whose signals are integrated by the hypothalamus. Effectors are:

– *Eccrine sweat glands in the skin*: heat is lost as a result of the latent heat of evaporation.

– *Cutaneous vasodilatation*: heat is lost by conduction.

Following the onset of exercise:

– There is an initial transient fall in core temperature of 1°C as venous return increases from the limbs.

– As exercise continues, there is net heat generation. Heat loss mechanisms (sweating and peripheral vasodilatation) commence. Further heat is lost as a result of the large increase in $\dot{V}_E$ (through the latent heat of evaporation as dry inhaled gases are humidified), although this mechanism is less important in humans than in animals that pant.

– In hot, humid climates, heat loss mechanisms are impaired. When the environmental temperature is greater than body temperature, there is no net gradient for heat loss by conduction; sweating becomes the only heat loss mechanism. In humid conditions, evaporation of sweat is impaired. Thermoregulation thus fails, leading to increased core temperature. Heat stroke (a core body temperature greater than 40.6°C) may result, with a variety of symptoms, including confusion and syncope. Rapid external cooling is required.

What is meant by the term '$\dot{V}O_2$ $_{max}$'?

O_2 consumption ($\dot{V}O_2$) increases linearly with exercise intensity, but reaches a plateau at $\dot{V}O_2$ $_{max}$ (Figure 42.2). $\dot{V}O_2$ $_{max}$ is the maximum capacity of a person's body to transport and use O_2 during incremental exercise (units: mLO_2/kg of body weight/min) and is used as a measure of a person's physical fitness – athletes have much greater $\dot{V}O_2$ $_{max}$ than normal individuals. $\dot{V}O_2$ $_{max}$ is one of the main

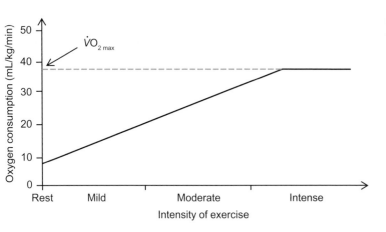

Figure 42.2 Effect of exercise intensity on O_2 consumption.

measurements attained by cardiopulmonary exercise testing[1] (CPET) (see Chapter 43).

What happens to oxygen consumption after a patient stops exercising?

A person continues to breathe deeply for a period of time after exercise has ceased. $\dot{V}O_2$ remains high during the recovery phase – this is known as the excess post-exercise O_2 consumption (EPOC) or O_2 debt. There are two distinct phases to the EPOC (Figure 42.3):

- **The alactacid phase**, which is rapid and involves:
  - *Replenishment of high-energy phosphocreatine and ATP stores* that were depleted in the early phase of exercise;
  - *Replenishment of O_2 to myoglobin;*
  - *Replenishment of muscle and liver glycogen stores.*

- **The lactacid phase**, which takes much longer and involves the conversion of lactate back to pyruvate, mostly in the liver.

In the longer term, high catecholamine levels and raised temperature cause a global increase in metabolic rate. Anabolic processes (e.g. muscle fibre repair and hypertrophy) may occur over days to weeks of repeated exercise.

The time taken to repay the O_2 debt depends on the duration and intensity of exercise: following a short walk, $\dot{V}O_2$ may be raised for a few minutes, but it may take more than a day to fully recover metabolically after running a marathon.

How do elite athletes differ from the 'normal' population?

Unsurprisingly, the main changes that occur with physical training are to the cardiovascular system:

- **Stroke volume** (SV). Physical training causes cardiac hypertrophy,[2] which results in an increase in SV of up to 40%.
- **HR**. Maximum HR does not change, but the resting HR of athletes is often lower than that of the general population due to increased vagal tone. As the resting SV is increased, resting CO remains approximately the same. The increase in vagal tone often results in the sinus arrhythmia of childhood extending into adulthood.
- **CO**. The increased SV means that the maximal CO is increased in athletes.
- $\dot{V}O_2$ $_{max}$ may increase by up to 25% with training. This is thought to be due to an increase in O_2 delivery as a result of increased muscle vascularisation.

In addition, there are changes in:

- **The lungs**. Maximum breathing rate increases, the volume of the lungs increases and the number of pulmonary capillaries also increases. Altogether, maximal $\dot{V}_E$ may increase by up to 15 L/min with training.

---

[1] Strictly, it is $\dot{V}O_2$ $_{peak}$ rather than $\dot{V}O_2$ $_{max}$ that is measured in CPET. $\dot{V}O_2$ $_{peak}$ is the maximum $\dot{V}O_2$ achieved within the time period of the CPET. Many of the patients referred for CPET never achieve the plateau shown in Figure 42.2.

[2] This is structurally and metabolically different from pathological cardiac hypertrophy resulting from, for example, aortic stenosis.

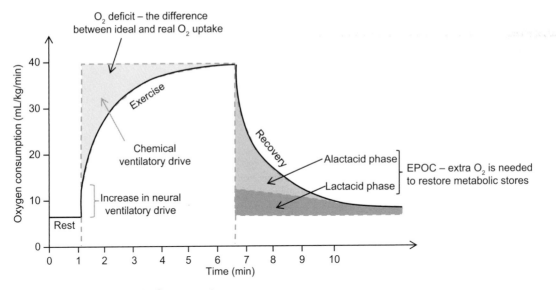

Figure 42.3 Excess post-exercise O_2 consumption.

- **Skeletal muscle.** Hypertrophy occurs as a result of training (an effect of the resistive work done by the muscles rather than aerobic training). Endurance training increases the diameter of type I muscle fibres and encourages the formation of muscle capillaries, increases the density of mitochondria and increases the activity of oxidative metabolic enzymes. Exercise carried out in repetitive, intense episodes increases the diameter of type IIb muscle fibres and increases the activity of anaerobic metabolic enzymes.

- **Bone mineral density.** Weight-bearing exercise increases bone mineral density. Exercise is a particularly important means of reducing the risk of fractures in the elderly.

Further reading

D. A. Burton, K. Stokes, G. M. Hall. Physiological effects of exercise. *Continuing Educ Anaesth Crit Care Pain* 2004; 4(6): 185–8.

N. Agnew. Preoperative cardiopulmonary exercise testing. *Continuing Educ Anaesth Crit Care Pain* 2010; 10(2): 33–7.

Exercise Testing

How can we assess a patient's fitness for surgery?

Surgery places a person's body under physiological stress: the magnitude of the stress response is proportional to the severity of the surgical trauma. The surgical stress response increases an individual's O_2 consumption ($\dot{V}O_2$). Patients who are less physiologically fit will be less able to increase their O_2 delivery and may therefore be unable to match the increase in $\dot{V}O_2$. Respiratory and cardiovascular co-morbidities place a major limitation on the cardiovascular response to major surgery, but physical deconditioning also plays a significant role.

When a patient is assessed for a surgical procedure, a number of factors must be considered:

- The invasiveness and surgical difficulty of the proposed surgical procedure;
- The patient's co-morbidities, which may be previously known or newly diagnosed, and may be well controlled, poorly controlled or uncontrolled;
- The patient's physical fitness, which may be quantified using exercise testing.

Ultimately, the aim of the preoperative assessment process is to identify those individuals at significant risk of perioperative complications in order to:

- Better inform the patient of their individual risk so as to help them with their decision-making.
- Inform decision-making by the multidisciplinary team; for example, an alternative, less invasive surgical procedure may instead be offered to a patient (e.g. endovascular aortic aneurysm repair in place of open repair).
- Plan post-operative care; for example, a high-dependency bed may be required.

How can you clinically assess exercise capacity?

Exercise capacity can be assessed by asking the patient a series of questions relating to their everyday activities, such as 'How far can you walk on the flat?' or 'How many stairs can you climb without stopping?' The problem is that these questions are very subjective, and patients often overestimate their exercise tolerance.

Are there any more objective methods of assessing exercise capacity?

There are a number of more objective methods available:

- **Questionnaire based**, such as the Duke Activity Status Index (DASI). DASI is a 12-question self-assessment in which patients are asked about whether they can complete certain physical tasks. Each task is weighted according to its metabolic cost (in metabolic equivalents, METs). A patient who is unable to complete physical tasks of at least 4 METs is at higher risk of perioperative complications.
- **Incremental shuttle walk test**, in which patients are asked to walk continuously between two cones set 9 m apart, with a progressively decreasing time permitted to reach the next cone. Patients who are unable to walk at least 250 m are at increased perioperative risk of complications. While this test is cheap and easy to carry out, there are groups of patients who may be unable to perform a walk test: lower limb amputees, those with peripheral vascular disease or those with hip or knee osteoarthritis.
- **Cardiopulmonary exercise testing** (CPET), which is considered the gold-standard exercise test. During a CPET test, the patient's expired gases are measured whilst the patient carries out a continually increasing amount of work on an electromagnetically braked cycle ergometer. Over 5000 measurements are taken during the 10-minute test, including:
  - *The work rate* (in Watts);

- *Metabolic gas exchange measurements*: $\dot{V}O_2$, CO_2 production ($\dot{V}CO_2$) and respiratory exchange ratio ($=\dot{V}CO_2/\dot{V}O_2$).
- *Ventilatory measurements*: oxygen saturations, $\dot{V}_E$, V_T, respiratory rate, ventilatory equivalents for O_2 ($\dot{V}_E/\dot{V}O_2$) and CO_2 ($\dot{V}_E/\dot{V}CO_2$).
- *Cardiovascular parameters*: heart rate, electrocardiogram (ECG) ST-segment changes and non-invasive blood pressure.

The data points are graphically represented in a standard format, known as the nine-panel plot. Two important values can be determined through analysis of CPET data:

- *Anaerobic threshold* (AT), the $\dot{V}O_2$ above which aerobic metabolism is supplemented by anaerobic metabolism. An AT < 10.2 mL kg^{-1} min^{-1} is associated with a greater risk of perioperative complications.
- *Peak oxygen consumption* ($\dot{V}O_{2\ peak}$), the maximum $\dot{V}O_2$ achieved by the patient in the test. 'Normal' $\dot{V}O_{2\ peak}$ measurements are typically 25–40 mL kg^{-1} min^{-1}; $\dot{V}O_{2\ peak}$ < 15 mL kg^{-1} min^{-1} is associated with a higher risk of perioperative complications.

One of the advantages of CPET is that useful data can often be obtained for individuals who cannot complete other exercise testing due to diseases such as peripheral vascular disease.

What normally happens to $\dot{V}O_2$ during a CPET?

In a normal patient, $\dot{V}O_2$ increases linearly with exercise intensity until the end of the test,[1] when the patient is either unable to continue or exhibits adverse signs such as ST-segment elevation on the ECG. Clinically, $\dot{V}O_{2\ peak}$ gives a useful measure of cardiopulmonary 'physiological reserve' in order to predict how well a patient will cope with the additional metabolic demands of surgery.

---

[1] When testing elite athletes, $\dot{V}O_2$ initially increases linearly before reaching a plateau (see Chapter 42, Figure 42.2). $\dot{V}O_2$ at the plateau is termed $\dot{V}O_{2\ max}$. The highest measured $\dot{V}O_{2\ max}$ is 97.5 mL kg^{-1} min^{-1}, recorded in an elite cyclist.

Exercise limitation is usually multifactorial:

- Factors involved in delivery of O_2 to the muscles include:
  - *O_2-carrying capacity* of the blood; thus, anaemia reduces $\dot{V}O_{2\ peak}$.
  - *The capillary density* of the muscles themselves. This is likely to be the limiting factor in normal exercise and in athletes.

    Athletes train at altitude to increase their performance; the resulting hypoxaemia is a strong inducer of vascular endothelial growth factor, which induces muscle vascularisation and thus increases $\dot{V}O_{2\ peak}$. Additionally, hypoxaemia results in erythropoietin secretion and increased haematocrit.
- In patients with cardiovascular disease, exercise capacity may be limited if the heart cannot increase cardiac output (CO) sufficiently to match the increased demand of the muscles. Additionally, patients who take medication that limits CO (e.g. β-blockers) have a correspondingly lower $\dot{V}O_{2\ peak}$.
- With the exception of severe lung disease, the respiratory system almost never limits exercise capacity. The increase in $\dot{V}_E$ usually far exceeds the increase in CO, and transfer of O_2 across the alveolar–capillary barrier is usually not diffusion limited (see Chapter 10).

How are METs related to $\dot{V}O_2$?

The MET of a task is another method of expressing the energy cost of a particular physical activity (see Chapter 77). One MET – the basal metabolic rate of a fasted, resting patient – is associated with a $\dot{V}O_2$ of 3.5 mL kg^{-1} min^{-1}. Therefore, METs can be related to $\dot{V}O_2$:

- A patient who is unable to climb one flight of stairs (an activity of approximately 3 METs, equivalent to a $\dot{V}O_2$ of 9.5 mL kg^{-1} min^{-1}) is at higher risk of perioperative mortality.
- The ability to climb two flights of stairs without stopping (an activity of approximately 4 METs, equivalent to a $\dot{V}O_2$ of 14 mL kg^{-1} min^{-1}) is associated with a lower perioperative mortality risk.
- Climbing five flights of stairs (an activity of around 8 METs, equivalent to a $\dot{V}O_2 > 20$ mL kg^{-1} min^{-1}) is associated with minimal perioperative mortality.

Further reading

D. J. Chambers, N. Wiseley. Cardiopulmonary exercise testing – a beginner's guide to the nine-panel plot. *BJA Education* 2019; in press.

D. Z. H. Levett, S. Jack, M. Swart, et al. Perioperative cardiopulmonary exercise testing (CPET): consensus clinical guidelines on indications, organisation, conduct, and physiological interpretation. *Br J Anaesth* 2018; **120**(3): 484–500.

P. O. Older, D. Z. H. Levett. Cardiopulmonary exercise testing and surgery. *Ann Am Thorac Soc* 2017; **14**(Suppl. 1): S74–83.

J. Moran, F. Wilson, E. Guinan, P. McCormick, J. Hussey, J. Moriarty. Role of cardiopulmonary exercise testing as a risk-assessment method in patients undergoing intra-abdominal surgery: a systematic review. *Br J Anaesth* 2016; **116**(2): 177–91.

R. A. Hartley, A. C. Pichel, S. W. Grant, et al. Preoperative cardiopulmonary exercise testing and risk of early mortality following abdominal aortic aneurysm repair. *Br J Surg* 2012; **99**(11): 1539–46.

Neuronal Structure and Function

What are the functions of the nervous system?

The nervous system is a complex network of specialised cells called neurons, which coordinate and control the other organ systems.

The nervous system has three basic functions:

- **Sensory input.** Sensory receptors detect changes in the external and internal environments. In response to a stimulus, the sensory receptor generates an electrical signal – an action potential – which is then relayed to the brain and spinal cord (collectively known as the central nervous system, CNS).
- **Integration.** Sensory input is received and processed by the CNS. Decisions are made on the basis of this sensory integration.
- **Motor output.** Neurons relay action potentials from the CNS to the muscles and glands. Motor output is the only way we can interact with our external environment; even salivation requires smooth muscle contraction. Much of the nervous system is therefore dedicated to producing movement.

Neurons communicate between themselves and other organs through two forms of signalling:

- **Neural.** An action potential is conducted from the cell body of a presynaptic neuron to its terminus. The signal is then transmitted from the presynaptic neuron to a postsynaptic cell (which may be another neuron, a muscle cell or a gland) by means of an electrical or chemical synapse. Whilst nerve conduction is relatively rapid (up to 120 m/s in large myelinated nerves), conduction across a chemical synapse is slower.
- **Endocrine.** The brain synthesises and releases hormones into the circulation, which conveys them to the target organ. Endocrine signalling is therefore much slower than neural signalling.

Describe the structure of a neuron

The neuron is the functional unit of the nervous system. Although neurons vary in their detailed cellular structure, all include the following components (Figure 44.1):

- **The cell body,** which in common with other cell types contains cytoplasm, a nucleus and organelles. The cell body is involved in protein synthesis and the generation of ATP. However, as mature neurons lack a centriole, which is necessary for cell division, neurons cannot undergo mitosis. The cell bodies form the grey matter in the brain and spinal cord. Groupings of cell bodies are termed nuclei in the CNS and ganglia in the peripheral nervous system (PNS).
- **Dendrites** are branched projections that receive signals from other neurons through synapses and propagate them towards the cell body.
- **The axon** is a long projection originating at the cell body. Action potentials are generated at the axon hillock[1] and conducted along the axon, away from the cell body. The axon may be either unmyelinated or myelinated. Myelin is made up of multiple layers of electrically insulating lipid and protein, produced by the Schwann cells in the PNS or oligodendrocytes in the CNS. Lipid gives axons a white colour and therefore forms the 'white matter' of the brain and spinal cord. Myelin increases the speed of action potential propagation (see Chapter 52).
- **An axon terminal,** the distal end of the axon. At the axon terminal, the neuron communicates with another cell through a synapse. In a motor neuron, this synapse is the neuromuscular junction.

---

[1] The axon hillock has the lowest threshold for action potential generation in the cell, owing to its high density of voltage-gated Na^+ channels. It is usually the first site of action potential generation, even when inputs are received on the dendrites.

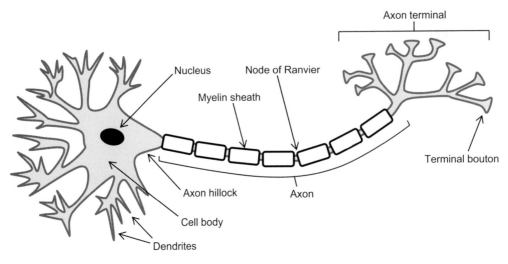

Figure 44.1 Basic structure of a neuron.

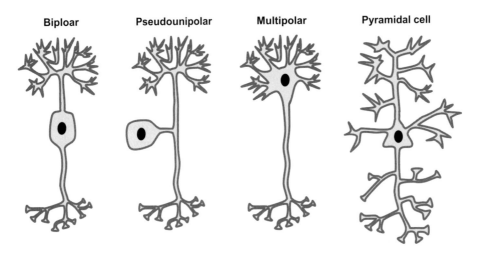

Figure 44.2 Common types of neuron.

These components can be arranged to give differing nerve morphologies. The major neuron classes are (Figure 44.2):

- **Unipolar**. These neurons have an axon projecting from a cell body. They are not common in humans, but are found in the cochlear.
- **Bipolar**. These neurons have a cell body between the dendrites and the axon. Bipolar cells are found in the retina and the olfactory neurons.
- **Pseudounipolar**. Some bipolar neurons may look unipolar – the axon is interrupted by the cell body approximately midway down. Most sensory neurons are pseudounipolar.

- **Multipolar**. The dendrites insert directly into the cell body without coalescing. The classical example of a multipolar neuron is a motor neuron.
- **Anaxonic**. Dendrites and axons are indistinguishable, looking like a large tree of insertions into a cell body. These are exemplified by amacrine cells in the retina.
- **Pyramidal cells**. These have a triangular cell body (hence the name), a single axon and a large number of dendrites – through these dendrites, pyramidal cells can integrate many afferent signals. They are commonly found in the cerebral cortex and hippocampus.

How is the nervous system divided?

All of the elements of the nervous system work together holistically. However, the nervous system has traditionally been divided into:

- **The CNS**, consisting of the brain and spinal cord:
  - *The brain* is the site of higher integration of sensory inputs, motor output, thinking and learning.
  - *The spinal cord* contains long sensory and motor pathways that convey information between the periphery and the CNS, as well as local integrative networks. Interneurons (e.g. Renshaw,[2] multipolar and pyramidal cells) provide connections between neurons within the CNS.

- **The PNS**, whose cell types are:
  - *Sensory (afferent) neurons*, which relay information from the external environment and viscera to the CNS. Most have a pseudounipolar structure with the cell body on a process to the side of the axon (Figure 44.2) located in the dorsal root ganglion.
  - *Motor (efferent) neurons*, also known as somatic motor neurons, are under voluntary control. Motor neurons transmit action potentials from the CNS to skeletal muscle. These neurons are typically multipolar; they receive many inputs through multiple dendrites, with the resultant action potential propagated through a single axon (Figure 44.2).
  - *Enteric neurons* form a large network around the gastrointestinal tract. The enteric nervous system is sometimes referred to as a 'second brain', as it operates with relative independence from the CNS. The brain can still influence the enteric nervous system through the action of autonomic neurons.

  - *Autonomic neurons* deal with the more primitive 'housekeeping' functions of the viscera, as well as the body's emergency responses. The autonomic nervous system is involuntary and divided into two subsystems, the sympathetic and parasympathetic nervous systems, discussed in more detail in Chapter 59.

What are the component tissue layers of peripheral nerves?

A peripheral nerve is a bundle of many nerve axons. Connective tissue physically separates and electrically insulates the axons from one another. The result is a layered structure, rather like an onion skin, containing:

- **Schwann cells.** Myelinated nerve axons are surrounded by a layer of myelin produced by the Schwann cells. An axon surrounded by a myelin sheath is often referred to as a nerve fibre.
- **Endoneurium.** Each nerve fibre is surrounded by a thin layer of connective tissue called endoneurium.
- **Perineurium.** Many nerve fibres are bundled together into groups called fascicles. Each fascicle is wrapped in a layer of connective tissue called perineurium, which supports the fascicles.
- **Epineurium.** This is the thick outer layer of the peripheral nerve. The epineurium encloses the multiple fascicles, together with their blood vessels.

For local anaesthetic to exert its effects on the nerve axons, it must therefore diffuse through three layers: the epineurium, the perineurium and the endoneurium.

Further reading

E. Pannese. *Neurocytology: Fine Structure of Neurons, Nerve Processes and Neuroglial Cells, 2nd edition*. Stuttgart, Thieme Publishing Group, 2016.

---

[2] Renshaw cells are simple inhibitory interneurons.

Chapter 45

The Brain

Describe the gross anatomy of the brain

The brain performs complex sensory, motor and higher functions, coordinating the activity of other body systems. It has a high metabolic activity, receiving 15% of the resting cardiac output, a much greater proportion than would be predicted on the basis of its weight. It can be divided into five regions:

- **The telencephalon** (cerebrum) is the largest part of the human brain, occupying the anterior and middle cranial fossae. It comprises three sub-regions:

  - *The right and left cerebral hemispheres* perform higher functions of memory, thinking, planning and language, in addition to being essential for sensory perception and the initiation of voluntary movement.
  - *The basal ganglia*, a collection of nuclei located deep within the cerebral hemispheres, has classically been regarded as part of the extrapyramidal system which coordinates fine motor control, muscle tone and posture.
  - *The limbic system*, a collection of structures located on either side of the thalamus, is involved in a number of higher functions, including long-term memory, emotion and behaviour.

The right and left cerebral hemispheres are connected by a thick bundle of myelinated nerve axons called the corpus callosum. The cerebral cortex – the outer layer of the cerebrum – is made up of grey matter, reflecting the relatively large number of nerve cell bodies. The deeper layers of the cerebrum are composed of white matter, reflecting the greater proportion of myelinated nerve axons. The cerebral cortex has a large surface area shaped into numerous folds with ridges (gyri) and troughs (sulci). Each cerebral hemisphere has four lobes:

- *Frontal lobe*. The majority of the frontal lobe is involved in higher functions: problem-solving, reasoning, planning, language generation and complex social and sexual behaviour. The premotor and primary motor cortices, located in the posterior frontal lobe, are involved in the planning and initiation of movement.
- *Parietal lobe*, the area of the brain involved in sensory integration. The post-central gyrus – the most anterior part of the parietal lobe – contains the primary somatosensory cortex. The left and right parietal lobes have slightly different functions. The dominant hemisphere (the left hemisphere in 97% of the population) is concerned with structure and order; for example, reading and mathematics involve ordering letters and numbers, respectively. The non-dominant hemisphere is concerned with spatial awareness.
- *Temporal lobe*, which controls hearing, language and memory. The left temporal lobe contains the primary auditory cortex. Wernicke's area – an area of cortex important in receptive language – lies between the temporal and frontal lobes of the dominant hemisphere.
- *Occipital lobe*, the area of the brain that interprets visual stimuli.

- **The diencephalon**, which includes:

  - *The thalamus*, which acts as a relay station. Sensory afferent neurons, with the exception of the olfactory neurons, synapse in the lateral thalamic nuclei before relaying to the cerebral cortex. The medial structures of the thalamus have roles in pain perception, awareness and the regulation of sleep.

- *The hypothalamus*, a specialised area of the brain that regulates autonomic function and links the nervous system to the endocrine system. The hypothalamus exerts control over the pituitary gland, a major endocrine gland (see Chapter 80). In addition, the hypothalamus has roles in appetite and satiety, thirst and control of osmolarity, thermoregulation and circadian rhythm.
- *The subthalamus* contains the subthalamic nucleus, which is thought to be part of the basal ganglia.
- *The metathalamus* contains the lateral geniculate nucleus, which relays visual information from the optic nerve to the primary visual cortex, and the medial geniculate nucleus, which relays auditory information to the primary auditory cortex.

- **The mesencephalon** (midbrain) joins the hindbrain to the cerebral hemispheres. The midbrain contains the cerebral aqueduct of Sylvius, which connects the third ventricle to the fourth ventricle (see Chapter 46). The midbrain also contains the third (oculomotor) and fourth (trochlear) cranial nerve nuclei and the red nuclei, which relay extrapyramidal tracts from the cerebellum and cerebral cortex to the spinal cord. The medulla oblongata, pons and midbrain are collectively referred to as the brainstem.
- **The cerebellum** (meaning 'little brain') occupies the posterior cranial fossa. Although it makes up only 10% of the brain's volume, the cerebellum contains over 50% of the brain's neurons, reflecting its central role in the refinement of movement. The cerebellum does not initiate movements (this is the role of the motor cortex). Instead, it modifies movements to ensure they are smooth, coordinated and accurate. The cerebellum is also responsible for learning motor movements: it builds a 'working model' of the environment based on experience. Damage to the cerebellum therefore does not result in paralysis, but in ataxia and poor motor learning. The cerebellum is divided into two main parts:

  - *The vermis*, the central part, is concerned with motor and postural control of the trunk.
  - *The cerebellar hemispheres*, located on either side of the vermis, are concerned with

coordinated motor control of the limbs. Damage to the right cerebellar hemisphere causes limb ataxia on the right side (i.e. the ipsilateral side) and vice versa. This is in contrast to damage to the right side of the motor cortex, which causes a left-sided hemiplegia.

On each side, afferent and efferent nerve impulses are carried between the cerebellum and the brainstem through three nerve bundles:

- *The superior and middle cerebellar peduncles* connect the cerebellum to the pons.
- *The inferior cerebellar peduncle* connects the cerebellum to the medulla.

- **The rhombencephalon** consists of the following structures:

  - *The pons* ('bridge') connects the cerebellum to the brainstem and the medulla oblongata to the midbrain. The nuclei of cranial nerves V to VIII are also located in the pons. The pneumotaxic and apneustic centres – nuclei that form part of the respiratory centre – are located at the border between the pons and medulla.
  - *The medulla oblongata* connects the brain to the spinal cord. Most descending motor tracts of the pyramidal system decussate (cross over to the contralateral side) in the medulla, at the bulges known as the pyramids. Ascending sensory tracts of the dorsal column–medial lemniscal pathway also decussate in the medulla. The medulla contains the nuclei involved in the physiological functions most essential to life: the respiratory and vasomotor centres and extrinsic regulation of the heart through the autonomic nervous system. The medulla controls many stereotyped reflexes, including the vomiting, swallowing, sneezing, gag and cough reflexes.

What are the meninges?

The meninges are membranes that cover the brain and spinal cord, providing protection to the central nervous system (CNS). The meninges consist of three layers:

- **The dura mater**, a thick outer membrane. The dura consists of an outer periosteal layer and an inner meningeal layer and has four infoldings:
  - *Falx cerebri*, which separates the cerebral hemispheres;
  - *Tentorium cerebelli*, which separates the occipital lobes from the cerebellum;
  - *Falx cerebelli*, which lies inferior to the tentorium, separating the cerebellar hemispheres;
  - *Diaphragma sellae*, a circular fold of dura that envelops the pituitary gland in the sella turcica.
- **The arachnoid mater**, a thin membrane with a spider-like appearance.
- **The pia mater**, a very thin and highly vascular membrane that adheres to the surface of the brain and spinal cord. Beyond the terminus of the spinal cord, the pia continues as the filum terminale, which (along with the dura) tethers the spinal cord to the coccyx.

Some features of the meninges are common to both the brain and spinal cord:

- **The subdural space** is a potential space located between the dura and arachnoid. The two meningeal layers may be separated by blood as a result of a tear in a bridging vein – this is referred to as a subdural haematoma.
- **The subarachnoid space** contains cerebrospinal fluid and is located between the arachnoid and pia.

Other features are unique to the brain or spinal cord:

- **In the brain**, venous blood drains into the dural venous sinuses (e.g. the superior and inferior sagittal, carvernous, sigmoid and transverse), which are located between the two layers of dura mater.
- **In the spinal cord**, the spinal dura mater is separated from the ligamenta flava and the periosteum of the vertebral bodies, pedicles and laminae by the epidural (or extradural) space. The epidural space contains lymphatics, spinal nerve roots, loose connective tissue and the epidural venous plexus. The epidural space extends from the sacrococcygeal membrane to the foramen magnum.

What are the neuroglia?

The neurons of the CNS are supported by four types of cell, known collectively as the neuroglia. Unlike neurons, which cannot replicate, neuroglia continue to divide throughout life. The neuroglial cell types are:

- **Astrocytes**, the most abundant of the neuroglia. Astrocytes anchor neurons to blood vessels and form the blood–brain barrier, providing the neurons with a constant external environment (see Chapter 47).
- **Oligodendrocytes**, which have an equivalent role to that of Schwann cells in the peripheral nervous system, coating the nerve axons in myelin, an electrical insulator (see Chapter 52).
- **Ependymal cells**, which form the epithelial lining of the ventricles of the brain and the central canal of the spinal cord.
- **Microglia**, the specialised macrophages of the CNS.

Describe the cerebral arterial blood supply

The cerebral arterial blood supply is derived from four main arteries: the right and left internal carotid arteries (ICAs) and the right and left vertebral arteries. Two-thirds of cerebral blood comes from the ICAs.

The unique feature of the cerebral circulation is the 'circle of Willis', an anastomosis of the following cerebral vessels (Figure 45.1):

- **Right and left anterior cerebral arteries** (ACAs), branches of the ICAs that supply the superior and medial portions of the cerebral hemispheres.
- **Anterior communicating artery** (ACom), a small artery that connects the left and right ACAs.
- **Right and left middle cerebral arteries** (MCAs), which arise from the ICAs and supply the lateral aspect of the cerebral hemispheres.
- **Basilar artery**, a single artery that arises from the amalgamation of the two vertebral arteries. Branches of the basilar artery supply the brainstem.
- **Right and left posterior cerebral arteries** (PCAs), which are formed when the basilar artery divides. The PCAs supply the occipital lobes and the medial portion of the temporal lobes.
- **Right and left posterior communicating arteries** (PComs), which connect the PCA to the ICA on either side of the brain.

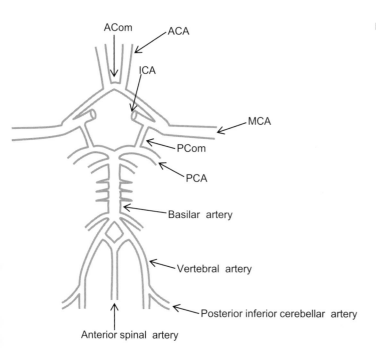

Figure 45.1 The circle of Willis.

The cerebral vessels supplied by the ICAs (ACAs, ACom and MCAs) are referred to as the anterior circulation, whilst the cerebral vessels supplied by the vertebral arteries (basilar artery, PCAs and PComs) are called the posterior circulation.

Describe the venous drainage of the brain

The cerebral venous system can be subdivided into superficial and deep systems:

- **Superficial**, comprising the dural venous sinuses: venous channels located between the two layers of dura mater (see above). Blood from the dural sinuses ultimately drains into the paired internal jugular veins. The venous sinuses are different from veins elsewhere in the body: as they are formed from dura, they lack valves and are not collapsible, which in part explains the higher risk of air embolus during neurosurgery.
- **Deep**, consisting of traditional veins that drain blood from the deep structures of the brain. These veins merge to form the vein of Galen, which drains into the inferior sagittal sinus.

Clinical relevance: stroke

The Bamford classification divides ischaemic stroke into categories based on the affected cerebral circulation:

- **Anterior circulation infarct** (ACI; subclassified as total or partial), in which a thrombus or embolus obstructs blood flow in the anterior circulation of the circle of Willis, resulting in a large cortical infarct. The vessel most commonly affected is the MCA. As discussed above, the anterior circulation supplies the medial, superior and lateral portions of the cerebral hemispheres. ACI is therefore associated with three categories of clinical signs:

  - *Contralateral weakness* when the motor cortex is affected;
  - *Homonymous hemianopia* when the optic tract is affected;
  - *Higher cerebral dysfunction*; for example, dysphasia or visuospatial disorder, depending on whether the dominant or non-dominant parietal lobe is affected.

- **Posterior circulation infarct**. Thrombus or embolus obstructing blood flow in the vertebrobasilar circulation results in infarction of the downstream areas of the brain, causing:

- *Cerebellar dysfunction*: ataxia, nystagmus;
- *Cranial nerve palsies or loss of consciousness* as a result of brainstem involvement;
- *Homonymous hemianopia* as a result of occipital lobe involvement.

- **Lacunar infarct**, due to occlusion of a small subcortical vessel. The resulting clinical effects (e.g. a motor hemiparesis) are out of proportion to the small size of the infarct. This is because the infarct affects important structures deep in the cerebral hemisphere through which motor or sensory nerve axons pass, such as the lateral thalamus or the posterior limb of the internal capsule. Lacunar infarcts are not associated with higher cerebral dysfunction and as such have a much better prognosis than an anterior or posterior circulation infarct.

Theoretically, the circle of Willis should provide a collateral circulation if a vessel becomes occluded. However, the circle is often anatomically incomplete, resulting in stroke being the third leading cause of death in the UK.

What is an electroencephalogram?

The electroencephalogram (EEG) is a recording of the electrical activity of the brain, measured using 19 scalp electrodes. The electrical potential generated by depolarisation of a single neuron is far too small to be detected at the scalp. In the heart, the electrocardiogram records simultaneous depolarisation of all the atrial then ventricular myocytes. In a similar way, the EEG records patterns representing the synchronised depolarisation of groups of neurons. However, the complexity of the brain's electrical activity makes interpretation of the EEG a very difficult task. Electrical activity in the brain is categorised based on its frequency:

- δ-*waves*: 0–4 Hz;
- θ-*waves*: 4–8 Hz;
- α-*waves*: 8–13 Hz;
- β-*waves*: >13 Hz.

In anaesthetic practice, the clinical uses of the EEG are:

- **Diagnosis of epilepsy**. Seizure activity results in organised, simultaneous activity in neurons, which can be identified on the EEG. Non-convulsive status epilepticus is an important differential diagnosis in a critical care patient who fails to wake following a sedation hold.

- **Diagnosis of encephalopathy**. This is characterised by a progressive increase in slow-wave activity.
- **As an adjunct test of brain death**. This is not required to diagnose brain death under UK law, but is used elsewhere in the world to confirm brain death. The EEG of a brain-dead patient is isoelectric, reflecting the lack of electrical activity.
- **As a measure of depth of anaesthesia**, both in theatre anaesthetics (see below) and in critical care; for example, burst suppression of the EEG in barbiturate coma.
- **Somatosensory-evoked potentials** (SSEPs). During spinal surgery, SSEPs are used to reduce the risk of damage to the spinal cord. SSEP monitoring involves stimulating a peripheral nerve and detecting a response in the somatosensory cortex through appropriately placed scalp electrodes. SSEPs are usually combined with motor-evoked potentials. During spinal surgery, a loss of amplitude or increased latency of the SSEP signal suggests neurological injury.

Clinical relevance: monitoring depth of anaesthesia

General anaesthesia is associated with a change in the raw EEG from the fast-wave, small-amplitude (β-wave) trace of wakefulness to a slow-wave, large-amplitude (δ-wave) pattern. The bispectral index (BIS) is an attempt to simplify the highly complex EEG into a simple dimensionless number to help the anaesthetist assess depth of anaesthesia and prevent intraoperative awareness. BIS converts the frontal EEG to a number between 0 (no brain electrical activity) and 100 (fully awake), where 40–60 is considered to be an appropriate level of anaesthesia for surgery.

There are a number of potential problems with using BIS:

- BIS demonstrates a dose–response relationship with some anaesthetic agents, such as propofol, inhalational agents and midazolam. But other agents that are clinically synergistic have no effect on the BIS number, such as N_2O and opioids.
- In contrast to other anaesthetic agents, ketamine increases EEG activity, increasing the BIS number.
- Studies assessing the efficacy of BIS are contradictory:

- The B-Aware study found that BIS-guided anaesthesia reduced the risk of awareness with recall by 82%.
- The B-Unaware trial found that BIS-guided anaesthesia provided no greater reduction in intraoperative awareness than using end-tidal volatile concentration.

Further reading

S. Waxman. *Clinical Neuroanatomy, 28th edition.* New York, McGraw-Hill Medical, 2017.

S. Hagihira. Changes in the electroencephalogram during anaesthesia and their physiological basis. *Br J Anaesth* 2015; **115**(Suppl. 1): i27–31.

A. Raithatha, G. Pratt, A. Rash. Developments in the management of acute ischaemic stroke: implications for anaesthetic and critical care management. *Continuing Educ Anaesth Crit Care Pain* 2013; **13**(3): 80–6.

M. S. Avidan, L. Zhang, B. A. Burnside, et al. Anesthesia awareness and the bispectral index. *N Engl J Med* 2008; **358**(11): 1097–108.

P. S. Myles, K. Leslie, J. McNeil, et al. Bispectral index monitoring to prevent awareness during anaesthesia: the B-Aware randomised controlled trial. *Lancet* 2004; **363**(9423): 1757–63.

C. Macchi, R. M. Lova, B. Miniati, et al. The circle of Willis in healthy older persons. *J Cardiovasc Surg (Torino)* 2002; **43**(6): 887–90.

46

Cerebrospinal Fluid

What are the functions of cerebrospinal fluid?

Cerebrospinal fluid (CSF) is the transcellular fluid located within the cerebral ventricles and subarachnoid space that bathes the brain and spinal cord. CSF has a number of functions:

- **Buoyancy and cushioning.** The adult brain weighs around 1400 g. However, when suspended in CSF, the brain has an effective weight of less than 50 g. Sudden head movement produces potentially damaging acceleration and deceleration forces – the lower effective weight of the brain reduces its inertia, protecting it from damage. CSF also cushions the brain, protecting it from damage, especially from the ridged skull base.
- **Maintenance of a constant ionic environment.** Neurons are highly sensitive to changes in their external environment; maintaining a constant ionic and osmotic environment is essential for normal neuronal activity.
- **Buffering changes in intracranial pressure** (ICP). Displacement of CSF from the cranium is an important, but limited, compensatory mechanism that occurs following an increase in ICP (see Chapter 49).
- **Control of respiration.** As a small, lipid-soluble molecule, CO_2 can freely diffuse from the blood to the CSF. The CSF has a much lower protein concentration than plasma and therefore has a reduced buffering capacity, making the CSF pH very sensitive to changes in blood PCO_2. The central chemoreceptors detect changes in CSF pH, causing the respiratory centre to make corresponding adjustments in $\dot{V}_E$ (see Chapter 22).
- **Glymphatic system.** Outside the central nervous system (CNS), the lymphatic system is responsible for removing extracellular proteins, excess fluid

and some metabolic waste products. The brain also produces waste products that need to be cleared, but it lacks a lymphatic system. Instead, the glymphatic system allows CSF to circulate in paravascular channels between the blood vessels and the astrocyte foot processes, where it collects and removes waste products. The name 'glymphatic' comes from astrocytes (a type of glial cell) performing the role of the lymphatic system in the CNS.

Where is CSF produced?

CSF is produced by the choroid plexus, located in the ventricles of the brain: the two lateral ventricles, third ventricle and fourth ventricle. CSF is produced by a combination of filtration and active secretion of water and solutes at a rate of 0.3 mL/min, equivalent to 500 mL/day. The choroid plexus is formed by modified ependymal cells, ciliated cells that line the surface of the ventricles of the brain and the central canal of the spinal cord. Ciliary action propels CSF through the ventricles:

- From the lateral ventricles, CSF flows through the two foramina of Monro into the third ventricle, located between the right and left thalamic nuclei.
- CSF travels through the aqueduct of Sylvius, located within the midbrain, to the fourth ventricle, located within the pons.
- From the fourth ventricle, CSF flows into the subarachnoid space via the two lateral foramina of Luschka and the midline foramen of Magendie.[1] Most of the CSF flows around the cerebral hemispheres, whilst the remainder flows around the spinal cord.

Overall, the total volume of CSF is 100–150 mL, around half of which is located within the ventricular system and half is located within the subarachnoid space.

---

[1] Mnemonic: *l*ateral = *L*uschka, *m*idline = *M*agendie.

Where is CSF absorbed?

CSF is absorbed by the arachnoid granulations, villi that project from the arachnoid mater to the dural venous sinuses:

- 90% of CSF is absorbed by the arachnoid villi of the sagittal and sigmoid dural sinuses.
- 10% of CSF is absorbed through the spinal arachnoid villi.

CSF absorption depends on the pressure difference between CSF (typically 15 cmH$_2$O) and venous blood (typically 8 cmH$_2$O) and the difference between plasma (typically 25 mmHg) and CSF oncotic pressure (effectively 0 mmHg). An increase in CSF pressure (e.g. following traumatic brain injury) results in an increase in CSF absorption (see Chapter 49).

How do the constituents of CSF differ from those of plasma?

As discussed above, CSF is produced by a combination of filtration and active secretion. Despite their common origin, CSF and plasma have a number of important differences (see Table 46.1).

Note: CSF contains very little protein or cellular material, which accounts for its very low oncotic pressure and reduced buffering ability.

What is hydrocephalus?

Hydrocephalus is an abnormal resistance to the circulation of CSF or the impaired absorption of CSF. The rate of CSF production exceeds the rate at which CSF can circulate past the obstruction or the rate of CSF absorption, resulting in a local increase in CSF pressure within the ventricles. The increase in CSF

Table 46.1 Comparison of CSF and plasma.

	CSF	Plasma
Sodium, Na$^+$ (mmol/L)	140	140
Glucose (mmol/L)	4	6
Chloride, Cl$^-$ (mmol/L)	120	110
Bicarbonate, HCO$_3^-$ (mmol/L)	24	24
pH	7.32	7.4
Protein (g/L)	0.2–0.4	70
White blood cells (cells/mm^3)	0–5	4000–11,000

pressure compresses brain parenchymal tissue, resulting in enlargement of the ventricles, referred to as ventriculomegaly. Persistent compression of brain parenchyma results in irreversible damage. Hydrocephalus may be classified by site of obstruction to flow of CSF:

- **No obstruction.** Where there is no obstruction to the circulation or absorption of CSF, overproduction is the likely pathology. This rare situation can result from a choroid plexus papilloma.
- **Foramina of Monro.** These may be blocked as a result of compression by a tumour.
- **Aqueduct of Sylvius.** This narrow channel may be blocked as a result of congenital stenosis, subarachnoid haemorrhage or compression by a tumour.
- **The outlets of the fourth ventricle.** These may be obstructed by subarachnoid haemorrhage, chronic meningitis or as a result of the congenital Arnold–Chiari malformation type II.
- **Arachnoid granulations.** The absorption of CSF may be obstructed by blood clots caused by a subarachnoid haemorrhage.

The management of hydrocephalus is twofold: removal of the obstructing lesion (if this is surgically possible) and diversion of CSF flow to relieve the pressure on the ventricles by means of the following:

- **An external ventricular drain** (EVD), a temporary means of draining CSF. An EVD also allows CSF to be sampled, CSF pressure to be measured and intrathecal drugs to be administered.
- **A ventricular shunt**, a more permanent device that diverts CSF to the peritoneal cavity or the right atrium.
- **An endoscopic third ventriculostomy**, in which a hole is made in the floor of the third ventricle to allow CSF to pass directly into the basal cisterns, thus bypassing an obstruction in the aqueduct of Sylvius or fourth ventricle.

Further reading

D. N. Irani. *Cerebrospinal Fluid in Clinical Practice*. Philadelphia, Saunders, 2009.

H. L. Rekate. The definition and classification of hydrocephalus: a personal recommendation to stimulate debate. *Cerebrospinal Fluid Res* 2008; 5: 2.

47

Blood–Brain Barrier

What are the functions of the blood–brain barrier?

The blood–brain barrier (BBB) is a physiological, cellular and metabolic barrier at the level of the cerebral capillaries. Their permeability properties restrict the free movement of substances between the capillaries and the extracellular fluid (ECF) of the brain. The BBB has several functions:

- To maintain a constant extracellular environment within the central nervous system (CNS). This is arguably the most important feature. The concentration of solutes in blood varies considerably, and neuronal function may be adversely affected if neurons are directly exposed to this variation. For example, exercise produces changes in plasma pH and K^+ concentration that may depress neuronal activity if transmitted to the CNS.
- To protect the brain from harmful or neuroactive blood-borne substances.
- To prevent the release of CNS neurotransmitters into the systemic circulation.

What are the anatomical layers of the BBB?

The BBB comprises three layers:

- **Capillary endothelial cells**, interconnected by tight junctions, restricting the passage of substances from the capillaries to the brain ECF. The capillaries of the BBB differ from extracerebral capillaries in having a high density of mitochondria.
- **A thick basement membrane**, which lies beneath the endothelial cells.
- **Astrocyte foot processes**. Astrocytes are a type of supportive glial cell with projections called foot processes that encircle and are closely

applied to the capillaries. Astrocytes secrete chemicals that reduce the permeability of the capillary endothelial cells. In contrast, the choroid plexus is not surrounded by astrocytes, and its endothelial cells are therefore highly permeable.

These three layers form a virtually impenetrable barrier to lipophobic molecules, comparable to a continuous capillary.

How do substances cross the BBB?

Some signalling and nutritional substances gain entry to the brain ECF through a number of mechanisms:

- **Simple diffusion**. Small, lipid-soluble molecules can cross the phospholipid bilayers of the BBB by simple diffusion, in common with cellular barriers elsewhere in the body. Examples include O_2, CO_2, ethanol and steroid hormones.
- **Active transport**. The passage of small ions across the BBB, such as Na^+, K^+, Mg^{2+}, Ca^{2+}, Cl^-, HCO_3^- and H^+, is controlled by the membrane, including transport processes. This means that blood and CSF may differ in pH and ion concentrations. The high density of mitochondria in the cerebral capillaries reflects the high metabolic activity of this process.
- **Facilitated diffusion**. Some small molecules are transported across the BBB by facilitated diffusion along their concentration gradients:
  - *Glucose* is transported by GLUT1 transporters, whose transport function does not require ATP.
  - *Water* is transported through pores called aquaporins.
- **Pinocytosis**. Other molecules (e.g. insulin) are thought to cross the BBB by pinocytosis (see Chapter 4).

Which substances are important to exclude from the brain?

Importantly, a number of substances do not permeate the BBB:

- **Catecholamines**, such as noradrenaline and dopamine, which act as neurotransmitters in the CNS. Note: whilst dopamine cannot cross the BBB, its precursor, L-dihydroxyphenylalanine (L-DOPA), is transported by facilitated diffusion. Patients with Parkinson's disease, in which there is a dopamine deficiency of the substantia nigra, are therefore treated with L-DOPA rather than dopamine.
- **Amino acid** transport across the BBB is tightly regulated. A number of amino acids also act as neurotransmitters in the CNS, such as glycine and glutamic acid.
- **Ammonia** (NH_3), a small, lipophilic molecule that is potentially neurotoxic, might be expected to cross the BBB. However, it is rapidly metabolised in the astrocytes to glutamine and does not normally reach the neurons in significant concentrations.

Clinical relevance: drug transport across the BBB

The tight junctions of the BBB prevent not only endogenous molecules from entering the brain ECF, but also exogenous molecules. The BBB therefore represents a major obstacle to the delivery of drugs to the CNS. Drugs may cross the BBB through a variety of mechanisms:

- **Simple diffusion** of lipid-soluble drugs. Examples are propofol, thiopentone, volatile anaesthetics, benzodiazepines and phenytoin.
- **Bypassing the BBB** by direct administration into the CNS. Examples are intrathecal methotrexate and intracerebral implantation of polymer-bound chemotherapy agents.
- **Transport by transmembrane carriers**. As discussed above, L-DOPA is transported into the CNS through a neutral amino acid transporter, where it is then converted to dopamine.
- **Increasing the lipophilicity of drugs**. The increased lipophilicity of diamorphine results in it crossing the BBB 100 times more easily than its parent compound, morphine.

The BBB is also weakened by inflammation: antibiotics, which do not normally cross the BBB, may become effective in meningitis.

Which CNS structures are located outside the BBB?

The BBB protects the brain from harmful blood-borne substances. However, it is important that the brain retains a direct connection with the systemic circulation in relation to two important functions:

- Detection of alterations in composition of the blood;
- Secretion of hormones.

Some structures are characterised by their lack of a normal BBB: their capillaries are fenestrated, making the BBB 'leaky'. These structures are located around the third ventricle, so are often referred to as the circumventricular organs, and they are said to be located outside the BBB:

- **The area postrema**, also known as the chemoreceptor trigger zone, sends afferent signals to the vomiting centre in the presence of noxious substances, triggering vomiting.
- **The hypothalamus**, within which hypothalamic osmoreceptors monitor the osmolarity of systemic blood.
- **The anterior and posterior lobes of the pituitary gland** secrete eight pituitary hormones directly into the systemic circulation, six from the anterior lobe and two from the posterior lobe.
- **The pineal gland**, which secretes melatonin directly into the systemic circulation.
- **The choroid plexus**, which uses plasma from systemic blood to produce CSF.

Whilst the BBB is deficient in the circumventricular organs, the blood–CSF barrier remains intact. Hence, substances can leak out of the capillaries and into the circumventricular organs, but are unable to enter the CSF and access the brain's neurons.

Further reading

R. Daneman, A. Prat. The blood–brain barrier. *Cold Spring Harb Perspect Biol* 2015; 7(1): a020412.

M. Tajes, E. Ramos-Fernández, X. Weng-Jiang, et al. The blood–brain barrier: structure, function and therapeutic approaches to cross it. *Mol Membr Biol* 2014; **31**(5): 152–67.

R. Daneman. The blood–brain barrier in health and disease. *Ann Neurol* 2012; **72**(5): 648–72.

B. K. Lawther, S. Kumar, H. Krovvidi. Blood brain barrier. *Continuing Educ Anaesth Crit Care Pain* 2011; **11**(4): 128–32.

Cerebral Blood Flow

What proportion of the cardiac output is directed to the brain?

In the adult, cerebral blood flow (CBF) is typically 15% of the resting cardiac output (approximately 750 mL/min). CBF is commonly expressed in terms of the weight of brain parenchyma – normal CBF is 50 mL/ 100 g brain tissue/min. It is determined by the ratio of the cerebral perfusion pressure (CPP) and cerebral vascular resistance (CVR).

What is CPP?

CPP is the net pressure gradient driving blood flow through the cerebral circulation, resulting in the CBF. It is dependent upon both the mean arterial pressure (MAP) and the intracranial pressure (ICP). It is related to the remaining key parameters as follows:

Key equation: CPP

- *In relation to ICP:*

  $$CPP = MAP - ICP$$

- *In relation to CVR:*

  $$CPP = CBF \times CVR$$

What is cerebral autoregulation?

CBF is remarkably constant, remaining close to 50 mL/100 g/min across a wide range of cerebral perfusion pressures, ranging from 50 to 150 mmHg (Figure 48.1). This property of the brain is known as autoregulation.

Autoregulation is thought to take place through a myogenic mechanism in which the cerebral arterioles vasoconstrict in response to an increase in wall tension, and they vasodilate in response to a decrease in wall tension, thereby increasing or decreasing CVR (see Chapter 34).

Outside the autoregulatory range:

- When CPP is greater than 150 mmHg, CBF becomes directly proportional to CPP.
- When CPP falls below 50 mmHg, CBF falls below the 'normal' value of 50 mL/100 g/min, resulting in brain ischaemia.

The autoregulation curve (Figure 48.1) is shifted to the right in patients with chronic hypertension and to the left in neonates.

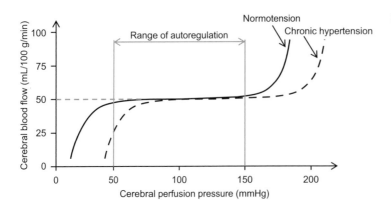

Figure 48.1 Cerebral autoregulation.

What happens to neurons when CBF falls below 50 mL/100 g/min?

The brain is more sensitive to even short periods of ischaemia than any other organ in the body. For example, a reduction in CBF to 30 mL/100 g/min for just 5 s, as may occur during a vasovagal episode, results in loss of consciousness. As CBF decreases, there is a corresponding reduction in cerebral O_2 delivery, which leads to cellular ischaemia:

- CBF < 50 mL/100 g/min results in cellular acidosis.
- CBF < 40 mL/100 g/min results in impaired protein synthesis.
- CBF < 30 mL/100 g/min results in cellular oedema.
- CBF < 20 mL/100 g/min leads to failure of cell membrane ion pumps, with loss of transmembrane electrochemical gradients.
- CBF < 10 mL/100 g/min results in cellular death.

What is meant by the term 'flow–metabolism coupling'?

Although the overall CBF remains close to 50 mL/100 g/min, blood is preferentially routed to the most metabolically active brain regions. For example, CBF to grey matter is 70 mL/100 g/min, whereas CBF to white matter is only 20 mL/100 g/min. Areas of metabolically active brain have higher concentrations of vasodilatory metabolites (e.g. CO_2, H^+, K^+ and adenosine), thereby increasing local blood flow and O_2 delivery.

Which other factors affect global CBF?

Just as local CBF is closely matched to local cerebral metabolic rate (CMR), total brain CBF is matched to total brain metabolism. An increase in overall CMR, as occurs in status epilepticus or pyrexia, results in a corresponding increase in CBF. Likewise, a decrease in CMR, as occurs with general anaesthesia or hypothermia, results in a corresponding fall in CBF.

In addition to locally produced metabolites, cerebral vessel tone (and therefore CVR) is affected by a number of blood constituents:

- CO_2. An increase in the P_aCO_2 results in cerebral arteriolar vasodilatation. CVR is reduced, resulting in a corresponding increase in CBF. Likewise, hypocapnoea results in cerebral arteriolar vasoconstriction and a corresponding reduction in CBF. CBF shows an approximately linear relationship with P_aCO_2 between 3.5 and 8 kPa (Figure 48.2a). Outside these limits:
  - $P_aCO_2 > 8$ kPa: the cerebral arteries are already maximally vasodilated. Any further increase in P_aCO_2 has no effect on CVR or CBF.

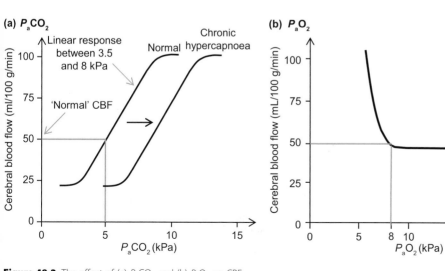

Figure 48.2 The effect of (a) P_aCO_2 and (b) P_aO_2 on CBF.

- $P_aCO_2 < 3.5\ kPa$: the cerebral arteries are already maximally vasoconstricted. A further reduction in P_aCO_2 causes no additional vasoconstriction, but the resulting alkalosis may shift the oxyhaemoglobin curve to the left, reducing the offloading of O_2 to the brain. The resulting brain tissue hypoxia causes cerebral arterial vasodilatation and thus an increase in CBF (see below).

- **O_2.** This has little effect on the cerebral arterioles at 'normal' P_aO_2. However, a fall in P_aO_2 below 8 kPa triggers an early vasodilatation of the cerebral arterioles, resulting in a significant increase in CBF (Figure 48.2b).

- **Blood haematocrit.** According to the Hagen–Poiseuille equation (see Chapter 34), flow increases as viscosity decreases. Marked reductions in haematocrit cause a decrease in blood viscosity, and this can lead to an increase in CBF. However, blood of lower haematocrit contains less haemoglobin (Hb) and can therefore deliver less O_2 to the brain parenchyma. The optimum balance between CBF and cerebral O_2 delivery is said to occur at a haematocrit of 0.3.

- **Autonomic nervous system.** Under normal physiological conditions, neurogenic control appears to exert little influence on cerebral autoregulation in relationship to the remaining vasomotor, chemical, and metabolic control mechanisms.

Clinical relevance: effect of drugs on CBF

A number of anaesthetic drugs have important effects on CBF:

- **Intravenous induction agents**:
  - Propofol, thiopentone and etomidate all reduce CMR. Owing to flow–metabolism coupling, these drugs all accordingly reduce CBF.
  - In contrast, ketamine increases CMR and thus may increase CBF.

- **The volatile anaesthetic agents** are unique in uncoupling CMR and CBF. Whilst they decrease CMR, which would be expected to decrease CBF, they also cause cerebral arteriolar vasodilatation, which has the effect of increasing CBF. Which of these two effects is predominant depends on the volatile agent and its partial pressure:

  - *Below approximately 1 MAC* (minimum alveolar concentration), both effects are approximately equal; CBF is unchanged.
  - *Above approximately 1 MAC*, the reduction in CMR is already maximal, and CBF increases due to cerebral arteriolar vasodilatation.

Of the available volatile anaesthetic agents, sevoflurane has the lowest propensity for cerebral arteriolar vasodilatation.

- **N_2O** is a potent cerebral arteriolar vasodilator and also increases CMR. As a result of both effects, its use is associated with a significant increase in CBF.

- **Opioids** have no significant effect on either CMR or CBF.

How can CBF be measured?

CBF can be measured by a number of methods. The two methods most commonly encountered in clinical practice are:

- **Transcranial Doppler ultrasonography.** This is by far the most common clinical method of measuring CBF. An ultrasound probe is placed on the temple and the Doppler principle is used to determine the velocity of blood in the middle cerebral artery. From this, CBF in one half of the brain can be estimated. Transcranial Doppler is also used to detect emboli during carotid endarterectomy and to diagnose vasospasm following subarachnoid haemorrhage.

- **Jugular bulb catheterisation.** The jugular bulb is a dilatation of the internal jugular vein, just below the base of the skull. The jugular bulb can be catheterised by using a Seldinger technique similar to inserting a central line, but instead the needle is directed cranially. Once the tip of the catheter is within the jugular bulb, blood can be sampled for O_2 tension, Hb O_2 saturation and lactate. This method estimates the overall adequacy of CBF on the ipsilateral side of the brain, but does not give any information about regional blood flow within the brain.

- **Functional magnetic resonance imaging** (fMRI) and **positron emission tomography** (PET) rely on flow–metabolism coupling to identify areas of increased activity in the brain. fMRI analyses the brain for areas of O_2-rich blood and O_2-poor blood, whilst PET utilises a radioactive analogue of glucose.

The following are primarily research methods:

- **Kety–Schmidt technique**, which applies the Fick principle using arterial and jugular venous N_2O concentrations. Only global CBF can be measured using this method.
- **Radioactive xenon-133**. The radioactive decay of injected radioactive isotope ^{133}Xe can be detected by a gamma-camera, giving information about regional CBF.

Further reading

M. ter Laan, J. M. C. van Dijk, J. W. J. Elting, et al. Sympathetic regulation of cerebral blood flow in humans: a review. *Br J Anaesth* 2013; **111**(3): 361–7.

C. Ayata. Spreading depression and neurovascular coupling. *Stroke* 2013; **44**(6 Suppl. 1): S87–9.

E. C. Peterson, Z. Wang, G. Britz. Regulation of cerebral blood flow. *Int J Vasc Med* 2011; **2011**: 823525.

Intracranial Pressure and Head Injury

What is intracranial pressure? How is it measured?

The intracranial pressure (ICP) is simply the hydrostatic pressure within the skull, reflecting the pressure of the cerebrospinal fluid (CSF) and brain parenchyma. At rest in a normal supine adult, ICP is 5–15 mmHg; ICP varies throughout the cardiac and respiratory cycles. Even in a normal brain, coughing, straining and sneezing can transiently increase ICP to as high as 50 mmHg.

Unfortunately, ICP cannot be estimated, only invasively measured. ICP may be measured by a variety of devices, each with their advantages and disadvantages:

- **External ventricular drain** (EVD): a catheter inserted into the lateral ventricle, which is considered the 'gold standard' for measuring ICP. In addition to ICP measurement, an EVD can be used to remove CSF for diagnostic and therapeutic purposes (to reduce ICP – see later) and for the administration of intrathecal medication. However, to measure ICP, the EVD must be 'clamped'; that is, CSF cannot be simultaneously drained. An EVD may be surgically challenging to insert, especially if the ventricles are small or displaced. Also, EVDs are frequently complicated by blockage and are associated with an infection risk of up to 5%.
- **Intraparenchymal probe**: a fibre-optic-tipped catheter placed within the brain parenchyma through a small burr hole. An intraparenchymal probe is much easier to insert than an EVD and can be used in situations where the ventricles are compressed or displaced. Measurement of ICP using an intraparenchymal probe is almost as accurate as an EVD, and infection rates are substantially lower. However, there are concerns about the accuracy of intraparenchymal catheters used for prolonged periods: the catheter is zeroed at the time of insertion and cannot be recalibrated in situ.[1] An intraparenchymal probe only measures the pressure of the brain parenchyma in which it is located, which may not represent global ICP.
- **Subarachnoid and subdural probes**: now considered relatively obsolete. Although associated with a low rate of infection, these probes are less accurate, prone to blockage and require regular flushing.

What is the Monro–Kellie hypothesis?

The Monro–Kellie hypothesis states that the cranium is a rigid box of fixed volume, which contains:

- **Brain tissue**, 1400 g or approximately 80% of the intracranial volume;
- **CSF**, 150 mL or approximately 10% of intracranial volume;
- **Arterial and venous blood**, 150 mL or approximately 10% of intracranial volume.

An increase in the volume of any of these intracranial contents will increase ICP, unless there is also a corresponding reduction in the volume of one or both of the other contents. For example:

- An increase in the volume of brain tissue may be localised (e.g. a brain tumour or abscess) or generalised (as occurs with cerebral oedema).
- The volume of CSF may be increased in hydrocephalus (see Chapter 46).
- The volume of intracranial blood may be increased following haemorrhage (extradural, subdural or intraparenchymal) or venous sinus thrombosis.

---

[1] However, drift has been shown to be as little as 1 mmHg after 5 days' use.

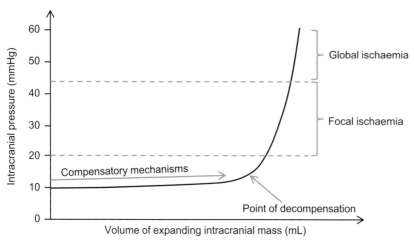

Figure 49.1 Change in intracranial pressure with increasing intracranial volume.

When one of the intracranial contents increases in volume, there is a limited capacity for displacement of the other contents:

- Some CSF is displaced from the cranium into the spinal subarachnoid space. Whilst the rate of CSF production remains approximately the same, CSF absorption by the arachnoid villi is increased.
- Dural venous sinuses are compressed, displacing venous blood into the internal jugular vein, thus reducing the volume of intracranial blood.

After these small compensatory changes have occurred, ICP will rise. The only options left are then potentially disastrous: a reduction in arterial blood volume or displacement of brain parenchyma through the foramen magnum (Figure 49.1).

- **Symptoms suggesting raised ICP** include:
  - A headache that is worse in the morning and is exacerbated by straining and lying flat;
  - Nausea and vomiting.
- **Signs of raised ICP** include:
  - A bulging, tense fontanelle in infants and neonates;
  - Papilloedema;
  - Altered consciousness.
- **Severe intracranial hypertension** may result in additional signs as a result of brain displacement:
  - *Cranial nerve palsies*: most commonly the abducens (cranial nerve VI) due to its lengthy course through the skull.

  - *Pupillary dilatation*: caused by compression of the oculomotor nerve (cranial nerve III).
  - *Cushing's triad*:

    - Systemic hypertension;
    - Bradycardia;
    - Abnormal respiratory pattern.

Can you explain Cushing's triad?

As discussed in Chapter 48, cerebral perfusion pressure (CPP) is related to mean arterial pressure (MAP) and ICP:

$$CPP = MAP - ICP$$

According to this equation, an increase in ICP results in a decrease in CPP, unless MAP also increases.

The Cushing response is a late physiological response to increasing ICP. When CPP falls below 50 mmHg, the cerebral arterioles are maximally vasodilated and cerebral autoregulation fails. Cerebral blood flow (CBF) falls below the 'normal' value of 50 mL/100 g/min, resulting in cellular ischaemia (Chapter 48, Figure 48.1).

In the event of brainstem ischaemia, the brain has an 'emergency' hypertensive mechanism: the vasomotor area dramatically increases sympathetic nervous system outflow, triggering an intense systemic arteriolar vasoconstriction that results in systemic hypertension. The rise in MAP restores perfusion, and hence CBF, to the brainstem. In response to systemic hypertension, the arterial baroreceptors induce a reflex bradycardia.

If ICP continues to rise, the brain parenchyma starts to be displaced downwards. The cerebellar tonsils are pushed through the foramen magnum, a process referred to as 'tonsillar herniation' or 'coning'. The cerebellar tonsils compress the brainstem, causing the failure of brainstem functions:

- *Irregular breathing and apnoea* through compression of the respiratory centre;
- *Decreased consciousness*: Glasgow Coma Scale (GCS) of 3–5 is usual;
- *Hypotension*, as the vasomotor centre is compressed.

The Cushing reflex is a desperate attempt to maintain CPP (and therefore CBF) in the face of substantially increased ICP. Unless swift action is taken (and often despite this being done), brainstem death is inevitable.

How may ICP be reduced?

The Monro–Kellie hypothesis states that an increase in the volume of one of the three intracranial contents will cause an increase in ICP, unless there is also a reduction in the volume of one or both of the other components. It therefore follows that ICP may be reduced if the volume of one or more of the intracranial contents is reduced:

- **Reduction in the volume of CSF** by means of an EVD. This method can be used to reduce ICP even when hydrocephalus is not the cause. Even the removal of a few millilitres of CSF can result in a significant decrease in ICP.
- **Reduction in the volume of blood**: if the cause of raised ICP is a haematoma, this should be urgently evacuated. Otherwise, in the context of raised ICP, intracranial venous and arterial blood can be considered as two entirely different entities:
  - *Venous blood*. Intracranial venous blood serves no useful purpose and should be permitted to drain from the cranium. As ICP increases, the dural venous sinuses are compressed, displacing blood into the internal jugular vein, thereby reducing the volume of intracranial venous blood. As the dural venous sinuses do not have valves, venous drainage from the cranium is entirely dependent on the venous pressure gradient between the venous sinuses and the right atrium and is therefore promoted by:

- Keeping the head in a neutral position and removing neck collars and tight-fitting endotracheal tube (ETT) ties, which prevent kinking or occlusion of the internal jugular veins.
- Nursing the patient in a 30° head-up tilt.
- Using minimal positive end-expiratory pressure (PEEP). Positive intrathoracic pressure reduces the venous pressure gradient. Therefore, in ventilated patients, PEEP should be reduced to the lowest value required to achieve adequate oxygenation.
- Using muscle relaxants to prevent coughing and straining, both of which transiently increase intrathoracic pressure.

  - *Arterial blood*. An adequate volume of well-oxygenated arterial blood is essential to meet the metabolic demands of the brain, but CBF in excess of that required merely serves to increase ICP. Therefore, the goal is to provide just sufficient CBF to meet the brain's metabolic needs. Two main strategies are employed:

    - **Reducing cerebral metabolic rate** (CMR). Owing to flow–metabolism coupling, CBF is related to CMR. Seizure activity substantially increases CMR, which in turn increases CBF and consequently increases ICP – seizures should be rapidly treated with benzodiazepines and anti-epileptic drugs. CMR may be reduced to subnormal levels through the use of drugs (propofol, thiopentone or benzodiazepines such as midazolam).
    - **Preventing hypoxaemia or hypercapnoea**. As discussed in Chapter 48, hypoxaemia and hypercapnoea both trigger cerebral arteriolar vasodilatation, which increases CBF and consequently increases ICP. In situations of raised ICP, P_aO_2 should be maintained above 10 kPa and P_aCO_2 between 4.5 and 5.0 kPa.

- **Reduction in the volume of brain parenchyma**:
  - Severely raised ICP may be temporarily reduced by decreasing brain extracellular fluid volume through osmotherapy, following intravenous administration of an osmotic diuretic: mannitol or hypertonic saline.

- When raised ICP is caused by a brain tumour, the volume of surrounding oedema may be reduced by using dexamethasone, or surgical excision may be considered.
- The volume of a cerebral abscess may be reduced by surgical drainage and by antibiotic therapy.

Finally, if all other measures have failed to control a raised ICP, then a decompressive craniectomy may be performed. A decompressive craniectomy is a neuro-surgical procedure whereby a bone flap is removed from the cranium and the overlying skin closed, thus allowing the brain to herniate upwards through the skull defect.

How is head injury classified?

Head injury is defined as any trauma to the head, whether or not brain injury has occurred. Head injury may be classified by:

- **Mechanism of injury**, which may be blunt (road traffic collision or fall) or penetrating (gunshot or stab injury). In the military setting, blast injury can also occur. Blunt head injury may be:
    - *Closed*, where the dura mater remains intact;
    - *Open*, where the dura mater is breached, exposing the brain and CSF to environmental microorganisms. Penetrating head injury is, by definition, open.
- **Presence of other injuries**. Following trauma, patients may have an isolated head injury or there may be accompanying traumatic injuries.

Where a head injury results in a traumatic brain injury (TBI), further classifications can be made:

- **Severity of injury**. On arrival to hospital, the severity of TBI is commonly assessed using the post-resuscitation GCS:
    - *Mild TBI* corresponds to a GCS score of 13–15.
    - *Moderate TBI* corresponds to a GCS score of 9–12.
    - *Severe TBI* corresponds to a GCS score of 3–8.

Patients presenting with mild TBI have a good prognosis with a mortality rate of 0.1%. However, patients with moderate and severe TBI have much higher mortality rates of around 10% and 50%, respectively. Many survivors are left with severe disability.

- **Area of brain injury**. Brain injury can be focal (e.g. extradural haematoma, contusions) or diffuse (e.g. diffuse axonal injury, hypoxic brain injury), but both types of injury commonly coexist.

What is the difference between primary and secondary brain injury?

Brain injury may be classified as primary or secondary:

- **Primary brain injury** is damage to the brain during the initial injury caused by mechanical forces: stretching and shearing of neuronal and vascular tissue. Neuronal tissue is more susceptible to damage than blood vessels; this is why diffuse axonal injury frequently accompanies injuries where there has been vessel disruption, such as extradural haematoma or traumatic subarachnoid haemorrhage.
- **Secondary brain injury** refers to the further cellular damage caused by the pathophysiological consequences of the primary injury. Cells injured in the initial trauma trigger inflammatory reactions, resulting in cerebral oedema and an increase in ICP. Secondary brain injury occurs hours to days after the primary injury through a number of different mechanisms:
    - Damage to the blood–brain barrier;
    - Cerebral oedema;
    - Raised ICP;
    - Seizures;
    - Ischaemia;
    - Infection.

Once primary brain injury has occurred, it cannot be reversed. Prevention of trauma is the best method of reducing primary brain injury: reducing speed limits, safer driving strategies, and so on. The impact of trauma on the brain can be reduced by the use of airbags and seatbelts in cars, and of helmets for cyclists and motorcyclists. Medical and surgical efforts are concentrated on preventing secondary brain injury: preserving as many neurons as possible.

How would you approach the management of a patient with TBI?

Patients with TBI frequently present with other, more immediately life-threatening injuries. The broad principles of initial trauma management are the same whether in the emergency department or the prehospital setting: with a multidisciplinary team following an airway–breathing–circulation–disability–exposure (ABCDE) approach, ensuring spinal immobilisation and treating life-threatening injuries first.

Following the initial resuscitation phase, patients with suspected TBI will require rapid transfer for brain imaging, the results of which will help guide further medical and surgical management.

What are the main principles of medical management in a patient with TBI?

The medical management of TBI is concerned with preventing secondary brain injury and reducing ICP. It is divided into maintenance of:

- **Normoxia.** Hypoxaemia (defined as $P_aO_2 < 8$ kPa) is associated with a worse outcome following TBI due to its detrimental effects on CBF and hence ICP. Hypoxaemia may occur for a number of reasons, such as airway obstruction, associated chest injuries and aspiration pneumonitis. In the initial resuscitation phase, all trauma patients should have high-flow O_2 administered, and patients with the potential to develop hypoxaemia (e.g. those with a low GCS) should be intubated at an early stage.

- **Normotension.** A fall in CPP below 50 mmHg leads to failure of cerebral autoregulation, reduced CBF and cellular ischaemia. Therefore, in the neurointensive care unit, when ICP is being measured, CPP should be kept above 60 mmHg. Unfortunately, trauma patients do not arrive in hospital with ICP monitoring *in situ* – the Association of Anaesthetists of Great Britain and Ireland (AAGBI) recommends maintaining MAP > 80 mmHg. This should be achieved initially using fluid resuscitation, or blood if significant haemorrhage is suspected. Even a single episode in which systolic blood pressure is <90 mmHg has been shown to worsen outcome.

  Hypertension can also be detrimental: the hypertensive response to laryngoscopy can cause a surge in MAP, exceeding the upper limit of autoregulation, which causes a surge in CBF and consequently an increase in ICP. Therefore, when intubating a patient with suspected TBI, some means of attenuating the sympathetic response to

laryngoscopy should be used, such as pretreatment with a strong opioid.

- **Normocapnoea.** As discussed in Chapter 48, CBF varies linearly with P_aCO_2 (see Chapter 48, Figure 48.2a). Hypercapnoea causes cerebral arteriolar vasodilatation, increasing CBF above 50 mL/100 g/min, which consequently increases ICP. Hypocapnoea causes cerebral arteriolar vasoconstriction, reducing CBF to below 50 mL/100 g/min, inducing cellular ischaemia. The AAGBI recommends maintaining P_aCO_2 between 4.5 and 5.0 kPa following TBI.

- **Normoglycaemia.** Normally, the brain uses glucose as its sole metabolic substrate. The stress response to TBI commonly results in hyperglycaemia, which is associated with a worse overall outcome. Insulin therapy is indicated when plasma glucose rises and is typically instituted at a plasma glucose concentration of 11 mmol/L.

  Hypoglycaemia is rarely the direct result of TBI, but a hypoglycaemic episode in an insulin-dependent diabetic may have been the cause of the traumatic incident. Hypoglycaemia further exacerbates cellular acidosis within the brain; prolonged hypoglycaemia may result in neuronal cell death.

- **Normothermia.** Pyrexia (defined as core body temperature > 37.6°C) increases CMR, which leads to an increase in CBF and consequently an increase in ICP. Hyperthermia should therefore be treated promptly using an antipyretic (such as paracetamol) and external cooling devices.

- **Venous drainage.** This is promoted by nursing the patient in a 30° head-up tilt, with a neutral head position and ensuring that ETT ties are loose. Minimal PEEP should be used.

Further reading

M. D. Wiles. Blood pressure in trauma resuscitation: 'pop the clot' vs. 'drain the brain'? *Anaesthesia* 2017; **72**(12): 1448–55.

R. T. Protheroe, C. L. Gwinnutt. Early hospital care of severe traumatic brain injury. *Anaesthesia* 2011; **66**(11): 1035–47.

K. Pattinson, G. Wynne-Jones, C. H. E. Imray. Monitoring intracranial pressure, perfusion and metabolism. *Continuing Educ Anaesth Crit Care Pain* 2005; **5**(4): 130–3.

The Spinal Cord

Describe the anatomy of the spinal cord

The spinal cord is part of the central nervous system (CNS), located within the spinal canal of the vertebral column. The spinal cord begins at the foramen magnum, where it is continuous with the medulla oblongata. The spinal cord is much shorter than the vertebral column, ending at a vertebral level of L1/2 in adults, but at a lower level of around L3 in neonates.

Like the brain, the spinal cord is enveloped in three layers of the meninges: pia, arachnoid and dura mater. Cerebrospinal fluid (CSF) surrounds the spinal cord in the subarachnoid space and extends inferiorly within the dural sac to approximately the S2 level. After the spinal cord terminates, the pia and dura merge to form the filum terminale, which tethers the cord to the coccyx.

The spinal cord is divided into 31 segments, each emitting a pair of spinal nerves. There are:

- Eight cervical segments. Note: there is one more pair of cervical nerves emitted than there are cervical vertebrae.
- Twelve thoracic segments.
- Five lumbar segments.
- Five sacral segments.
- One coccygeal segment.

With the exception of C1 and C2, the spinal nerves exit the spinal canal through the intervertebral foramina.

The spinal cord enlarges in two regions:

- **The cervical enlargement at C4–T1,** corresponding to the brachial plexus, which innervates the upper limbs;
- **The lumbar enlargement at L2–S3,** corresponding to the lumbar plexus, which innervates the lower limbs.

At the terminal end of the spinal cord:

- **The conus medullaris** is the tapered terminal portion of the cord.
- **The cauda equina** is the collection of spinal nerves that continue inferiorly in the spinal canal after the cord has ended, until they reach their respective intervertebral foramina.

Describe the cross-sectional anatomy of the spinal cord

In cross-section, the spinal cord is approximately oval, with a deep anterior median sulcus and a shallow posterior median sulcus. The centre of the cord contains an approximately 'H'-shaped area of grey matter, surrounded by white matter:

- The grey matter contains unmyelinated axons and the cell bodies of interneurons and motor neurons. Located in the centre of the grey matter is the CSF-containing central canal. The points of the 'H' correspond to the dorsal and ventral (posterior and anterior) horns. There are also lateral horns in the thoracic region of the cord, which correspond to pre-ganglionic sympathetic neurons.
- The white matter contains columns of myelinated axons, called tracts. These tracts are organised into:

  - *Ascending tracts*, containing sensory axons;
  - *Descending tracts*, containing motor axons.

The most important ascending tracts are shown in Figure 50.1:

- **The dorsal (posterior) columns** contain axons of nerves concerned with proprioception (position sense), vibration and two-point discrimination (fine touch).
- **The anterior and lateral spinothalamic tracts** carry sensory information about pain, temperature, crude touch and pressure.

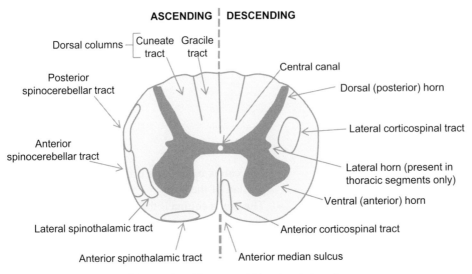

Figure 50.1 Cross-section of the spinal cord (extrapyramidal tracts not shown).

- **The anterior and posterior spinocerebellar tracts** carry proprioceptive information from the muscles and joints to the cerebellum.

The most important descending tracts are (Figure 50.1):

- **The anterior and lateral corticospinal tracts**, also known as the pyramidal tracts, carry the axons of upper motor neurons. In the ventral horn of the spinal cord, these axons relay to α-motor neurons (or lower motor neurons) that innervate muscle.
- **The extrapyramidal tracts**: rubrospinal, tectospinal, vestibulospinal, olivospinal and reticulospinal tracts. The extrapyramidal neurons originate at brainstem nuclei and do not pass through the medullary pyramids. Their primary role is in the control of posture and muscle tone.

Describe the blood supply to the spinal cord

The spinal cord is supplied by three arteries, derived from the posterior circulation of circle of Willis (see Chapter 45). However, the blood flow through these vessels is insufficient to perfuse the cord below the cervical region – an additional contribution from radicular arteries is essential. The three spinal arteries are:

- **One anterior spinal artery**, which arises from branches of the right and left vertebral artery (see Chapter 45, Figure 45.1). The anterior spinal artery descends in the anterior median sulcus and supplies the anterior two-thirds of the spinal

cord – essentially all of the structures, with the exception of the dorsal columns. The anterior spinal artery is replenished along its length by several radicular arteries, the largest of which is called the artery of Adamkiewicz. The location of this vessel is variable, but is most commonly found on the left between T8 and L1.

- **Two posterior spinal arteries**, which arise from the posterior inferior cerebellar arteries (see Chapter 45, Figure 45.1). The posterior spinal arteries are located just medial to the dorsal roots and supply the posterior third of the cord. Again, the posterior spinal arteries are replenished by radicular arteries.

Blood from the spinal cord is drained via three anterior and three posterior spinal veins located in the pia mater, which anastomose to form a tortuous venous plexus. Blood from this plexus drains into the epidural venous plexus.

Clinical relevance: anterior spinal artery syndrome
The artery of Adamkiewicz most commonly arises from the left posterior intercostal artery, a branch of the aorta. Damage or obstruction of the artery can occur through atherosclerotic disease, aortic dissection or surgical clamping during aortic aneurysm repair. As the anterior spinal artery supplies the anterior two-thirds of the spinal cord, cessation of blood flow can have profound consequences (Figure 50.4).

Signs and symptoms of anterior spinal artery syndrome are:

- **Paraplegia**, as a result of involvement of α-motor neurons within the anterior horn of the cord (i.e. a lower motor neuron deficit at the level of the lesion) and the corticospinal tracts carrying the axons of upper motor neurons (i.e. an upper motor neuron deficit below the level of the lesion).
- **Loss of pain and temperature sensation** due to involvement of the spinothalamic tracts.
- **Autonomic dysfunction** involving the bladder or bowel due to disruption of the sacral parasympathetic neurons.

Crucially, proprioception and vibration sensation remain intact. These sensory modalities are carried in the dorsal columns, which are supplied by the posterior spinal arteries and thus remain unaffected.

Describe the main sensory afferent pathways

The somatosensory nervous system consists of:

- **Sensory receptors**, which encode stimuli by repetitive firing of action potentials. The different sensory receptor types are specific to their sensory modalities: proprioceptors, nociceptors, thermoreceptors and mechanoreceptors relay sensory information concerning limb position, tissue damage (potentially causing pain), temperature and touch, respectively. The perception of the stimulus is dependent upon the neuronal pathway rather than the sensory receptor itself. For example, pressing on the eye activates the optic nerve and gives the impression of light, despite the stimulus being pressure rather than photons.
- **First-order neurons** transmit action potentials from sensory receptors to the spinal cord, where they synapse with second-order neurons. These neurons are pseudounipolar, with their cell bodies located in the dorsal root ganglion, a swelling of the dorsal root just outside the spinal cord.
- **Second-order neurons** conduct action potentials to the thalamus, where they synapse with third-order neurons.
- **Third-order neurons** relay action potentials to the cerebral cortex via the internal capsule.

- **The primary somatosensory cortex** is the area of the cerebral cortex that receives and performs an initial processing of the sensory information. It is organised in a somatotropic way with specific areas of cortex dedicated to specific areas of the body, known as the sensory homunculus. Of note: the hands and lips make up a major component, reflecting their tactile importance.

There are two major pathways by which sensory information ascends in the spinal cord:

- **The dorsal column–medial lemniscal (DCML) pathway** carries sensory information about two-point discrimination, vibration and proprioception (Figure 50.2a). The name of the pathway comes from the two structures through which the sensory signals pass: the dorsal columns of the spinal cord and the medial lemniscus in the brainstem:

  - The first-order neuron is extremely long. It enters the dorsal root of the spinal cord and ascends in the dorsal columns on the same side (ipsilateral). Sensory neurons from the lower body travel in the medial gracile tract and synapse in the gracile nucleus in the medulla oblongata, whilst sensory neurons from the upper body travel in the lateral cuneate tract and synapse in the cuneate nucleus.[1]
  - In the medulla, first-order neurons synapse with second-order neurons, which then cross over to the contralateral side and ascend to the thalamus. After this sensory decussation, the fibres ascend through the brainstem in a tract called the medial lemniscus.

- **The spinothalamic tract** carries sensory information about crude touch, pressure, temperature and pain (Figure 50.2b). In contrast to the DCML pathway, the spinothalamic tract crosses the midline at the level of the spinal cord rather than the medulla:

  - The first-order neurons enter the dorsal root of the spinal cord and may ascend or descend one or two vertebral levels (along Lissauer's tract) before synapsing with second-order neurons in the dorsal horn.

---

[1] Remember: the 'foot' treads on the 'grass' (gracile)

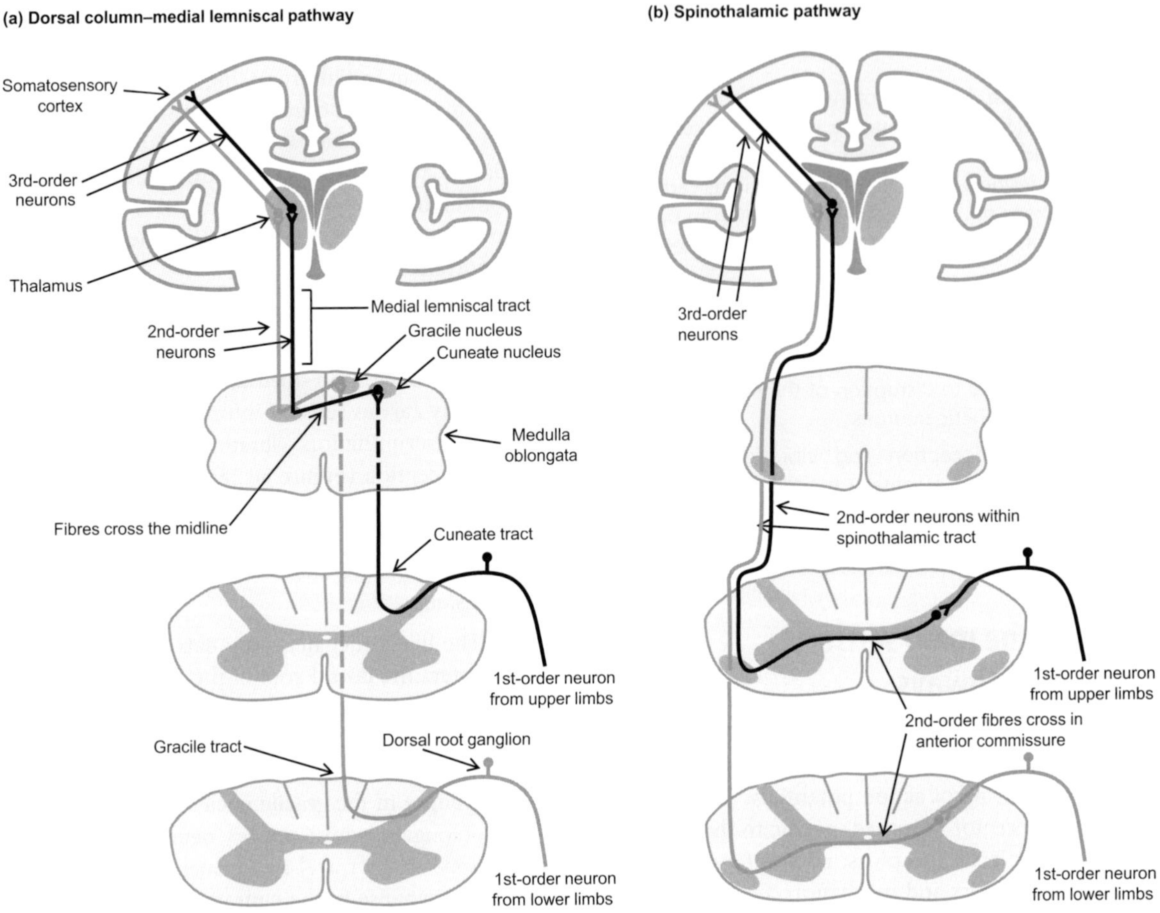

(a) Dorsal column–medial lemniscal pathway

(b) Spinothalamic pathway

Figure 50.2 The two major sensory pathways: (a) dorsal column–medial lemniscal and (b) spinothalamic.

The axons of the second-order neurons decussate anterior to the central canal of the spinal cord, in an area called the anterior commissure, before ascending to the thalamus in the contralateral spinothalamic tract.

Clinical relevance: dissociated sensory loss

Dissociated sensory loss is a relatively rare pattern of neurological injury characterised by the selective loss of two-point discrimination, vibration sense and proprioception without the loss of pain and temperature, or vice versa. This is due to the different points of decussation of the DCML and spinothalamic tracts. Causes of dissociated sensory loss include:

- **Brown-Séquard syndrome**, in which a hemi-section of the spinal cord causes ipsilateral motor weakness, ipsilateral loss of two-point discrimination, proprioception and vibration sensation with contralateral loss of pain and temperature sensation below the level of the lesion (see Figure 50.4). Hemi-section of the cord may be the result of trauma (e.g. a gunshot wound), inflammatory disease (e.g. multiple sclerosis) or by local compression: spinal cord tumour or infection (e.g. tuberculosis).

- **Syringomyelia**, a condition in which the central canal of the spinal cord expands over time (referred to as a syrinx), destroying surrounding structures. The axons of the spinothalamic tract that decussate at the anterior commissure are usually the first to be damaged. The clinical consequence is loss of pain and temperature sensation at the level of the syrinx, usually involving the upper limbs, with preservation of

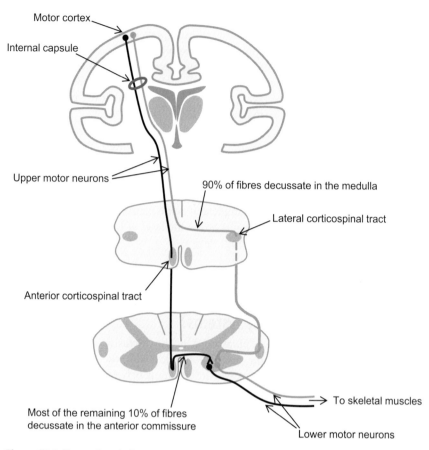

Figure 50.3 The corticospinal tract.

two-point discrimination, proprioception and vibration sensation.

- **Lateral medullary syndrome**, a brainstem stroke in which occlusion of the posterior inferior cerebellar artery causes infarction of the lateral medulla, a very important area containing, amongst other structures,[2] the spinothalamic tracts from the contralateral side of the body and the trigeminal nerve nuclei. Clinically, therefore, lateral medullary syndrome is characterised by loss of pain and temperature sensation on the contralateral side of the body and the ipsilateral side of the face.

---

[2] Other important structures affected are the vestibular nuclei (resulting in nystagmus and vertigo), the inferior cerebellar peduncle (resulting in ataxia), the nucleus ambiguus (affecting cranial nerves IX and X, resulting in dysphagia and hoarseness) and the sympathetic chain (resulting in an ipsilateral Horner's syndrome).

Describe the course of the corticospinal tract

The corticospinal tract, also known as the pyramidal tract, is the most important descending tract as it is the primary route for somatic motor neurons. The corticospinal tract is composed of (Figure 50.3):

- **The motor cortex**, located in the pre-central gyrus. This area is the brain's final common output, resulting in the initiation of movement.
- **An upper motor neuron**, which originates in the motor cortex and descends through the spinal cord within the corticospinal tract:

  - Upper motor neurons travel through the posterior limb of the internal capsule.
  - At the level of the pons, a significant proportion of upper motor neurons synapse in the pontine nuclei, forming the ventral part of the pons. These postsynaptic fibres then travel

posteriorly to reach the cerebellum through the middle cerebral peduncle.

- At the medullary pyramids, 90% of the remaining nerve fibres decussate and descend in the lateral corticospinal tract of the spinal cord.
- The 10% of nerve fibres that do not decussate descend in a separate ipsilateral tract: the anterior corticospinal tract.[3]
- When they have reached their intended vertebral level in the spinal cord, the upper motor neurons synapse with lower motor neurons in the ventral horn of the spinal cord.

- **A lower motor neuron**, which leaves the CNS to innervate skeletal muscle. There are two types of lower motor neuron:

- *α-motor neurons* leave the anterior horn, forming the spinal nerve. The spinal nerve exits the spinal canal via the intervertebral foramen, becoming a peripheral nerve. Ultimately, the α-motor neuron innervates extrafusal fibres of skeletal muscle, causing muscle contraction.
- *γ-motor neurons* innervate the intrafusal fibres of skeletal muscle (the 'muscle spindles'), which are involved in proprioception (see Chapter 55).

How can acute spinal cord injury be classified?

Spinal cord injury is often devastating – permanent neurological injury is common. Spinal cord injury can be classified in a number of ways:

- **Level of injury**. The majority of injuries occur in the cervical and thoracic regions of the spinal cord – lumbar cord injuries are much less common. A higher level of the cord injury results in a greater loss of neurological function.
- **Stability of vertebral column**. The vertebral column is anatomically divided into anterior, middle and posterior columns. Unstable vertebral fractures (those potentially involving anything

other than solely the anterior column) require immobilisation to prevent further damage to the spinal cord. The high mobility of the cervical spine makes it especially vulnerable to unstable fractures; fortunately, the spinal cord has more space within the spinal canal at the cervical level than elsewhere.

- **Extent of neurological injury**. Approximately half of spinal cord injuries involve complete transection of the cord, with an absence of motor and sensory neurological function below the level of injury. A spinal cord injury is said to be 'incomplete' if some neurological function remains below the level of injury (e.g. sacral sparing).

How does the level of a complete spinal cord injury affect the different body systems?

The spinal cord is the exclusive relay of sensory, motor and autonomic (with the exception of the vagus nerve) information between the CNS and the peripheries. The level of spinal cord injury determines whether individual organs will remain in communication with the brain:

- **Respiratory system**. Respiratory failure is common after spinal cord injury; respiratory complications are the most common cause of death. The higher the spinal cord lesion, the greater the impact on ventilation:

- *Injury above T8 vertebral level* will cause intercostal muscle weakness or paralysis. The 'bucket-handle' mechanism for respiratory movements is abolished and diaphragmatic contraction becomes the sole mechanism of inspiration. The loss of intercostal muscle tone reduces the outward spring of the chest wall. The functional residual capacity, which reflects the volume at which the inward elastic recoil of the lung equals the outward spring of the chest wall, is therefore reduced.
- *Injury below C5 vertebral level* does not directly affect diaphragmatic contraction (the phrenic nerve is formed by the C3, C4 and C5 nerve roots). However, diaphragmatic contraction is indirectly affected as a result of intercostal muscle paralysis: the loss of intercostal muscle tone results in paradoxical

---

[3] Most of these upper motor neurons decussate in the spinal cord (through the anterior commissure) before synapsing with a lower motor neuron.

movement of the chest wall – it is drawn inwards during diaphragmatic contraction. As a result, vital capacity reduces by up to 50%.

- *Injury at C3 vertebral level and above* will result in paralysis of all respiratory muscles. Patients have gross ventilatory impairment requiring immediate ventilatory support. These patients usually require long-term mechanical ventilation or phrenic nerve stimulation.

Spinal cord injury also alters lung mechanics in other ways:

- Paralysis of the external intercostal muscles and the abdominal muscles results in markedly reduced forced expiratory gas flows. Forced expiratory volume in 1 s is significantly reduced and cough is severely impaired, leading to impaired clearance of respiratory secretions.
- Impaired inspiration results in basal atelectasis, reduced lung compliance and $\dot{V}/\dot{Q}$ mismatch.
- As a consequence of the lower lung volume, the production of pulmonary surfactant is reduced. Lung compliance is further decreased, which increases the work of breathing.
- Rarely, neurogenic pulmonary oedema can result from cervical cord injury, though the mechanism for this is unclear.

- **Cardiovascular system.** Like the respiratory system, the cardiovascular consequences of spinal cord injury are more significant with higher spinal cord lesions. Adverse cardiovascular effects result from the interruption of the sympathetic nervous system:

- *Injury above T6 vertebral level* results in hypotension, known as 'neurogenic shock'. Sympathetic nervous outflow to the systemic arterioles is interrupted, resulting in arteriolar vasodilatation. Similarly, venodilatation leads to venous pooling, which increases the risk of thromboembolic disease and reduces venous return to the heart, further contributing to hypotension.
- *Lesions above T1 vertebral level* can result in bradycardia; the sympathetic cardioacceleratory nerves are disconnected

from the heart, allowing unopposed parasympathetic activity. Cardiac output cannot be increased by the normal mechanism of sympathetic stimulation of heart rate. Stroke volume must therefore be maintained by adequate cardiac preload; hypovolaemia is poorly tolerated in high spinal cord injury.

- **Peripheral nervous system.** Spinal cord injury results in disruption of the motor, sensory and autonomic fibres:

- Initially, there is flaccid paralysis and loss of reflexes below the level of the spinal cord lesion; this is referred to as 'spinal shock'.
- Over the next 3 weeks, spastic paralysis and brisk reflexes develop.
- Below the level of injury, somatic and visceral sensation is absent.

- **Gastrointestinal system.** Though the enteric nervous system is semi-autonomous, it is still affected by the sudden disruption of sympathetic fibres, resulting in unopposed parasympathetic input via the vagus nerve:

- Delayed gastric emptying and paralytic ileus are common. Abdominal distension may further impair ventilation.
- In high spinal cord lesions, gastric ulceration is almost inevitable without gastric protection (e.g. by an H_2 receptor antagonist such as ranitidine). Gastric ulceration is thought to be due to the unopposed vagal stimulation of gastric acid secretion.
- Patients usually become constipated as the sensations of defecation are lost; regular laxatives and bowel care regimes are important to prevent faecal impaction.

- **Metabolic.** Spinal cord injury has several metabolic consequences:

- Thermoregulation may be impaired due to the loss of sympathetic outflow below the level of the spinal cord injury:

  - Arteriolar vasodilatation in the skin may result in heat loss.
  - Overzealous attempts to warm patients may cause hyperthermia, as sweating is impaired.

– Hyperglycaemia is common following spinal cord injury as a result of the stress response; good glycaemic control is needed to prevent exacerbation of ischaemic cord injury.

Describe the common patterns of incomplete spinal cord injury

Incomplete spinal cord injury describes a situation in which there is partial damage to the spinal cord: some motor and sensory function remains below the level of the cord lesion. Important patterns of incomplete cord injury are shown in Figure 50.4:

- **Anterior spinal artery syndrome**, which, as described above, results in paraplegia, loss of pain and temperature sensation and autonomic dysfunction below the level of the lesion. Crucially, proprioception and vibration sensation remain intact.

- **Central cord syndrome**, the most common incomplete spinal cord injury:

  – Central cord syndrome results from hyperextension of the neck, usually in older patients with cervical spondylosis, but sometimes in younger patients involved in high-force trauma.

  – Signs and symptoms are upper and lower limb weakness below the level of the lesion, with a varying degree of sensory loss. Autonomic

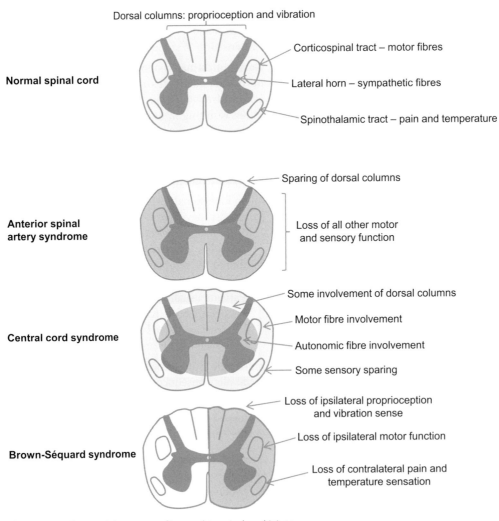

Figure 50.4 Characteristic patterns of incomplete spinal cord injury.

disturbance is common, especially bladder dysfunction.

- Central cord syndrome is now thought to be due to selective axonal disruption of the lateral columns at the level of the injury, with relative preservation of grey matter.

- **Brown-Séquard syndrome**, which, as described above, results in three characteristic clinical features: ipsilateral motor weakness, ipsilateral loss of two-point discrimination, proprioception and vibration sensation with contralateral loss of pain and temperature sensation below the level of the lesion.

- **Cauda equina syndrome**. Although cauda equina syndrome is not strictly speaking a spinal cord injury, it is sufficiently similar to be included:

  - In adults, the spinal cord ends at L1/2 vertebral level, where it gives rise to the 'horse-tail' of L1 to S5 nerve roots: the cauda equina. A lesion at or below the level of L2 therefore compresses these nerve roots rather than the spinal cord; this is called cauda equina syndrome.

  - The nerve roots carry sensory afferent nerves, parasympathetic nerves and lower motor neurons.

  - Patients typically present with severe leg weakness, with at least partially preserved sensation. 'Saddle anaesthesia' (sensory loss around the anus, buttocks, perineum and genitals) is the most common sensory disturbance. Autonomic disturbance is extremely common; urinary retention is almost universal.

  - The most common cause of cauda equina syndrome is an acute central intervertebral disc herniation – a surgical emergency requiring lumbar discectomy. Other causes are metastatic disease, trauma and epidural abscess. Of particular interest to the anaesthetist: there is an association between cauda equina syndrome and the technique of continuous spinal anaesthesia with fine-bore spinal catheters. It is not clear whether this is due to the hyperbaric 5% lignocaine that was used in the technique or the introduction of small amounts of neurotoxic chlorhexidine cleaning solution into the CSF.

Describe the initial management of acute spinal cord injury

Trauma patients frequently have multiple injuries; for example, 25% of patients with a cervical spine injury also have a traumatic brain injury. Unfortunately, nothing can be done to reverse the mechanical aspects of a spinal cord injury, such as an axonal injury due to rotational and shearing forces. The aim of medical management is the prevention of secondary spinal cord damage. The most common cause of secondary damage is cord ischaemia resulting from systemic hypoxaemia or cord hypoperfusion due to vascular damage, cord oedema or systemic hypotension.

The anaesthetic management of patients with spinal injury frequently starts in the resuscitation room of the emergency department and increasingly occurs in the prehospital setting. Patients should be managed following an airway–breathing–circulation–disability–exposure (ABCDE) approach, treating life-threatening problems first. Whenever spinal trauma is suspected, spinal immobilisation must be maintained throughout to prevent any further mechanical spinal cord injury. The cervical spine is traditionally immobilised by means of a hard collar, sandbags on either side of the head and straps holding the patient's head to a backboard.[4] The thoracic and lumbar spine are immobilised simply by the patient lying still on a flat surface. If the patient needs to be moved, the spine is kept in alignment by 'log-rolling'.

Aspects of anaesthetic management specific to spinal injuries are:

- **Airway**. The head tilt manoeuvre should be avoided, as it may worsen a cervical fracture; jaw thrust is thought to be a safer airway manoeuvre. Oxygenation should be maintained – either by high-flow O_2 administration in a conscious patient or by intubation and ventilation in an unconscious patient. If intubation is likely to be required, this should take place at an early stage to

---

[4] However, the routine use of hard collars has been questioned due to increasing evidence of harm associated with their use. Applying spinal immobilisation delays transfer to hospital, and poorly fitting collars may not adequately immobilise the cervical spine and may actually promote spinal cord injury with certain fracture types. Finally, the need to maintain spinal immobilisation makes laryngoscopy much more difficult, risking hypoxaemia at induction of anaesthesia.

prevent hypoxaemia-related secondary cord damage. A difficult intubation should be anticipated owing to:

- Suboptimal positioning of the patient;
- Rapid sequence induction (RSI) with cricoid pressure;
- Manual in-line stabilisation of the cervical spine;
- Associated maxillofacial injuries;
- Blood and debris in the oral cavity.

Nasal intubation and high-flow nasal O_2 therapy should be avoided owing to the possibility of associated basal skull fractures.

- **Induction of anaesthesia.** The risk of pulmonary aspiration necessitates an RSI.[5] The best intravenous induction agent is a matter of debate, but in the setting of trauma, a cardio-stable drug (e.g. ketamine) may be required. Suxamethonium may be used as the muscle relaxant for the initial RSI, but 24 h following the injury, the use of suxamethonium is contraindicated: a significant rise in plasma K^+ may occur due to the depolarisation of the newly developed extra-junctional acetylcholine receptors (see Chapter 53). If head injury is suspected, some means of obtunding the sympathetic response to laryngoscopy should be used to avoid a rise in intracranial pressure; for example, by co-administering a fast-acting, strong opioid.
- **Breathing.** In the acute phase, P_aO_2 should be kept above 10 kPa. Oxygenation may be impaired by associated chest injuries (e.g. flail chest, haemothorax), which should be dealt with promptly. As discussed above, the respiratory consequences of cervical spine injury make hypoxaemia particularly common; if a conscious patient is unable to maintain adequate arterial oxygenation or becomes hypercapnoeic, intubation and ventilation are indicated.
- **Circulation.** Hypovolaemia should be treated promptly with fluids to minimise secondary ischaemic damage of the spinal cord. In a trauma patient, hypotension is most likely to be the result of haemorrhage – the search for the site of bleeding is both clinical and radiological: chest and pelvic X-rays, abdominal ultrasound and computed tomography. Bradycardia with hypotension may be due to spinal cord injury with unopposed parasympathetic innervation of the heart – atropine or glycopyrrolate should be given.
- **Disability.** A basic neurological assessment should include an assessment of conscious level using the Glasgow Coma Scale or the 'alert, voice, pain, unresponsive' (AVPU) scale, pupil size and reactivity and tendon reflexes. Patients with a reduced level of consciousness will almost inevitably require imaging of their brain in addition to their spine.
- **Everything else.** Plasma glucose and electrolytes should be tested and abnormalities corrected. A full secondary survey should be carried out when the patient has been stabilised – this includes log-rolling the patient to examine the spine, flanks and anal motor tone. Care should be taken to keep the patient warm; hypothermia is common, due to prolonged exposure to the environment at the scene of trauma, cold intravenous fluids and blood and removal of clothes for clinical examination.

Further reading

J. A. Kiernan, R. Rajakumar. *Barr's The Human Nervous System: An Anatomical Viewpoint, 10th edition.* Philadelphia, Lippincott Williams & Wilkins, 2013.

J. H. Martin. *Neuroanatomy Text and Atlas, 4th edition.* New York, McGraw-Hill Medical, 2012.

G. Hadjipavlou, A. M. Cortese, B. Ramaswamy. Spinal cord injury and chronic pain. *BJA Education* 2016; **16**(8): 264–8

M. Denton, J. McKinlay. Cervical cord injury and critical care. *Continuing Educ Anaesth Crit Care Pain* 2009; **9**(3): 82–6.

J. Šedy, J. Zicha, J. Kuneš, et al. Mechanisms of neurogenic pulmonary edema development. *Physiol Res* 2008; **57**: 499–506.

P. Veale, J. Lamb. Anaesthesia and acute spinal cord injury. *Continuing Educ Anaesth Crit Care Pain* 2002; **2**(5): 139–43.

---

[5] Have a low threshold for removing cricoid pressure if it is impeding laryngoscopic view – avoiding hypoxaemia at induction is paramount.

51

Resting Membrane Potential

How is the membrane potential produced?

The cell membrane provides a selectively permeant electrical barrier between the intracellular and extracellular compartments. The membrane potential of a cell is the electrical voltage of its interior relative to its exterior. The electrical potential across the membrane will be zero when there are exactly equal numbers of positively and negatively charged ions on either side of the cell membrane. A non-zero membrane potential arises from inequalities in the distribution of charged ions across the cell membrane.

The distribution of ions across a cell membrane results from a combined effect of:

- The different ionic compositions of the intracellular fluid (ICF) and extracellular fluid (ECF).
- The selective permeability of the cell membrane to the different ions.
- The presence of negatively charged intracellular proteins, whose large molecular weight and charge mean that they are unable to cross the cell membrane. These proteins tend to bind positively charged ions and repel negatively charged ions.

Thus:

- A *negative* membrane potential is produced when there is a greater number of positively charged ions on the *outside* of the cell membrane relative to the inside.
- A *positive* membrane potential is produced when there is a greater number of positively charged ions on the *inside* of the cell membrane relative to the outside.

A quiescent cell typically has a negative resting membrane potential (RMP). RMP is more negative in excitable cells (-70 mV in nerve cells, -90 mV in skeletal muscle cells) than non-excitable cells (around -30 mV).

Cell excitation results in an action potential (see Chapter 52), a transient change in the membrane potential from the RMP to a positive value; the cell membrane has been briefly depolarised.

The RMP is particularly influenced by the concentrations and membrane permeability of three major ions:

- K^+: the intracellular K^+ concentration is normally greater (150 mmol/L) than the extracellular K^+ concentration (5 mmol/L). The phospholipid bilayer of the cell membrane itself is impermeable to K^+ ions, as they are polar. However, the cell membrane contains open K^+ leak channels[1] that permit K^+ to pass down its concentration gradient from the ICF to the ECF.
- Na^+: the extracellular Na^+ concentration is higher (140 mmol/L) than the intracellular Na^+ concentration (20 mmol/L). Na^+ ions are polar and therefore do not traverse the cell membrane, and Na^+ channels present in the membrane are normally closed at RMP, leaving the resting cell membrane impermeable to Na^+.[2]
- Cl^-: membrane permeability varies with cell type:
  - *In neurons*, the cell membrane is relatively impermeable to Cl^-: permeability to Cl^- is about 1000 times less than that of K^+, and therefore its contribution is often ignored.
  - *Muscle* contains open membrane Cl^- channels. Cl^- therefore distributes itself across the cell membrane passively according to its electrochemical gradient. At RMP, Cl^- is driven out of the cell by the negatively charged cell interior. However, membrane

---

[1] These are also called two-pore-domain K^+ channels.
[2] In reality, the resting cell membrane is not completely impermeable to Na^+, as the K^+ leak channels are not completely specific to K^+. Overall, Na^+ permeability is about 100 times less than that of K^+.

depolarisation results in a positively charged cell interior, producing a Cl⁻ influx. Therefore, in most cells, Cl⁻ movement does not influence the RMP; rather, the membrane potential passively influences Cl⁻ movement. Passive Cl⁻ movements do, however, act like a 'ballast', making changes to the RMP more difficult, thus increasing membrane stability.

What is the Nernst equation?

Consider a particular membrane-permeant ion, X:

- X will distribute on either side of a cell membrane according to its chemical (i.e. concentration) and electrical gradients across the membrane.
- The movement of X ceases when the net chemical and electrical gradients of X across the membrane are zero; that is, at electrochemical equilibrium.
- The contribution that ion X makes to the RMP may be calculated using the Nernst equation from its valency, the concentration difference across the membrane and the temperature:

Key equation: the Nernst equation

$$E_X = \frac{RT}{zF} \ln \frac{[X]_o}{[X]_i}$$

where E_X (mV) is the Nernst potential for a particular ion, R is the universal gas constant (8.314 J K⁻¹ mol⁻¹), T (K) is the absolute temperature, F is the Faraday constant (the electrical charge per mole of electrons – 96,500 C/mol), z is the valency of the ion, $[X]_o$ (mmol/L) is the ion concentration outside the cell and $[X]_i$ (mmol/L) is the ion concentration inside the cell.

For example, the Nernst potential for K⁺ is calculated as follows:

Assuming a temperature of 37°C (i.e. 310 K) with ICF and ECF K⁺ concentrations as above:

$$E_K = \frac{RT}{zF} \ln \frac{[K^+]_o}{[K^+]_i}$$

$$E_K = \frac{8.314 \times 310}{1 \times 96500} \ln \frac{5}{150}$$

$$E_K \approx -90\,\text{mV}$$

Similarly:

- The Nernst potential for Na⁺ is calculated as +50 mV.
- The Nernst potential for Cl⁻ is calculated as –70 mV.

How may the Nernst equation be applied to explain the RMP?

The resting membrane has a significantly higher K⁺ permeability than Na⁺ permeability. This permits a net efflux of positively charged K⁺ from the cell interior down its concentration gradient, driving the membrane potential towards the Nernst potential for K⁺. As K⁺ ions exit, the cell interior becomes increasingly negatively charged, thus generating an opposing electrical gradient that limits further K⁺ efflux.

In contrast, there is a considerably lower resting membrane permeability to Na⁺ ions, and so there is little contribution from the transmembrane distribution of Na⁺ to the resting potential.

Accordingly, the measured neuronal RMP (–70 mV) is close to the calculated Nernst potential for K⁺, which reflects the major contribution that K⁺ makes to the RMP due to the high membrane K⁺ permeability and the low membrane Na⁺ and Cl⁻ permeability.

What is the Goldman equation?

As discussed above, the Nernst equation is used to calculate the membrane potential for a single ion, assuming that the cell membrane is completely permeable to that ion. However, the cell membrane has differing permeability to a number of ions. The RMP can be more precisely quantified by considering all of the ionic permeabilities and concentrations using the Goldman–Hodgkin–Katz equation.

Key equation: the Goldman–Hodgkin–Katz equation

$$E_m = \frac{RT}{F} \ln \frac{P_K[K^+]_o + P_{Na}[Na^+]_o + P_{Cl}[Cl^-]_i}{P_K[K^+]_i + P_{Na}[Na^+]_i + P_{Cl}[Cl^-]_o}$$

where E_m (mV) is the calculated membrane potential and P_X is the permeability of the membrane to ion X.

> Note:
> - If the membrane is permeable only to K$^+$, then P_{Na} and P_{Cl} equal zero and the equation reduces to the Nernst equation for K$^+$.
> - There is no valency term, as only monovalent ions are considered.
> - The concentrations of Cl$^-$ are shown opposite to those of K$^+$ and Na$^+$ to account for its negative valency.

How does the Na$^+$/K$^+$-ATPase contribute to the RMP?

The Na$^+$/K$^+$-ATPase causes the efflux of three Na$^+$ ions in exchange for the influx of two K$^+$ ions, with the following consequences:

- **Na$^+$ and K$^+$ concentration gradients.** The Na$^+$/K$^+$-ATPase is responsible for maintaining the high extracellular relative to intracellular Na$^+$ concentration, and conversely the high intracellular relative to extracellular K$^+$ concentration, which ultimately generate the RMP.
- **The osmotic effect** of the high extracellular concentration of impermeant Na$^+$ balances the osmotic effect of the high intracellular concentration of negatively charged protein, thereby ensuring an osmotic balance across the cell membrane.
- **Electrogenic effect.** Each cycle of Na$^+$/K$^+$-ATPase activity results in the net loss of one positive charge from the cell, making the cell interior

slightly more negative (i.e. hyperpolarisation) by around –3 to –6 mV, depending on the overall cell membrane resistance.

> **Clinical relevance: the effect of electrolyte disturbances**
>
> As discussed above, the RMP depends on the relative concentrations of ions on either side of the cell membrane. Changes in extracellular ionic concentration may therefore alter the RMP (Figure 51.1):
>
> - **K$^+$.**
>   - *Hyperkalaemia* depolarises the RMP. From the Nernst equation, an increase in extracellular K$^+$ concentration from 4.0 to 7.5 mmol/L changes the Nernst potential for K$^+$ from –90 to –80 mV. The RMP approaches threshold potential (the potential at which an action potential is triggered), transiently making spontaneous generation of action potentials more likely. Changes in extracellular K$^+$ also alter other channel kinetics involved in the action potential, notably those in the repolarisation phase of the cardiac action potential (resulting in tall-tented T-waves). In the heart, dangerous arrhythmias such as ventricular fibrillation may occur.
>   - *Hypokalaemia* causes the opposite effect: the cell membrane becomes hyperpolarised. It becomes harder to generate and propagate action potentials, causing weakness in skeletal muscle. In cardiac muscle, hypokalaemia directly inhibits K$^+$ channels, producing pro-arrhythmic increases in the QT interval.

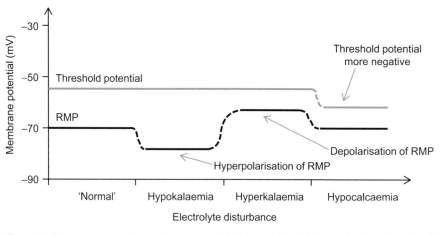

Figure 51.1 Changes to resting membrane potential (RMP) and threshold potential with electrolyte disturbances.

- **Na^+**. As discussed above, the cell membrane is relatively impermeable to Na^+ at rest. Therefore, changes to the Na^+ extracellular concentration would be expected to make little difference to the RMP. However, hyponatraemia alters the distribution of water in the body (see Chapter 69). The reduced ECF osmolarity causes cells to swell; for example, severe hyponatraemia leads to cerebral oedema. The additional intracellular water causes a fall in intracellular K^+ concentration, which in turn leads to cell membrane depolarisation towards threshold potential; spontaneous action potentials are more likely to be generated. This partially explains why cerebral oedema secondary to hyponatraemia is associated with seizure activity.
- **Ca^{2+}**. As discussed above, K^+ is the major determinant of the RMP – Ca^{2+} plays no direct role, as the membrane is largely impermeable to Ca^{2+} at rest. However, Ca^{2+} has a membrane-stabilising effect due to the 'surface charge hypothesis'. Ca^{2+} binds to the outside of the cell membrane by becoming attached to glycoproteins. This increases the amount of local positive charge directly apposed to the extracellular side of the membrane, which hyperpolarises the membrane relative to the overall RMP. Hypocalcaemia increases excitability of the membrane, bringing the threshold potential nearer to the RMP. This predisposes to spontaneous action potential generation, leading to tetany, parasthesias and arrhythmia.

  Ca^{2+} may be given for cardioprotection in hyperkalaemia, allowing time for the underlying cause to be dealt with.

Further reading

R. D. Keynes, D. J. Aidley, C. L.-H. Huang. *Nerve and Muscle, 4th edition*. Cambridge, Cambridge University Press, 2011.

S. H. Wright. Generation of resting membrane potential. *Adv Physiol Educ* 2004; **28**: 139–42.

Chapter

52

Nerve Action Potential and Propagation

What is an action potential?

An action potential is a transient reversal of the membrane potential that occurs in excitable cells, including neurons, muscle cells and some endocrine cells. The action potential is an 'all-or-nothing' event: if the triggering stimulus is smaller than a threshold value, the action potential does not occur. But once triggered, the action potential has a well-defined amplitude and duration. Action potential propagation allows rapid signalling within excitable cells over relatively long distances.

Describe the events that result in the nerve action potential

Action potentials usually begin at the axon hillock of motor neurons or at sensory receptors in sensory afferent neurons. Events proceed as follows (Figure 52.1a):

- As discussed in Chapter 51, the neuronal resting membrane potential (RMP) of approximately –70 mV is relatively close to the Nernst equilibrium potential for K^+ of around –90 mV.
- An initial depolarisation of a sensory receptor, synapse or another part of the nerve results in Na^+ and K^+ movements, producing a net depolarisation of the cell membrane:
  - *If the stimulus is small*, the Na^+ influx is exceeded by K^+ efflux through K^+ leak channels primarily responsible for the RMP (see Chapter 51). The cell membrane returns to –70 mV.
  - *If the stimulus is large enough*, depolarising the cell membrane to approximately –55 mV[1] results in a significant activation of transmembrane voltage-gated Na^+ channels;

Na^+ influx then exceeds K^+ efflux. This is known as the 'threshold potential'.

- The resulting membrane depolarisation leads to further opening of voltage-gated Na^+ channels, thus further increasing the membrane permeability to Na^+ (Figure 52.1b). This further increases the Na^+ influx, which in turn produces further membrane depolarisation, resulting in the rapid upstroke of the action potential. This drives the membrane potential towards the Nernst equilibrium potential for Na^+ of approximately +50 mV. However, the action potential never reaches this theoretical maximum, as two further events intervene:

  - *Inactivation of voltage-gated Na^+ channels*: the voltage-gated Na^+ channels make a further transition from the open state to an inactivated (refractory) state; membrane Na^+ permeability decreases.
  - *Delayed activation of voltage-gated K^+ channels*: membrane depolarisation slowly opens voltage-gated K^+ channels (Figure 52.1b). Membrane K^+ permeability increases and the resulting K^+ efflux acts to drive the membrane potential back towards the Nernst equilibrium potential for K^+ of approximately –90 mV.

- The membrane potential briefly becomes more negative than the RMP. This after-hyperpolarisation occurs because of the gradual closure of the voltage-gated K^+ channels, which results in the membrane being briefly more permeable to K^+ than at the RMP, thus achieving a value closer to the E_K.

In summary, the action potential results from a brief increase in membrane conductance to Na^+ followed by a slower increase in membrane conductance to K^+ (Figure 52.1b).

---

[1] Threshold potential is dependent on a number of factors, but is commonly between –55 and –40 mV.

(a) Nerve action potential

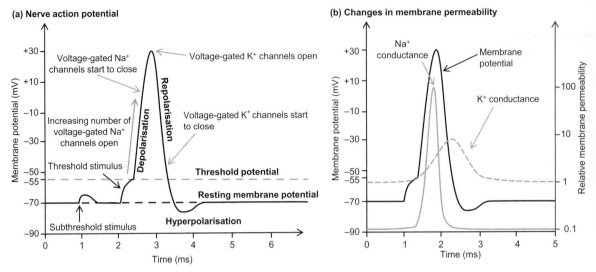

(b) Changes in membrane permeability

Figure 52.1 (a) The nerve action potential and (b) changes in the membrane permeability of Na$^+$ and K$^+$ throughout the action potential.

How are action potentials propagated along nerve axons?

Electrical depolarisation propagates by the formation of local circuits (Figure 52.2):

- The intracellular surface of a resting portion of cell membrane is negatively charged.
- Following an action potential, a portion of cell membrane depolarises, resulting in the intracellular surface becoming positively charged. The action potential is limited to a small portion of cell membrane; neighbouring segments remain quiescent.
- Ion movement at the edges of the depolarised cell membrane results in current flow; the neighbouring quiescent portions of cell membrane become depolarised.
- Current decays exponentially along the length of the nerve axon with a length constant of a few millimetres.[2] Nevertheless, provided the propagated depolarisation in the previously quiescent cell membrane is sufficient to reach threshold potential, an action potential is generated.

This process of local circuit propagation and action potential generation is continued until the action potential reaches its destination (Figure 52.2).

The velocity of action potential conduction is affected by several factors:

- **The axon diameter.** Just like a copper wire, the intracellular fluid within a larger-diameter nerve axon has a smaller resistance to the longitudinal flow of current, thereby permitting a higher conduction velocity.
- **The transmembrane resistance.** This determines how easily current may flow out of the nerve and into the extracellular fluid (ECF). A higher transmembrane resistance reduces the leak of current out of the cell, thereby maximising the longitudinal flow of current. Myelination increases the transmembrane resistance as the myelin sheath is made of insulating lipids.
- **The membrane capacitance.** The greater the capacitance of the membrane, the longer it takes to alter the membrane polarity,[3]

---

[3] As $\tau = RC$, where τ is the time constant, R the transmembrane resistance and C is the capacitance. As myelination actually increases transmembrane resistance (as this increases longitudinal flow), the decrease in membrane capacitance offsets this effect on the overall time constant.

---

[2] Longitudinal current is reduced by a deposition of charge on intervening membrane, as well as its leak across the membrane into the extracellular fluid.

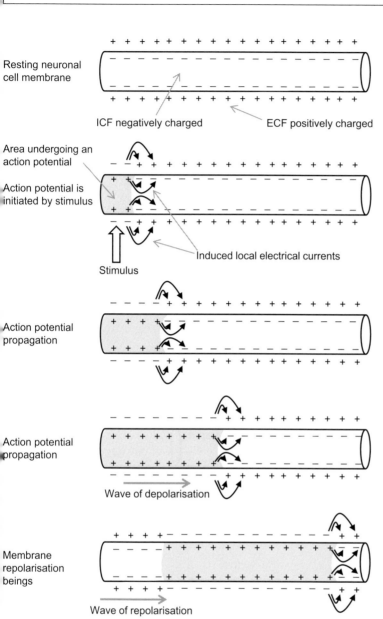

Figure 52.2 Action potential propagation in unmyelinated neurons (ECF = extracellular fluid; ICF = intracellular fluid).

Resting neuronal cell membrane

ICF negatively charged   ECF positively charged

Area undergoing an action potential

Action potential is initiated by stimulus

Induced local electrical currents

Stimulus

Action potential propagation

Action potential propagation

Wave of depolarisation

Membrane repolarisation beings

Wave of repolarisation

thus slowing action potential propagation. Myelination decreases membrane capacitance.

• **Temperature.** Like enzymes, the activity of ion channels is very dependent on temperature. The rate of ion channel opening increases around three- or four-fold with a 10°C increase in temperature. Therefore, the voltage-gated Na^+ channels open more rapidly, increasing the velocity of action potential propagation.

How does myelination alter the nature of action potential propagation?

Larger-diameter nerve axons are coated in a white, lipid-rich insulating material called myelin. The myelin sheath is produced by Schwann cells in the peripheral nervous system (PNS) and by oligodendro-cytes in the central nervous system (CNS). The myelin sheath covers the nerve axon except at regularly spaced gaps known as 'nodes of Ranvier'. These

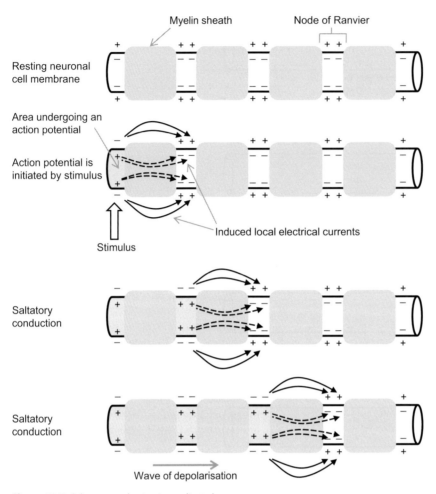

Figure 52.3 Saltatory conduction in myelinated axons.

exposed regions of membrane are densely populated with voltage-gated Na$^+$ channels.

The electrical impulse propagates passively across the internode (where the axon is covered by the myelin sheath) by local circuit conduction, as in Figure 52.2. Passive propagation is rapid as it does not require protein interactions at the surface membrane. As discussed above, the myelin sheath insulates the nerve axon, preventing loss of current to the ECF and decreasing the membrane capacitance. This ensures that the membrane is depolarised in excess of the threshold potential at the adjacent node of Ranvier. The action potential therefore appears to 'jump' from node to node; this is known as saltatory conduction (Figure 52.3). Action potential conduction velocity increases from 2 m/s in unmyelinated nerves to up to 120 m/s in myelinated axons.

Clinical relevance: demyelination

Myelination is an extremely important determinant of nerve conduction velocity. The myelin sheath is especially important in nerves that require the rapid conduction of action potentials for their function, such as motor and sensory nerves.

There are two important diseases in which there is autoimmune destruction of the myelin sheath: multiple sclerosis (where CNS neurons demyelinate) and Guillain–Barré syndrome (where demyelination occurs in the PNS).

A demyelinated neuron differs in its disposition of Na$^+$ channels from normally unmyelinated neurons.

Myelinated neurons have Na^+ channels clustered at high density at the nodes of Ranvier, but not in surface membrane beneath the myelin sheath. Upon demyelination, the abnormally exposed areas of cell membranes do not have adequate numbers of Na^+ channels to ensure effective action potential conduction. In contrast, whilst unmyelinated axons conduct action potentials slowly, they are reliably conducted along the entire length of the neuron.

The clinical features of demyelinating disease are therefore deficiencies in sensation, motor function, autonomic function or cognition depending on the type and location of the nerves involved.

How are nerve fibres functionally classified?

Nerves can be classified based on their diameter and conduction velocity:

- **Type A fibres** are myelinated fibres of large diameter (12–20 μm) with a conduction velocity of 70–120 m/s. Type A fibres are subdivided into α, β, γ and δ in order of decreasing nerve conduction velocity:
    - *Aα motor fibres* supply extrafusal muscle fibres; that is, those involved in skeletal muscle contraction.
    - *Aβ sensory fibres* carry sensory information from receptors in the skin, joints and muscle.
    - *Aγ motor fibres* supply intrafusal muscle spindle fibres.
    - *Aδ sensory fibres* relay information from fast nociceptors and thermoreceptors.
- **Type B fibres** are narrow (diameter < 3 μm) myelinated fibres. Their conduction velocity is correspondingly lower, at 4–30 m/s. The preganglionic neurons of the autonomic nervous system (ANS) are type B fibres.
- **Type C fibres** have narrow (diameter 0.4–1.2 μm) unmyelinated axons with a correspondingly slow conduction velocity (0.5–4.0 m/s). Post-ganglionic neurons of the ANS and slow pain fibres are type C fibres.

Clinical relevance: local anaesthetics

Local anaesthetics act by blocking fast voltage-gated Na^+ channels, thereby preventing further action

potentials being propagated. The mechanism of action is:

- Local anaesthetics are weak bases.
- Only unionised local anaesthetic can diffuse across the phospholipid bilayer of the neuronal cell membrane.
- The lower pH within the axoplasm means that as soon as the local anaesthetic has crossed the cell membrane, it is protonated (becomes ionised) and therefore cannot diffuse back into the ECF.
- The ionised local anaesthetic blocks the voltage-gated Na^+ channels by binding to the inner surface of the ion channels when they are in their inactive state.
- In other words, local anaesthetics indefinitely prolong the absolute refractory period (ARP); further action potentials are prevented.

Some nerves are more sensitive to local anaesthetics than others. In general:

- Small nerve fibres are more sensitive to local anaesthetics than are large nerve fibres.
- Myelinated fibres are more sensitive to local anaesthetics than are unmyelinated fibres of equivalent diameters. This likely reflects myelinated fibres having only small areas of cell membrane exposed (nodes of Ranvier), in which the Na^+ channels are densely packed.

The overall clinical effect is:

- Intermediate-sized myelinated fibres are the easiest to block, such as Aδ fibres (which relay fast nociceptive signals) and B fibres (pre-ganglionic autonomic fibres).
- Larger Aα, Aβ and Aγ fibres (which relay touch, pressure and proprioception) are the next easiest to block.
- Unmyelinated C fibres are the most resistant to local anaesthetics.

What is meant by the term 'refractory period'?

The refractory period describes the time following an action potential when a further action potential either cannot be triggered whatever the size of the stimulus (i.e. ARP) or only with application of a stimulus of increased size (i.e. relative refractory period, RRP):

- **The ARP** starts from the moment the voltage-gated Na^+ channels open and typically lasts around 1 ms. The basis of the ARP is:

- Shortly after the voltage-gated Na^+ channels have opened, they become refractory.
- The Na^+ channels remain in their refractory state and are incapable of reopening until the membrane regains its negative potential.

- **The RRP** continues for 2–3 ms after the ARP has ended. The mechanism behind the RRP is as follows:

  - An insufficient proportion of Na^+ channels have recovered from their refractory period to generate significant inward current on stimulation.
  - During the repolarisation phase, both the K^+ leak channels and voltage-gated K^+ channels are open. The membrane K^+ permeability is therefore at its highest.
  - During this period, the threshold potential is higher, as a greater stimulus is required to counteract the increased K^+ efflux (Figure 52.4).

The refractory period is important for two reasons:

- **To ensure unidirectional propagation of action potentials**. When a segment of a cell membrane depolarises, the trailing region of cell membrane is in its refractory state, whilst the leading segment of cell membrane is in its resting state.
- **Limiting the frequency of action potentials**. The refractory period limits the number of

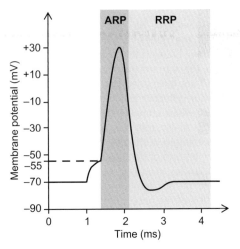

Figure 52.4 Absolute refractory period (ARP) and relative refractory period (RRP).

action potentials that can be generated in a given time period.

Further reading

R. D. Keynes, D. J. Aidley, C. L.-H. Huang. *Nerve and Muscle, 4th edition.* Cambridge, Cambridge University Press, 2011.

A. Scholz. Mechanisms of (local) anaesthetics on voltage-gated sodium and other ion channels. *Br J Anaesth* 2002; **89**(1): 52–61.

Chapter 53

Synapses and the Neuromuscular Junction

What is a synapse?

A synapse is the functional point of contact between two excitable cells, across which a signal can be transmitted. There are two types of synapse:

- **Chemical synapse**, in which the signal is relayed by means of a chemical messenger called a neurotransmitter. Arrival of an action potential triggers neurotransmitter release into the synaptic cleft, a narrow (20–50-nm) gap between the pre- and post-synaptic membranes, which excites or inhibits the postsynaptic cell. An example of a chemical synapse is the neuromuscular junction (NMJ): the terminal bouton of an α-motor neuron forms a synapse with the motor end plate of a skeletal muscle cell. Action potential transmissions at chemical synapses are typically unidirectional: the signal can only be transmitted from pre- to post-synaptic cells. Transmission of an action potential across a chemical synapse is associated with a synaptic delay, as it takes time for each of the processes of neurotransmitter release, diffusion and combination with postsynaptic receptors to occur.

- **Electrical synapse**, in which the pre- and post-synaptic cells are electrically connected by gap junctions that allow electric current to pass; an action potential in the presynaptic cell induces a local current in the postsynaptic cell, which triggers an action potential. Signals are transferred from neuron to target cell without a synaptic delay, and therefore this occurs more rapidly than when the cells are connected by a chemical synapse. This is exemplified by cardiac muscle, where gap junctions are essential for the rapid conduction of action potentials (see Chapter 57). Electrical synapses are bidirectional: the signal can be transmitted from pre- to post-synaptic cells, or vice versa.

What are neurotransmitters?

A neurotransmitter is a substance released by a neuron at a synapse, which then acts upon the post-synaptic cell. Neurotransmitters are classified as:

- **Small molecules**, of which there are three main classes:
  - *Amines*: acetylcholine (ACh), histamine, serotonin (5-HT), catecholamines (noradrenaline, adrenaline, dopamine);
  - *Amino acids*: γ-amino butyric acid (GABA), glycine, glutamate;
  - *Purines*: ATP, adenosine.

- **Large molecules**; over 50 neuroactive peptides are known, including:
  - *Opioids*: β-endorphin, enkephalins;
  - *Tachykinins*: substance P, neurokinins;
  - *Secretins*;
  - *Somatostatins*.

Most neurotransmitters exert excitatory effects on the target cell, which may result in the triggering of an action potential (if the target cell is a nerve or muscle) or secretion (if the target cell is a gland). The most widespread excitatory neurotransmitter is glutamate, which is present in over 90% of synapses in the brain. Some neurotransmitters are inhibitory, causing either increased K^+ conductance resulting in hyperpolarisation or increased Cl^- conductance at the postsynaptic membrane, thereby reducing the likelihood of an action potential being generated. GABA, the second most prevalent neurotransmitter in the brain, is the major inhibitory neurotransmitter. Glycine is an inhibitory neurotransmitter that is particularly widespread in the spinal cord and brainstem.

Occasionally, neurotransmitters have an excitatory effect at one synapse whilst having an inhibitory effect at another. For example, ACh is an excitatory neurotransmitter at the nicotinic receptors of the

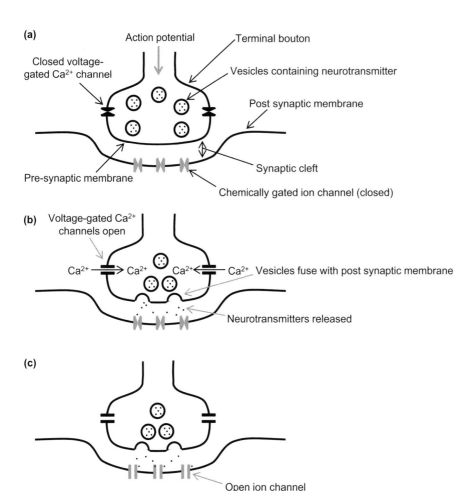

Figure 53.1 The mechanism of a chemical synapse.

NMJ, but it produces an inhibitory response at the muscarinic M_2 receptors of the heart.

How are neurotransmitters released into the synaptic cleft?

Neurotransmitters are stored in packets called vesicles, which are docked at the active zone of the presynaptic membrane. When the action potential propagates down the axon and into the terminal bouton (Figure 53.1a), a well-defined sequence of events occurs:

- **Increase in presynaptic Ca^{2+} concentration.** Depolarisation results in the opening of voltage-gated Ca^{2+} channels (N-type). Ca^{2+} diffuses down its electrochemical gradient from the extracellular fluid (ECF) to the cell interior (Figure 53.1b).

- **Exocytosis.** Periodically, vesicles in the active zone spontaneously fuse with the presynaptic membrane, releasing their neurotransmitter contents into the synaptic cleft. Axonal Ca^{2+} binds to a vesicular membrane protein called synaptotagmin, which, in conjunction with proteins known as SNAREs,[1] triggers 50–100 vesicles to undergo exocytosis. Thus, a very large number of neurotransmitter molecules are released into the synaptic cleft following an action potential.

- **Diffusion across the synaptic cleft.** The neurotransmitters diffuse down their concentration gradient, travelling the short distance to the postsynaptic membrane.

---

[1] **SNAP** (soluble *N*-ethylmaleimide-sensitive fusion attachment protein) **Receptor**.

- **Binding to postsynaptic receptors.** Neurotransmitters that reach the postsynaptic membrane bind to specific receptors, resulting in excitation or inhibition of the membrane (Figure 53.1c).

What is the difference between an ionotropic and a metabotropic receptor?

At the postsynaptic membrane, neurotransmitters encounter two types of receptor:

- *Ionotropic receptors* are ligand-gated postsynaptic ion channels. Binding of a neurotransmitter and the resulting alteration of their conformation directly results in ion channel opening.
- *Metabotropic receptors.* Binding of a neurotransmitter also causes the receptor to change its conformation. However, metabotropic receptors are indirectly linked to membrane ion channels through intermediate intracellular chemical messengers, usually involving a G protein. An important example of a metabotropic synapse is the muscarinic (M_2) ACh receptor of the pacemaker cells in the heart (see Chapter 57).

What is the mechanism for ionotropic receptor signalling?

Ionotropic signalling may produce either an excitatory postsynaptic potential (EPSP) or an inhibitory postsynaptic potential (IPSP) depending on the flow of ions at the postsynaptic ion channel:

- **In an EPSP**, binding of neurotransmitter at the postsynaptic membrane opens non-specific cation channels.

  - Na^+ and K^+ diffuse along their electrochemical gradients: Na^+ flows into the postsynaptic cell from the synaptic cleft, whilst K^+ diffuses out of the cell. Overall, Na^+ influx is greater than K^+ efflux; the net intracellular movement of positively charged ions causes a depolarisation of the postsynaptic membrane – the EPSP.
  - There is usually an excess of postsynaptic ion channels; the size of the EPSP is therefore dependent on the number of neurotransmitter vesicles released:

    - The spontaneous exocytosis of a single vesicle of neurotransmitter results in a miniature 0.5-mV depolarisation. This depolarisation is not large enough to reach threshold potential and the EPSP will fade back to the resting membrane potential (RMP).
    - Following an action potential, a large number of neurotransmitters are released into the synaptic cleft. The depolarising effect of each vesicle's contents at the postsynaptic membrane is additive; to exceed threshold potential and generate an action potential at the postsynaptic cell, many vesicles must be released simultaneously (Figure 53.2a).

- **In an IPSP**, the postsynaptic membrane contains either ligand-gated K^+ or Cl^- channels.

  - K^+-mediated IPSPs: binding of neurotransmitter opens specific K^+ channels. K^+ ions diffuse along their electrochemical gradient from the postsynaptic cell to the synaptic cleft. The efflux of positively charged ions hyperpolarises the cell membrane, making it more difficult to reach threshold potential (Figure 53.2b).
  - Cl^--mediated IPSP: binding of neurotransmitter opens Cl^- channels. The resulting intracellular movement of Cl^- ions usually makes little difference to the postsynaptic membrane potential, as the Nernst potential of Cl^- (–70 mV) is approximately the same voltage as the RMP. However, to reach threshold, an excitatory signal must trigger sufficient Na^+ influx to exceed the combined effects of Cl^- influx and K^+ efflux, making it much more difficult to depolarise the cell membrane; this is known as the 'chloride clamp'.

Clinical relevance: mechanism of action of general anaesthetics

Despite general anaesthetics having been administered since 1846, their exact mechanism of action remains a matter of debate. The most likely explanation involves a receptor theory, whereby general anaesthetics interact with two main transmembrane proteins in the central nervous system (CNS):

(a) Excitatory post-synaptic potential

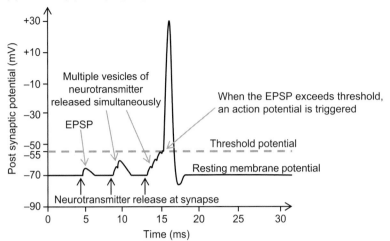

Figure **53.2** (a) Excitatory and (b) inhibitory postsynaptic potentials.

(b) Inhibitory post-synaptic potential

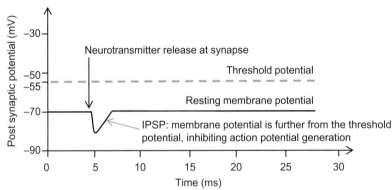

- **The GABA$_A$ receptor** utilises the inhibitory neurotransmitter GABA. The receptor has five subunits arranged around a Cl$^-$ channel. A number of drugs act at this receptor:

  - *Benzodiazepines*: a subset of GABA$_A$ receptors bind benzodiazepines in addition to GABA. The benzodiazepine binding site is located at a different site from that of GABA, between the α- and γ-subunits. Following the binding of a benzodiazepine, the GABA$_A$ receptor changes its conformation, which increases its affinity for GABA.
  - *Propofol, thiopentone and etomidate*: all of these drugs act, at least in part, at the GABA$_A$ receptor. Like the benzodiazepines, all bind at a site distant to the GABA binding site and act by increasing the conductance of Cl$^-$.

The exact binding site and why their effects differ from those of the benzodiazepines are not yet known.

- **The *N*-methyl-D-aspartate (NMDA) receptor** is a tetrameric receptor that utilises the excitatory neurotransmitter glutamate. A number of anaesthetic agents are thought to act by antagonising this excitatory receptor, thus reducing neurotransmission:

  - *Ketamine* binds at a site distant to the glutamate binding site. A conformation change occurs in the NMDA receptor that prevents the subsequent binding of glutamate.
  - *N$_2$O, Xe*: both are also thought to exert their anaesthetic effects through antagonism of the NMDA receptor.

How is neurotransmission terminated?

Once released, neurotransmitters are rapidly removed from the synaptic cleft. This prevents repetitive and unwanted stimulation of the postsynaptic cell. There are three possible mechanisms by which this takes place:

- **Diffusion**. Neurotransmitters may diffuse out of the synaptic cleft along their concentration gradients. This is a minor and relatively slow mechanism.
- **Degradation**. Specific enzymes within the synaptic cleft may inactivate the neurotransmitters. An important example is the hydrolysis of ACh by acetylcholinesterase (AChE) into acetic acid and choline.
- **Neuronal reuptake**. Neurotransmitters may be actively transported back into the presynaptic membrane. Instead of synthesising large amounts of new neurotransmitter, the presynaptic nerve recycles the neurotransmitter molecules, storing them in vesicles ready for release. This occurs with catecholamine neurotransmitters such as noradrenaline and dopamine, which are metabolically expensive to produce. In clinical practice, the action of neurotransmitters may be prolonged through the use of reuptake inhibitors. Examples include selective serotonin reuptake inhibitors, which prevent the reuptake of serotonin in the CNS, and cocaine, which blocks the reuptake of dopamine in the CNS.

What is the NMJ?

The NMJ is the chemical synapse between an α-motor neuron and a muscle cell. The transmission of motor action potentials – or indeed their prevention – is of obvious importance to anaesthetists. The NMJ exemplifies many of the features of synapses discussed above, but its importance makes it worth reiterating the key features.

The α-motor neuron originates in the ventral horn of the spinal cord. Its axon is myelinated, as the conduction of motor action potentials needs to be rapid. Before the axon reaches the NMJ, it branches to innervate several muscle cells. A motor unit consists of an α-motor neuron and the muscle cells that it innervates.

The NMJ itself consists of (Figure 53.3):

- **The terminal boutons of the nerve axon**, within which are located vesicles containing the neurotransmitter ACh.
- **The synaptic cleft**, across which ACh must diffuse.

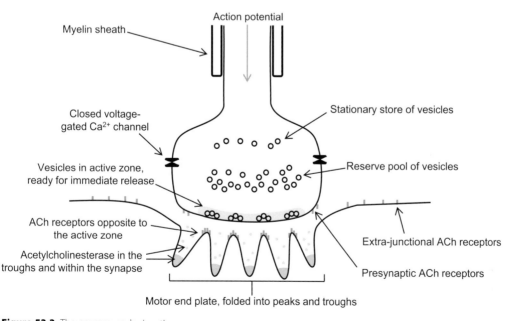

Figure 53.3 The neuromuscular junction.

- **The motor end plate** (postsynaptic membrane), which is folded into peaks and troughs; the peaks are densely packed with ACh receptors (AChRs), whilst the troughs contain the enzyme AChE. There are estimated to be in excess of 1,000,000 AChRs at each motor end plate.

Before the action potential arrives, the NMJ must be ready for neurotransmission to occur:

- **ACh synthesis**. In the axoplasm of the nerve terminal, ACh is synthesised from choline and acetyl-CoA, a reaction catalysed by the enzyme choline-O-acetyltransferase. Choline originates from the diet or by hepatic synthesis, whilst acetyl-CoA is produced in the axon mitochondria.
- **ACh storage**. Once synthesised, ACh is packaged into vesicles. Each vesicle contains around 5000 ACh molecules, known as a 'quantum'. There are functionally three types of vesicle:
  - *Vesicles in the active zone* (1% of vesicles): these vesicles are 'docked' at the presynaptic membrane, ready for immediate release.
  - *Vesicles in the reserve pool* (around 80% of vesicles): these vesicles move forward to replace the vesicles in the active zone as they are used.
  - *Vesicles in the stationary store* (around 20% of vesicles): these vesicles cannot release their ACh.

Neurotransmission occurs as follows:

- **ACh release**. When an action potential reaches the terminal bouton, it causes voltage-gated Ca^{2+} channels to open:
  - Ca^{2+} ions diffuse from the ECF to the nerve axoplasm.
  - An increase in intracellular Ca^{2+} concentration triggers the vesicles of the active zone to fuse with the presynaptic membrane, releasing their contents by exocytosis. Typically, 50–100 vesicles release >250,000 ACh molecules into the synaptic cleft.
- **The AChR** is a nicotinic receptor, a ligand-gated, non-specific cation channel. It has some important features:
  - AChRs are densely packed into the peaks of the postsynaptic membrane, directly opposite

to the active zone of the presynaptic membrane.
  - The AChR is composed of five subunits: two α-, one β-, one δ- and one ε-subunit. The subunits are arranged in a cylinder, forming a central ion channel.
  - To open the ion channel, two ACh molecules must bind to the two α-subunits. Na^+ and K^+ may then diffuse along their electrochemical gradients; the net influx of cations depolarises the postsynaptic membrane. The AChR ion channel stays open for a very brief period, around 1 ms.
  - Following an action potential, a significant excess of ACh molecules is released; the resulting postsynaptic depolarisation (the end-plate potential) easily exceeds threshold potential, thereby triggering an action potential in the muscle cell. This safety margin is clinically important: 70–80% of AChRs must be blocked by muscle relaxants to prevent neurotransmission.
- **Termination of neurotransmission**. ACh is rapidly removed from the synaptic cleft, mainly by degradation:
  - ACh is rapidly hydrolysed by the enzyme AChE to choline and acetic acid. These breakdown products are actively transported into the presynaptic membrane for the re-synthesis of ACh.
  - AChE is mainly found in the junctional folds of the synaptic cleft.
  - The structure of AChE is of pharmacological importance. The active site of the enzyme has two binding sites: anionic and esteratic. Anticholinesterases, drugs that inhibit the AChE enzyme, reversibly or irreversibly bind to these binding sites.

Clinical relevance: drugs acting at the NMJ

Neurotransmission at the NMJ may be blocked by a number of means, not just muscle relaxants:

- **Inhibition of ACh synthesis**: hemicholinium blocks the uptake of choline in the nerve axon, preventing ACh synthesis.
- **Inhibition of vesicle exocytosis** may occur through two mechanisms:

- *Mg^{2+} and aminoglycosides* block the presynaptic voltage-gated Ca^{2+} channels. Without Ca^{2+} influx, vesicles cannot release their contents into the synaptic cleft. This is why patients receiving prolonged Mg^{2+} infusions (e.g. in pre-eclampsia) are at risk of muscle weakness.
- *Botulinum toxin* degrades a protein called SNAP-25 that is required for vesicle docking at the presynaptic membrane. If vesicles cannot dock, ACh cannot be released into the synaptic cleft.

- **Blockage of the AChR**. There are, of course, two classes of drug that act at the AChR:

  - *Depolarising muscle relaxants*, such as suxamethonium. Chemically, suxamethonium is two ACh molecules joined end to end. The spacing between the ACh components is exactly right for both to bind to the two α-subunits of the AChR. Because it acts like ACh, suxamethonium opens the AChR cation channel, causing depolarisation of the postsynaptic membrane. In contrast to ACh, however, suxamethonium is not hydrolysed by AChE. The AChR remains open for a prolonged period, and the muscle membrane remains depolarised. The muscle action potential can only fire once: the fast voltage-gated Na^+ channels that open during cell membrane depolarisation become inactivated and cannot return to their resting state until the cell membrane repolarises, which cannot happen until suxamethonium diffuses away from the AChR. Clinically, depolarising block is characterised by muscle fasciculations followed by flaccid paralysis.
  - *Non-depolarising muscle relaxants*, such as aminosteroids and benzylisoquinoliniums. These drugs compete with ACh for its binding site at the AChR. Non-depolarising muscle relaxants have no intrinsic activity at the AChR – they merely antagonise ACh. Insufficient ACh reaches the AChRs to trigger an action potential in the muscle cell. Clinically, non-depolarising muscle relaxants cause flaccid paralysis without any initial muscle contraction.

Where else are ACh receptors found?

In addition to the postsynaptic membrane, AChRs are found:

- **At the presynaptic membrane**. Following ACh exocytosis, some ACh binds to presynaptic AChRs, which allows Na^+ ions to enter the terminal bouton. This triggers the mobilisation of vesicles from the reserve pool to the active zone, ready for release.
- **Outside the NMJ**, where they are known as extra-junctional AChRs. In health, only a small number of AChRs are present on areas of the muscle cell membrane outside the motor end plate. However, following denervation, extra-junctional AChRs proliferate over the entire muscle cell membrane, with significant implications for the anaesthetist.

Clinical relevance: myasthenia gravis

Myasthenia gravis (MG) is an autoimmune condition characterised by fatigable weakness, in which immunoglobulin G autoantibodies are directed at the nicotinic AChR of the NMJ:

- Autoantibody attack of AChRs results in inflammation that not only reduces the number of AChRs, but also flattens the folds of the postsynaptic membrane, widening the distribution of AChRs and AChE.
- The overall effect is a reduction in the number of ACh–AChR interactions, which reduces the size of the end-plate potential and decreases the likelihood of an action potential being triggered in the muscle cell, leading to weakness.
- There is also autoimmune destruction of presynaptic AChRs. Therefore in MG, when action potentials are repeatedly fired, fewer vesicles are moved from the reserve pool to the active zone. Consequently, as fewer vesicles are available for release, fewer molecules of ACh are released into the synaptic cleft. This is the basis of the fatigability associated with MG.

Note: 10% of patients with MG are seronegative; that is, they do not raise autoantibodies against the nicotinic AChR. Instead, they generate autoantibodies against another protein at the postsynaptic membrane: MuSK. This causes inflammation at the motor end plate, with the same clinical effects.

Clinical relevance: denervation hypersensitivity

Extra-junctional AChRs are structurally different from those at the motor end plate: they also have five subunits, but the adult ε-subunit is replaced by the foetal γ-subunit. Classic examples of acute denervation include burns and acute spinal cord injury. However, chronic denervation also leads to proliferation of extra-junctional AChRs (e.g. motor neuron disease and some peripheral neuropathies such as Charcot–Marie–Tooth disease).

Extra-junctional AChRs are not just of academic interest. Following administration of the depolarising muscle relaxant suxamethonium, a potentially fatal hyperkalaemia can occur. This is due to:

- Suxamethonium binding to both junctional and extra-junctional AChRs, opening their non-specific cation channels. Owing to the sheer number of AChRs activated, the K^+ efflux is significantly greater.
- Once open, extra-junctional AChRs remain open for up to 10 ms, which is much longer than their junctional counterparts.

The combination of these two effects has the potential for a life-threatening increase in plasma K^+ concentration.

Following acute denervation, extra-junctional AChRs take a little time to develop – clinically significant hyperkalaemia is a risk from 24 h post-injury. Therefore, suxamethonium can safely be administered for up to 24 h following the insult. After around 100 days, the risk of hyperkalaemia is thought to reduce sufficiently to permit the cautious use of suxamethonium. In chronic denervation, suxamethonium has an unpredictable response depending on the numbers of extra-junctional AChRs formed.

Further reading

J. M. Hunter. Reversal of residual neuromuscular block: complications associated with perioperative management of muscle relaxation. *Br J Anaesth* 2017; **119**(Suppl. 1): i53–62.

T. Thevathasan, S. L. Shih, K. C. Safari, et al. Association between intraoperative non-depolarising neuromuscular blocking agent dose and 30-day readmission after abdominal surgery. *Br J Anaesth* 2017; **119**(4): 595–605.

M. Naguib, S. J. Brull, K. B. Johnson. Conceptual and technical insights into the basis of neuromuscular monitoring. *Anaesthesia* 2017; **72**(Suppl. 1): 16–37.

R. Khirwadkar, J. M. Hunter. Neuromuscular physiology and pharmacology: an update. *Continuing Educ Anaesth Crit Care Pain* 2012; **12**(5): 237–44.

C. J. Weir. The molecular mechanisms of general anaesthesia: dissecting the $GABA_A$ receptor. *Continuing Educ Anaesth Crit Care Pain* 2006; **6**(2): 49–53.

M. Thavasothy, N. Hirsch. Myasthena gravis. *Continuing Educ Anaesth Crit Care Pain* 2002; **2**(3): 88–90.

Chapter

54

Skeletal Muscle

What are the functions of skeletal muscle?

- **Locomotion**: contraction of muscle reduces the distance between its sites of origin and insertion, thereby producing movement.
- **Maintenance of posture and joint stability**: this is achieved through tonic contraction of multiple synergistic and opposing muscle groups.
- **Support of soft tissues**: the muscles of the abdominal wall and pelvic floor support and protect their underlying viscera.
- **Sphincteric function in the gastrointestinal tract and urinary tracts**: skeletal muscle provides voluntary control over swallowing, defecation and micturition.
- **Heat production**: this occurs through alterations in background muscle metabolic rate and shivering (repeated muscle contraction and relaxation).
- **Venous return**: contraction of leg muscles aids in the generation of local pressure gradients to move venous blood towards the heart.

Describe the macroscopic and microscopic anatomy of skeletal muscle

Skeletal muscles are made up of many muscle fibres (myocytes). They are served by blood vessels and nerves and are supported by a number of connective tissue layers:

- **Endomysium**, the thin layer of connective tissue surrounding each myocyte.
- **Perimysium** – bundles of around 100 myocytes surrounded by perimysium are called fascicles.
- **Epimysium**, the thick layer of connective tissue that encases the entire muscle.

At each end of the muscle, the layers of connective tissue (endomysium, perimysium and epimysium) merge to form a tendon or an aponeurosis, which usually connects the muscle to bone.

Myocytes have a number of unusual anatomical features:

- **Size**. A muscle fibre may span the entire length of the muscle and have a diameter of up to 50 μm.
- **Nuclei**. Myocytes are multinucleate. Nuclei are located peripherally, unlike in cardiac and smooth muscle.
- **Striations**. Skeletal and cardiac muscle, but not smooth muscle, have a striped or 'striated' appearance due to regularly repeating sarcomeres (see below).

Myocytes have a number of specialised cellular features in addition to the usual complement of Golgi apparatus, mitochondria and ribosomes:

- **The sarcoplasmic reticulum** (SR) is a modified endoplasmic reticulum (ER) that acts as an intracellular store of Ca^{2+} and can rapidly release and sequester Ca^{2+}.
- **The transverse (T)-tubules** are invaginations of the muscle surface membrane, or sarcolemma, capable of relaying action potentials deep into the myocyte interior.
- **Myofibrils**, the contractile apparatus of the cell, are arranged in parallel with one another spanning the entire length of the myocyte. Because myofibrils are anchored to the sarcolemma at either end of the myocyte, the whole myocyte shortens when they contract.
- **Myofilaments** – within the myofibrils are bundles of myofilaments, containing the contractile proteins actin and myosin.
- **Glycogen stores**, which release glucose to provide energy for muscle contraction.

(a) Sarcomere

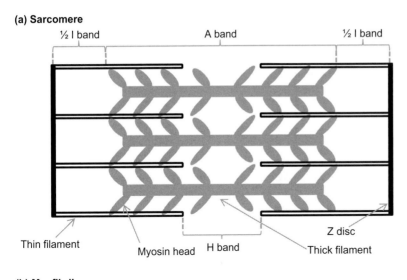

(b) Myofibril

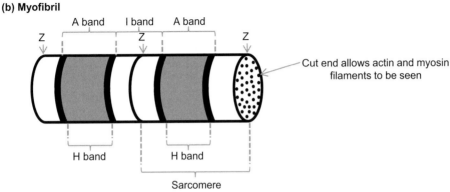

Figure 54.1 Structure of (a) the sarcomere and (b) the myofibril.

What is a sarcomere?

A sarcomere is the functional unit of a skeletal muscle fibre. It contains interdigitating thick, myosin-containing and thin, actin-containing filaments (Figure 54.1a). These are arranged in a regular, repeating, overlapping pattern, giving an alternating sequence of dark and light bands, resulting in a striated appearance. Key features of the sarcomere are:

- *Z disc,* located at either end of the sarcomere, bisecting the I band.
- *Thick and thin filaments.* The thin filaments are joined at one end to the Z disc. The thick filaments are at the centre of the sarcomere, interdigitating with thin filaments.
- *I (isotropic) or light band,* containing the portion of the thin filament that does not overlap with the thick filament.

- *A (anisotropic) or dark band,* the entire length of the thick filament, including regions that overlap the thin filament.
- *H (Heller) band,* the part of the A band that contains only myosin.

Each mammalian sarcomere therefore contains one A band and two half I bands (Figure 54.1b).

Describe the key structural features of the thick and thin filaments

Key features are:

- **Thick filament.** Each thick filament contains myosin, a large protein that has two globular 'heads' and a long 'tail'. The myosin heads have distinct binding sites for actin and ATP (Figure 54.2a). Each thick filament is surrounded

(a) Thick filament

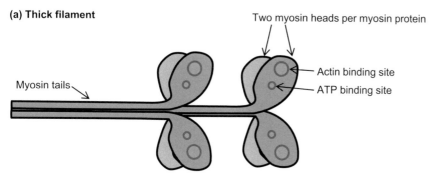

(b) Thin filament

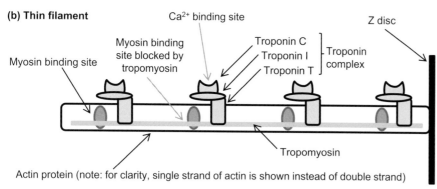

Figure 54.2 Structure of (a) the thick and (b) the thin filament.

by six thin filaments in an approximately hexagonal arrangement

- **Thin filament.** Each thin filament is composed of three proteins: the contractile protein actin and the regulatory proteins tropomyosin and troponin (Figure 54.2b):
  - *Actin* is a globular protein that forms chains that are twisted together in double strands. Each thin filament contains around 300–400 actin molecules with regularly spaced myosin binding sites along its length.
  - *Tropomyosin* is a fibrous protein chain that lies in the groove between the two strands of actin. Tropomyosin obstructs access to the myosin binding site, preventing crossbridges forming between actin and myosin.
  - *Troponin.* This protein complex is located at regularly spaced intervals along the tropomyosin protein chain. The troponin complex is made up of three subunits:
    - *Troponin T* binds the troponin complex to tropomyosin (hence 'T').

    - *Troponin I* has an uncertain role. It may inhibit myosin ATPase activity (hence 'I').
    - *Troponin C* contains the Ca^{2+} binding site (hence 'C' for Ca^{2+}). Binding of Ca^{2+} to troponin C causes tropomyosin to roll deeper into the actin groove, which uncovers the myosin binding site, allowing crossbridges to form between actin and myosin.

What is meant by 'excitation–contraction coupling'?

Excitation–contraction coupling refers to the processes linking depolarisation of the muscle cell membrane to the initiation of myocyte contraction.

In common with neurons, the sarcolemma has excitable properties:

- The myocyte resting membrane potential is typically –90 mV (see Chapter 51).
- The sarcolemma has the capacity to fire action potentials (see Chapter 52): synaptic activity at the motor end plate causes depolarisation of the

sarcolemma, triggering an action potential that propagates along the myocyte surface membrane.

Excitation–contraction coupling occurs as follows:

- **The T-tubules** transmit the action potential deep into the myocyte interior and close to the sarcoplasmic reticular Ca^{2+} store.
- **The dihydropyridine receptor** (DHPR) senses the depolarisation of a T-tubule. The DHPR is a modified subtype of the voltage-gated L-type Ca^{2+} channel; depolarisation causes a conformation change, but allows little Ca^{2+} to pass.[1]
- **The ryanodine receptor** (RyR). The DHPR is in allosteric (physical) contact with the cytoplasmic portion of another important Ca^{2+} channel, the RyR. The RyR also contains an intramembrane portion embedded within the SR membrane. Following a conformation change in the DHPR, these physical connections cause the RyR to open and release Ca^{2+} from the SR, where Ca^{2+} is present at high concentration, to the sarcoplasm, where the Ca^{2+} concentration is low.[2]
- **Release of Ca^{2+} from the SR** increases the intracellular Ca^{2+} concentration by a factor of 2000.
- **Ca^{2+} binds to troponin C**, causing a conformational change of the whole troponin–tropomyosin complex. The myosin binding site is uncovered, which allows actin–myosin interaction.

Clinical relevance: malignant hyperthermia

Malignant hyperthermia (MH) is an inherited disorder of skeletal muscle that may produce a potentially fatal combination of hypermetabolism (with a consequent hyperthermia), muscle rigidity and rhabdomyolysis. MH is a condition of particular relevance

---

[1] A very small quantity of Ca^{2+} passes through the DHPR, but this Ca^{2+} influx is of insufficient quantity and has a time course that is too slow to trigger muscle contraction; therefore, its function remains unclear. Some studies suggest it may be important in controlling gene expression within the muscle fibre (so-called 'excitation–transcription coupling').

[2] Note: the mechanism of excitation–contraction coupling is different in cardiac muscle. Here, Ca^{2+} enters the cardiac myocyte during the plateau phase of the action potential, triggering Ca^{2+}-induced Ca^{2+} release at the SR (see Chapter 57).

to anaesthetists, as the only universally accepted triggering agents are the halogenated volatile anaesthetics and suxamethonium.

It is now known that the genetic defect in MH is an RyR mutation. Once triggered, the abnormal RyR allows uncontrolled Ca^{2+} release from the SR. Clinically, this results in tetanic muscle contraction, which consumes ATP and generates heat. Prolonged muscle tetany may result in rhabdomyolysis. Meanwhile, the SR has increased activity, sequestering cytosolic Ca^{2+} through its Ca^{2+}-ATPase, which exacerbates this ATP consumption. The resulting hypermetabolic state increases total O_2 consumption and CO_2 production and generates a metabolic acidosis.

In addition to supportive measures, the only specific treatment for MH is administration of dantrolene, which is thought to bind to and block the Ca^{2+}-permeant properties of the RyR, inhibiting further Ca^{2+} release. Untreated, the mortality rate for MH is very high, in the order of 80%. However, the introduction of dantrolene together with a greater awareness of the condition has led to a much lower mortality rate of 2–3%.

How does skeletal muscle contract?

Exposure of the myosin binding site on the actin filament permits the process of crossbridge cycling, which in turn generates mechanical force:

- The myosin heads bind ATP (Figure 54.3a). The ATP molecule is hydrolysed to ADP and inorganic phosphate (P_i), and the released bond energy is transferred to the myosin head. Energised myosin heads are now able to bind to their neighbouring actin molecules, forming crossbridges (Figure 54.3b).
- The energised myosin head flexes on its actin binding site, and the action of this on the myosin tail gives rise to the 'power stroke' that moves the actin filament closer to the centre of the sarcomere (Figure 54.3c). In this process, ADP and P_i dissociate from the energised myosin head.
- A fresh ATP molecule binds to the myosin head. The myosin–ATP complex has a low affinity for its binding site on the actin filament and dissociates from it (Figure 54.3d). ATP is then hydrolysed to ADP, and the whole process repeats.

During contraction, the movement of the actin filament results in the following changes:

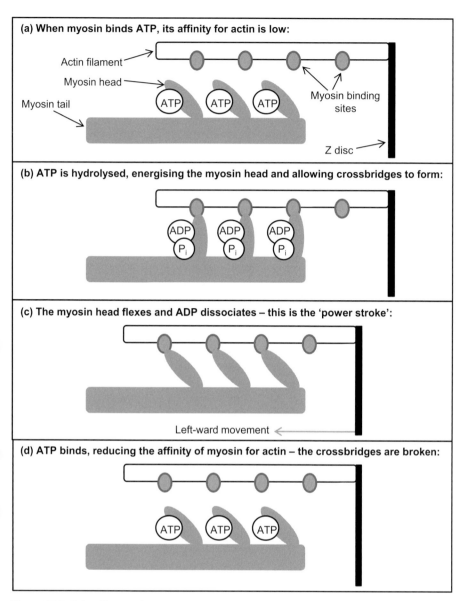

Figure 54.3 Sliding filament theory.

- The Z lines move closer together – the overall width of the sarcomere decreases.
- The width of the I band decreases, as thin filaments overlap thick filaments to a greater extent.
- There is no change in the width of the A band, as thick filaments do not shorten.

Actin–myosin crossbridge cycling continues until the intracellular Ca^{2+} concentration decreases. This occurs when Ca^{2+} is re-sequestered into the SR by means of the SR/ER Ca^{2+}-ATPase (SERCA). As sarcoplasmic Ca^{2+} concentration decreases:

- Ca^{2+} dissociates from troponin C.
- Troponin T and tropomyosin return to their resting configurations. Tropomyosin covers the myosin binding sites: crossbridges can no longer form between actin and myosin. The muscle relaxes and the sarcomere returns to its original length.

Overall, ATP therefore has three crucial roles in skeletal muscle contraction:

- **Energising the myosin head**: the hydrolysis of ATP energises the myosin head, providing the energy for the power stroke.
- **Detachment of crossbridges**: following the power stroke, binding of ATP causes dissociation of the myosin head from the actin filament.
- **Muscle relaxation**: Ca^{2+} is sequestered in the SR by the SERCA.

After death, muscle ATP stores are rapidly depleted. There is no longer sufficient ATP to power the SERCA. Ca^{2+} therefore remains bound to troponin C and thus actin–myosin crossbridges cannot detach, resulting in a high skeletal muscle tone known as rigor mortis.

What is the motor unit?

The motor unit consists of a single α-motor neuron, its axon and the many muscle cells that it innervates. A single action potential in an α-motor neuron results in the contraction of all the myocytes within the motor unit. Motor units have some key features:

- Each motor unit innervates only one myocyte type, such as type I muscle fibres (see Chapter 42).
- Groups of motor units often work together to coordinate the contraction of a single muscle. The force of contraction within a muscle is controlled by the number of motor units activated.
- The number of muscle fibres within each motor unit varies considerably between muscles:

  - Large, powerful muscles, like the quadriceps femoris, perform gross movements. The quadriceps therefore contain >1000 myocytes per motor unit.
  - Some muscles require fine control and thus have proportionally more motor units that contain fewer myocytes. The extraocular muscles have as few as 10 myocytes per motor unit.

How is the force of muscle contraction determined?

Three main factors determine muscle tension:

- **Recruitment of motor units**. The force of contraction of a whole muscle depends on the number of contracting myocytes. Initially, the smallest motor units are recruited; larger motor units are additionally recruited as greater muscle tension is required.

- **Frequency of action potentials**. The duration of the refractory period in nerve and skeletal muscle is shorter than the time course of both the relaxation of muscle tension and Ca^{2+} uptake into the SR. Delivery of action potentials at a high frequency therefore results in a progressive accumulation of Ca^{2+} in the cytoplasm and thus an increased and sustained muscle tension, or tetanus.
- **Initial muscle length**. The tension generated within a single muscle fibre is related to the number of actin–myosin crossbridges formed (see Chapter 30 and Figure 30.2):

  - At the optimal sarcomere length, the myosin heads have the greatest possible overlap with actin filaments.
  - Excessive sarcomere stretch can completely remove actin–myosin overlap; no crossbridges can then form.
  - Excessive sarcomere shortening results in filament collisions, leading to an increase in frictional forces and distortion of the sarcomere, which precludes further contraction.

Normally, the sarcomeres within skeletal muscles are arranged near to their optimal length, so the initial muscle length usually contributes little to muscle tension.

Clinical relevance: disorders of skeletal muscle

Skeletal muscle disorder is a broad term encompassing dystrophies, myotonias, myopathies and metabolic disorders. The most common are:

- **Duchenne's muscular dystrophy** (DMD), an X-linked recessive disorder that causes a deficiency of dystrophin, a protein that anchors actin via a support protein to the sarcolemma. Clinically, patients present between the ages of 3 and 5 with proximal muscle weakness. The sarcomeres are inadequately tethered to the cell membrane and become replaced by fibrous tissue, which clinically results in pseudohypertrophy. DMD is usually fatal by late adolescence from respiratory or cardiac failure.
- **Becker's muscular dystrophy** (BMD), also an X-linked recessive disorder affecting the dystrophin protein. In BMD, the amount of dystrophin protein is reduced and structurally abnormal. Clinically, BMD is less severe than

DMD, presenting in adolescence, with death in the fourth or fifth decade.

- **Myotonic dystrophy**, is an autosomal dominant trinucleotide repeat disorder that may show anticipation. Mutations in either dystrophia myotonica protein kinase (DMPK, in DM1) or cellular nucleic acid binding protein (CNBP, in DM2) result in the abnormal expression of Na^+ or Cl^- channels in the muscle sarcolemma. The myocytes exist in an abnormal hyperexcitable state, resulting in repetitive action potentials and sustained muscle contraction. The resulting clinical features include myotonia (abnormally prolonged or repetitive muscle contraction after voluntary relaxation or percussion), muscle wasting, insulin resistance, cardiomyopathy and cardiac conduction defects.
- **Myotonia congenita**, an autosomal dominant disorder characterised by an abnormal sarcolemma ClC-1 chloride channel. Like myotonic dystrophy, the myocytes become hyperexcitable, leading to myotonia. However, the two conditions differ: myotonia congenita is not associated with generalised muscle weakness, but may cause palatopharyngeal dysfunction, leading to dysphagia.

Clinical relevance: muscle atrophy

Muscle atrophy refers to a decrease in muscle mass, which may be caused by:

- **Muscle inactivity**, such as immobilisation of a fractured limb, extended bed rest and space travel.
- **Neurogenic atrophy**, where muscle denervation leads to atrophy.
- **Cachexia**, which accompanies a range of illnesses, including cancer, cystic fibrosis, chronic obstructive pulmonary disease and human immunodeficiency virus. Cachexia is probably caused by inflammatory cytokines such as tumour necrosis factor-α, interferon-γ and interleukin-6.
- **Drugs**, such as corticosteroids, which cause preferential wasting of the proximal muscles though increased muscle catabolism.

- **Starvation**, due to catabolism of skeletal muscle.
- **Ageing**, which is associated with a generalised decrease in muscle mass and function known as sarcopenia.

Intensive care unit-acquired weakness (ICUAW) is common cause of morbidity in critically ill patients, characterised by symmetric, flaccid muscle weakness, which classically affects all muscle groups with relative sparing of the cranial nerves. ICUAW is classified into the overlapping syndromes of critical illness polyneuropathy, critical illness myopathy and critical illness neuromyopathy. The pathophysiology of ICUAW is complex and includes the use of corticosteroids and neuromuscular blockers, circulating cytokines as a result of severe sepsis and immobilisation. Patients lose an average of 2–4% of muscle mass per day, which causes difficulty in weaning from mechanical ventilation and increased risk of ventilator-associated pneumonia and venous thromboembolism.

Further reading

J. Xiao. *Muscle Atrophy*. Singapore, Springer Verlag, 2018.

R. D. Keynes, D. J. Aidley, C. L.-H. Huang. *Nerve and Muscle, 4th edition*. Cambridge, Cambridge University Press, 2011.

P. K. Gupta, P. M. Hopkins. Diagnosis and management of malignant hyperthermia. *BJA Education* 2017; 17(7): 249–54.

C. L.-H. Huang, T. H. Pedersen, J. A. Fraser. Reciprocal dihydropyridine and ryanodine receptor interactions in skeletal muscle activation. *J Muscle Res Cell Motil* 2011; 32(3): 171–202.

R. Appleton, J. Kinsella. Intensive care unit-acquired weakness. *Continuing Educ Anaesth Crit Care Pain* 2012; 12(2): 62–6.

S. Marsh, N. Ross, A. Pittard. Neuromuscular disorders and anaesthesia. Part 1: generic anaesthetic management. *Continuing Educ Anaesth Crit Care Pain* 2011; 11(4): 115–18.

S. Marsh, A. Pittard. Neuromuscular disorders and anaesthesia. Part 2: specific neuromuscular disorders. *Continuing Educ Anaesth Crit Care Pain* 2011; 11(4): 119–23.

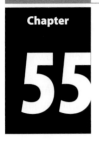

Chapter

Muscle Spindles and Golgi Tendon Organs

What is proprioception?

Proprioception refers to the detection of stimuli relating to body position in space and postural equilibrium. Mechanoreceptors within muscle, joints and tendons relay sensory information about joint position, movement, vibration and pressure to the central nervous system. The major sensory receptors involved include:

- **Muscle spindles**, which detect changes in muscle length;
- **Golgi tendon organs**, which detect muscle tension.

What is a muscle spindle?

The muscle spindle is an encapsulated structure containing between 3 and 12 specialised intracapsular muscle fibres, known as intrafusal fibres. Intrafusal fibres are arranged in parallel with contractile extrafusal fibres; stretch of the extrafusal fibres therefore alters the intrafusal fibre length. An intrafusal fibre consists of a central non-contractile elastic portion with outer contractile ends.

There are two morphologically distinct types of intracapsular muscle fibre (Figure 55.1):

- **Nuclear bag fibres**, in which the nuclei are collected in a central dilated portion of the fibre;
- **Nuclear chain fibres**, in which the nuclei are distributed along the fibre without a dilatation.

How are muscle spindles innervated?

Muscle spindles have their own dedicated afferent and efferent nerve supplies (Figure 55.1):

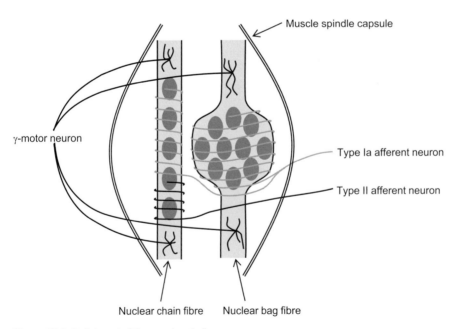

Figure 55.1 Basic layout of the muscle spindle.

- **Afferent nerve supply**: sensory afferent neurons wind around the central portion of the intrafusal fibres. There are two types:

  - *Type Ia afferent neurons* receive inputs from both nuclear bag and nuclear chain fibres. Electrical activity in type Ia fibres reflects changes in both static intrafusal fibre length and rate of such change.
  - *Type II afferent neurons* receive inputs from nuclear chain fibres only. Type II neurons relay information only about the static intrafusal fibre length.

- **Efferent nerve supply**: γ-motor neurons innervate the contractile outer portions of the intrafusal fibres. Each γ-motor neuron innervates a number of muscle spindles.

Voluntary contraction involves the simultaneous activation of both α- and γ-motor neurons. Contraction of the outer portions of the intrafusal fibres prevents slackening of the spindle, despite the shortening of the extrafusal fibres. The sensitivity of the muscle spindles is therefore maintained despite skeletal muscle shortening and variations in its load.

What is a Golgi tendon organ?

Golgi tendon organs are stretch receptors located at the junction between skeletal muscle and tendon. Golgi tendon organs are arranged in series rather than in parallel with the extrafusal muscle fibres and therefore sense muscle tension. Each Golgi tendon organ is innervated by a single type Ib afferent neuron. They have no motor innervation.

What is a reflex arc?

A reflex is an automatic, predictable response to a stimulus that is generally not under voluntary control. The simplest reflexes involve a sensory receptor, an afferent neuron, one or more synapses, an efferent neuron and an effector organ.

Reflex arcs may be classified by their number of synapses:

- **Monosynaptic reflex arcs**. The classical example is the knee-jerk (see below).
- **Polysynaptic reflex arcs**. For example, the withdrawal reflex: when a limb touches a hot object, the whole limb moves away through the coordinated contraction and relaxation of many muscle groups.

Reflex arcs may also be classified by the origin of the sensory signal:

- **From a peripheral sensory afferent neuron** – for example, the knee-jerk.
- **From the autonomic nervous system** – for example, the baroreceptor reflex.
- **From a cranial nerve** – for example, the gag reflex.

Describe the knee-jerk reflex

Striking the patellar tendon with a tendon hammer results in a predictable response: contraction of the quadriceps muscle and extension of the knee – this is known as the knee-jerk or patellar reflex. The knee-jerk is classically regarded as a monosynaptic reflex[1] involving (Figure 55.2):

- **Sensory receptors** – muscle spindles of the quadriceps muscle. When the patellar tendon is struck, the quadriceps muscle is stretched along with its embedded muscle spindles.
- **An afferent neuron** – type Ia afferent neurons from the muscle spindles relay information about the degree of muscle stretch to the ventral horn of the spinal cord through the dorsal root.
- **A synapse** – in the ventral horn of the spinal cord, the afferent neuron synapses directly with an α-motor neuron. This synapse is excitatory (utilising glutamate as the neurotransmitter).
- **An efferent neuron** – the α-motor neuron leaves the ventral horn in a spinal nerve and travels to the quadriceps muscle, where it innervates several muscle fibres.
- **An effector organ** – the quadriceps muscle contracts in response to α-motor neuron activity.

As the knee-jerk is a monosynaptic pathway, the latency period between muscle spindle activation and quadriceps contraction is relatively short.

However, other processes contribute to the knee-jerk reflex:

- The type Ia afferent neurons branch within the spinal cord, synapsing through interneurons with α-motor neurons of antagonistic muscles, which in this case would oppose knee flexion

---

[1] Note: although classical descriptions refer to the knee-jerk as a monosynaptic reflex, there is also a relaxation of the antagonistic hamstring muscles through a polysynaptic mechanism.

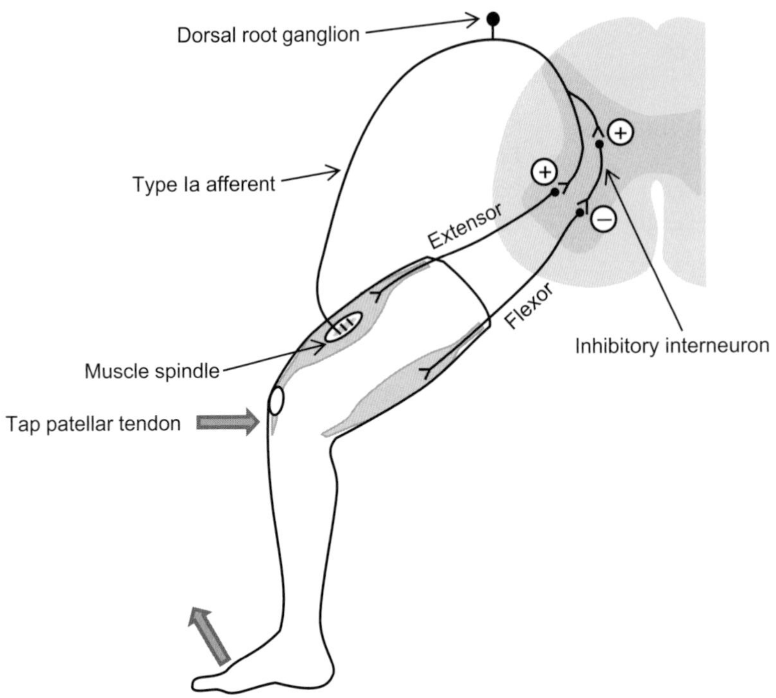

Figure 55.2 The knee-jerk reflex.

(e.g. the hamstrings). This synapse is inhibitory, utilising glycine as neurotransmitter. Inhibition of antagonistic muscles allows the quadriceps muscle to contract unopposed (Figure 55.2).

- Additionally, descending inputs from the brain may modulate the intensity of reflexes:
  - The knee-jerk reflex is lost following repeated rapid strikes of the patellar tendon.
  - The Jendrassik manoeuvre, where the patient clenches their teeth or pulls their interlocked hands apart, results in an increased level of γ-motor neuron firing, thereby increasing the background stretch in the spindle, which results in an accentuation of the knee-jerk reflex.

How is muscle tone controlled?

Muscle tone reflects a continuous, basal level of muscle contraction. Muscle tone is controlled by descending extrapyramidal supraspinal neurons, which innervate the γ-motor neurons of the muscle spindles. γ-motor neuron activation leads to:

- Shortening of the contractile ends of the intrafusal fibres, which in turn stretches the central non-contractile portion of the fibre, increasing

the level of action potentials firing in the type Ia afferent fibres.

- Type Ia afferent activity in turn activates α-motor neurons through the monosynaptic reflex arc, causing contraction of the extrafusal fibres, thereby increasing the tone of the skeletal muscle.

Clinical relevance: spinal shock

As discussed above, muscle tone is primarily determined by extrapyramidal supraspinal neurons. In acute spinal cord injury, these supraspinal pathways are interrupted. The γ-motor neurons become inactive and the muscles become hypotonic or flaccid, which is termed spinal shock.

After around 2 weeks, the activity in the γ-motor neurons becomes excessive, which results in increased muscle tone. This hypertonicity is known as muscle spasticity. The exact mechanism behind the increase in γ-motor neuron activity is not known.

Further reading

U. Proske, S. C. Gandevia. The proprioceptive senses: their roles in signaling body shape, body position and movement, and muscle force. *Physiol Rev* 2012; **92**(4): 1651–97.

56

Smooth Muscle

Where is smooth muscle found in the body?

Smooth muscle is a type of involuntary muscle, innervated by the autonomic nervous system (ANS). In contrast to skeletal and cardiac muscle, smooth muscle is non-striated. Smooth muscle is found within the walls of hollow organs and tubes. The following are important examples:

- **The uterus** is primarily composed of smooth muscle. Uterine smooth muscle contraction provides the driving force for parturition. Smooth muscle contraction is also essential in the immediate post-partum period in securing uterine haemostasis following delivery; uterine atony is a common cause of post-partum haemorrhage.
- **The arteries** contain layers of vascular smooth muscle within their tunica media. Contraction of vascular smooth muscle reduces the vessel radius, increasing its resistance to blood flow.
- **The respiratory tract**, where bronchiolar smooth muscle contraction results in bronchoconstriction.
- **The gastrointestinal (GI) tract** – coordinated contraction of longitudinal and circular smooth muscle (segmentation and peristalsis) in the intestinal wall mixes and propels the luminal contents along the gut.

What are the two types of smooth muscle?

Smooth muscle is classified into two types:

- **Single-unit smooth muscle** occurs in the viscera and the blood vessels, except the large elastic arteries, as sheets of smooth muscle cells forming syncytial units. The ANS innervates a single cell within the sheet, with action potentials rapidly propagated to neighbouring cells through gap junctions, leading to synchronous contraction.

- **Multi-unit smooth muscle** is found in the large elastic arteries, the trachea and the iris. These smooth muscle cells are not connected by gap junctions. A single autonomic nerve branches to innervate many smooth muscle cells, in a similar way to the motor unit in skeletal muscle.

How do smooth muscle cells differ from skeletal muscle cells?

Smooth muscle and skeletal muscle have a number of anatomical and functional differences:

- **Size**: skeletal muscle cells are large, cylindrical cells that span the entire length of the muscle. Smooth muscle cells are much smaller, spindle-shaped cells that are arranged in sheets, or syncytia.
- **Nuclei**: skeletal muscle cells are multi-nucleate, whilst smooth muscle cells have only one nucleus.
- **Sarcomeres**: like skeletal muscle, the primary function of smooth muscle is contraction. In both skeletal and smooth muscle, actin and myosin are the main contractile proteins: actin is arranged in thin filaments and myosin in thick filaments. However, in smooth muscle, the thick and thin filaments are not organised into sarcomeres – smooth muscle is therefore not striated.
- **Troponin complex**: whilst tropomyosin is present in both smooth and skeletal muscle, troponin is absent in smooth muscle.
- **Transverse (T)-tubules**: the tube-like invaginations of the skeletal muscle sarcolemma are absent in smooth muscle. Instead, smooth muscle has shallower, rudimentary invaginations known as caveolae, which increase the surface area-to-volume ratio of the muscle cell.
- **The sarcoplasmic reticulum** (SR): an intracellular store of Ca^{2+}. Despite the important role of the SR in skeletal muscle excitation–contraction coupling (see Chapter 54), the SR is poorly developed in smooth muscle.

Describe how smooth muscle is excited

Smooth muscle cells receive both excitatory and inhibitory signals: excitatory signals depolarise whilst inhibitory signals hyperpolarise the smooth muscle cell membrane. If the net effect of these signals is depolarisation to threshold potential, contraction occurs. Like skeletal muscle, multi-unit smooth muscle can only be stimulated by nerve impulses. However, single-unit smooth muscle cells may be stimulated in a number of ways:

- **Autonomic neuronal input.** Single-unit smooth muscle is often innervated by two neurons: sympathetic (releasing noradrenaline as the neurotransmitter) and parasympathetic (releasing acetylcholine). These two autonomic inputs are usually antagonistic: one tends to excite whilst the other tends to inhibit the smooth muscle cell.
- **Hormones and other circulating molecules.** Smooth muscle cells may be excited or inhibited by circulating molecules, including O_2, CO_2, NO, adrenaline, noradrenaline, histamine, prostaglandins and serotonin.
- **Stretch** of the smooth muscle sheets triggers smooth muscle contraction. In the arterial system, this is referred to as the 'myogenic response', responsible for the autoregulation of blood flow (see Chapter 34). In the GI tract, peristalsis may be triggered when the luminal contents stretch the smooth muscle of the gut wall.
- **Pacemaker activity.** Like the heart, the GI tract contains pacemaker cells (the interstitial cells of Cajal) whose cell membrane spontaneously depolarises, triggering an action potential. The spontaneous oscillation in the pacemaker cell membrane potential is called the 'slow wave'. The frequency of slow waves differs throughout the GI tract. For example, around 12 action potentials are generated per minute in the duodenum, compared with only three per minute in the colon.

Describe how excitation–contraction coupling occurs in smooth muscle

Smooth muscle excitation–contraction coupling differs from skeletal muscle in several respects:

- **Lack of T-tubules:** action potentials are propagated rapidly between cells through gap junctions, but are not relayed directly to the cell interior. Caveolae increase the surface area-to-volume ratio, which facilitates Ca^{2+} entry.
- **Ca^{2+}:** like skeletal muscle, an increase in intracellular Ca^{2+} concentration triggers muscle contraction. But smooth muscle cells lack T-tubules and have an absent or poorly developed SR. Smooth muscle cells have various mechanisms to increase Ca^{2+} influx:
  - *Voltage-gated Ca^{2+} channels;*
  - *Ligand-gated Ca^{2+} channels;*
  - *Stretch-responsive Ca^{2+} channels.*

  Smooth muscle cells with a functional SR augment the increase in sarcoplasmic Ca^{2+} by releasing further Ca^{2+}.
- **Calmodulin:** as discussed above, the thin filaments of smooth muscle do not contain troponin. Instead, calmodulin regulates smooth muscle contraction. When the sarcoplasmic Ca^{2+} concentration rises, Ca^{2+} binds to calmodulin. The resulting Ca^{2+}–calmodulin complex then activates smooth muscle contraction through three pathways:
  - *Myosin light-chain kinase* (MLCK). The sarcoplasmic enzyme MLCK is activated by the Ca^{2+}–calmodulin complex. MLCK phosphorylates the myosin light-chains, allowing myosin to form crossbridges with actin filaments.
  - *Caldesmon.* In skeletal muscle, the troponin complex positions tropomyosin over the myosin binding site, preventing actin–myosin interaction. Troponin is absent in smooth muscle – this role is instead played by a protein called caldesmon. The Ca^{2+}–calmodulin complex causes a conformational change in caldesmon that leads to tropomyosin movement, unblocking the myosin binding site and permitting actomyosin crossbridge cycling.
  - *Calponin.* This protein inhibits the ATPase activity of the myosin head. It may be activated either by the Ca^{2+}–calmodulin complex or directly by Ca^{2+}.

There are thus more points of biochemical regulation in smooth muscle contraction than in skeletal muscle contraction, reflecting the greater importance of hormones and neurotransmitters in controlling smooth muscle activity.

How does smooth muscle contract?

The mechanism of contraction is similar to that of skeletal muscle (Chapter 54), involving ATP binding to the myosin head, ATP hydrolysis, the 'power stroke' and the release of ADP and inorganic phosphate followed by binding of a new ATP molecule.

The rate of smooth muscle contraction is much slower than that of skeletal muscle:

- Smooth muscle action potentials are typically slower and more prolonged than those of skeletal muscle: smooth muscle sarcoplasmic Ca^{2+} concentration increases and decreases slowly.
- Enzymatic phosphorylation is required before myosin can bind to actin.
- Crossbridge cycling is also much slower than that of skeletal muscle.

Smooth muscle also relaxes much more slowly than skeletal muscle due to slower Ca^{2+} removal from the sarcoplasm in the absence of an efficient SR. Overall, contraction occurs up to ten times slower and lasts up to 30 times longer in smooth muscle, but the muscle tension generated is equal to that of skeletal muscle.

How is smooth muscle adapted for its function?

Compared with skeletal muscle, smooth muscle must be energy efficient and often needs to maintain tension for long durations. This is achieved in two ways:

- **Slow contraction consumes less energy**, as the power of contraction is equal to the force multiplied by the velocity.
- **Latch bridge formation**. If myosin is dephosphorylated whilst still attached to actin, the crossbridge remains in place. This is known as latch bridge formation. The tension in smooth muscle therefore remains high without further consumption of ATP. This type of activity is common in sphincter control where the muscle must remain tonically active for long periods.

Smooth muscle is therefore well suited to contract for sustained periods of time whilst using ATP economically.

Further reading

R. D. Keynes, D. J. Aidley, C. L.-H. Huang. *Nerve and Muscle, 4th edition*. Cambridge, Cambridge University Press, 2011.

K. M. Sanders. Regulation of smooth muscle excitation and contraction. *Neurogastroneterol Motil* 2008; 20(Suppl. 1): 39–53.

Cardiac Muscle

Describe the structural features of cardiac muscle

The primary function of the heart is ejection of blood into the vascular system. Individual cardiomyocytes are specialised in the generation of spontaneous activity (automaticity), transmission of the resulting excitable activity and contraction in response to such excitation. Thus:

- **Atrial and ventricular myocardial cells** are capable of both contraction and conduction of action potentials.
- **Pacemaker and conducting cells** are excitable but non-contractile:
  - *Pacemaker cells*, found in the sinoatrial (SA) and atrioventricular (AV) nodes, generate spontaneous cardiac action potentials.
  - *Conducting cells*, known as Purkinje fibres, spread the cardiac action potentials around the ventricles.

Cardiac myocytes share a number of structural features with skeletal muscle:

- **A striated appearance**, owing to organised rows of thick and thin filaments within the sarcoplasm.
- **A sarcotubular system** – ventricular myocytes have both T-tubules and sarcoplasmic reticulum (SR), although they are often less developed than in skeletal muscle.

However, cardiac myocytes also share a number of similarities with smooth muscle:

- **Involuntary control**. Like smooth muscle, the autonomic nervous system (ANS) and endocrine axes modulate the function of cardiac myocytes.
- **Cells connected by gap junctions**. These low-resistance electrical connections allow the rapid conduction of action potentials throughout the myocardium through connexin channels. Thus, the cardiac myocytes contract as a single unit or functional syncytium.

What is the resting membrane potential in cardiac muscle cells?

Like the neuronal resting membrane potential (RMP) discussed in Chapter 51, the cardiac myocyte RMP is due to:

- A large difference between intracellular and extracellular K^+ and Na^+ ion concentrations.
- The resting cell membrane having a higher permeability to K^+ than to Na^+.
  - *In neurons*, K^+ permeability is predominantly due to membrane K^+ leak channels (two-pore-domain K^+ channels), which are constitutively open.
  - *In cardiac myocytes*, K^+ permeability is due to the presence of inward rectifying K^+ channels (K_{ir} channels), which are open at negative membrane potentials, but close with depolarisation.
- K^+ diffuses down its electrochemical gradient, resulting in the cell interior becoming negatively charged with respect to the cell exterior.

The RMP varies depending on the cardiac region:

- SA node, approximately –50 mV, but unstable;
- Atrial myocyte, –70 mV;
- Purkinje fibre, –90 mV;
- Ventricular myocyte, –90 mV.

How do cardiac and nerve action potentials differ?

There are a number of important differences between nerve and cardiac action potentials:

- **RMP**. As discussed above, the RMP of cardiac myocytes varies with cardiac region. Ventricular myocytes and Purkinje fibres have an RMP that is more negative (–90 mV) than the neuronal RMP (–70 mV).
- **Duration**. The nerve action potential is very short (1–2 ms), whilst the cardiac action potential has a

much longer duration, depending on myocardial cell type (200–400 ms in ventricular myocytes and Purkinje fibres).

- **Shape**. Morphologically, the nerve action potential is a single spike, whilst the cardiac action potential varies from having a triangular waveform (atrial muscle) to having a long plateau phase (ventricular myocytes and Purkinje fibres).
- **The role of Ca^{2+}**. In cardiac cells, Ca^{2+} influx prolongs the duration of the action potential, resulting in the characteristic plateau phase of ventricular myocytes. Ca^{2+} plays no role in the nerve action potential.

Outline the phases of the cardiac action potential

The cardiac action potential has five phases (Figure 57.1):

- **Phase 0, rapid depolarisation**.
  - The threshold potential for cardiac myocytes is around –65 mV. The threshold potential is reached by the depolarising action of local currents conducted through gap junctions from neighbouring myocytes.
  - Stimuli that exceed threshold potential trigger the opening of fast voltage-gated Na^+ channels, thereby increasing membrane Na^+ permeability.
  - The resultant increased Na^+ influx causes a further membrane depolarisation, which triggers further opening of voltage-gated Na^+ channels; a positive-feedback loop is created.
  - The end result is rapid depolarisation to approximately +20 mV.
- **Phase 1, early rapid repolarisation**. Following the membrane depolarisation of phase 0:
  - Voltage-gated Na^+ channels inactivate, resulting in a rapid decrease in the membrane Na^+ permeability.
  - Fast voltage-gated K^+ channels transiently open, resulting in a transient outward K^+ current I_{to} (Figure 57.2).

The overall effect is a brief phase of repolarisation.

- **Phase 2, plateau**. Membrane depolarisation is maintained for a prolonged period (around 200 ms) through a balance of inward and outward currents:

  - *Inward current*: voltage-gated L-type Ca^{2+} channels slowly open following membrane depolarisation. Ca^{2+} ions flow down their concentration gradient from the extracellular fluid (ECF), where the ionised Ca^{2+} concentration is around 1.2 mmol/L, to the intracellular fluid (ICF), which has a considerably lower ionised Ca^{2+} concentration (around 500 nmol/L).
  - *Outward current*: as discussed above, K_{ir} channels are predominantly responsible for generating the RMP, but close following membrane depolarisation. At the same time, membrane depolarisation causes slow delayed rectifier K^+ channels to open.

  Overall, there is a net inward current that maintains the plateau.

- **Phase 3, repolarisation**. A gradual inactivation of voltage-gated Ca^{2+} channels reduces the inward Ca^{2+} current. Additional outward K^+ currents[1] return the membrane to its RMP (Figure 57.2).
- **Phase 4, electrical diastole**. During this phase, the membrane is maintained at RMP due to K^+ efflux through K_{ir} channels. There is also a correction of the small net fluxes of Na^+, K^+ and Ca^{2+} that took place during the action potential through Na^+/K^+-ATPase and Na^+/Ca^{2+}-exchanger activity.

In summary (Figure 57.2):

- *Phase 0* – a brief, rapid increase in Na^+ conductance results in rapid depolarisation.
- *Phase 1* – K^+ conductance increases transiently.
- *Phase 2* – the increase in Ca^+ conductance results in an inward Ca^{2+} current, which opposes the tendency of the outward K^+ current to restore the membrane potential, resulting in the action potential plateau.
- *Phase 3* – a decrease in Ca^{2+} conductance and a progressive increase in K^+ conductance results in membrane repolarisation.
- *Phase 4* – Ca^{2+}, Na^+ and K^+ conductance have returned to resting levels, with K^+ conductance exceeding Ca^{2+} and Na^+ conductance, resulting in the RMP.

---

[1] Rapid and slow delayed rectifier K^+ channels produce outward K^+ currents I_{Kr} and I_{Ks}, respectively. As the cell membrane develops an increasingly negative potential, K_{ir} channels reopen, which further increases membrane K^+ permeability and thus K^+ efflux.

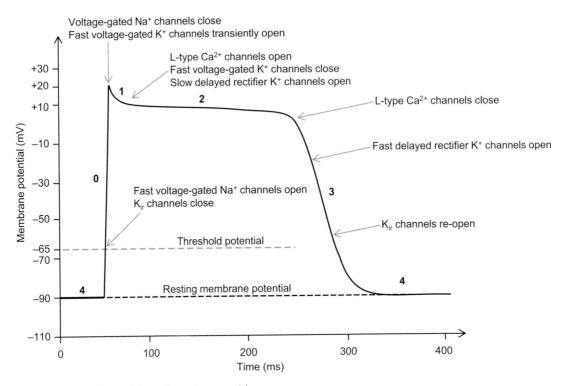

Figure 57.1 The phases of the cardiac action potential.

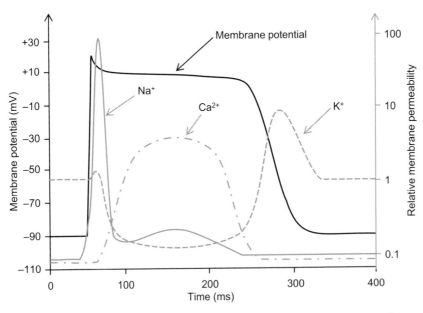

Figure 57.2 Changes in membrane permeability to ions during the cardiac action potential.

At a heart rate (HR) of 75 bpm, the ventricular action potential lasts for around 250 ms:

- Phases 0 and 1 have a total duration of 1–2 ms, similar to that of the nerve action potential. The summed activity of phase 0 and 1 across the septum and ventricular wall corresponds to the QRS complex of the electrocardiogram (ECG).

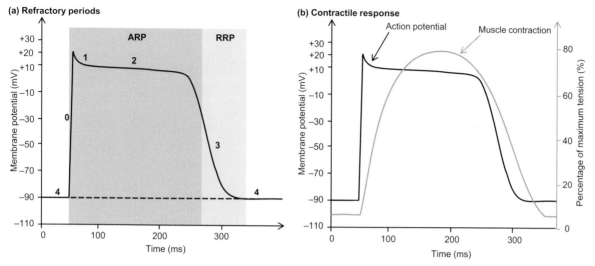

Figure 57.3 (a) The absolute refractory period (ARP) and relative refractory period (RRP) of the cardiac action potential and (b) Relationship between the cardiac action potential and the contractile response of cardiac muscle.

- Phase 2 lasts for around 200 ms and corresponds to the ST-segment of the ECG.
- Phase 3 takes around 50 ms, and corresponds to the T-wave of the ECG.

The duration of the action potential decreases with increasing HR: at a rate of 200 bpm, the action potential lasts for only 150 ms. This is why QT intervals must be corrected (QTc) to make values comparable across a range of HRs.

What are the refractory periods of the cardiac action potential?

In common with the nerve action potential (Chapter 52), the cardiac action potential has two refractory periods (Figure 57.3a):

- **The absolute refractory period** (ARP), where a further action potential cannot be initiated, no matter how large a stimulus is applied. Following membrane depolarisation, the fast voltage-gated Na^+ channels become inactivated. Inactivated Na^+ channels cannot return to their resting state until membrane repolarisation has occurred. The prolonged plateau phase of the cardiac action potential means that the ARP is 200 ms, which is considerably longer than that of the nerve action potential. The long ARP of cardiac muscle means that further action potentials cannot be triggered until muscle contraction is nearly complete (Figure 57.3b). A short ARP could potentially lead

to tetany of the cardiac muscle, which would be incompatible with diastolic filling.

- **The relative refractory period** (RRP), when a further action potential can be initiated, but it requires a greater stimulus than normal.

Clinical relevance: antiarrhythmic drugs

The Singh–Vaughan Williams classification (Table 57.1) categorises antiarrhythmic drugs into four classes on the basis of their ionic mechanism. Later, Class V was added to include antiarrhythmic drugs with mechanisms dissimilar to the other four classes. However, few antiarrhythmic drugs are specific to one class. For example, flecainide (Class 1C) also blocks K^+ channels, amiodarone (Class III) also blocks Na^+ and Ca^{2+} channels and sotalol (Class III) is also a β-blocker. It is also important to note that relatively few drugs are effective in the treatment of ventricular fibrillation; cardioversion is therefore indicated.

Where are action potentials generated in the heart?

Pacemaker cells are specialised cardiac myocytes whose spontaneous activity results in the regular generation of action potentials. The rate at which action potentials are produced by the pacemaker cells determines the frequency of cardiac contraction. Several sites within the heart may act as pacemakers:

Table 57.1 Classification of antiarrhythmic drugs (see also Vaughan Williams, 1975).

Class	Mechanism	Examples	Use	Physiological effect
1	Na^+ channel blockers			↓ membrane excitability and conduction velocity
1A	Intermediate kinetics	Quinidine, procainamide	AF, SVT	↑ APD and ERP
1B	Fast kinetics	Lidocaine	Digoxin toxicity (VF)	↓ APD and ERP
1C	Slow kinetics	Flecainide	AF, SVT	Normal APD
II	β-blockers	Propranolol, bisoprolol	VT, AF, SVT	↓ sympathetic drive and AVN conduction
III	K^+ channel blockers	Amiodarone, sotalol	VT, AF, SVT, (VF)	↑ APD and ERP
IV	Ca^{2+} channel blockers	Verapamil	AF, SVT	↓ AVN conduction without affecting sympathetic drive
V	Other	Adenosine, digoxin, M_gSO_4	SVT, AF, Tdp	↓ AVN conduction ↓ AVN conduction and HR ↓ Ca^{2+} influx and EADs

VT = ventricular tachycardia; AF = atrial fibrillation; SVT = supraventricular tachycardia; VF = ventricular fibrillation; Tdp = torsades de pointes (polymorphic ventricular tachycardia); AVN = atrioventricular node; APD = action potential duration; ERP = effective refractory period; EAD = early afterdepolarisation.

- **The SA node**, located at the junction between the superior vena cava and right atrium. The SA node generates action potentials at a higher frequency than the other pacemaker cells and therefore normally sets the HR.
- **The AV node**, located between the atrial septum and tricuspid valve, just above the opening of the coronary sinus.
- **The bundle of His**, located within the interventricular septum.
- **The Purkinje fibres**, a specialised network of cardiac myocytes that conduct electrical impulses to the ventricles.

What is meant by the term 'pacemaker potential'?

The pacemaker potential refers to the spontaneous decay of the membrane potential of a pacemaker cell, from a membrane potential of approximately –60 mV (in the SA node) to threshold potential (approximately –40 mV in the SA node), thereby initiating an action potential. The rate at which the pacemaker potential decays to threshold determines the HR; this

property of the pacemaker potential is called automaticity.

Historically, the pacemaker potential was called the 'funny' current I_f. It is now known that the slow depolarisation of the membrane potential is due to the intracellular movement of Na^+ ions exceeding the extracellular movement of K^+ ions (see below).

Describe the action of the pacemaker currents

- The action potential in pacemaker cells (Figure 57.4) includes contributions from hyperpolarisation-activated cyclic nucleotide-gated (HCN) channels. These channels are permeable to both Na^+ and K^+.
- Following an action potential, membrane hyperpolarisation opens HCN channels, allowing Na^+ and K^+ to diffuse along their electrochemical gradients. Overall, Na^+ influx slightly exceeds K^+ efflux, resulting in a slow depolarisation of the cell membrane from its initial voltage of –60 mV.
- When the membrane potential reaches approximately –50 mV, T-type (transient) Ca^{2+}

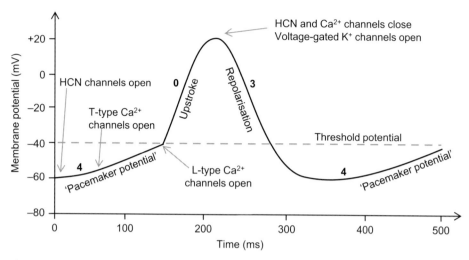

Figure 57.4 The pacemaker action potential.

channels open in the pacemaker cell membrane, resulting in inward Ca^{2+} current from the ECF, where the concentration of ionised Ca^{2+} is approximately 1.2 mmol/L, to the ICF, where the Ca^{2+} concentration is ~500 nmol/L. The influx of Ca^{2+} ions enhances membrane depolarisation.

- The action of both is to cause a spontaneous decay of the membrane potential to the threshold potential of –40 mV.

How are action potentials conducted through the heart?

An efficient conducting system is essential to ensure the synchronous contraction of the ventricular myocytes. Action potentials generated in the SA node are relayed as follows:

- **The internodal pathways.** Action potentials are relayed from the SA node to the AV node through three specific internodal pathways:

  - *Anterior*, the Bachmann pathway, which also relays action potentials to the left atrium via the Bachmann bundle;

  - *Middle*, the Wenckebach pathway;

  - *Posterior*, the Thorel pathway.

- **The AV node** is the only physiological means of transmitting action potentials between the atria and the ventricles; elsewhere, the junction between the chambers is insulated by the annulus

fibrosus.[2] The AV node delays transmission of the action potential between atria and ventricles, allowing the atria time to contract. AV nodal delay is a major component of the PR interval of the ECG.

- **The bundle of His.** Shortly after leaving the AV node, the bundle of His divides into the right and left bundle branches. The left bundle branch divides again into the left anterior and left posterior fascicles.

- **The Purkinje fibres.** The branches of the bundle of His divide to form the Purkinje fibres, which rapidly conduct action potentials throughout the right and left ventricles, thereby synchronising ventricular contraction. The Purkinje fibres terminate just below the endocardium; thereafter, action potential conduction is performed by the cardiac myocytes themselves.

- **The cardiac myocytes** have both mechanical and electrical connections. The myocytes are connected end to end by intercalated discs, which

---

[2] The existence of congenital accessory conduction pathways between the atria and ventricles (collectively known as the 'bundle of Kent') can result in action potential conduction bypassing the AV node, with arrhythmic consequences referred to as the Wolff–Parkinson–White syndrome. Similar accessory pathways with the AV node itself result in AV node re-entrant tachycardia.

allow them to contract as a single unit or functional syncytium. Adjacent to the intercalated discs are gap junctions, which allow the action potential to pass from one myocyte to the next.

Describe the process of excitation–contraction coupling in a cardiac myocyte

Excitation–contraction coupling in cardiac muscle is slightly different from that of skeletal muscle (see Chapter 54). In cardiac muscle, intracellular Ca^{2+} concentration is increased through Ca^{2+}-induced Ca^{2+} release rather than as a result of a physical connection between the T-tubule, the ryanodine receptor (RyR) and the dihydropyridine receptor (DHPR).

The process of excitation–contraction coupling in cardiac muscle is as follows:

- Ventricular and atrial myocytes differ in the anatomy of their cell membranes:
  - Ventricular myocytes have T-tubules, which contain L-type Ca^{2+} channels (i.e. DHPRs). The T-tubules conduct action potentials deep into the myocyte interior.
  - The atrial myocyte cell surface membrane contains L-type Ca^{2+} channels. The surface area of the cell membrane is increased by small invaginations called caveolae.
- In both cell types, membrane depolarisation causes L-type Ca^{2+} channels to open. Ca^{2+} diffuses through the open Ca^{2+} channels from the ECF to the sarcoplasm.
- Like skeletal muscle, the SR of cardiac muscle contain RyRs. Ca^{2+} influx opens the RyR, causing the SR to release Ca^{2+}. This process is known as Ca^{2+}-induced Ca^{2+} release.

Therefore, excitation–contraction coupling in cardiac muscle involves both DHPRs and RyRs, but unlike in skeletal muscle, there is no physical connection between the two.

How does cardiac muscle contract?

Cardiac muscle contraction starts shortly after depolarisation and continues until about 50 ms after repolarisation is complete; that is, contraction has a duration of around 300 ms (Figure 57.3b). Once Ca^{2+} has been released from the SR, activation of

crossbridge cycling follows a similar ATP-dependent mechanism to that of skeletal muscle (see Chapter 54):

- Binding of sarcoplasmic Ca^{2+} to troponin C causes tropomyosin to roll deeper into the groove between actin filaments.
- This conformation change leads to the uncovering of myosin binding sites on the actin filament, allowing myosin to form crossbridges with actin.
- The myosin head pulls the actin filament towards the centre of the sarcomere in the power stroke.
- Crossbridge cycling continues until the cytoplasmic Ca^{2+} concentration decreases during repolarisation.

How is cardiac contraction terminated?

Crossbridge cycling is terminated by actively removing Ca^{2+} from the cell. As the sarcoplasmic concentration of Ca^{2+} decreases, Ca^{2+} dissociates from troponin C. Tropomyosin re-covers the actin binding site; myosin can no longer bind to actin and relaxation occurs.

In diastole, the intracellular Ca^{2+} concentration is extremely low (around 0.1 μmol/L). This is achieved through three mechanisms:

- **The plasma membrane Ca^{2+}-ATPase pump,** which uses energy (from ATP hydrolysis) to actively remove Ca^{2+} ions from the cell (i.e. primary active transport).
- **The Na^+/Ca^{2+}-exchanger,** which removes one Ca^{2+} ion from the cell in exchange for the influx of three Na^+ ions. The efflux of Ca^{2+} occurs against its concentration gradient and is driven by the low intracellular concentration of Na^+, itself maintained by the Na^+/K^+-ATPase pump (i.e. secondary active transport).
- **Sarcoplasmic/ER Ca^{2+}-ATPase pump,** which uses energy (from ATP hydrolysis) to sequester Ca^{2+} in the SR.

Diastolic relaxation is therefore an ATP-dependent process, as ATP is required to actively remove Ca^{2+} from the sarcoplasm by either primary or secondary active transport or by sequestration in the SR.

How does the ANS influence the heart?

The HCN channels give the heart the property of automaticity: action potentials can be generated independently of the nervous system. However, the ANS and endocrine axes can modulate both the rate (chronotropic effects) and force (inotropic effects) of contraction:

- **Parasympathetic nervous system.** The right vagus nerve supplies the SA node, whilst the left vagus nerve supplies the AV node. Atrial muscle is also innervated by parasympathetic neurons, but ventricular muscle is not (and is therefore unaffected). Parasympathetic nervous system activity therefore affects HR and conduction, but has little effect on the force of contraction:

  - *Negative chronotropy* (decreased HR). The intrinsic rate of the SA node is 90–120 bpm. At rest, there is continuous parasympathetic nervous discharge at the SA node, known as vagal tone, which decreases the resting HR to 60–80 bpm. The mechanism behind this is:

    - Acetylcholine (ACh) is released by the presynaptic neuron (parasympathetic post-ganglionic neuron) and binds to an inhibitory G protein-coupled receptor in the postsynaptic membrane.
    - The associated G protein becomes activated, triggering the division of its $G_{\alpha i}$ and $G_{\beta\gamma}$ subunits.
    - The $G_{\alpha i}$ subunit inhibits the intracellular enzyme adenylate cyclase, which leads to a decrease in the intracellular concentration of cyclic AMP (cAMP). HCN channels, as the name suggests, are activated by cyclic nucleotides. Therefore, decreased cAMP leads to decreased Na^+ influx, and thus reduces the gradient of the pacemaker potential, resulting in a reduced HR (Figure 57.5a).
    - The $G_{\beta\gamma}$ subunit activates G protein-coupled, inwardly rectifying K^+ channels. The resulting additional K^+ efflux causes membrane hyperpolarisation (Figure 57.5a) that counteracts the pacemaker current, thereby decreasing HR.

  - *Decreased conduction velocity through the AV node.* AV nodal delay is increased. Sometimes, marked parasympathetic nervous activity may prevent transmission of electrical impulses through the AV node altogether. If this occurs, the pacemaker cells within the bundle of His

and Purkinje system generate action potentials at the much slower rate of 15–40 bpm – this is referred to as a ventricular escape rhythm.

- **The sympathetic nervous system.** The heart is innervated by post-ganglionic sympathetic fibres from the upper thoracic sympathetic chain (mainly T1–T3). Increased sympathetic nervous system activity causes release of noradrenaline at sympathetic nerve endings and release of adrenaline from the adrenal medulla. Both noradrenaline and adrenaline act at the cardiac β_1-adrenergic receptor, a G protein-coupled receptor whose activation increases the intracellular concentrations of cAMP and protein kinase A, resulting in:

  - *Positive chronotropy:* in the SA node, cAMP opens HCN channels, which increases Na^+ influx, thereby increasing the gradient of the pacemaker potential (Figure 57.5b). Threshold potential is reached more quickly, which increases the HR.
  - *Positive inotropy* (increased myocardial contractility): in the cardiac myocytes, protein kinase A phosphorylates L-type Ca^{2+} channels, which increases Ca^{2+} influx during the plateau phase. Intracellular Ca^{2+} concentration rises, which increases the force of contraction.
  - *Shorter action potential duration:* protein kinase A increases the opening of delayed rectifier K^+ channels that open during phase 3 of the cardiac action potential, shortening the repolarisation time.
  - *Increased rate of transmission through the AV node:* the opposite effect of parasympathetic activity.

Clinical relevance: local anaesthetic toxicity

The potential for toxicity when using local anaesthetics has been known for more than 100 years. It is hardly surprising:

- Local anaesthetics are extremely effective at blocking the fast voltage-gated Na^+ channels of peripheral nerves.
- Similar fast voltage-gated Na^+ channels are also found in central nervous system (CNS) neurons and cardiac myocytes.

Clinical signs and symptoms of local anaesthetic toxicity fall into three categories:

(a) Parasympathetic stimulation – HR decreases

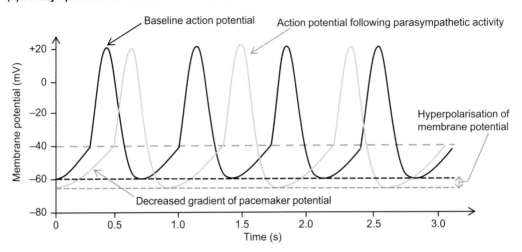

(b) Sympathetic stimulation – HR increases

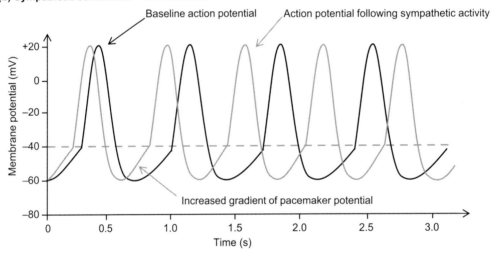

Figure 57.5 The effects of (a) parasympathetic and (b) sympathetic nervous system activity on the pacemaker action potential.

- **Immunological.** Local anaesthetics can cause allergy, especially ester-based local anaesthetics whose metabolite, para-aminobenzoic acid, is especially allergenic. Allergy may be local (urticaria) or systemic (anaphylaxis).
- **CNS toxicity.** High plasma concentrations of local anaesthetic may result in CNS toxicity, which occurs in two phases:

  - *Excitatory phase.* Initially, blockade of Na^+ channels in inhibitory interneurons causes excitatory phenomena: tinnitus, circumoral parasthesias, seizures.

  - *Depressive phase.* This is followed by blockade of Na^+ channels in excitatory interneurons, resulting in global CNS depression: coma, respiratory depression.

- **Cardiac toxicity.** In addition to Na^+ channels, local anaesthetics block K^+ and Ca^{2+} channels in the heart. Initial signs of cardiotoxicity are those of direct myocardial depression and bradycardia; higher plasma concentration may lead to refractory ventricular fibrillation. Important points to note are:

– *Ion channels are stereospecific*: one enantiomer of local anaesthetic has much greater toxicity than the other enantiomer. For example, levobupivacaine, the pure S-enantiomer of bupivacaine, has a lower cardiac and CNS toxicity than racemic bupivacaine.

– *Bupivacaine is particularly cardiotoxic* when compared with other local anaesthetics. In addition, signs of cardiac toxicity may occur before CNS toxicity; that is, there is potentially no 'warning' before the onset of cardiovascular collapse. This marked cardiotoxicity is thought to be due to the high affinity of bupivacaine for Na^+ channels in the heart and due to the fact that bupivacaine also binds Ca^{2+} channels, inhibiting Ca^{2+} release from the SR.

In addition to supportive management, a specific treatment of local anaesthetic toxicity is administration of Intralipid®. Intralipid is thought to act as a 'lipid sink', drawing the lipophilic bupivacaine out of the plasma and away from cardiac ion channels (though this mechanism has recently been disputed – see Further reading).

Clinical relevance: heart transplant

A transplanted donor heart is denervated – it has neither sympathetic nor parasympathetic innervation. In the resting state, this is relatively well tolerated owing to automaticity, intrinsic regulation via Starling's law and hormonal regulation via circulating adrenaline. However, there are a number of physiological consequences:

- **Loss of resting vagal tone**, resulting in a resting HR of around 100 bpm.
- **Loss of cardiovascular reflexes** – the usual cardiovascular responses to, for example, laryngoscopy and peritoneal traction are lost. The fall in systemic vascular resistance caused by anaesthetic drugs is poorly tolerated, with the potential for dramatic hypotension if cardiac preload is not maintained.
- **Blunted cardiovascular response to exercise** – the HR gradually increases with exercise, followed by a gradual decrease with rest (the normal response involves rapid changes in HR – see Chapter 42). This is because β_1-adrenergic

receptors on the transplanted heart are still able to respond to the circulating catecholamines released from the adrenal medulla. There may also be a contribution from the Bainbridge reflex.

Heart transplants also have pharmacological implications, including:

- **Atropine and glycopyrrolate have no effect** – these drugs are competitive antagonists of the muscarinic M_2 ACh receptor. The transplanted heart has no parasympathetic innervation and therefore no ACh to antagonise. Instead, isoprenaline may be used to increase HR in the transplanted heart.
- **Adrenaline and noradrenaline have an increased effect** – sympathetic denervation causes upregulation of β_1-adrenergic receptors. Therefore, the transplanted heart has an exaggerated response to these catecholamines.

Further reading

R. D. Keynes, D. J. Aidley, C. L.-H. Huang. *Nerve and Muscle, 4th edition*. Cambridge, Cambridge University Press, 2011.

E. Litonius, P. Tarkkila, P. J. Neuvonen, et al. Effect of intravenous lipid emulsion on bupivacaine plasma concentration in humans. *Anaesthesia* 2012; **67**(6): 600–5.

M. E. Stone, B. Salter, A. Fischer. Perioperative management of patients with cardiac implantable electronic devices. *Br J Anaesth* 2011; **107**(Suppl. 1): i16–26.

AAGBI Safety Guideline. Management of Severe Local Anaesthetic Toxicity, Association of Anaesthetists of Great Britain and Ireland, 2010; www.aagbi.org/sites/default/files/la_toxicity_2010_0.pdf.

J. Pinnell, S. Turner, S. Howell. Cardiac muscle physiology. *Continuing Educ Anaesth Crit Care Pain* 2007; **7**(3): 85–8.

J. M. Dippenaar. Local anaesthetic toxicity. *S Afr J Anaesth Analges* 2007; **13**(3): 23–8.

S. Rohr. Role of gap junctions in the propagation of the cardiac action potential. *Cardiovasc Res* 2004; **62**(2): 309–22.

N. J. Morgan-Hughes, G. Hood. Anaesthesia for a patient with a cardiac transplant. *Continuing Educ Anaesth Crit Care Pain* 2002; **2**(3): 74–8.

E. Vaughan. Williams classification of antidysrhythmic drugs. *Pharmacol Ther B* 1975; 1: 115–38.

B. Singh. Beta-blockers and calcium channel blockers as anti-arrhythmic drugs. In: D. Zipes, J. Jalife. *Cardiac Electrophysiology from Cell to Bedside*. Philadelphia: Saunders, 2004; 918–31.

Chapter 58

The Electrocardiogram

The electrocardiogram (ECG) represents a summation of electrical activity in the heart, derived from extracellular electrode recordings obtained from the body surface. Although a detailed description of ECG analysis for detecting cardiac pathology is beyond the scope of this book, this chapter provides a simplified outline of the electrical basis of the normal ECG.

Describe the normal ECG

The normal ECG, as recorded using lead II, is shown in Figure 58.1. Heart rate (HR) may be calculated from the ECG most simply by dividing 300 by the number of large squares between adjacent QRS complexes. For example, if there are five large squares between adjacent QRS complexes, the HR is 60 bpm (note: this shortcut is only valid for regular heart rhythms and standard UK paper speeds).

- **The P wave** represents atrial depolarisation. The smaller muscle mass of the atria compared with the ventricles results in the P wave having a smaller amplitude than the QRS complex. The duration of the P wave is normally <100 ms, or <2.5 'small squares'.[1] P waves are absent in atrial fibrillation, where there is uncoordinated atrial depolarisation. In mitral stenosis, left atrial hypertrophy results in a larger, and sometimes bifid, P wave.

- **The PR interval** is the time between the onset of atrial and ventricular depolarisation, which represents atrioventricular (AV) nodal delay. It is conventionally measured as time from the beginning of the P wave to the beginning of the Q wave rather than the R wave. The normal PR interval is 0.12–0.2 s; that is, three to five small squares. First-degree AV nodal block is characterised by a prolonged PR interval, whilst the δ-wave of Wolff–Parkinson–White syndrome characteristically shortens the PR interval.

- **The QRS complex** represents ventricular depolarisation and its propagation. The normal QRS complex is <0.12 s; that is, three small squares. A widened QRS complex may occur in a bundle branch block – a conduction defect in either the right or left bundle branches. Pathological Q waves may result from a pulmonary embolus, which classically gives an $S_1Q_3T_3$ pattern, or a previous myocardial infarction. Pathological Q waves have a duration >40 ms (one small square) or an amplitude ≥25% of the subsequent R wave.

- **The ST segment** is the isoelectric segment that follows the QRS complex. The ST segment corresponds to the plateau phase of the cardiac action potential. Myocardial ischaemia or infarction may cause the ST segment to become depressed or elevated respectively.

- **The T wave** represents the wave of ventricular repolarisation. Repolarisation of cardiac myocytes is not nearly as rapid as depolarisation; the T wave is therefore wider than the QRS complex. Inverted T waves may be caused by ventricular ischaemia.

- **The QT interval** is the time from the onset of ventricular depolarisation to the completion of ventricular repolarisation. The QT interval therefore represents the duration of the cardiac action potential. As discussed in Chapter 57, the duration of the cardiac action potential shortens with increasing HR. The QT interval is therefore routinely 'corrected' (QTc) for HR using an algorithm, the most popular of which is Bazett's formula (QT interval divided by the square root of the R–R interval, the time between consecutive

---

[1] At the standard UK ECG recording speed of 25 mm/s, each 1-mm 'small square' represents 40 ms. One large square contains five small squares and thus represents 0.2 s. The voltage is calibrated so that +1 mV is represented by a positive deflection of 10 mm.

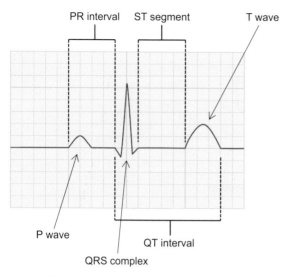

PR interval   ST segment   T wave

P wave

QT interval

QRS complex

Figure 58.1 The normal ECG.

R waves). Normal QTc is <0.44 s; that is, 11 small squares. A prolonged QTc interval is associated with a propensity to ventricular tachyarrhythmias.

How does cardiac electrophysiological activity generate ECG signals?

The ECG signals are generated from the changing electrical fields around the heart as the cardiac myocytes undergo a coordinated depolarisation, followed by a coordinated repolarisation:

- The exterior of the normal resting membrane is positive relative to the interior (see Chapter 51).
- When an action potential is triggered, the exterior of the membrane becomes negative relative to the interior (see Chapter 52).
- Following the action potential, the cell membrane returns to its resting state, where its exterior is positive relative to its interior.
- Each time the cell membrane changes polarity, local currents are generated.

An 'observer' watching this process take place from a vantage point outside the cell would see a 'waveform of depolarisation' sweep over the cell membrane, switching the polarity of charge from positive to negative, followed by a 'waveform of repolarisation', switching the polarity of the membrane back to positive (Figure 58.2).

In the case of the ECG, the observer is a series of electrodes placed at defined points on the skin surface:

- The local currents generated during each change in membrane polarity are conducted through the extracellular fluid to the skin surface.
- 'Exploring' electrodes measure the small changes in voltage at the skin surface.
- The change in voltage produced by a single cardiac myocyte is far too small to be measured at the skin surface. Electrical signals are detectable because large numbers of cardiac myocytes depolarise and repolarise simultaneously and their electrical signals are additive. The strength of the signal (voltage) is proportional to the number of cardiac myocytes that depolarise simultaneously – this is why the QRS (representing ventricular depolarisation) is of a greater amplitude (voltage) than the P wave (representing atrial depolarisation).

What is meant by an ECG lead?

The potential difference between pairs of electrodes in different body areas is referred to as a lead. Each lead views electrical activity in the heart from a different angle. A standard 12-lead ECG consists of:

- **The limb leads** (I, II and III) use electrodes on the right arm, left arm and left leg:
    - Lead I records the potential difference between right and left arm electrodes.
    - Lead II records the potential difference between right arm and left leg electrodes.
    - Lead III records the potential difference between left arm and left leg electrodes.
- **The augmented limb leads** (aVF, aVR and aVL) are derived from the same three electrodes, but offer additional angles to those provided by leads I, II and III. For example, aVF records the potential difference between the left leg electrode and the average of the right arm and left arm electrodes.
- **The six chest or precordial leads** (V_1–V_6) measure the potential difference between chest leads and a voltage given by the average of the three limb leads. Whereas the limb leads and augmented limb leads view the heart in the coronal plane, the chest leads view the heart in cross-section, thus facilitating the use of the 12-lead ECG as a diagnostic tool.

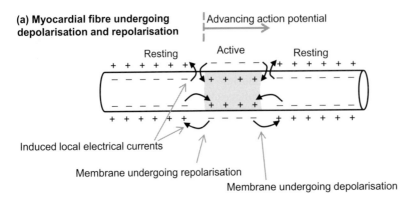

(a) Myocardial fibre undergoing depolarisation and repolarisation

Advancing action potential

Resting   Active   Resting

Induced local electrical currents

Membrane undergoing repolarisation

Membrane undergoing depolarisation

(b) Waveform of depolarisation

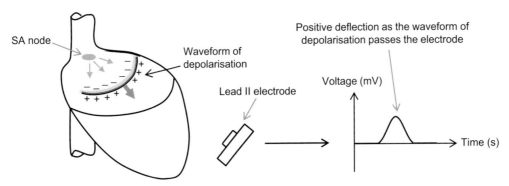

SA node

Waveform of depolarisation

Lead II electrode

Positive deflection as the waveform of depolarisation passes the electrode

Voltage (mV)

Time (s)

Figure 58.2 Generation of electrical signals by the heart: (a) myocardial fibre undergoing propagation of an action potential wave and (b) representation of a depolarising waveform and the resultant change in voltage of the recording electrode (SA = sinoatrial).

Explain the waveform of the QRS complex

The wave of cardiac depolarisation (Figure 58.3):

- Starts from the sinoatrial (SA) node.
- Spreads through the atria to the atrioventricular (AV) node.
- In the interventricular septum, as the wave of depolarisation propagates towards the apex, cardiac myocytes depolarise from left to right.
- Finally, the wave of depolarisation spreads from the apex to the base of the ventricles.

The active electrode (lead II is shown in Figure 58.3) measures the change in potential as ventricular myocytes depolarise. Positive and negative deflections indicate net electrical current flow towards and away from the electrode, respectively:

- Septal depolarisation produces a small negative deflection known as a Q wave (Figure 58.3a).

- As the remaining ventricular muscle begins to depolarise, net current flows towards the electrode, resulting in a large positive deflection known as the R wave (Figure 58.3b).
- The wave of depolarisation then flows towards the bases of the ventricles, away from the electrode (Figure 58.3c), returning the electrical potential to zero.
- Finally, the base of the left ventricle depolarises (Figure 58.3d), resulting in a small negative deflection known as the S wave.

What is the cardiac axis?

The leads that view the heart in the coronal plane (the six limb leads and augmented limb leads) can be used to determine the cardiac axis: the net direction (or vector) of the depolarisation wave (Figure 58.4).

Owing to the large mass of ventricular excitable tissue, the net direction of depolarisation normally

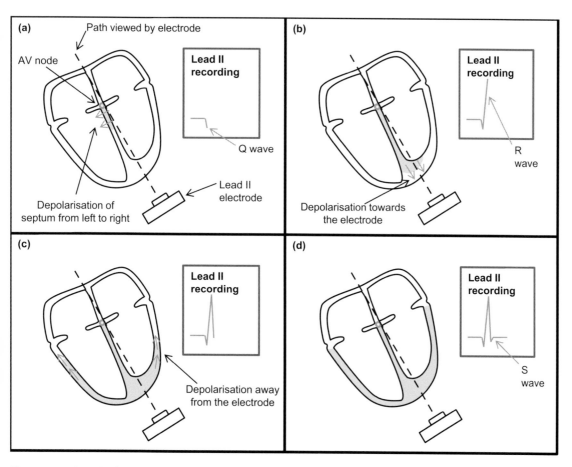

Figure 58.3 The path of ventricular depolarisation (atrial depolarisation not shown).

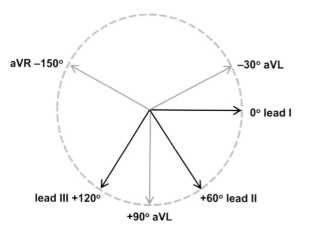

Figure 58.4 Vectors of the ECG leads.

- An axis more negative than −30°, termed left axis deviation, may result from left ventricular hypertrophy or the leftward displacement of the heart during pregnancy.
- An axis greater than +90°, termed right axis deviation, may result from right ventricular hypertrophy.

The cardiac axis of an ECG can be estimated from the QRS complexes of leads I, II, III, aVF and aVL:

- Identify the isoelectric lead, the one in which the QRS has equal positive and negative deflections.
- The cardiac axis is 90° (i.e. at right angles) to this lead.

For example, if lead II (which represents a vector of +60°) is the isoelectric lead, the cardiac axis is at 90° to lead II. The cardiac axis is therefore either −30° or +150°. Referring to the deflection in aVF (which represents a vector of −30°) will confirm the cardiac axis:

runs diagonally from the SA node to the apex, giving a typical cardiac axis of around 45°. A normal cardiac axis is considered to be between −30° and +90°.

- If the QRS complex of lead aVL has a predominantly positive deflection, the cardiac axis is −30° and therefore just within the normal range.
- If the QRS complex of lead aVL has a predominantly negative deflection, the cardiac axis is +150°; that is, extreme right axis deviation.

Further reading

F. Kusumoto. *ECG Interpretation: From Pathophysiology to Clinical Application.* Berlin, Springer, 2009.

M. K. Das, D. P. Zipes. *Electrocardiography of Arrhythmias: A Comprehensive Review.* New York, Elsevier, 2012.

59

Autonomic Nervous System

What is the autonomic nervous system?

The autonomic nervous system (ANS) is the portion of the nervous system that innervates smooth muscle and glands, thus influencing the function of internal organs that regulate heart rate (HR), arterial blood pressure, digestion, micturition, defecation, sweating and sexual function.

Describe the two divisions of the ANS

The ANS is subdivided into two separate nervous systems – sympathetic and parasympathetic – which usually have antagonistic effects. Most viscera are innervated by both divisions of the ANS. Some authorities separately identify the enteric nervous system as a distinct ANS subdivision. The ANS comes under the control of the hypothalamus (see Chapter 80).

The function of the sympathetic nervous system is often summarised by *fight, flight or fright.* Its role is concerned with preparing the body for stressful situations: increasing cardiac output (by increasing HR, stroke volume and myocardial contractility), vasoconstriction, venoconstriction, mobilising glucose stores and pupillary dilatation.

The function of the parasympathetic nervous system is often summarised by *rest and digest.* It carries out the basic functions required for life, including decreasing HR, salivation, stimulating peristalsis in the gut, urination and pupillary constriction.

Name some of the effects of sympathetic and parasympathetic nervous system activity on the viscera

The effects of sympathetic and parasympathetic activity on the viscera are perhaps best described in a table (see Table 59.1).

Describe the anatomy of the ANS in more detail

Irrespective of the ANS subdivision, action potentials reach the viscera through two sets of neurons: pre-ganglionic and post-ganglionic. The sympathetic and parasympathetic nervous systems differ in the length of these neurons, the location of their synapses (ganglia) and the neurotransmitter utilised (Figure 59.1).

- **Sympathetic nervous system**:
  - Sympathetic pre-ganglionic neurons originate from the lateral horn of the spinal cord between T1 and L2/3, the so-called thoracolumbar outflow of the ANS.
  - Pre-ganglionic nerves emerge from the spinal cord with the spinal nerves in white rami communicantes,[1] but separate shortly afterwards to form either paravertebral or prevertebral ganglia. The paravertebral ganglia form the sympathetic chain; important named prevertebral ganglia are the coeliac, the superior mesenteric and the inferior mesenteric (Figure 59.1).
  - The sympathetic chain is often divided into four parts:

    - *Cervical*, which supplies the head and neck.
    - *Thoracic*: the upper thoracic sympathetic chain (T1–5) supplies the heart, lungs and aorta, whilst the lower thoracic sympathetic chain (T6–12) supplies the foregut and midgut viscera.
    - *Lumbar* (or abdominal), which supplies the hindgut viscera.
    - *Sacral* (or pelvic), which supplies the pelvic viscera.

---

[1] Referred to as 'white' because there are more myelinated fibres than unmyelinated. Pre-ganglionic fibres are type B neurons.

Table 59.1 Comparison of sympathetic and parasympathetic effects on viscera.

Organ	Sympathetic nervous stimulation	Parasympathetic nervous stimulation
Heart	Increased HR, increased contractility	Reduced HR[3]
Lung	Bronchodilatation	Bronchoconstriction, increased mucus production
Pupils	Pupillary dilatation	Pupillary constriction
Salivary glands	Inhibition of salivation	Stimulation of salivation
Arterioles	Vasoconstriction	No effect[4]
Sweat glands	Activates sweating	No effect
Adrenal gland	Release of adrenaline and noradrenaline	No effect
Gastrointestinal tract	Inhibits peristalsis	Stimulates peristalsis
Bladder	Relaxes bladder	Contracts bladder
Penis	Ejaculation	Erection

– In the ganglia, pre-ganglionic neurons synapse with post-ganglionic neurons. The neurotransmitter at this synapse is acetylcholine (ACh), which acts upon nicotinic postsynaptic membrane receptors.

– Post-ganglionic neurons leave the ganglia through grey rami communicantes[2] and travel within peripheral nerves to synapse with their target organ. The neurotransmitter at this synapse is noradrenaline, which acts upon post-ganglionic adrenergic receptors.

There are three major exceptions to the system outlined above:

– *The adrenal medulla* is directly innervated by pre-ganglionic neurons, with ACh as the neurotransmitter. This is because the adrenal gland is effectively a modified sympathetic ganglion that releases its neurotransmitter directly into the blood.

– *The sweat glands* are innervated by sympathetic cholinergic neurons, which release ACh but act through muscarinic receptors.

– *Metarterioles in skeletal muscle beds* are also innervated by sympathetic cholinergic fibres. These metarterioles cause functional arteriovenous shunting, thus preventing excessive increases in mean arterial pressure at the onset of exercise.

Clinical relevance: sympathetic blockade

The sympathetic nervous system has long been implicated in the development of chronic neuropathic, vascular and visceral pain. The sympathetic chain may be pharmacologically blocked, either temporarily with local anaesthetic or semi-permanently with phenol or alcohol, for the diagnosis or treatment of sympathetically mediated pain.

- **Stellate ganglion blockade**. The stellate ganglion is a fusion of the inferior cervical sympathetic ganglion with the first thoracic ganglion located at C7. Stellate ganglion blockade may be used to treat sympathetically mediated pain of the upper limbs (e.g. Raynaud's syndrome), complex regional pain syndrome, certain sympathetically driven arrhythmias (such as long QT syndrome) and hyperhydrosis.

- **Coeliac plexus blockade**. The coeliac plexus is located at either side of the L1 vertebral body and provides the sympathetic supply to most of the abdominal viscera. Pain associated with pancreatic carcinoma and chronic pancreatitis may be treated by semi-permanent blockade of the coeliac plexus using phenol under fluoroscopic guidance.

- **Lumbar sympathectomy**. The lumbar portion of the sympathetic chain may be blocked through

---

[2] Referred to as 'grey' because they are unmyelinated. Post-ganglionic fibres are type C neurons.

[3] The ventricular muscle of the heart receives very little parasympathetic innervation (see Chapter 57).
[4] The arterioles have insignificant parasympathetic innervation, aside from in the penis.

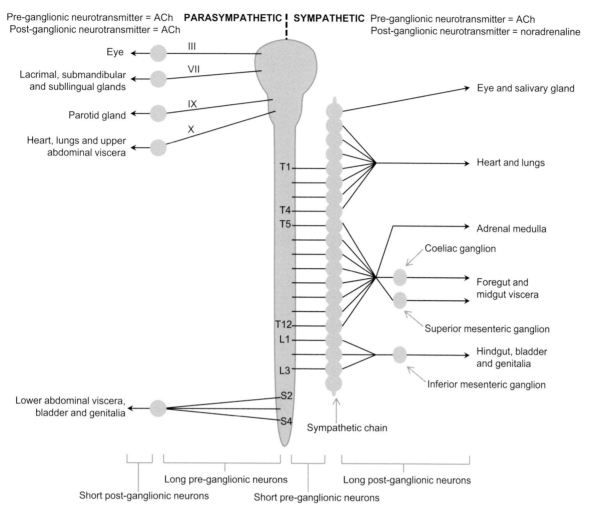

Pre-ganglionic neurotransmitter = ACh **PARASYMPATHETIC | SYMPATHETIC** Pre-ganglionic neurotransmitter = ACh
Post-ganglionic neurotransmitter = ACh   Post-ganglionic neurotransmitter = noradrenaline

Eye

Lacrimal, submandibular and sublingual glands

Parotid gland

Heart, lungs and upper abdominal viscera

III

VII

IX

X

Eye and salivary gland

Heart and lungs

Adrenal medulla

Coeliac ganglion

Foregut and midgut viscera

Superior mesenteric ganglion

Hindgut, bladder and genitalia

Inferior mesenteric ganglion

Lower abdominal viscera, bladder and genitalia

Sympathetic chain

Long pre-ganglionic neurons

Long post-ganglionic neurons

Short post-ganglionic neurons

Short pre-ganglionic neurons

Figure 59.1 Layout of the autonomic nervous system.

an injection anterolateral to the L3 vertebral body under fluoroscopic guidance. Lumbar sympathectomy is used in the diagnosis and management of sympathetically mediated pain of the lower limbs.

In addition, there is increasing evidence of the importance of sympathetic blockade in the management of acute pain and in reducing the risk of developing chronic pain. In clinical practice, this is usually achieved by using spinal, epidural or paravertebral blocks.

- **Parasympathetic nervous system:**
  - Parasympathetic neurons are carried with cranial nerves III, VII, IX and X and with

spinal nerves S2–4. This forms the so-called craniosacral outflow of the ANS.

- The axons of the pre-ganglionic neurons are often long. They synapse in ganglia close to their target organs. The post-ganglionic neurons are therefore relatively short.

- The cranial parasympathetic nerves supply viscera in the upper half of the body, up to the junction of the midgut and hindgut (just before the splenic flexure of the transverse colon). The sacral parasympathetic outflow supplies the viscera of the lower half of the body.

- In the ganglia, pre-ganglionic neurons release ACh, which acts upon postsynaptic nicotinic receptors.

Table 59.2 Comparison of sympathetic and parasympathetic nervous system anatomy.

Feature	Division of ANS	
	Sympathetic	Parasympathetic
Location of pre-ganglionic neuron cell bodies	Lateral horn of spinal segments T1–L3	Brainstem, lateral grey areas of spinal segments S2–4
Length of pre-ganglionic neuron	Short	Long
Location of post-ganglionic cell bodies	Sympathetic chain; prevertebral ganglion	Ganglia close to the target organ
Pre-ganglionic neurotransmitter, post-ganglionic receptor	ACh, nicotinic receptor	ACh, nicotinic receptor
Length of post-ganglionic neuron	Long	Short
Post-ganglionic neurotransmitter, target organ receptor	Noradrenaline, adrenergic receptor (exceptions described in text)	ACh, muscarinic receptor

- At the target organ, the post-ganglionic neuron releases ACh, which acts upon postsynaptic muscarinic receptors.

These features are summarised in Table 59.2.

Outline the types of ACh receptor

As suggested above, there are two types of ACh receptor:

- **Nicotinic ACh receptors** are directly linked to an ion channel; that is, they are ionotropic. Nicotinic ACh receptors are found in the postsynaptic membrane of the neuromuscular junction (NMJ) within autonomic ganglia and within the brain. The receptor is referred to as nicotinic because, in addition to ACh, nicotine acts as an agonist. Nicotinic ACh receptors in the NMJ (foetal: $\alpha_2\beta\gamma\delta$; adult: $\alpha_2\beta\epsilon\delta$) and autonomic ganglia ($\alpha_2\beta_3$) have different subunit isoforms and are thus acted upon by different drugs.

- **Muscarinic ACh receptors** are G protein-coupled receptors and act through an intracellular second messenger system; that is, they are metabotropic. The fungal alkaloid muscarine also acts on these receptors. There are five subtypes of muscarinic receptors:

  - M_1 *receptors* are commonly found in secretory glands (e.g. the salivary glands) and the central nervous system (CNS).

  - M_2 *receptors* are found in the heart.
  - M_3 *receptors* are found in smooth muscle of the bronchioles and arterioles.
  - M_4 and M_5 *receptors* are found in the CNS.

What are the subtypes of adrenergic receptors?

Adrenergic receptors, or adrenoceptors, are G protein-coupled receptors whose ligands are catecholamines. Adrenoceptors are therefore metabotropic, exerting their effects through intracellular second messenger systems. There are four main subtypes:

- α_1-*adrenoceptors* are G_q-coupled receptors found in arteriolar smooth muscle and the urethral sphincter. The vasoconstrictors noradrenaline, metaraminol and phenylephrine are all α_1-adrenoceptor agonists. Doxazosin and tamsulosin are examples of selective α_1-adrenoceptor antagonists used to treat hypertension and benign prostatic hypertrophy.

- α_2-*adrenoceptors* are presynaptic G_i-coupled receptors found in the pancreas, arterioles and CNS. Both noradrenaline and adrenaline activate α_2-adrenoceptors, resulting in vasodilatation, inhibition of insulin release from the pancreas, sedation and analgesia. Clonidine, an α_2-agonist, is used as a sedative and analgesic.

- β_1-*adrenoceptors* are G_s-coupled receptors found in the heart and kidney. Activation by adrenaline and noradrenaline results in positive chronotropy and inotropy and renin secretion. Bisoprolol, a β_1-adrenoceptor antagonist, is used to reduce myocardial contractility and HR in ischaemic heart disease.

- β_2-adrenoceptors are also G_s-coupled receptors. They are found in the smooth muscle of the bronchioles and uterus. β_2-adrenoceptors are predominantly activated by adrenaline, resulting in bronchodilatation and uterine relaxation. Salbutamol, a β_2-agonist, is used as a bronchodilator in acute asthma and as a tocolytic in premature labour.

Further reading

D. Robertson, I. Biaggioni, G. Burnstock, P. A. Low, J. F. R. Paton. *Primer on the Autonomic Nervous System.* Cambridge, MA, Academic Press, 2012.

M. H. Andreae, D. A. Andreae. Regional anaesthesia to prevent chronic pain after surgery: a Cochrane systematic review and meta-analysis. *Br J Anaesth* 2013; **111**(5): 711–20.

J. G. McDonnell, O. Finnerty, J. G. Laffey. Stellate ganglion blockade for analgesia following upper limb surgery. *Anaesthesia* 2011; **66**(7): 611–14.

R. Menon, A. Swanepoel. Sympathetic blocks. *Continuing Educ Anaesth Crit Care Pain* 2010; **10**(3): 88–92.

60

Pain Physiology

What is the definition of pain?

Pain is defined by the International Association for the Study of Pain as 'an unpleasant sensory and emotional experience associated with actual or potential tissue damage or described in terms of such damage.'

How does pain differ from nociception?

Nociception is the process by which noxious signals are encoded as action potentials and transmitted from the periphery to the central nervous system (CNS). Pain results from the brain's interpretation of these nociceptive signals, resulting in the perception of an unpleasant sensory and emotional experience.

How is pain classified?

Traditionally, pain has been classified as either acute or chronic based on a duration of <12 weeks or >12 weeks, respectively. This arbitrary distinction has been replaced, and chronic pain is now defined as pain that extends beyond the expected period of healing following tissue injury.

Pain may be arbitrarily classified as nociceptive (caused by stimulation of nociceptors) or neuropathic (caused by damage to the neurons themselves). Nociceptive pain may be classified as:

- **Superficial or cutaneous pain** due to skin damage and characterised by sharp, well-localised pain.
- **Deep pain**, a dull, aching and poorly localised pain arising from structures such as muscles, tendons and ligaments.
- **Visceral pain**, a dull, diffuse and poorly localised pain arising from the viscera; for example, spasm or overdistension of a hollow viscus.

What is a nociceptor?

A nociceptor is a free, unmyelinated nerve ending capable of generating action potentials in response to a variety of stimuli that are generated by cellular damage. For example:

- **K^+** is released from damaged cells.
- **Histamine** is released from mast cells near to the site of tissue damage.
- **Bradykinin** is increased at the site of injury as a result of inflammation.
- **Leukotrienes** and **prostaglandins** are synthesised in response to cellular damage as part of the inflammatory process.
- **Serotonin** is released by platelets in response to vascular injury.

What nerve fibre types carry pain sensation?

There are two types of nociceptor fibre, classified by fibre structure (see Chapter 52):

- **Type Aδ fibres** carry impulses produced in response to mechanical and thermal stimuli. These neurons have myelinated axons of large diameter and have a relatively high conduction velocity of around 20 m/s. As a consequence of the higher conduction velocity, nociceptive impulses carried by type Aδ fibres produce the first sensation of pain, often perceived as being sharp and well localised in character.
- **Type C fibres** carry impulses produced in response to thermal, mechanical and chemical stimuli. These neurons have unmyelinated axons of small diameter, which results in a relatively low action potential conduction velocity (0.5–4.0 m/s). Firing of their associated nociceptors produces a sensation of dull, poorly localised

pain that often follows the early sharp pain mediated by Aδ fibres.

What are the pathways by which pain signals are relayed to the brain?

As discussed in Chapter 50, the afferent neurons that relay nociceptive impulses from the peripheries travel in the spinothalamic tract:

- A first-order neuron (C or Aδ fibre) relays action potentials from a nociceptor to the substantia gelatinosa (Rexed lamina II) or nucleus proprius (Rexed laminae III, IV and V) in the dorsal horn of the spinal cord. Here, the first-order neuron synapses with a second-order interneuron, with substance P as the neurotransmitter.
- The second-order interneuron decussates in the anterior commissure, before ascending the length of the spinal cord in the spinothalamic tract. The second-order neuron synapses with a third-order neuron in the thalamus.
- The third-order neuron relays nociceptive action potentials to the somatosensory cortex.

Sensation from the face is relayed to the brain through the trigeminal pathway:

- A first-order neuron (C or Aδ fibre) relays action potentials from the face to the trigeminal nucleus. Most of this sensory information is relayed to the brain through the trigeminal nerve, but a small number of sensory afferent neurons from the oropharynx and ear travel in the facial, glossopharyngeal and vagus nerves. Irrespective of the cranial nerve, all sensory afferent fibres synapse with second-order neurons in the trigeminal nucleus, the equivalent of the dorsal horn of the spinal cord. Again, substance P is thought to be the neurotransmitter at this synapse.
- The trigeminal nucleus (also known as the Gasserian ganglion) is large, extending from the medulla to the midbrain. Three parts of the trigeminal nucleus receive different sensory modalities:
  - *The spinal trigeminal nucleus* receives pain and temperature information.
  - *The main trigeminal nucleus* receives touch and proprioception information from the face and mouth.

  - *The mesencephalic trigeminal nucleus* receives proprioceptive information from the jaw.
- Like the spinothalamic pathway, the second-order neurons immediately decussate and ascend through the brainstem to the thalamus, where they synapse with third-order neurons.
- The third-order neurons relay action potentials to the somatosensory cortex.

How is pain modulated?

It has long been known that the pain associated with an injury may not always correlate with the severity of that injury. For example, soldiers with severe battle wounds may experience little or no pain. Clearly, the traumatic amputation of a limb will result in activation of peripheral nociceptors. This suggests an existence of mechanisms by which nociceptive signals received by the brain are modulated. Three mechanisms contribute to pain modulation:

- **Segmental inhibition.** It is well known that rubbing an injured area or the external application of heat or ice reduces the sensation of pain. This led to the gate theory of pain control (1965). At the time, it was thought that only C fibres carried pain, whereas Aδ fibres carried touch, pressure and vibration sensory modalities. The gate control theory hypothesised that both type C and Aδ fibres converge on the same second-order neuron and that greater activity of the Aδ fibres reduced the transmission of pain through C fibres (Figure 60.1).

  Gate theory has now largely been disproved by the subsequent identification of interneurons dedicated to carrying nociceptive impulses from Aδ fibres alone. This does not exclude alternative mechanisms for segmental inhibition that may explain phenomena such as transcutaneous electrical nerve stimulation, in which electrical stimulation of Aδ fibres using skin electrodes reduces pain intensity in some patients.
- **Endogenous opioid system.** Opioid receptors are located throughout the CNS, but especially in the periaqueductal grey matter, the ventral medulla and the spinal cord. Opioid receptors are G protein-coupled receptors of three classes: μ, κ and δ. When endogenous opioids (enkephalins, endorphins and dynorphin) bind to opioid

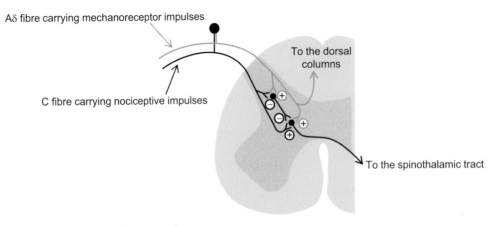

Figure 60.1 Gate theory of pain control.

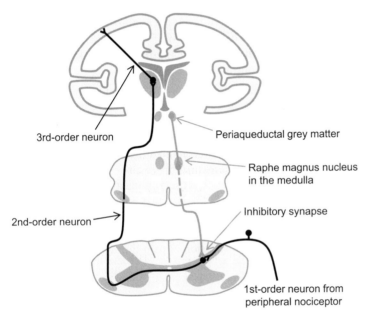

Figure 60.2 Descending inhibition.

receptors, there is reduced transmission of nociceptive impulses along the second-order neurons; that is, activation of opioid receptors inhibits pain transmission. Opioid receptors achieve this by either:

- Opening K^+ channels on the postsynaptic membrane, thus hyperpolarising the second-order neuronal membrane;
- Inhibiting Ca^{2+} influx into the presynaptic terminal, thus reducing neurotransmitter release (substance P).

- **Descending inhibition.** Neurons from the periaqueductal grey matter project to the dorsal horn of the spinal cord via the raphe nuclei in the

brainstem, where they influence the activity of ascending second-order nociceptive neurons (Figure 60.2). By inhibiting neurotransmission at the synapse between the first- and second-order nociceptive neurons, the perception of pain is reduced. Serotonin and noradrenaline are thought to be the main neurotransmitters of the descending inhibition pathway, which in part explains the analgesic properties of selective serotonin reuptake inhibitors and tricyclic antidepressant drugs. The analgesic effects of clonidine, an α_2-adrenergic agonist, are thought to occur through augmentation of activity in the descending inhibitory pathway.

Define hyperalgesia and allodynia. How do they occur?

Hyperalgesia is defined as increased pain from a stimulus that normally provokes pain. Hyperalgesia is of two types:

- **Primary hyperalgesia** occurs in damaged tissues. For example, areas of sunburnt skin have a greater sensitivity to pain than normal areas of skin. Primary hyperalgesia is due to release of substance P, bradykinin and histamine at the site of tissue damage, which sensitise the nociceptors, decreasing their threshold potential for the generation of action potentials.
- **Secondary hyperalgesia** occurs in the tissues surrounding the areas of tissue damage. Secondary hyperalgesia is thought to result from the increased release of substances (e.g. substance P, calcitonin gene-related peptide and glutamate) by activated second-order interneurons, which sensitise neighbouring second-order interneurons. Because neurons in the brain and spinal cord are somatotropically organised, these neighbouring neurons correspond to the tissue surrounding the site of tissue damage.

Allodynia is defined as pain due to a stimulus that does not normally provoke pain; for example, light touch or a cold breeze may be perceived as pain. Whilst hyperalgesia can be thought of as a protective mechanism, preventing an area of damaged tissue becoming further damaged, allodynia serves no useful purpose. Allodynia is often a feature of neuropathic pain, such as trigeminal neuralgia.

The physiological mechanism behind the development of allodynia is far from clear. One possible mechanism involves reorganisation of the circuitry of the spinal cord, so that the interneurons serving nociceptors are exchanged with the interneurons transmitting mechanoreceptor impulses.

What is neuropathic pain?

Neuropathic pain is pain caused by a lesion or disease of the somatosensory nervous system. Neuropathic pain may originate from either the peripheral nervous system (PNS) or the CNS. For example:

- The PNS may be damaged by diabetes, infections such as herpes zoster or invasion by cancer.
- Central neuropathic pain may result from multiple sclerosis or spinal cord injury.

Neuropathic pain differs from nociceptive pain. Whilst nociceptive pain is usually sharp or aching, neuropathic pain may be an episodic pain, like an electric shock, or a burning pain. Abnormal sensations are common, such as parasthesias and allodynia.

Neuropathic pain may result from a number of mechanisms; for example:

- In diabetic neuropathy, ischaemia of a myelinated nerve fibre causes demyelination. The newly exposed axon fires ectopic action potentials, which are perceived as a shooting or burning pain.
- Transected nerve axons attempt to regrow with the aid of nerve growth factor released from the supporting Schwann cells. However, axon regrowth may be disorganised: sprouting nerve endings may spontaneously generate action potentials or may have altered threshold potentials.

How is the sympathetic nervous system involved in the development of pain?

Trauma to the tissues damages not only somatic nerves, but also sympathetic nerves. For reasons as yet unknown, a small number of patients develop chronic sympathetic nervous system dysfunction following tissue trauma, resulting in complex regional pain syndrome (CRPS). Patients with CRPS develop chronic abnormalities at the site of injury:

- *Vasomotor changes* – the affected limb may be hotter or colder than the other limb.
- *Sudomotor changes* – reduced sweating.
- *Reduced hair or nail growth.*
- *Osteoporosis* of the underlying bone.
- *Neuropathic pain* – hyperalgesia and allodynia are common.

The significance of the sympathetic nervous system in the development of acute pain is a matter of debate (see Chapter 59).

Further reading

A. R. Moller. *Pain: Its Anatomy, Physiology and Treatment.* Dallas, Moller Publishing, 2014.

P. Brook, T. Pickering, J. Connell. *Oxford Handbook of Pain Management.* Oxford, Oxford University Press, 2011.

E. Albrecht, K. R. Kirkham, S. S. Liu, et al. Perioperative intravenous administration of magnesium sulphate and postoperative pain: a meta-analysis. *Anaesthesia* 2013; **68**(1): 79–90.

J. Sandkühler. Models and mechanisms of hyperalgesia and allodynia. *Physiol Rev* 2009; **89**(2): 707–58.

R. D'Mello, A. H. Dickenson. Spinal cord mechanisms of pain. *Br J Anaesth* 2008; **101**(1): 8–16.

The Eye and Intraocular Pressure

Describe the anatomy of the globe of the eye

The globe is an approximately spherical structure made up of three layers (Figure 61.1):

- **Sclera**, the dense, fibrous outer layer that provides structure and protection to the eye. There are two gaps in the sclera – one anteriorly for the cornea and one posteriorly for the optic nerve.
- **Choroid**, the middle vascular layer whose main role is the supply of nutrients to the sclera and retina.
- **Retina**, the inner neural layer of the globe that contains the photosensitive cells – the rods and cones:
  - *Rods* are the most numerous photoreceptor and are extremely light sensitive. Rods perform their visual function mainly in dim light, but cannot distinguish between different wavelengths of light.

  - *Cones* primarily function in bright light. There are three types of cones, each responding to the wavelength of a different primary colour (red, green and blue), resulting in colour perception.
  - *Retinal ganglion cells* relay signals from the rods and cones to the brain: their axons form the optic nerve. The optic nerve (cranial nerve II) then transmits visual information to the occipital lobe of the brain (via a synapse in the lateral geniculate nucleus).

An important structure within the retina is the fovea, a small indentation with a high density of cone cells, which provides the necessary visual acuity for activities such as reading.

The globe is divided anatomically into three chambers:

- **Anterior chamber**, the space between the cornea and the iris;
- **Posterior chamber**, the triangular space between the iris, the lens and the ciliary body;
- **Vitreous chamber**, the space behind the lens.

The three chambers contain two intraocular fluids:

- **Aqueous humour**, within the anterior and posterior chambers. Aqueous humour is a watery, optically clear solution of water and electrolytes, similar to extracellular fluid.
- **Vitreous humour**, within the vitreous chamber. Vitreous humour is a transparent gel consisting of a three-dimensional collagen network, hyaluronic acid and water.

Describe the blood and nerve supply to the eye

The blood supply to the globe is from a single source – the ophthalmic artery. Arterial blood enters the globe through branches of the ophthalmic artery: the central retinal artery, the anterior ciliary arteries and

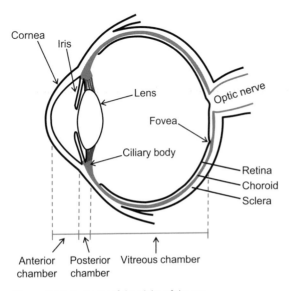

Figure 61.1 Anatomy of the globe of the eye.

the posterior ciliary artery. Venous drainage of the eye is via the central retinal vein and vortex veins.

In addition to the visual information carried by the optic nerve:

- **Sensory innervation** of the globe takes place through the ophthalmic division of the trigeminal nerve (cranial nerve V_1): the lacrimal branch innervates the conjunctiva and the nasociliary branch innervates the cornea, sclera, iris and ciliary body.
- **Parasympathetic pre-ganglionic neurons** originate in the Edinger–Westphal nucleus of the brainstem and travel along the outside of the oculomotor nerve (cranial nerve III) to the ciliary ganglion. From here, post-ganglionic neurons travel in the short ciliary nerve to innervate two muscles: the sphincter pupillae of the iris, resulting in pupil constriction (meiosis), and the ciliaris, changing the shape of the lens (accommodation).
- **Sympathetic pre-ganglionic neurons** originate from the T1 nerve root and synapse in the superior cervical ganglion. From here, the post-ganglionic sympathetic neurons ascend on the outside of the internal carotid artery and enter the orbit along with the ophthalmic division of the trigeminal nerve to supply the dilator pupillae muscle of the iris, resulting in pupil dilatation (mydriasis), and the superior tarsal muscle of the upper eyelid.
- **Motor innervation** of the extraocular muscles is provided by the oculomotor, trochlear and abducens nerves (cranial nerves III, IV and VI, respectively). The lateral rectus muscle (which brings about eye abduction) is innervated by the abducens nerve, whilst the superior oblique muscle (which results in eye intorsion) is innervated by the trochlear nerve. The remaining extraocular muscles (superior and inferior rectus, medial rectus and inferior oblique) are innervated by the oculomotor nerve. The facial nerve (cranial nerve VII) innervates the main upper eyelid retractor, the levator palpebrae superioris.

Clinical relevance: sympathetic blockade

The stellate ganglion is a collection of sympathetic nerves formed by the fusion of the inferior cervical and first thoracic ganglion, just anterior to the C7 vertebral body. A stellate ganglion local anaesthetic block may be performed to manage sympathetically mediated chronic pain originating from the arm, neck, face and heart or to decrease the symptoms of Raynaud's syndrome. A confirmatory sign of a successful stellate ganglion block is the onset of Horner's syndrome, a triad of:

- **Meiosis**, caused by blockade of the sympathetic innervation of the dilator pupillae muscle.
- **Partial ptosis**, caused by blockade of the sympathetic supply to the superior tarsal muscle. The ptosis is only partial because the major muscle responsible for raising the upper eyelid – the levator palpebrae superioris – is innervated by the facial nerve.
- **Anhydrosis** (absence of sweating), caused by interruption of sympathetic innervation of sweat glands.

What is the optic disc?

The optic disc is the head of the optic nerve, the point at which ganglion cell axons leave the retina, and it can be seen on fundoscopy as a pale orange disc. There are no rods or cones overlying the optic disc, resulting in a physiological 'blind spot', a small gap in the visual field of each eye. We do not usually perceive the blind spot, as the brain 'fills in' the missing information based on the surrounding colours and patterns.

What is intraocular pressure and how is it related to aqueous humour production?

Intraocular pressure (IOP) is the tissue pressure of the intraocular contents and is normally measured as between 10 and 20 mmHg. Because the volume of vitreous humour is relatively fixed, IOP is primarily determined by the balance of production and drainage of aqueous humour:

- **Aqueous humour is produced** in the ciliary bodies by active transport of Na^+ into the posterior chamber, dependent on activity of the Na^+/K^+-ATPase pump (80%) and ultrafiltration of plasma (20%).
- **In the posterior chamber**, aqueous humour passes through the narrow space between the lens and iris and enters the anterior chamber through the pupil.

- **In the anterior chamber**, aqueous humour circulates and drains through the trabecular meshwork into the canal of Schlemm. The canal communicates directly with the episcleral veins – absorption is directly related to the difference between IOP and venous pressure.

Clinical relevance: penetrating eye injury

An acute increase in IOP may cause expulsion of globe contents through a traumatic opening. Acute increases in IOP may be caused by:

- **Laryngoscopy**, which can increase IOP by 10–20 mmHg. This response can be avoided by obtunding the sympathetic response to laryngoscopy (e.g. by co-administering a strong opioid) or by avoiding intubation altogether (e.g. using a laryngeal mask airway, LMA).
- **Increases in venous pressure**, which increase episcleral venous pressure, thus reducing aqueous humour drainage, which increases IOP. Notably, coughing, straining and vomiting can increase IOP by 30–40 mmHg through this mechanism. This is of particular importance at emergence, where deep extubation or exchange of an endotracheal tube (ETT) for an LMA may reduce the risk of coughing. It is also wise to secure an ETT or LMA with tape, as jugular venous drainage may be obstructed by tight tube ties. Positioning the patient with head-up tilt further decreases episcleral venous pressure.
- **Suxamethonium administration**, which increases IOP by up to 10 mmHg for 5–10 min through an unknown mechanism. Patients presenting for surgery with a penetrating eye injury are often not adequately starved – rocuronium may therefore be the best choice of muscle relaxant for a rapid sequence induction.
- **Hypercapnoea**, which causes choroidal vasodilatation with an associated small increase in IOP.

NB: with the exception of suxamethonium, the causes of increases in IOP mirror those of intracranial pressure (Chapter 49).

Further reading

P. L. Kaufman, A. Alm, L. A. Levin, et al. *Adler's Physiology of the eye, 11th edition*. Philadelphia, Saunders Elsevier, 2011.

H. Murgatroyd, J. Bembridge. Intraocular pressure. *Continuing Educ Anaesth Crit Care Pain* 2008; **8**(3): 100–3.

S. Roth. Perioperative visual loss: what do we know, what can we do? *Br J Anaesth* 2009; **103**(Suppl. 1): i31–40.

Saliva, Oesophagus and Swallowing

What are the functions of saliva?

A volume of 500–1000 mL of saliva is secreted by the parotid, submandibular and sublingual glands per day in response to the thought, smell, taste and presence of food in the mouth or stomach. Saliva is 98% water, with the remaining 2% made up of:

- **Electrolytes.** Saliva is hypotonic – it has a lower Na^+ concentration but a higher K^+ concentration than plasma. Resting salivary pH is 7.0, but when HCO_3^- secretion is increased, the pH rises to 8.0.
- **Proteins and enzymes**, including mucin, haptocorrin, α-amylase and lingual lipase.
- **Bactericidal substances**, including thiocyanate, lysozyme, lactoferrin and immunoglobulin A.

Unsurprisingly, the functions of saliva are reflected by its constituents:

- **Lubrication of food**: saliva protects the pharyngeal and oesophageal mucosa from damage during swallowing. Mucin is primarily responsible for the lubrication properties of saliva.
- **Digestion**:
  - *α-amylase* is an enzyme identical to pancreatic amylase, which catalyses the breakdown of carbohydrate polymers. It works optimally at pH 7 – the pH of saliva – and manages to cleave up to 75% of starch before becoming denatured by the acidic environment of the stomach.
  - *Lingual lipase* commences the digestion of dietary triglyceride. It is particularly important in neonates, whose pancreatic lipase is immature and not particularly effective at digesting milk fats.
  - *Haptocorrin* is a protein that binds to vitamin B_{12}, protecting it from the low-pH environment of the stomach.

- **Neutralisation of acid**: the HCO_3^--containing saliva dilutes and neutralises gastric acid when the contents of the stomach either:
  - *Reflux into the oesophagus.*
  - *Enter the oral cavity during vomiting.* There is a large increase in salivation immediately before vomiting, which protects tooth enamel against acid erosion.
- **Antibacterial effects**: despite the many bactericidal constituents of saliva, there is little evidence of any significant bacteriostatic action in humans.

How is saliva produced?

Salivary glands are composed of acinar cells and ducts surrounded by contractile myoepithelial cells. Production of saliva occurs in two phases:

- **The acinar cells** produce the primary secretion by the active transport of electrolytes, followed by the passive movement of H_2O. The primary secretion is approximately isotonic: Na^+, Cl^- and HCO_3^- concentrations approximately resemble those of plasma.
- **The duct cells** modify the primary secretion to give a secondary secretion. Na^+ and Cl^- are reabsorbed, whereas K^+ and HCO_3^- are secreted. Reabsorption takes place at a greater rate than secretion – saliva therefore becomes more hypotonic as it progresses through the duct.

The rate of saliva production affects its composition. At higher rates saliva is rich in Na^+ and HCO_3^-, whilst at lower rates it has a greater proportion of K^+ and Cl^-. Aldosterone increases Na^+ reabsorption and K^+ secretion, similar to its effect in the kidney.

How are the salivary glands innervated?

The basic secretory unit of the salivary gland is the acinus. The acini of the parotid, submandibular and sublingual glands have both:

- **Parasympathetic innervation** – stimulation produces vasodilatation of blood vessels supplying the acini and myoepithelial cell contraction, resulting in the secretion of a mainly serous, electrolyte-rich saliva.
- **Sympathetic innervation** – stimulation produces vasoconstriction of blood vessels supplying the acini and myoepithelial cell contraction. This results in a brief increase in the secretion of mainly mucous saliva that is rich in amylase, followed by a period of decreased saliva production.

The origin of the parasympathetic fibres differs between the salivary glands:

- **The parotid gland** is supplied by the glossopharyngeal nerve (cranial nerve IX); pre-ganglionic fibres synapse at the otic ganglion.
- **The submandibular and sublingual glands** are supplied by the facial nerve (cranial nerve VII); pre-ganglionic fibres synapse at the submandibular ganglion, whilst post-ganglionic fibres travel in the lingual nerve.

What are the phases of swallowing?

Swallowing is a complex process involving the coordination of a number of muscles, both voluntary and involuntary. Swallowing involves passing a food bolus from the oral cavity to the oesophagus via the pharynx, with closure of the larynx to prevent pulmonary aspiration. The swallowing reflex is controlled by the swallowing centre in the medulla oblongata. Swallowing is divided into three phases:

- **The oral phase**, the only voluntary phase of swallowing. A food bolus is pushed against the hard palate by the tongue. Sensory information from the hard palate is fed back to the medulla via the glossopharyngeal nerve, which triggers the initiation of the involuntary phases of swallowing.
- **The pharyngeal phase**, which is under involuntary control. The medulla coordinates:
  - *Closure of the nasopharynx* by the soft palate.
  - *Protection of the laryngeal inlet* by adduction of the vocal cords (lateral cricoarytenoid, oblique and transverse arytenoid muscles) followed by adduction of the aryepiglottic folds (aryepiglottic muscles). All of these laryngeal muscles are supplied by the recurrent laryngeal nerve.
  - *Elevation of the hyoid* (by the digastric and stylohyoid muscles), which moves the larynx superiorly and anteriorly. In addition, the epiglottis moves downwards to direct the food bolus towards the posterior pharynx and away from the larynx.

The food bolus is propelled towards the oesophagus by successive contractions of the superior and middle pharyngeal constrictor muscles. The inferior pharyngeal constrictor muscle (cricopharyngeus), which is normally closed, relaxes to allow the food bolus to pass. Cricopharyngeus is also known as the upper oesophageal sphincter.

During the pharyngeal phase of swallowing, the larynx is involuntarily closed by the true and false vocal cords and covered by the epiglottis, only re-opening once the food bolus has passed. It is therefore impossible to breathe during the pharyngeal phase; the respiratory centre in the medulla coordinates a 1–2-s period of apnoea during swallowing.

- **The oesophageal phase**, which is also involuntary.
  - Once the food bolus has entered the oesophagus, the upper oesophageal sphincter closes and the lower oesophageal sphincter (LOS) partially relaxes.
  - The food bolus is then propelled along the oesophagus by peristalsis. There are two types of peristaltic waves propagated by the enteric nervous system:
    - *A primary peristaltic wave* is initiated by the medullary swallowing centre during swallowing and continues from the beginning of the oesophagus to the LOS regardless of the location of the food bolus.
    - *Secondary peristaltic waves* are initiated by the food bolus stretching the oesophageal wall.
  - By the time the peristaltic wave reaches the LOS, it has fully relaxed to allow the food bolus to pass. The smooth muscle of the LOS then contracts to prevent gastric contents refluxing into the oesophagus.

Clinical relevance: aspiration pneumonia

Aspiration pneumonia occurs when foreign materials (usually vomit, food, fluids or oral or nasal secretions) enter the tracheobronchial tree, causing infection and inflammation in the lungs. Aspiration pneumonia has many causes, including:

- **Decreased conscious level**, causing depression of the cough reflex. Examples include alcohol intoxication, drug overdose and general anaesthesia.
- **Disorders of the oesophagus**, such as gastro-oesophageal reflux, oesophageal stricture and tracheoesophageal fistula.
- **Problems with swallowing**. These can be:
  - *Generalised weakness of pharyngeal muscles*, such as myasthenia gravis, motor neurone disease, Guillain–Barré syndrome and critical illness polyneuropathy.
  - *Damage to the swallowing centre or its neural connections*, such as multiple sclerosis and stroke.

Describe the functional anatomy of the oesophagus

The oesophagus is a muscular tube that transmits food from the pharynx to the stomach. It has some important features:

- The upper third of the oesophagus has skeletal (striated) muscle, whereas the lower two-thirds has smooth muscle. Despite the two different muscle types, peristalsis occurs smoothly along the length of the oesophagus.
- The LOS is formed by the tonic contraction of smooth muscle in the distal 2–4 cm of the oesophagus, just as it passes through the diaphragmatic hiatus. Diaphragmatic contraction assists the oesophageal smooth muscle contraction.
- The oesophagus follows an acute angle at the point where it passes through the diaphragm, which further reduces the reflux of gastric contents into the oesophagus.
- While the upper oesophageal sphincter has a high resting pressure (up to 100 mmHg), the LOS has a much lower resting pressure. 'Barrier pressure' is defined as the difference between the LOS pressure (normally 20–30 mmHg) and intragastric pressure (normally 5–10 mmHg). Barrier pressure is reduced by:
  - *Swallowing*. When a peristaltic wave reaches the LOS, the smooth muscle relaxes to allow the food bolus to pass.
  - *Pregnancy*. LOS tone is reduced by progesterone. In addition, the gravid uterus

increases intra-abdominal pressure, further reducing barrier pressure.
  - *Hiatus hernia*. Barrier pressure is reduced through two mechanisms:
    - The LOS is no longer anatomically aligned with its diaphragmatic opening, so the diaphragm can no longer assist oesophageal smooth muscle contraction.
    - The acute angle taken by the oesophagus as it passes through the diaphragm is lost.
  - *Drugs*. Many drugs reduce LOS tone, such as alcohol, volatile anaesthetics, propofol, thiopentone, opioids, atropine and glycopyrrolate. Important drugs that increase LOS tone are metoclopramide, suxamethonium and anticholinesterases (e.g. neostigmine and edrophonium). It is worth noting that the non-depolarising muscle relaxants have no significant effect on LOS tone.

Clinical relevance: gastro-oesophageal reflux disease

Gastro-oesophageal reflux disease occurs when gastric add enters the oesophagus. This causes damage to the mucosa, resulting in retrosternal pain. Gastro-oesophageal reflux disease is caused by:

- **Raised abdominal pressure** – obesity, gravid uterus, acute abdomen;
- **Reduced LOS barrier pressure** – see above;
- **Anatomical changes to the LOS** – hiatus hernia.

Mendelson's syndrome is a pneumonitis caused by pulmonary aspiration of gastric contents associated with general anaesthesia. Aspiration of >25 mL of gastric fluid of pH < 2.5 is said to be sufficient to cause a severe pneumonitis. Prevention of aspiration in high-risk patients is multifactorial:

- Preoperative fasting;
- A freely draining nasogastric tube for patients with intestinal obstruction, aspirated before induction of anaesthesia;
- Neutralisation of gastric add through premedication with:
  - An H_2-receptor antagonist (e.g. ranitidine);
  - A non-particulate antacid (e.g. sodium citrate);
- The use of a rapid sequence induction with cricoid pressure.
- Induction of anaesthesia in the semi-recumbent position.

Further reading

L. R. Johnson. *Gastrointestinal Physiology: Mosby Physiology Monograph Series, 9th edition.* St Louis, Mosby, 2018.

D. M. Jolliffe. Practical gastric physiology. *Continuing Educ Anaesth Crit Care Pain* 2009; **9**(6): 173–7.

H. J. Skinner, N. M. Bedforth, K. J. Girling, et al. Effect of cricoid pressure on gastro-oesophageal reflux in awake subjects. *Anaesthesia* 1999; **54**(8): 798–808.

Chapter 63

Stomach and Vomiting

What are the functions of the stomach?

The stomach has a range of functions:

- **Temporary storage of large meals** – releasing ingested food slowly into the small intestine.
- **Secretion of digestive enzymes** – for example, gastrin.
- **Mixing** – vigorous contraction of gastric smooth muscle helps mix and liquefy ingested food.
- **Secretion of gastric acid** – in part to defend against ingested microorganisms.
- **Secretion of intrinsic factor** (IF) – which aids the absorption of vitamin B_{12}.
- **Endocrine** – secreting hormones to control gastric emptying.

Which substances are secreted by the stomach?

A total of 2 L of gastric fluid is produced by the stomach per day. There are five important substances secreted by the stomach:

- **Hydrochloric acid** (HCl). The parietal cells secrete HCl to concentrations of up to 150 mmol/L (equivalent of a pH of 0.8). HCl secretion is increased by three stimuli:
  - *Histamine*, which stimulates H_2 receptors – the most important stimulus for gastric acid secretion.
  - *Parasympathetic stimulation* through the vagus nerve. Acetylcholine (ACh) acts as the neurotransmitter at muscarinic M_3 receptors.
  - *Gastrin*, the least important direct stimulus of the parietal cells. However, gastrin has an important indirect effect, as it triggers histamine release from neighbouring enterochromaffin-like (ECL) cells.
- **Pepsinogen**, a proenzyme secreted by the chief cells, is converted into pepsin by the acidic environment of the stomach. Pepsin is an

important peptidase that starts the process of protein breakdown. Pepsinogen secretion is triggered by:

  - *Gastrin*;
  - *Parasympathetic nervous activity* through the vagus nerve.
- **Gastrin**, a peptide hormone secreted by G cells in the stomach in response to:
  - *Parasympathetic nervous activity* through the vagus nerve;
  - *Distension of the stomach*;
  - *The presence of partially digested proteins* in the stomach.
- Gastrin has three main roles:
  - *Stimulation of parietal cells to secrete HCl*, both directly and through stimulation of histamine release by the ECL cells;
  - *Stimulation of chief cells to secrete pepsinogen*;
  - *Stimulation of gastric motility*.

  Gastrin secretion is controlled by negative feedback: high acid concentration releases somatostatin from δ cells, which inhibits further release of gastrin from G cells.
- **IF**, a glycopeptide secreted by parietal cells. IF has an important role in vitamin B_{12} absorption:
  - Vitamin B_{12} is released from ingested animal proteins as they are broken down in the stomach.
  - In the low-pH environment of the stomach, IF has a low binding affinity for vitamin B_{12}, so very little is bound. Released vitamin B_{12} is instead bound by haptocorrin, a vitamin B_{12} binding protein. This protects the acid-sensitive structure of vitamin B_{12}.
  - In the duodenum, vitamin B_{12} is re-released as haptocorrin is digested by trypsin. In contrast, IF is resistant to trypsin.
  - In the higher-pH environment of the duodenum, IF avidly binds vitamin B_{12}.

- In the terminal ileum, IF receptors allow absorption of the IF–vitamin B_{12} complex.

In pernicious anaemia, autoimmune destruction of parietal cells leads to an IF deficiency. Vitamin B_{12} therefore cannot be absorbed, resulting in a megaloblastic anaemia.

- **Mucus.** Mucous cells secrete an HCO_3^--rich mucus that covers the gastric mucosa. It has two main roles:

    - Protection of the gastric mucosa from the highly acidic contents of the stomach lumen;
    - Lubrication of the stomach wall, protecting it from frictional damage due to vigorous peristalsis and mixing of partially digested food.

How do the parietal cells secrete gastric acid?

The parietal cells are triangular-shaped epithelial cells of the gastric mucosa (Figure 63.1). Key features are:

- Their close proximity to ECL cells;
- An extensive network of secretory canaliculi;
- The H^+/K^+-ATPase pump;
- Three stimulatory receptors: histamine H_2, ACh and gastrin;
- One inhibitory receptor: somatostatin;

- Carbonic anhydrase (CA) within the cell cytoplasm.

The main stimulus for the secretion of gastric acid is histamine, synthesised and stored by neighbouring ECL cells that release histamine in response to gastrin or parasympathetic stimuli. Histamine acts by increasing the cyclic AMP (cAMP) concentration within the parietal cell. Gastrin and ACh also directly stimulate the parietal cell, but to a lesser extent than histamine.

The mechanism for gastric acid secretion is:

- CO_2 diffuses into the parietal cell from the blood.
- CO_2 reacts with water to give H_2CO_3 in a reaction catalysed by CA.
- H_2CO_3 dissociates into H^+ and HCO_3. These ions then go their separate ways:

    - *In the apical membrane*: the H^+/K^+-ATPase actively pumps H^+ into the secretory canaliculi in exchange for K^+. The H^+/K^+-ATPase is known as the proton pump.
    - *In the basolateral membrane*: HCO_3^- is exchanged for Cl^-. HCO_3^- enters the blood, where it causes a measurable increase in blood pH whenever gastric acid secretion is stimulated; this is referred to as the alkaline tide.

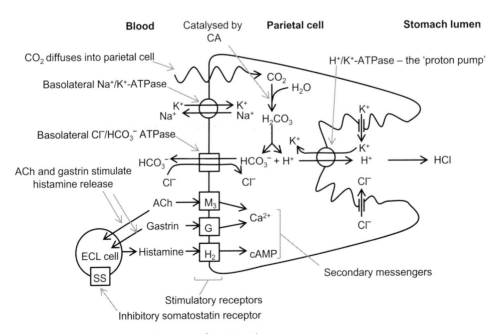

Figure 63.1 The parietal cell and secretion of gastric acid.

- Cl^- diffuses down its concentration gradient through a Cl^- channel to the secretory canaliculi.
- K^+ also diffuses down its electrochemical gradient, back into the secretory canaliculi through a K^+ channel.

The overall effect is HCl secretion into the stomach lumen and $NaHCO_3$ secretion into the bloodstream.

Clinical relevance: neutralisation of gastric acid

Neutralisation of gastric acid is a key part of the management of gastro-oesophageal reflux disease and of gastric and duodenal ulcers. Gastric acid can also be neutralised prior to induction of general anaesthesia in patients at risk of aspiration pneumonia, such as in cases of acute abdomen and pregnancy.

The neutralisation of gastric acid can achieved by:

- **Antacids**. These alkaline drugs react directly with HCl in the gastric fluid. Gastric acid is rapidly neutralised, resulting in prompt resolution of symptoms. Antacids include:
  - *Particulate antacids*: for example, aluminium hydroxide, magnesium hydroxide and calcium carbonate. Particulate antacids are so called because the aluminium, magnesium and calcium salts produced are non-absorbable, resulting in particulate matter. The importance of this is that, despite a higher pH, pulmonary aspiration of the salts of particulate antacids still cause pulmonary damage.
  - *Non-particulate antacids*: for example, sodium citrate, commonly used immediately prior to caesarean section because of its speed of action and non-particulate nature.
- **Gastric acid inhibitors**. These drugs prevent gastric acid being secreted. They therefore take longer to act than antacids but have a much longer duration of action. They target some of the steps in the synthesis of gastric acid discussed above:
  - *Histamine H_2 receptor antagonists* (e.g. ranitidine) block the action of histamine on the parietal cell, thus decreasing the production of gastric acid. Some gastric acid is still secreted due to the direct effects of gastrin and ACh on the parietal cell.
  - *Proton-pump inhibitors* (PPIs; e.g. omeprazole). PPIs act by irreversibly inhibiting the H^+/K^+-ATPase (the proton pump), the final common pathway of gastric acid secretion. They are more effective than H_2 receptor antagonists at increasing gastric pH, but longer-term use carries a greater risk of *Clostridium difficile* infection, osteoporosis, vitamin B_{12} deficiency and iron-deficiency anaemia.

What are the phases of gastric secretion?

There are three phases of gastric secretion:

- **Cephalic phase.** Around 30% of the total gastric acid secreted per meal is produced in response to the anticipation, smell and sight of food. Vagus nerve activity results in the secretion of HCl, gastrin and pepsinogen.
- **Gastric phase.** Gastric distension triggers gastrin release from G cells, which in turn stimulates pepsinogen release from the chief cells, histamine release from the ECL cells and HCl secretion by the parietal cells. Some 60% of gastric acid is secreted during the gastric phase.
- **Intestinal phase.** Once the acidic chyme enters the duodenum, secretin is released from the duodenal mucosa. Secretin reduces the acidity of the chyme by:
  - *Stimulating pancreatic ductal cells to secrete* HCO_3^-, thus increasing the pH of chyme (see Chapter 64);
  - *Inhibiting gastrin release* from G cells, which in turn reduces the amount of acid produced by the parietal cells.

How is gastric emptying controlled?

It is important that the stomach is gradually emptied into the duodenum. Following gastric surgery, a condition called 'gastric dumping syndrome' may occur in which rapid gastric emptying leads to chyme passing into the small intestine largely undigested. This causes:

- **Duodenal distension.** Large amounts of hyperosmolar chyme enter the duodenum, causing the osmotic movement of water from the extracellular fluid to the duodenal lumen. The rapid increase in duodenal volume causes cramping pains, nausea and bloating. This is called 'early' dumping syndrome, because it occurs soon after ingestion of a meal.

- **Hypoglycaemia.** Rapid absorption of a large amount of carbohydrate triggers the β-cells of the islets of Langerhans in the pancreas to secrete large amounts of insulin. Plasma glucose is rapidly taken up by the cells; plasma insulin concentration takes longer to fall back to normal, resulting in hypoglycaemia. This is referred to as 'late' dumping syndrome, as it occurs 1–3 h after a meal.

The rate of gastric emptying into the duodenum depends on:

- **The consistency of the chyme.** Liquids pass through the stomach much faster than solids. The pyloric sphincter constricts when solids come close, preventing them from leaving the stomach until they are essentially liquefied.
- **The volume of chyme.** Increased gastric volume promotes gastric emptying.
- **The content of the chyme.** Protein enters the small intestine the most rapidly, followed by carbohydrate. High-fat meals are associated with the slowest gastric emptying.

The rate of gastric emptying is primarily controlled by the duodenum – chyme passes through the pylorus and into the small bowel at an optimal rate for digestion and absorption of food. The four main duodenal factors that slow the rate of gastric emptying are:

- **Duodenal distension.** This results in a reflex inhibition of the enteric nervous system, reducing gastric emptying.
- **Acid.** Low duodenal pH triggers the release of secretin from the duodenal mucosa. As discussed above, secretin promotes pancreatic HCO_3^- secretion and inhibits gastrin secretion. As gastrin is responsible for stimulating gastric motility, reduced gastrin concentration slows gastric emptying.
- **Fat.** Cholecystokinin (CCK) is secreted by the duodenal mucosa in response to the presence of duodenal lipid. CCK increases the tone of the pylorus, thereby reducing gastric emptying, which allows the small intestine more time to digest the lipids that have already passed from the stomach.
- **Hyperosmolarity.** Hyperosmolar chyme passing into the duodenum inhibits gastric emptying through a complex enteric nervous system reflex.

In addition, there are a number of other factors that inhibit gastric emptying:

- Sympathetic nervous system activity;
- Pain;
- Drugs (e.g. opioids);
- Diseases such as diabetic autonomic neuropathy, acute abdomen and ileus.

How long does gastric emptying take?

As discussed above, gastric emptying depends on whether gastric contents are solid or liquid:

- **Solids.** After consuming a typical meal, there is a 20–30-min period where there is minimal gastric emptying. This lag period allows time for mixing of food with gastric secretions and for pepsin to start the breakdown of proteins. After 30 min, the rate of gastric emptying is approximately linear, resulting in a steady decrease in gastric volume (Figure 63.2).
- **Liquids.** Unlike solids, clear liquids empty from the stomach at rates showing an exponential time course, without a lag phase (Figure 63.2). However, if the fluid is hyperosmolar, acidic or contains fats, the rate of gastric emptying will be slower and may mirror the non-exponential pattern of solid food.

Clinical relevance: preoperative fasting

The aim of preoperative fasting is to reduce the volume and acidity of gastric fluid, thereby reducing the risk of pulmonary aspiration. However, there is increasing evidence of the harms of excessive starvation periods, including:

- Patient discomfort;
- Dehydration;
- Electrolyte disturbance;
- Increased incidence of post-operative nausea and vomiting (PONV);
- Glycaemic disturbance in patients with diabetes;
- Increased body muscle catabolism following major surgery.

The risk of pulmonary aspiration is related to the volume of gastric contents: at a given time after ingestion, gastric volume is considerably less for liquids than solids. Therefore, liquids can be ingested much nearer to the time of general anaesthesia than solids can.

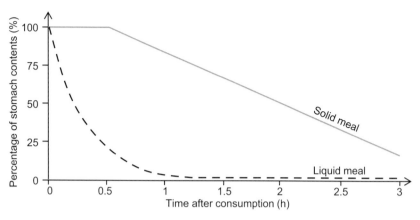

Figure 63.2 Gastric emptying of solids and liquids.

There has been much debate over the last few decades regarding guidelines for perioperative fasting. The latest European evidence-based recommendations for perioperative fasting are:

- 6 h for solids;
- 4 h for breastfeeding infants (formula milk counts as 'solid food');
- 2 h for clear fluids, which include:

  - Carbohydrate drinks;
  - Tea or coffee with milk (up to one-fifth of the total volume).

What is vomiting? Where is vomiting controlled?

Vomiting is the involuntary, forceful, rapid expulsion of gastric contents through the mouth. Vomiting is usually preceded by nausea, an unpleasant upper abdominal sensation, though nausea commonly occurs without vomiting.

Vomiting is coordinated by the vomiting centre, an anatomically ill-defined area in the medulla oblongata. The vomiting centre is in close contact with (but not part of) three important structures:

- **The respiratory centre;**
- **The nucleus tractus solitarius,** which receives afferent information from various cranial nerves;
- **The chemoreceptor trigger zone** (CTZ), located on the floor of the fourth ventricle of the medulla in the 'area postrema'.

Crucially, the CTZ receives blood directly from the systemic circulation; it is located outside the blood–brain barrier (BBB), which provides a faster vomiting response to emetic stimuli. This is convenient, as antiemetic drugs do not have to cross the BBB to reach their target receptors.

Many inputs to the vomiting centre can trigger nausea and vomiting:

- **The CTZ,** which has many stimulatory receptors:

  - *Dopamine, D_2;*
  - *Serotonin, $5\text{-}HT_3$;*
  - *ACh;*
  - *Opioids;*
  - *Substance P* (NK-1).

- **Cranial nerve VIII,** which carries afferent information from the vestibular system and involves muscarinic and histamine H_1 receptors. This input to the vomiting centre is implicated in travel sickness.
- **Cranial nerve IX,** which carries afferent information from the pharynx. This input is involved in the gag reflex.
- **The enteric nervous system and cranial nerve X,** which carries afferent information from the gastrointestinal (GI) system. GI mucosal cells stimulate the vomiting centre through activation of serotonin $5\text{-}HT_3$ receptors in response to distension, infection (e.g. gastroenteritis), chemotherapy and radiotherapy.
- **Higher centres** (e.g. the limbic system) can also initiate vomiting in response to anxiety and extreme emotional states.

In response to emetic stimuli, the vomiting centre coordinates the parasympathetic nervous system, the sympathetic nervous system and motor neurons to produce a characteristic series of events that results in the expulsion of gastric contents through the mouth.

Describe the sequence of events involved in vomiting

Vomiting is a highly organised series of events, divided into three phases:

- **Pre-ejection phase**, consisting of:
  - *Nausea*;
  - *Decreased gastric motility*;
  - *Reverse peristalsis of the small intestine*, which pushes proximal small bowel contents back into the stomach;
  - *Secretion of HCO_3^--rich saliva* mediated by the parasympathetic nervous system;
  - *Sweating and tachycardia*, mediated by the sympathetic nervous system.

- **Retching phase**, consisting of:
  - *Deep inspiration followed by closure of the glottis*, which protects the trachea from aspiration of gastric contents.
  - *Rhythmic contraction* of the intercostal muscles, diaphragm and abdominal muscles against a closed glottis. The alkaline contents of the proximal small intestine are vigorously mixed with stomach contents, thereby increasing the pH of gastric fluid. The increased intrathoracic pressure compresses the oesophagus, preventing reflux of stomach contents.

- **Ejection phase**, consisting of:
  - *Continuation of glottic closure*.
  - *Contraction of the pylorus*, which pushes gastric contents into the body and fundus of the stomach.
  - *Relaxation of the LOS and the oesophagus*.
  - *Sudden dramatic increase in intra-abdominal pressure* resulting from contraction of abdominal muscles and descent of the diaphragm. This pushes the gastric contents completely out of the stomach and into the oesophagus.
  - *The soft palate occludes the nasopharynx* and reverse peristalsis in the oesophagus rapidly expels its contents upwards, out of the mouth.

Clinical relevance: antiemetic drugs

The aetiology of PONV is multifactorial, with anaesthetic, surgical and patient risk factors:

- **Anaesthetic factors**: use of volatile anaesthetics and/or N_2O, intraoperative or post-operative opioids and high-dose anticholinesterases;
- **Surgical factors**: longer duration of surgery, middle-ear surgery, laparoscopic surgery and neurosurgery;
- **Patient factors**: female, child, history of PONV, history of motion sickness and non-smoker.

Strategies in anaesthesia to reduce PONV include:

- **Avoidance of emetic drugs**: avoidance of opioids/use of short-acting opioids only, avoidance of volatile anaesthetics through the use of regional anaesthesia or total intravenous anaesthesia;
- **Intravenous fluid therapy**: to replace fluid losses resulting from preoperative fasting;.
- **Use of antiemetic drugs**.

Antiemetic drugs target the receptors of the CTZ, the vestibular apparatus and the GI tract. For example:

- Domperidone (a butyrophenone) antagonises dopamine D_2 receptors in the CTZ.
- Hyoscine is an antagonist of the muscarinic ACh receptor in the vestibular apparatus and is used as an antiemetic in motion sickness.
- Cyclizine is an antagonist of the histamine H_2 receptor in the vestibular apparatus and is also commonly used in motion sickness.
- Ondansetron is a serotonin $5\text{-}HT_3$ receptor antagonist and has a wide spectrum of uses as an antiemetic as it blocks $5\text{-}HT_3$ receptors in the CTZ and the GI tract.

Further reading

L. R. Johnson. *Gastrointestinal Physiology: Mosby Physiology Monograph Series*, 9th edition. St Louis, Mosby, 2018.

I. Smith, P. Kranke, I. Murat, et al. Perioperative fasting in adults and children: guidelines from the European Society of Anaesthesiology. *Eur J Anaesthesiol* 2011; **28**(8): 556–69.

K. Clark, L. T. Lam, S. Gibson, et al. The effect of ranitidine versus proton pump inhibitors on gastric secretions: a meta-analysis of randomised control trials. *Anaesthesia* 2009; **64**(6): 652–7.

Chapter

64

Gastrointestinal Digestion and Absorption

Which gastrointestinal organs are involved in digestion?

The gastrointestinal (GI) tract is a tube that extends from mouth to anus and is approximately 9 m in length. It consists of the mouth, oesophagus, stomach, small intestine and large intestine. In addition, there are a number of accessory organs of digestion:

- **The teeth and tongue** are involved in the initial mixing of food with saliva.
- **The salivary glands, liver, gallbladder and pancreas** secrete substances involved in the chemical and enzymatic breakdown of food.

How is the small intestine anatomically and histologically arranged?

The small intestine is divided into three parts:

- Duodenum;
- Jejunum;
- Ileum.

Most dietary nutrients are absorbed in the jejunum, but some are absorbed at other sites:

- Vitamin B_{12} and bile salts are absorbed in the terminal ileum.
- Iron is absorbed in the duodenum.
- Dietary fat and water are absorbed throughout the small intestine.

The small intestine is made up of four layers:

- **The adventitia,** the outermost layer, is composed of loose connective tissue.
- **The muscularis externa** consists of an outer layer of longitudinal smooth muscle and an inner layer of circular smooth muscle. Peristalsis results from coordinated contraction of the smooth muscle. The myenteric plexus, part of the enteric nervous system, lies between the muscle layers, where it coordinates smooth muscle contraction.

- **The submucosa** contains nerve cells making up Meissner's plexus (a secondary enteric nervous system plexus), blood vessels, lymphatic vessels and elastic connective tissue.
- **The mucosa,** the innermost layer, is divided into (from outermost to innermost):
  - *Muscularis mucosae,* a layer of smooth muscle that provides continuous agitation of the mucosa, increasing contact with the luminal contents and preventing their adherence.
  - *Lamina propria,* which contains blood vessels and collections of immune cells. In the ileum, the immune cells are organised into lymphoid nodules called Peyer's patches.
  - *Epithelium:* the absorptive cells of the intestine are called enterocytes.

Although the length of the small intestine is only 7 m, the absorptive surface area of the small intestine is enormous: over 250 m^2. The absorptive surface area is increased as a result of:

- **Valvulae conniventes,** mucosal folds that project into the lumen of the small intestine.
- **Villi,** tiny finger-like projections of the intestinal wall. In between the intestinal villi are goblet cells, which secrete mucus, and intestinal crypts, which secrete the brush border enzymes and contain stem cells.
- **Microvilli,** microscopic projections on top of the villi. The fuzzy microscopic appearance of the microvilli superimposed on the intestinal villi gives rise to the name brush border.

Each villus has three vessels:

- **A single arteriole.** This gives rise to a capillary network at the tip of the villus.
- **A single venule.** The capillary network drains into a single venule, which returns blood to the liver through the portal vein.

- **A single lacteal**. Each villus also has a single lymphatic capillary called a lacteal, which transports absorbed dietary fats as chylomicrons to the thoracic duct.

What are the three main classes of dietary nutrients?

The three main dietary nutrients are carbohydrates, amino acids and fats. Each is broken down and absorbed very differently.

How are carbohydrates digested and absorbed?

Dietary carbohydrate polymers (e.g. starch) must be broken down into their constituent monosaccharides before they can be absorbed:

- **In the mouth**. Salivary amylase breaks down complex carbohydrates into smaller carbohydrate polymers and monosaccharides.
- **In the duodenum**. Pancreatic amylase continues the breakdown of complex carbohydrates.
- **At the brush border**. Specific brush border enzymes (e.g. sucrase, maltase and lactase) hydrolyse the smaller carbohydrate polymers into their constituent monosaccharides. For example, sucrase hydrolyses the disaccharide sucrose into glucose and fructose. The brush border enzymes are integral membrane proteins attached to the villi. Individuals with brush border enzyme deficiencies cannot digest certain carbohydrates. For example, lactose intolerance is caused by brush border lactase enzyme deficiency. Some carbohydrates, such as cellulose, pass through the GI tract unchanged, as humans do not have the brush border enzymes necessary for hydrolysis.
- **At the enterocyte**, monosaccharides are absorbed:
  - *Glucose and galactose* can only be absorbed by secondary active transport through an Na^+ co-transporter. This co-transporter (called the sodium-glucose linked transporter, SGLT1) requires a low enterocyte intracellular Na^+ concentration, generated as a result of basolateral Na^+/K^+-ATPase pump activity.
  - *Fructose* is absorbed by facilitated diffusion, not by Na^+ co-transport.
  - *Pentose sugars* are absorbed by simple diffusion.

- **Within the enterocyte**. Once absorbed into the enterocyte, glucose and galactose travel down their concentration gradients. They pass through the basolateral membrane and into the capillary by facilitated diffusion (via the transmembrane glucose transporter, GLUT-2). As monosaccharides are osmotically active, their absorption across the enterocyte also results in the absorption of water.

Clinical relevance: oral rehydration therapy

Worldwide, diarrhoea is the second commonest cause of death in children under 5 years old. It is, of course, the complications of dehydration rather than diarrhoea that are to blame for this high mortality.

Oral rehydration therapy (ORT) is an effective method of rehydration in diarrhoeal illness, reducing the need for intravenous fluid therapy in cases of moderate and severe dehydration. Oral rehydration solution is essentially just water, salt (sodium chloride) and glucose. ORT exploits the intestinal Na^+–glucose co-transport system to facilitate the absorption of water:

- Both Na^+ and glucose are osmotically active, and their absorption into the enterocyte is accompanied by a significant amount of water.
- Because Na^+ is also absorbed with oral rehydration solutions, some of the Na^+ lost from the GI tract is replaced.

However, ORT does not contain potassium, so hypokalaemia can occur following prolonged diarrhoea and oral replacement.

How are proteins digested and absorbed?

Ingested proteins must be broken down into single amino acids, dipeptides and tripeptides before they can be absorbed:

- **In the stomach**, protein digestion begins. The proenzyme pepsinogen is released by chief cells in the stomach. The low-pH environment then converts pepsinogen into pepsin. Pepsin cleaves the peptide bonds of dietary protein, resulting in shorter polypeptides.
- **In the duodenum**, protein digestion continues. The two most important peptidases are trypsin and chymotrypsin, both of pancreatic origin. Polypeptides are progressively cleaved by these powerful peptidases, resulting in dipeptides and tripeptides (but not single amino acids).

- **At the brush border**, peptidases cleave dipeptides and tripeptides into single amino acids. Again, these brush border enzymes are integral membrane proteins attached to the villi.
- **At the enterocyte**, single amino acids are absorbed in a similar way to glucose, through Na^+-linked co-transport. There are different co-transporters for neutral, basic and acidic amino acids. Short peptides (two or three amino acids in length) are also absorbed by secondary active transport using an H^+-linked co-transport system.
- **Inside the enterocyte**, these short peptides are broken down into single amino acids, which then exit the enterocyte by facilitated diffusion across the basolateral membrane. Amino acids are osmotically active: as they are transported from the gut to the capillary, water molecules are also absorbed.

How are lipids digested and absorbed?

Most dietary lipid is triglyceride (a glycerol backbone with three fatty acid residues attached), with smaller amounts of phospholipid, cholesterol and fat-soluble vitamins. In common with carbohydrates and proteins, triglyceride must first be broken down into its constituent parts before absorption can take place.

- **Emulsification in the duodenum**. Lipids are insoluble in water. Triglyceride therefore tends to aggregate in large droplets when exposed to the aqueous environment of the GI tract. In a process called emulsification, bile acids (secreted by the liver and stored in and then released from the gallbladder) coat the lipid droplets, dividing them into smaller and smaller droplets.
- **Enzymatic breakdown of triglyceride**. Pancreatic lipase acts to hydrolyse each triglyceride molecule into two free fatty acid molecules and 2-monoglyceride. However, pancreatic lipase can only act on the surface of lipid droplets. This is why bile salts are required to divide large droplets into small ones, increasing the surface area upon which pancreatic lipase acts.
- **Micelle formation**. The free fatty acids and monoglycerides released from triglyceride combine with bile salts, forming micelles consisting of small balls of mixed lipids and bile salts.
- **At the enterocyte**. When a micelle makes contact with an enterocyte, the lipid contained within it is absorbed by simple diffusion. The bile salts

remain in the gut lumen and are absorbed in the terminal ileum, where they return to the liver and are recycled.

- **Within the enterocyte**. Monoglycerides and fatty acids travel to the endoplasmic reticulum, where they are recombined to form triglyceride. The triglyceride is packaged together with cholesterol, phospholipid and a cellular label called apolipoprotein to form lipid balls called chylomicrons. The chylomicrons are released from the enterocytes into lacteals, the lymphatic capillaries that service each villus. Chylomicrons flow through the lymphatic system until they are released into systemic circulation at the thoracic duct.

> **Clinical relevance: lipase inhibitors**
>
> The weight-reduction drug Orlistat is a lingual and pancreatic lipase inhibitor. It prevents dietary triglyceride being hydrolysed into free fatty acids and monoglyceride. Dietary triglyceride therefore remains undigested and is excreted in the faeces, resulting in steatorrhoea. Similarly, steatorrhoea is the main presenting symptom in pancreatic insufficiency.

What are the functions of the pancreas?

The pancreas has both endocrine and exocrine functions. Most of the pancreatic tissue is dedicated to the secretion of pancreatic fluid. Despite only occupying 1–2% of the pancreatic mass, the islets of Langerhans are the sole producers of glucagon (α-cells), insulin (β-cells) and pancreatic polypeptide (PP cells), and they are one of the main sites of somatostatin secretion (δ-cells).

How are pancreatic secretions involved in digestion?

A total of 1.5 L of pancreatic juice is produced per day, which drains into the duodenum through the pancreatic duct. The main cell types of the exocrine pancreas are:

- **Acinar cells**, which produce digestive enzymes;
- **Ductal cells**, which secrete HCO_3^- and water.

Acinar cells produce four main enzymes and proenzymes:

- **Trypsinogen and chymotrypsinogen**. On entering the duodenum, the proenzyme trypsinogen is cleaved by the duodenal enzyme enterokinase, resulting in trypsin, a powerful peptidase. Trypsin then cleaves both chymotrypsinogen and trypsinogen, resulting in chymotrypsin and more trypsin. The process of trypsin catalysing the formation of more trypsin is called autocatalysis, which, once initiated, results in an exponential increase in peptidase activity and therefore needs to be kept in check (see box below).

- **Pancreatic α-amylase.** This catalyses the hydrolysis of large polysaccharides to smaller carbohydrate polymers, such as starch to maltose. It has no activity against the polysaccharide cellulose.
- **Pancreatic lipase.** This catalyses the hydrolysis of dietary triglyceride to free fatty acid and 2-monoglyceride.

Clinical relevance: acute pancreatitis

Acute pancreatitis is inflammation of the pancreas, resulting in a wide spectrum of disease from a mild, self-limiting illness to a fulminant illness with multi-organ dysfunction. There are many causes of acute pancreatitis, the most common of which are alcohol and gallstones.

Whatever the precipitant, the problem is inappropriate activation of proenzymes within the pancreas. Trypsinogen is activated to produce trypsin, which then undergoes autocatalysis to produce more trypsin. Trypsin also activates other pancreatic proenzymes, such as prophospholipase A_2 and proelastase. One of the hallmarks of severe acute pancreatitis is haemorrhagic necrosis of the pancreas:

- Phospholipase A_2 digests pancreatic cell membrane phospholipids, causing necrosis.
- Elastase digests blood vessel walls, causing haemorrhage.

As pancreatic cells are digested, inflammatory mediators (most notably tumour necrosis factor-α and interleukin-1) are released, causing a severe systemic inflammatory response syndrome. Pancreatic lipase is released into the interstitium, where it digests retroperitoneal fat – the retroperitoneal haemorrhagic necrosis that results is the cause of Grey Turner's sign (discoloration of the flanks) and Cullen's sign (periumbilical discoloration).

The inorganic portion of pancreatic juice is produced by the ductal cells. HCO_3^- is an essential component of pancreatic juice: it neutralises the gastric acid that enters the duodenum. Without secretion of HCO_3^-, many of the pancreatic enzymes would become denatured by the acidic environment. HCO_3^- synthesis utilises the enzyme carbonic anhydrase (CA) in a similar manner to gastric acid secretion (Figure 64.1):

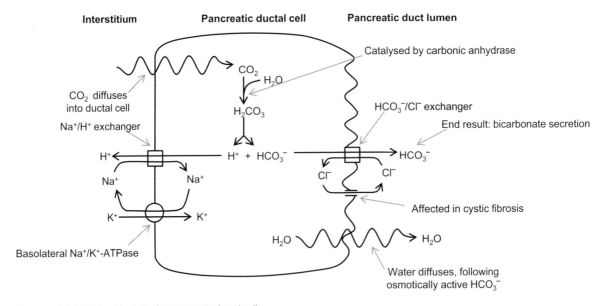

Figure 64.1 HCO_3^- synthesis in the pancreatic ductal cells.

- CO_2 diffuses into the ductal cells from the blood.
- CO_2 combines with water to form H_2CO_3, catalysed by CA.
- H_2CO_3 dissociates into H^+ and HCO_3^-. These two ions then go their separate ways:
  - HCO_3^- ions diffuse down their concentration gradient into the lumen of the pancreatic duct, crossing the luminal membrane by exchange with Cl^- ions. The Cl^- ions can then return to the lumen of the pancreatic duct through a separate Cl^- channel, CFTR. It is this Cl^- channel whose function is abnormal in cystic fibrosis.
  - H^+ is expelled from the ductal cell across the basolateral membrane into the capillary by exchange with Na^+. As with many cellular processes, the exchange of H^+ and Na^+ is driven by the low intracellular concentration of Na^+ generated by the Na^+/K^+-ATPase pump.
- HCO_3^- is osmotically active, and so its movement into the pancreatic duct is accompanied by water.

How are pancreatic secretions controlled?

Between meals, there is very little secretion of pancreatic fluid. However, when food enters the stomach, and especially when chyme enters the duodenum, secretion of pancreatic fluid is strongly stimulated. Secretion of pancreatic fluid has both neural and humoral control mechanisms:

- **Neural**. The pancreas is innervated by the vagus nerve; when activated during the cephalic phase of digestion (anticipation of a meal), there is a small increase in pancreatic acinar cell activity.
- **Gastrin**. This hormone is secreted by the G cells of the stomach in response to gastric distension. As well as stimulating gastric acid secretion by the parietal cells of the stomach, gastrin also stimulates pancreatic acinar cells to secrete digestive enzymes in preparation for the arrival of carbohydrates, proteins and fats.
- **Cholecystokinin** (CCK). This hormone is secreted by the duodenal mucosal cells in response to fat- or protein-rich chyme entering the duodenum. As well as increasing the production of bile in the liver, stimulating contraction of the gallbladder and slowing gastric emptying, CCK stimulates the pancreatic acinar cells to secrete digestive enzymes.
- **Secretin**. This hormone is secreted by the duodenal mucosa in response to the presence of acid-containing chyme in the duodenum. As well as slowing gastric emptying, secretin stimulates the duct cells of the pancreas to secrete HCO_3^- to neutralise the chyme.

How does intestinal motility differ in the fed and fasted states?

In the fed state, the contractions of the small intestine are designed to:

- Promote mixing of chyme with digestive enzymes and bile salts;
- Propel chyme along the small intestine to the large intestine.

The two types of contractions of the small intestine reflect these two functions:

- **Segmental contractions**. Contraction of the circular smooth muscle in neighbouring segments compartmentalises a section of bowel. This is followed by continuous contraction and relaxation of the longitudinal muscle, which results in the mixing of chyme with digestive enzymes rather than its propulsion along the GI tract. Segmental contractions also bring chyme into contact with the brush border, promoting nutrient absorption.
- **Propulsive contractions**. Highly coordinated contraction of the circular muscle behind the food bolus and longitudinal smooth muscle results in propulsion of chyme along the GI tract. Each peristaltic wave lasts only a few seconds, travelling at only a few centimetres per second.

In the fasted state, there are infrequent, irregular contractions of the small intestine. Every 90 min, there is a period of intense, coordinated intestinal contraction, spreading from the duodenum to the ileocaecal valve; this is known as the migrating motor complex (MMC). The contraction sweeps along the length of the small intestine, moving undigested chyme towards the colon.

How is intestinal motility controlled?

Like nerve cells, the smooth muscle cells of the small intestine have a negative resting membrane potential (–40 to –70 mV). Contraction of smooth muscle occurs when the membrane potential exceeds threshold potential; opening of voltage-gated channels permits a sudden influx of Na^+ and Ca^{2+}, which depolarises the cell membrane and stimulates contraction.

Normally, the smooth muscle cell membrane potential fluctuates 20–30 times per minute; these fluctuations are called slow waves. The fluctuations in cell membrane potential are insufficient to exceed threshold potential by themselves. Instead, they help to coordinate depolarisations and contractions of the GI tract. The presence of a food bolus stretches the intestinal walls and triggers the release of neurotransmitters, which cause a small depolarisation of the cell membrane. The threshold potential is exceeded when the next slow wave occurs, resulting in a spike potential: smooth muscle contraction is triggered.

Small intestinal motility is influenced by inputs from both the nervous and endocrine systems:

- **The enteric nervous system**. This extensive nervous system controls the GI tract. It consists of efferent and afferent neurons, converging on two types of ganglion: the myenteric (Auerbach's) plexus and the submucosal (Meissner's) plexus. The enteric nervous system operates semi-autonomously, with inputs from the autonomic nervous system:

  - *The sympathetic nervous system*, through synapses in the prevertebral ganglia, causes inhibition of the enteric nervous system, reducing intestinal motility and GI secretions. In addition, blood flow to the gut is reduced by splanchnic vasoconstriction.
  - *The parasympathetic nervous system*, through the vagus nerve, causes an increase in intestinal motility and stimulates GI secretions; the parasympathetic nervous system is thus often referred to as the 'rest and digest' system.

- **The endocrine system**. Whilst a number of hormones are involved in the modification of gastric motility (e.g. CCK and secretin), the endocrine control of intestinal motility is less well understood.

  - *Motilin* is a hormone released from the duodenal mucosa every 90 min during fasting and is responsible for stimulating the MMC. The stimulus for the release of motilin is unknown. Erythromycin is a motilin agonist, which is why it is used as a pro-kinetic in the intensive care unit.
  - *Vasoactive intestinal peptide* (VIP) has multiple effects on the GI tract. In the small intestine, it increases secretion of water and electrolytes and stimulates intestinal motility. This is why VIP overproduction due to a VIPoma usually presents with watery diarrhoea.

Further reading

L. R. Johnson. *Gastrointestinal Physiology: Mosby Physiology Monograph Series, 9th edition*. St Louis, Mosby, 2018.

K. Barrett. *Gastrointestinal Physiology, 2nd edition*. New York, McGraw-Hill Education, 2013.

L. G. Collis, D. J. Chambers, B. Carr. Hypertriglyceridaemia-induced acute pancreatitis: is plasmapheresis really indicated? *J Intensive Care Soc* 2014; **15**(1): 66–9.

Chapter 65

Liver: Anatomy and Blood Supply

Describe the blood supply to the liver

The liver is the largest solid organ in the body (the skin is overall the largest organ) and receives a large volume of blood. At rest, the liver receives around 25% of the cardiac output (approximately 1500 mL/min). Unlike other organs, the liver receives a dual blood supply:

- **The right and left hepatic arteries** contribute approximately a third of the liver's blood supply (500 mL/min) and half of its O_2 requirements.
- **The portal vein**[1] accounts for the majority of blood supplied to the liver (1000 mL/min). Because the blood has already passed through the abdominal organs, it has a lower oxygen saturation (S_aO_2):
  - In the fasting state, portal blood has an S_aO_2 saturation of approximately 85%.
  - In the fed state, portal blood has an S_aO_2 saturation of approximately 70%.

How is hepatic blood flow regulated?

Because of its dual blood supply, regulation of hepatic blood flow is more complicated than that of other organs. Hepatic blood flow is regulated by intrinsic and extrinsic mechanisms:

- **Intrinsic mechanisms.** In common with other arterial systems, hepatic arterial blood flow remains relatively constant despite changes in arterial pressure as a result of autoregulation (see Chapter 34). Below a mean arterial pressure of 60 mmHg, autoregulation fails and blood flow becomes pressure dependent.

In contrast, the portal vein has very little smooth muscle, so it cannot regulate blood flow in the same way. Instead, blood flow is proportional to the pressure gradient in the portal vein.

The two different sources of hepatic blood have a semi-reciprocal relationship, referred to as the 'hepatic arterial buffer response'. If portal vein blood flow falls, the hepatic arteries maintain overall liver blood flow through a vasodilatation response involving adenosine as the chemical mediator. However, if hepatic arterial blood flow falls, the portal vein cannot compensate (this is why the relationship is *semi*-reciprocal).

- **Extrinsic mechanisms.** The hepatic vessels are innervated by the sympathetic nervous system:
  - In the hepatic artery, increased sympathetic activity causes vasoconstriction.
  - More important is the effect of sympathetic nervous activity on the portal vein, portal venules and hepatic veins. Around 500 mL of blood is stored within these capacitance vessels. Sympathetic stimulation increases the tone of the vessels, resulting in around 250 mL of blood being returned to the circulation. Together with the splanchnic capacitance vessels, around 1000 mL of blood can be mobilised at times of physiological stress.

How does the respiratory cycle affect hepatic venous blood flow?

During spontaneous breathing, hepatic venous blood flow is increased during inspiration as a result of negative intrathoracic pressure. During expiration, the opposite occurs.

In contrast, positive-pressure ventilation causes a decrease in hepatic venous blood flow as a result of positive intrathoracic pressure. Likewise, positive end-expiratory pressure (PEEP) increases intrathoracic pressure, which results in a reduced hepatic venous blood flow.

---

[1] The term 'portal' refers to a vein that connects two capillary systems. Blood in the portal vein flows between the capillary networks of the abdominal organs (intestines, stomach, spleen and pancreas) and the liver.

Clinical relevance: intraoperative liver blood flow

Intraoperatively, liver blood flow is altered by both anaesthetic and surgical factors:

- **Anaesthetic factors**:

    - *Positive-pressure ventilation and PEEP*: as discussed above.
    - *Drugs*: volatile agents and vasopressors reduce hepatic arterial blood flow.
    - *Minute ventilation*: hypocapnoea reduces portal vein blood flow whilst hypercapnoea increases blood flow.
    - *Regional anaesthesia*: neuraxial blockade reduces hepatic blood flow to a similar extent as general anaesthesia.

- **Surgical factors**: intraoperative retraction and packing of the liver reduces hepatic blood flow significantly more than any of the above anaesthetic factors.

Describe the macroscopic anatomy of the liver

Liver anatomy is described in terms of either its morphological anatomy or its functional anatomy:

- **Morphological anatomy**. Based on the external appearance of the liver:

    - The liver is divided into the right anatomical lobe (much larger) and the left anatomical lobe by the falciform ligament.
    - When viewed from beneath, two additional small lobes can be seen between the right and left lobes. These are the caudate (posterior) and quadrate (inferior) lobes.

    This morphological anatomy is not particularly useful when it comes to hepatobiliary surgery.

- **Functional anatomy**. The Couinaud classification divides the liver into eight functionally independent lobes:

    - Each of the eight lobes has its own blood supply derived from branches of the hepatic artery and portal vein, along with its own hepatic venous drainage and biliary drainage.
    - The segments are numbered 1–8 in a clockwise direction, starting from the caudate lobe.
    - The point where the portal vein, common bile duct and hepatic artery enter the liver is known as the hilum or porta hepatis.

    - An imaginary line between the gallbladder fossa and inferior vena cava (called Cantlie's line) separates the functional right and left halves of the liver (this is not the falciform ligament). The vessels of the porta hepatis divide into right and left branches at this point.

From a surgical perspective, the Couinaud classification is much more useful: any given lobe can continue its normal function when neighbouring lobes are resected.

Describe the microscopic anatomy of the liver

Like the macroscopic anatomy, the liver microarchitecture can be considered in terms of either a classical histological or a functional description:

- **Histological approach**. The liver is composed of tens of thousands of lobules (Figure 65.1a). These are hexagon-shaped arrangements with a branch of the hepatic vein at the centre:

    - Radiating out from the central vein are columns of hepatocytes and hepatic sinusoids.
    - At each of the six corners of the lobule is a hepatic triad: a portal venule, hepatic arteriole and a bile duct.

However, this classical model was derived from studies of pig livers; human liver microarchitecture is more disorganised, with a large amount of connective tissue and fewer well-defined lobules.

- **Functional approach**. Current thinking considers the functional unit of the liver to be the acinus. The elliptical acinus has a terminal branch of the hepatic vein at either end, with two portal triads at the midpoint of the flattened sides (Figure 65.1b). Blood flows from the portal triad towards the terminal vein. The further a hepatocyte is positioned from the portal triad, the lower the O_2 tension. Each acinus is therefore said to have three zones of oxygenation – zones 1, 2 and 3:

    - **Zone 1** is the area of the acinus closest to the two portal triads and is therefore the best oxygenated. The most energy-consuming processes (e.g. gluconeogenesis and β-oxidation of fatty acids) occur in zone 1.
    - **Zone 2** is an intermediate area where hepatocytes carry out processes characteristic of both zone 1 and zone 3.

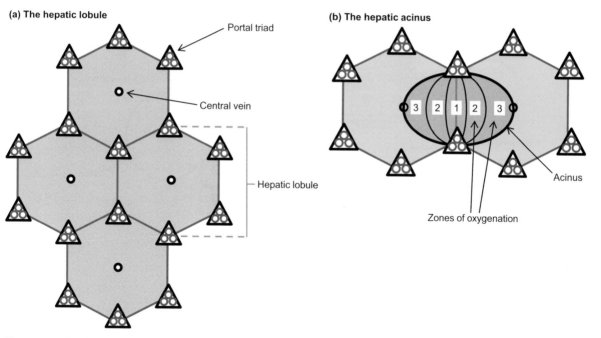

(a) The hepatic lobule

Portal triad

Central vein

Hepatic lobule

(b) The hepatic acinus

3 2 1 2 3

Acinus

Zones of oxygenation

Figure 65.1 (a) The hepatic lobule and (b) the hepatic acinus.

- **Zone 3** is the area of the acinus closest to the terminal vein and is therefore the area of lowest O_2 tension. The hepatocytes of zone 3 carry out the least energy-consuming processes (e.g. glycolysis and drug metabolism).

What are the different cell types within the liver?

The liver has two main cell types: hepatocytes (60% by mass) and Kuppfer cells (10% by mass). In addition, there are other non-parenchymal cells: sinusoidal, peri-sinusoidal and biliary epithelial cells.

- **Hepatocytes** are highly specialised cells that are arranged in columns, making up about 80% of the volume of the liver. They perform a wide range of metabolic, synthetic and exocrine functions (see Chapter 66). Within the column of hepatocytes are small channels called bile canaliculi (Figure 65.2). The hepatocytes secrete bile into the canaliculi. Bile flows from canaliculi to bile ductules and then to bile ducts. Bile ducts merge and exit the liver as the common hepatic duct. On either side of the hepatocyte columns are

blood-filled spaces called hepatic sinusoids. Oxygenated blood flows from the hepatic arteriole and portal venule towards a branch of the hepatic vein. The sinusoidal epithelial cells have very large fenestrations and lack tight junctions, making them highly permeable (see Chapter 36). Substances within the blood (nutrients, drugs, toxins, etc.) are filtered through the sinusoidal epithelial cells to the peri-sinusoidal space, where they come into contact with the hepatocytes (Figure 65.2).

- **Kuppfer cells** are specialised macrophages that line the walls of the hepatic sinusoids (Figure 65.2). Their role is to destroy bacteria or other foreign material contained within the venous blood flowing from the gastrointestinal tract. They also remove worn-out red blood cells and leukocytes from the circulation.

Clinical relevance: centrilobular necrosis

Centrilobular necrosis (zone 3 of the acinus) is a common histological finding in severe liver disease due to:

- **Hypoxic injury**. Owing to their distance from the portal triad, the hepatocytes of zone 3 are the

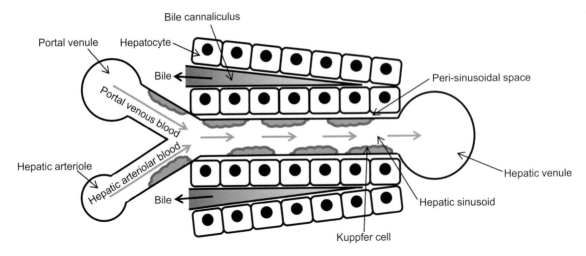

Figure 65.2 Hepatocytes, canaliculi and sinusoids.

most susceptible to hypoxic injury. Centrilobular necrosis is often found on liver biopsy of patients with severe sepsis complicated by hepatic dysfunction.

- **Drug metabolism**. Zone 3 is the main site of drug metabolism; toxic metabolites produced by the cytochrome P450 enzyme system may cause damage to local hepatocytes. Zone 3 is the site of accumulation of the toxic paracetamol metabolite N-acetyl-p-benzoquinone imine (NAPQI) in paracetamol overdose.

Halothane hepatitis exemplifies both of the above. Following halothane exposure, a patient can develop two types of hepatocyte injury:

- **Type I halothane hepatitis** is characterised by a mild, transient post-operative rise in serum liver enzymes. Halothane is metabolised in zones 2 and 3 by cytochrome P450, usually through an oxidative pathway resulting in the metabolite trifluoroacetic acid. A small amount of metabolism occurs through a reductive pathway;

this is favoured by the relatively hypoxic environment of zone 3. This reductive pathway generates free radicals, which damage hepatocytes.

- **Type II halothane hepatitis** is a rare complication of halothane anaesthesia with a mortality of 50%. The mechanism is thought to be autoimmune: trifluoroacetyl metabolites bind to hepatocyte proteins in zone 3, forming a hapten complex that activates the immune system. Antibodies are produced that target these hepatocyte–metabolite complexes, resulting in massive centrilobular necrosis and fulminant liver failure.

Further reading

K. Barrett. *Gastrointestinal Physiology, 2nd edition*. New York, McGraw-Hill Education, 2013.

J. A. Hinson, D. W. Roberts, L. P. James. Mechanisms of acetaminophen-induced liver necrosis. *Handb Exp Pharmacol* 2010; **196**: 369–405.

Chapter

66

Liver Function

The liver is responsible for a wide range of strategic biochemical functions, synthesising and eliminating a huge number of molecules for a variety of purposes. A healthy liver has some important features:

- **A huge physiological reserve**. Even if 80% of liver is removed, it can continue to carry out all of its physiological functions.
- **Regeneration**. In contrast to the other organs, following resection of up to three-quarters of the liver, active mitosis can regenerate a normal liver mass. This amazing ability of the liver has been used in transplantation medicine: living donor transplantation involves transplanting four segments of the right lobe (50–60% of the liver mass) from a live donor to a recipient. In the donor, the remaining liver regenerates to full size within 6–8 weeks; in the recipient, regeneration takes a little longer. Eventually, both donor and recipient have fully functioning, normal-sized livers.

Classify the functions of the liver

The functions of the liver are varied, and can be broadly classified as:

- Metabolic;
- Exocrine;
- Endocrine;
- Immunological;
- Synthetic;
- Hepatic clearance of drugs;
- A number of additional miscellaneous functions.

What are the metabolic functions of the liver?

The liver has a vast array of metabolic functions (see Chapter 77), the most important of which are:

- **Carbohydrate metabolism**. Many metabolic processes occur in the liver in order to maintain a normal plasma glucose concentration:

  - *Glycolysis*. Like all other cells, the liver produces energy by transforming glucose into pyruvate.
  - *Glycogenesis*. Following a meal, plasma glucose concentration rises, which causes insulin to be released from the pancreas. In the liver, insulin stimulates the polymerisation of excess glucose into its storage form, glycogen. Up to 100 g of glucose can be stored in this way.
  - *Glycogenolysis*. When plasma glucose concentration falls between meals, insulin secretion is reduced and glucagon is released from the pancreas. In response to glucagon secretion, the liver releases glucose by breaking down its glycogen store.
  - *Gluconeogenesis*. When plasma glucose concentration is low, glucagon also simulates the liver to synthesise glucose from non-carbohydrate precursors (e.g. amino acids, lactate and glycerol).

- **Fat metabolism**. Lipid is the body's most efficient method of energy storage. The liver is involved in lipid metabolism in a number of ways:

  - *Lipid breakdown*. Energy is extracted from free fatty acids as they are metabolised in a process called 'β-oxidation' within the hepatocyte mitochondria.
  - *Lipid synthesis*. The liver synthesises triglyceride from excess glucose. Cholesterol is also synthesised in the liver. Cholesterol is used as a structural component of cell membranes and as a precursor for steroid hormone and bile salt synthesis.
  - *Lipid processing*. Apolipoproteins are synthesised in the liver. These are involved in the packaging of cholesterol and triglyceride as low-density lipoprotein, very-low-density lipoprotein and high-density lipoprotein.

- **Protein metabolism:**
  - *Deamination.* Individual amino acids have their amino groups removed by the liver. The resulting carbon skeleton (a keto acid) can be used for energy in the citric acid cycle (see Chapter 77), transformed into another amino acid or used as a substrate for gluconeogenesis.
  - *Urea formation.* The other product of deamination is ammonia (NH_3). This is detoxified in the liver through conversion to urea or glutamine.
  - *Amino acid synthesis.* Keto acids can be transformed into non-essential amino acids by transamination, taking an amino group from one amino acid and transferring it to a keto acid, forming a new amino acid. Essential amino acids cannot be synthesised within the body and are only found in the diet.
  - *Protein synthesis.* The liver synthesises most plasma proteins, with the exception of immunoglobulins and some hormones (see below).

What are the exocrine functions of the liver?

The liver is an important exocrine organ as it secretes bile:

- Around 1000 mL of bile is produced by the hepatocytes per day. This is then concentrated to a fifth of its volume within the gallbladder.
- The main constituents of bile are water, electrolytes, bile salts, bile pigment, cholesterol and phospholipids.
- Bile acids are produced through the oxidation of cholesterol. Bile salts – the Na^+ and K^+ salts of bile acids – have an essential role in the emulsification of dietary lipid:
  - Bile salts are amphipathic: they are hydrophobic at one end and hydrophilic at the other.
  - Bile salts surround the dietary lipid, breaking up large fat droplets into a suspension of small fat droplets.
  - Formation of these micelles is essential; without them, pancreatic lipase is unable to act on the dietary lipid in their core.
  - The micelles then make contact with enterocytes, which absorb the lipid contents.

The fat-soluble vitamins (vitamins A, D, E and K) are also absorbed by this micelle-mediated mechanism.

The bile salts are left behind in the gut lumen and absorbed at the terminal ileum. The bile salts travel back to the liver through the portal vein, where they are reused.

- Bile is the main route of excretion of bilirubin metabolites, also known as bile pigment. The metabolism of bilirubin is complex (Figure 66.1):
  - Red blood cells (RBCs) are taken up by the spleen when they get old or damaged.
  - In the spleen, haemoglobin (Hb) is broken down (1) and its useful components recycled: the globin chain is broken down into its constituent amino acids and the Fe^{2+} ion is bound to transferrin and transported to the bone marrow for use in erythropoiesis (see Chapter 74). However, the body cannot make further use of the porphyrin ring.
  - Within the macrophages of the spleen, the porphyrin ring is oxidised to biliverdin and then reduced to bilirubin (2).
  - This unconjugated bilirubin is not water soluble, so is bound to albumin and transported to the liver for further processing (3).
  - In the liver, the hepatocytes take up bilirubin and conjugate it to glucuronic acid, making it water soluble (4). The enzyme responsible for this process is glucuronosyltransferase.
  - This conjugated bilirubin is excreted with the bile into the small intestine (5). Almost all of the conjugated bilirubin in the small intestine ends up being reabsorbed (6), transported to the liver in the portal vein and re-secreted into the small intestine; this is known as 'enterohepatic circulation'. However, some conjugated bilirubin inevitably passes into the large intestine.
  - In the large intestine, conjugated bilirubin is converted into urobilinogen by colonic bacteria (7). Urobilinogen has two fates: it may be oxidised further to urobilin and stercobilin (8) and excreted with faeces (stercobilin gives faeces its brown colour). Alternatively, urobilinogen may be reabsorbed by the gut (9) and transported via the portal vein to the liver

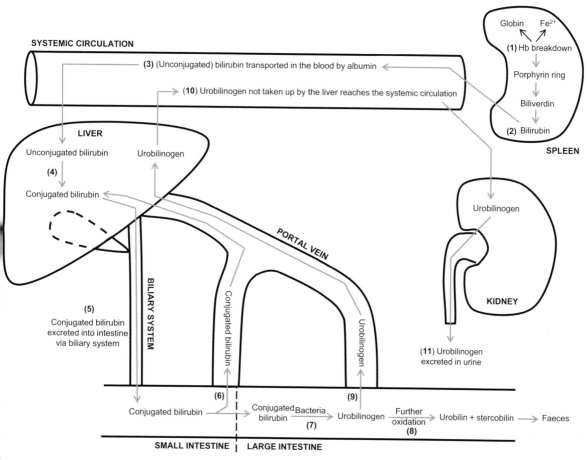

Figure 66.1 Bilirubin metabolism and excretion.

(i.e. enterohepatic circulation). Hepatic uptake of urobilinogen is incomplete, so some reaches the systemic circulation (10) and is excreted by the kidney (11), giving urine its yellow colour.

Clinical relevance: jaundice

Jaundice (plasma bilirubin concentration of >30 pmol/L) may be caused by excessive RBC breakdown or a failure of any of the excretory mechanisms described above:

- **Pre-hepatic jaundice** – increased bilirubin as a result of increased RBC breakdown; for example, haemolytic anaemia due to blood transfusion, sickle cell crisis or malaria. The large amount of bilirubin produced far exceeds the liver's capacity to conjugate – jaundice is therefore the result of a high plasma concentration of *unconjugated*

bilirubin. Because it is water insoluble, no unconjugated bilirubin is filtered by the glomerulus, so urinary dipstick is negative for bilirubin.

- Although anatomically within the liver, conditions involving the failure of bilirubin conjugation are often included with the 'pre-hepatic' causes of jaundice, such as neonatal jaundice (as a result of immature glucuronosyltransferase enzyme) and Gilbert's syndrome (a common genetic disorder where there is reduced activity of the glucuronosyltransferase enzyme). As the problem is conjugation of bilirubin, the plasma concentration of unconjugated bilirubin is high.
- **Post-hepatic jaundice** – failure of excretion of conjugated bilirubin in the bile; for example, as a result of a gallstone obstructing the common bile duct. When the normal route of bilirubin

excretion is blocked, *conjugated* bilirubin instead enters the systemic circulation, resulting in a high plasma concentration of conjugated bilirubin. As conjugated bilirubin is water soluble, it is freely filtered at the glomerulus and excreted in the urine; dipstick is therefore positive for bilirubin. As conjugated bilirubin does not enter the small intestine, urobilinogen and stercobilin are never formed; faeces is therefore pale in colour.

- **Hepatocellular jaundice** – hepatocyte necrosis and disruption of the biliary tree lead to a reduced ability to conjugate and excrete bilirubin. Causes include cirrhosis, acute viral hepatitis and paracetamol toxicity. Whether conjugated or unconjugated bilirubin predominates depends on the relative degrees of hepatocyte dysfunction compared with biliary duct disruption.

What are the endocrine functions of the liver?

The liver has an array of endocrine roles:

- **Secretion of hormones** – including angiotensinogen, thrombopoietin, hepcidin (see Chapter 74) and insulin-like growth factor 1 (IGF-1).
- **Synthesis of hormone binding proteins** – for example, thyroxine-binding globulin and sex hormone-binding globulin.
- **Activation of hormones** – thyroxine (T_4) is converted into either the activated thyroid hormone triiodothyronine (T_3) or inactivated (to reverse T_3; see Chapter 81). Vitamin D undergoes the initial part of its activation in the liver (the 25-hydroxylation of cholecalciferol).
- **Inactivation of hormones** – the liver inactivates many hormones, including aldosterone, antidiuretic hormone and oestrogen. Insulin is worth a special mention: up to half of the insulin released by the pancreas into the portal vein is inactivated by the liver before it passes into the systemic circulation.

What are the immunological functions of the liver?

The liver is an extremely important immunological organ, with a number of roles:

- **Phagocytosis.** Ingested bacteria, viruses and parasites in the gastrointestinal tract pass into the portal vein and must travel through the liver before reaching the systemic circulation. These microorganisms are phagocytosed by the Kuppfer cells, specialised macrophages that line the sinusoids (see Chapter 65).
- **Initiation of inflammation.** Like other macrophages, Kuppfer cells can initiate an inflammatory response by the secretion of proinflammatory cytokines.
- **Protein synthesis.** In addition, the liver is a key part of the innate immune system, synthesising the complement proteins and C-reactive protein.

Which substances are synthesised by the liver?

The liver is such an important synthetic organ that it would be much quicker to list the substances not synthesised by the liver! In addition to the substances already described above, the liver synthesises:

- **Haemostatic substances.** Clotting factors I (fibrinogen), II (prothrombin), V, VII, IX, X and XI, antithrombin III, protein C and protein S. Clotting factors II, VII, IX and X, protein C and protein S are referred to as the vitamin-K-dependent clotting factors because vitamin K is required as a cofactor in their synthesis, which involves vitamin K-catalysed γ-carboxylation.
- **Plasma transport proteins.** For example:
  - *Albumin* (see Chapter 76).
  - *α-globulins*: for example, haptoglobin binds free Hb released from RBCs as a result of haemolysis; caeruloplasmin transports copper; thyroxine-binding globulin transports thyroxine.
  - *β-globulins*: for example, transferrin binds iron in its ferric form (Fe^{3+}); sex hormone-binding globulin binds androgens and oestrogen.
  - *α₁-acid glycoprotein*: transports basic and neutrally charged drugs.

Of note is that immunoglobulins, the most important subgroup of the γ-globulins, are not synthesised in the liver. They are made by plasma cells (see Chapter 75).

- **Serine protease inhibitors.** α₁-antitrypsin is synthesised in the liver. It protects the body's tissues from the damaging enzymes released by activated inflammatory cells, such as neutrophil elastase. The importance of α_1-antitrypsin is seen when it is genetically deficient – the tissues of the lungs and liver are attacked by neutrophil elastase:

- In the lung, chronic destruction of elastic tissue results in chronic obstructive pulmonary disease, even in the absence of cigarette smoking.
- In the liver, chronic inflammation results in cirrhosis.

How does the liver metabolise drugs?

Drug metabolism is divided into three phases:

- **Phase 1: modification.** The hepatocytes use their cytochrome P450 enzyme system to make the drug more polar (and therefore more hydrophilic). The main chemical reactions involved are oxidation, reduction and hydrolysis. The resulting metabolites may be physiologically active – in some cases more active than the parent drug. If the metabolites are sufficiently water soluble, they can be excreted at this point. If not, they progress to undergo phase 2 reactions.
- **Phase 2: conjugation.** The drug, or the product of a phase 1 reaction, is attached to a polar molecule such as glucuronic acid, acetate or sulphate. The process is called glucuronidation, acetylation or sulphation, respectively. The consequence of conjugation is the production of water-soluble metabolites of the drug ready for excretion in bile or urine.
- **Phase 3: excretion.** This recently discovered phase involves ATP-dependent excretion of drug metabolites into the bile.

Clinical relevance: factors affecting drug metabolism

There is considerable inter-patient variability in the rate of drug metabolism, for a variety of reasons:

- Genetic differences in phase 1 and phase 2 reactions; for example:
  - Codeine is a prodrug that is metabolised to morphine by the enzyme CYP2D6 in the liver. Approximately 6% of Caucasians have an inactive or dysfunctional CYP2D6 enzyme; these patients do not gain any analgesic effects from codeine (but often still have the side effects of nausea and constipation). Conversely, 1–2% of patients are ultra-rapid metabolisers of codeine, rapidly resulting in a high plasma morphine concentration. A breastfeeding infant of an ultra-fast-metabolising mother receiving codeine may receive an opioid overdose through transfer in breast milk. For this reason, codeine is no longer recommended in breastfeeding mothers.
  - Patients fall into two categories of acetylation: fast and slow. Drugs that are metabolised by acetylation (e.g. isoniazid) have very different half-lives depending on whether the patient has fast or slow acetylation status.
  - Alcohol metabolism involves two phase 1 oxidation reactions; the enzymes involved are alcohol dehydrogenase and acetaldehyde dehydrogenase. Some 50% of patients of Chinese origin lack an effective acetaldehyde dehydrogenase enzyme, resulting in an increased incidence of acute alcohol intoxication and alcohol-flush reaction due to slow ethanol metabolism and increased plasma acetaldehyde concentration respectively.

- **Interaction of enzymes with other drugs.** Certain drugs increase (induce) or decrease (inhibit) the activity of the cytochrome P450 enzyme system:
  - *Drugs that induce hepatic enzymes*: phenytoin, carbamazepine, barbiturates (notably phenobarbitone), rifampicin, alcohol (chronic abuse), smoking (induces the enzyme CYP1A2, involved in the metabolism of drugs such as olanzapine and aminophylline). Mnemonic: PC BRAS.
  - *Drugs that inhibit hepatic enzymes*: omeprazole, allopurinol, disulfiram, erythromycin, valproate, isoniazid, cimetidine, ethanol (acute alcohol binge), sulphonamides. Mnemonic: OA DEVICES.

For example:
- The oral contraceptive pill is metabolised more quickly by patients taking enzyme inducers, leading to a risk of pregnancy.
- Ciclosporin metabolism may be slowed, potentially leading to toxicity, in patients who are given enzyme inhibitors, such as a course of the pro-kinetic erythromycin in intensive care.

Does the liver have any other physiological roles?

In addition to the many functions described above, the liver has a number of other functions:

- **Storage.** As well as storing glycogen, the liver is the main site of iron, copper and fat-soluble vitamin storage.
- **Haematological.** In the first trimester, the foetal liver is the main site of erythropoiesis. In addition, old or damaged RBCs are removed from the circulation by the liver's Kuppfer cells (though the spleen carries out the majority of this role).
- **Blood reservoir.** As discussed in Chapter 65, the liver can release up to 250 mL of venous blood into the systemic circulation in response to sympathetic stimulation.

What physiological changes occur in cirrhosis?

There are many causes of chronic liver failure, including viral hepatitis, alcohol, steatohepatitis, metabolic diseases (e.g. Wilson's disease, haemochromatosis), biliary disease (primary biliary cirrhosis, primary sclerosing cholangitis) and autoimmune hepatitis. Whatever the cause, chronic inflammation and scarring of the liver results in cirrhosis – a disorganised mixture of hepatocyte fibrosis and regeneration. Cirrhosis results in the following.

- **Alteration of liver function**, leading to:
  - *Disturbed carbohydrate metabolism*, resulting in hyper- or hypo-glycaemia;
  - *Decreased protein synthesis*, resulting in clotting abnormalities and hypoalbuminaemia, which predisposes to oedema and alters the protein binding of drugs;
  - *Altered drug metabolism*, which may be considerably slower;
  - *Inadequate clearance of NH_3*, leading to hepatic encephalopathy (see below).
- **Alteration of liver anatomy**, resulting in increased resistance to blood flow as fibrosis disrupts and obstructs the sinusoids. The portal vein is usually a low-pressure system, but in cirrhosis the increased resistance to blood flow increases portal vein pressure. Normal portal vein pressure is 5–10 mmHg – portal hypertension is

defined as a pressure > 12 mmHg. Portal hypertension results in:

- *Ascites*: high venous hydrostatic pressure leads to net fluid filtration into the peritoneal cavity. Ascites poses an especially high infection risk, as the fluid is relatively stagnant and patients with cirrhosis are relatively immunosuppressed.
- *Splenomegaly*: venous blood from the spleen drains into the portal vein. Therefore, if portal venous pressure were to rise, venous drainage of the spleen would become impaired and the spleen engorged – over time, splenomegaly occurs. An increased number of platelets and erythrocytes are removed from the circulation, resulting in thrombocytopaenia and anaemia, respectively.
- *Portocaval anastomoses*: high portal venous pressure opens collateral vessels between the portal and systemic circulations. These vessels become dilated and engorged, leading to oesophageal varices, rectal varices and caput medusae. These engorged veins, especially oesophageal varices, are liable to mechanical damage that may result in a potentially catastrophic haemorrhage. Nitrogen-containing molecules from the portal blood are able to pass directly into the systemic circulation without first traversing the liver, increasing the risk of hepatic encephalopathy.

What are liver function tests?

Liver function tests (LFTs) are laboratory tests that help to diagnose and monitor liver disease or damage. However, because of the large physiological reserve of the liver, LFTs may remain normal until a significant reduction in liver function has occurred. LFTs can divided into:

- **Tests of liver synthetic function**: albumin and prothrombin time (PT).
  - *Albumin* has a plasma half-life of 30 days. Hypoalbuminaemia may be a useful measure of liver function in chronic liver disease. However, the long half-life of albumin, capillary leakage and protein catabolism make serum albumin a poor marker of liver synthetic function in acute liver disease.

- *PT* is a test of the extrinsic pathway of coagulation (see Chapter 72). PT depends on clotting factors II, V, VII and X and fibrinogen. The liver is responsible for the synthesis of all of these factors. The half-life of these clotting factors is <24 h, which is considerably shorter than that of albumin. Therefore, PT acts as an effective measure of liver synthetic function in acute liver dysfunction.

- **Tests of hepatic clearance**: bilirubin (discussed above) and NH_3. Normally, NH_3 is converted to urea by the liver. In severe liver dysfunction, serum NH_3 concentration rises. NH_3 is implicated in hepatic encephalopathy; as it is a small, uncharged molecule, osmotically active NH_3 is able to cross the blood–brain barrier, leading to cerebral oedema and encephalopathy. However, serum NH_3 does not correlate particularly well with the clinical severity of hepatic encephalopathy.

- **Serum hepatic enzyme tests**: alkaline phosphatase (ALP), γ-glutamyl transpeptidase (γ-GT) and alanine aminotransferase (ALT). These tests are used to aid the exact diagnosis of hepatic dysfunction.

  - *ALP* is an enzyme concentrated in the biliary canalicular membrane of the hepatocyte. Disease of the biliary system causes release of ALP into the systemic circulation. Very high (greater than three times normal) ALP suggests either intrahepatic or extrahepatic biliary obstruction. Of note, ALP occasionally originates from sources other than the liver: kidney, bone and placenta.

  - *γ-GT* is also raised in biliary obstruction – this is because γ-GT is found in hepatocytes surrounding the biliary canaliculi. In fact, γ-GT is found in similar tissues to ALP, except it is only present in low concentrations in bone. This may be diagnostically useful,

distinguishing between bone and liver as the origin of a high ALP. γ-GT is often elevated by alcohol ingestion: a disproportionally raised γ-GT compared with ALP or ALT suggests alcohol abuse.

- *ALT* is present in the cytosol of hepatocytes. Therefore, generalised hepatocellular injury results in an increase in serum ALT. For example, ALT rises as a result of centrilobular necrosis in paracetamol overdose.

Clinical relevance: King's College Criteria for liver transplantation

Paracetamol overdose is relatively common, and liver transplantation subjects the patient to a lifetime of immunosuppression. Following a paracetamol overdose, it is important to be able to predict which patients are likely to deteriorate and require a life-saving liver transplant. LFTs play a part in this prediction. The King's College Criteria identify patients at risk of poor outcome following paracetamol overdose. Liver transplantation is considered if either:

- Arterial pH is <7.3;
- Or all three of PT > 100 s (equivalent to an international normalised ratio of >6.5), serum creatinine of >300 pmol/L and hepatic encephalopathy of grade III or IV.

Further reading

L. R. Johnson. *Gastrointestinal Physiology: Mosby Physiology Monograph Series, 9th edition*. St Louis, Mosby, 2018.

K. Barrett. *Gastrointestinal Physiology, 2nd edition*. New York, McGraw-Hill Education, 2013.

A. Kortgen, P. Recknagel, M. Bauer. How to assess liver function? *Curr Opin Crit Care* 2010; **16**(2): 136–41.

B. P. Sweeney, J. Bromilow. Liver enzyme induction and inhibition: implications for anaesthesia. *Anaesthesia* 2006; **61**(2): 159–77.

J. K. Limdi, G. M. Hyde. Evaluation of abnormal liver function tests. *Postgrad Med J* 2003; **79**(932): 307–12.

Chapter

67

Renal Function, Anatomy and Blood Flow

What are the functions of the kidney?

The kidney has an array of functions that can be classified as:

- **Homeostasis of blood composition**, including:
  - Regulation of plasma volume and electrolyte concentration.
  - Control of plasma osmolarity.
  - Removal of waste products and drugs or their metabolites.
  - Gluconeogenesis: the kidney is a major gluconeogenic organ.
  - Control of the metabolic aspects of acid-base balance.

- **Endocrine roles**:
  - Erythropoietin synthesis, which in turn controls erythrocyte production;
  - Activation of vitamin D to 1,25-dihydroxycholecalciferol;
  - Secretion of renin, the first hormone of the renin–angiotensin–aldosterone axis.

Describe the anatomy of the kidney

The kidneys are solid, 'bean-shaped' retroperitoneal organs located at vertebral levels T12 to L3. From inside to outside, the kidney is surrounded by the renal capsule, perirenal fat, renal fascia and pararenal fascia. At the midpoint of the concave medial border of each kidney is the hilum, the point of entry of the nerves, vessels and lymphatics. In cross-section, the kidney contains:

- An outer renal cortex.
- An inner renal medulla, interrupted by renal columns (extensions of the cortex) that penetrate deep into the renal medulla.
- Towards the hilum, minor calyces coalesce to form major calyces, which merge to form the renal pelvis and finally the ureter.

The blood supply to the kidneys is carried by the renal arteries, paired arteries that arise directly from the aorta. The right renal artery is longer, as the aorta is positioned slightly to the left of the midline. Sometimes there are also additional accessory arteries. Venous drainage of the kidneys is through the renal veins, which drain directly into the inferior vena cava (IVC). The left renal vein is longer than the right owing to the position of the IVC to the right of the midline.

Describe the structure of the nephron

The functional unit of the kidney is the nephron (Figure 67.1), of which there are around 1,000,000 per kidney. A nephron consists of:

- **The glomerulus**, a network of capillaries located in the renal cortex whose role is the filtration of plasma (see Chapter 68). The fluid is collected in Bowman's capsule and passes along a series of tubes.
- **The proximal convoluted tubule** (PCT) – a twisting tubule within the renal cortex where the majority of the filtered products are reabsorbed.
- **The loop of Henle** (LOH) – the tubule straightens and then enters the medulla to become the thin descending limb. This undergoes a hairpin bend to continue as the thin and then the thick ascending limb of the LOH. The main role of the LOH is to generate a longitudinal osmotic gradient in the renal medulla, which allows controlled water reabsorption from the collecting ducts.
- **The distal convoluted tubule** (DCT) – the thick ascending limb of the LOH returns to the renal cortex to form the DCT, the site of regulated reabsorption.
- **The collecting duct** (CD) – the DCT becomes the CD, before forming a minor calyx. The CD is an important site of water reabsorption.

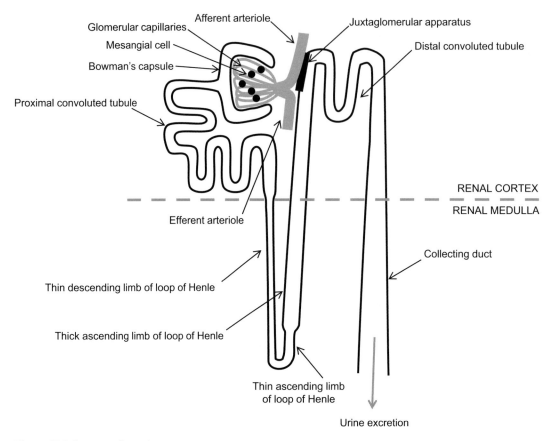

Figure 67.1 Structure of a nephron.

The arterial blood supply of the nephron is unique:

- The renal arterial tree divides as usual to give afferent arterioles, which in turn divide to give rise to the glomerular capillaries. These capillaries then unite to form efferent arterioles.
- By varying the relative resistances of the afferent and efferent arterioles, glomerular capillary hydrostatic pressure, which is the main driving force for glomerular filtration, can be modified. Glomerular filtration is therefore controllable (see Chapter 68).
- The vasa recta are an additional set of arterioles that arise from the efferent arterioles, whose role is to supply blood to the renal medulla. The vasa recta also have an unusual feature: they descend with the ascending limb of the LOH and ascend with the descending limb, providing a countercurrent flow of blood. This countercurrent arrangement is required to generate the high solute concentration gradients of the renal medulla (see Chapter 69).

It is important to note that this anatomy results in a well-vascularised renal cortex, but a relatively poor blood supply to the renal medulla. This latter feature prevents washout of solutes from the medullary interstitium that are required for water reabsorption.

What is the juxtaglomerular apparatus?

The DCT folds back to lie anatomically very close to its corresponding glomerulus. At this point are located a group of specialised cells that form the juxtaglomerular apparatus, consisting of three components:

- *Granular cells*, located within the wall of the afferent arteriole, whose role is renin secretion.
- *Macula densa cells*, located at the junction of the DCT and the thick ascending limb of the LOH. Macula densa cells sense tubular Na^+ and Cl^- concentration.
- *Extra-glomerular mesangial cells*. These interact with the macula densa via a purinergic signalling

mechanism to control the granular cells and the vascular smooth muscle of the afferent arterioles.

The juxtaglomerular apparatus regulates renal blood flow (RBF) (see p. 309) and the glomerular filtration rate (GFR) (see Chapter 68).

How is RBF regulated?

Despite only making up 1% of total body weight, the kidneys receive a blood flow of approximately 1000 mL/min, 20% of the cardiac output. Unlike tissues such as skeletal muscle, the kidneys receive far more blood than is required for their metabolic activity, reflecting their function of blood filtration. There is a greater proportion of blood flow to the glomerulus (500 mL/100 g of tissue/min) than the medulla (outer medulla: 100 mL/100 g/min; inner medulla: 20 mL/100 g/min).

RBF must be tightly controlled:

- Too high a flow results in end-organ damage due to high pressure. In addition, there is insufficient time for reabsorption processes to occur in the tubules, resulting in a pressure diuresis.
- Too low a flow results in ischaemia, particularly of the relatively poorly vascularised medulla and metabolically active PCTs, as well as a build-up of toxic metabolites in the blood due to reduced filtration.

For this reason, RBF is kept constant over a range of normal perfusion pressures (mean arterial pressure 75–165 mmHg; Figure 67.2). This phenomenon is called renal autoregulation (see Chapter 34).

What is the mechanism of renal autoregulation?

Both RBF and GFR are controlled through alterations in afferent and efferent arteriolar tone:

- Constriction of either the afferent or efferent arteriole increases the overall renal vascular resistance, which reduces RBF.
- Constriction of the afferent arteriole reduces glomerular capillary hydrostatic pressure and thus reduces GFR.
- Constriction of the efferent arteriole increases glomerular capillary hydrostatic pressure by causing a build-up of blood in the glomerulus, which in turn increases GFR.

Therefore, separate control of these vessels allows RBF and GFR to be determined independently.

The biological mechanism for autoregulation in the kidney is not completely elucidated. It is divided into myogenic and tubuloglomerular feedback mechanisms:

- **Myogenic mechanism:**
  - *When perfusion pressure increases*, the afferent arterioles are stretched. The arteriole responds by contracting its smooth muscle, which reduces the vessel diameter: vascular resistance increases, which keeps blood flow constant.[1]
  - *When perfusion pressure decreases*, the afferent arteriole responds by relaxing its smooth muscle: vascular resistance is reduced, which keeps blood flow constant.

- **Tubuloglomerular feedback**: this mechanism is more complex. The juxtaglomerular apparatus monitors the fluid flow through the DCT and adjusts glomerular filtration accordingly:
  - An increase in renal perfusion pressure leads to increased pressure within the glomerular capillaries and therefore increased glomerular filtration. This in turn increases tubular flow and therefore the rate of delivery of Na^+ and Cl^- ions to the macula densa.
  - The macula densa senses the Na^+ and Cl^- concentrations through its own $Na^+/K^+/2Cl^-$ co-transporter. The intracellular movement of

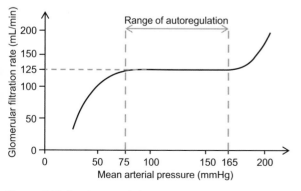

Figure 67.2 Renal autoregulation.

---

[1] Stretching of the arteriolar smooth muscle opens mechanically gated non-specific cation channels, which causes depolarisation of the arteriolar membrane, leading to smooth muscle contraction.

Na^+, K^+ and Cl^- ions is coupled with the osmotic movement of H_2O into the macula densa cell, causing cellular swelling in proportion to the GFR.

- An adenosine-based secondary messenger is released in proportion to the degree of cell swelling.[2]
- The secondary messenger acts at adenosine A_1 receptors located within the juxtaglomerular apparatus, resulting in a reduction in RBF and GFR:

  - *Afferent arterioles vasoconstrict*, which increases renal vascular resistance, thereby reducing RBF.
  - *Glomerular mesangial cells contract*, which reduces the surface area for filtration, thereby reducing GFR.
  - Granular cells are inhibited from secreting renin (see below).

The response to a decrease in renal perfusion pressure is the opposite: the afferent arteriole vasodilates, the mesangial cells relax and renin secretion is increased.

How does the renin–angiotensin–aldosterone axis regulate RBF?

Renin is released from the granular cells of the juxtaglomerular apparatus in response to:

- **Decreased tubular flow**, sensed by the macula densa as discussed above.
- **Low afferent arteriolar pressure**, which directly stimulates the release of renin. Granular cells effectively act as 'intra-renal baroreceptors'.
- **Sympathetic nervous system stimulation** through β_1-adrenoceptors.

Renin, a proteolytic enzyme, does not itself affect the vasculature. Renin cleaves the plasma protein angiotensinogen (produced by the liver) into angiotensin I, which is then converted into angiotensin II by angiotensin-converting enzyme. The renin-mediated proteolysis of

angiotensinogen forms the rate-determining, regulatory step in this sequence. Angiotensin II increases systemic blood pressure and therefore renal perfusion pressure through a number of mechanisms:

- **In the kidney**, angiotensin II causes vasoconstriction of both afferent and efferent arterioles, but has a greater effect on the efferent arterioles owing to their smaller basal diameter. The end result is an increase in systemic blood pressure due to the increased vascular resistance of the renal arterioles, but with a relatively preserved glomerular capillary hydrostatic pressure, and therefore GFR.[3]
- **In the systemic vasculature**, angiotensin II is a potent veno- and vaso-constrictor, thereby increasing the systemic blood pressure.
- **In the adrenal gland**, angiotensin II triggers the release of aldosterone from the zona glomerulosa in the adrenal cortex. Aldosterone acts at the DCT and CD of the kidney, promoting the reabsorption of Na^+ and water, thus expanding plasma volume (see Chapter 69).
- **In the brain**, angiotensin II acts on:

  - *The hypothalamus*, where it increases the sensation of thirst and triggers the release of antidiuretic hormone (ADH) from the posterior lobe of the pituitary gland. ADH increases water reabsorption at the CD.
  - *The sympathetic nervous system*, where it directly increases noradrenaline release at sympathetic neurons, resulting in arteriolar vasoconstriction.

How are eicosanoids involved in the regulation of RBF?

In situations where the concentrations of the circulating vasopressors noradrenaline and angiotensin II are persistently high, including haemorrhage and sepsis, prolonged afferent and efferent arteriolar vasoconstriction causes a significant reduction in RBF. In response, the vasodilatory prostaglandins (PGE_2 and PGI_2), which oppose the effects of the circulating vasoconstrictors, are produced locally within the kidney in an attempt to increase RBF and GFR.

---

[2] It is not clear whether the secondary messenger is ATP, ADP or AMP. One potential mechanism is that, in order to reduce cell swelling, the activity of the basolateral Na^+/ K^+-ATPase must be increased to remove Na^+. This in turn reduces the amount of intracellular ATP and increases ADP and AMP, which then leak from the cell.

---

[3] However, very high angiotensin II levels cause glomerular mesangial cells to contract, reducing the glomerular filtration area, which leads to a significant fall in GFR.

Patients who take non-steroidal anti-inflammatory drugs (NSAIDs) are less able to utilise this safety mechanism: NSAIDs inhibit the cyclo-oxygenase enzyme that is required for prostaglandin synthesis.

Clinical relevance: pathophysiology of acute kidney injury

Acute kidney injury (AKI) is defined as a rapid (<48-h) reduction in kidney function, as determined by a rise in serum creatinine or a reduction in urine output. The causes of AKI may be classified as:

- **Pre-renal**, in which severe hypovolaemia and hypotension compromise RBF. As a consequence of the reduction in glomerular capillary hydrostatic pressure, GFR falls. It is important to note that pre-renal AKI is potentially reversible, as glomerular and tubular function remain intact.
- **Intrinsic renal**, in which ischaemic, cytotoxic or inflammatory insults cause structural damage to the glomerulus or tubules. In contrast to pre-renal failure, this structural damage means that intrinsic renal failure is not immediately reversible once the causative factors have been removed. The main causes of intrinsic renal AKI may be classified according to anatomical location:
  - *Acute tubular necrosis* (ATN), the most common cause of intrinsic renal disease. The high metabolic activity and relatively poor blood supply make tubules particularly susceptible to ischaemia. Prolonged renal hypoperfusion results in tubular cell death. ATN may also be caused by tubular toxins such as myoglobin (due to rhabdomyolysis) and aminoglycosides.
  - *Glomerular inflammation* (glomerulonephritis) centred on:
    - The podocytes, known as minimal change disease;
    - The basement membrane, as occurs in Goodpasture's disease;
    - The mesangial cells; for example, immunoglobulin A (IgA) nephropathy, in which IgA deposits in the mesangial cells;
    - The glomerular capillaries, following antigen–antibody complex deposition in systemic lupus erythematosus and rheumatoid arthritis.
  - *Acute interstitial nephritis*, a hypersensitivity reaction to drugs such as NSAIDs, penicillins and allopurinol.

- **Post-renal**, in which there is obstruction to the flow of urine. Raised tubular pressure decreases glomerular filtration pressure, resulting in decreased GFR.

How can RBF be measured?

Measurement of RBF requires a substance that is both freely filtered and actively secreted into the tubule, so that all the substance entering the renal arteries passes into the urine, with none in the venous outflow. A substance that approaches these criteria is para-amino hippuric acid (PAH). PAH is a small enough molecule (194 Da) to be freely filtered, and is later secreted into the tubules through the organic anion transporter (OAT1). Renal plasma flow (RPF) is then calculated by the clearance of PAH:

$$\text{PAH amount entering the kidney} = \text{PAH amount appearing in urine}$$

Therefore:

$$RPF = \text{Clearance of PAH}$$

The clearance of a substance X is the volume of plasma completely cleared of X by the kidneys per unit time (see Chapter 69), calculated as:

$$\text{Clearance} = \frac{\text{Volume of urine excreted per unit time} \times [X]_{urine}}{[X]_{plasma}}$$

Therefore, for PAH:

$$RPF = \frac{\text{Volume}_{urine} \times [PAH]_{urine}}{[PAH]_{plasma}}$$

This method gives renal *plasma* flow, not renal *blood* flow. RBF can be calculated using the haematocrit:

$$RBF = \frac{RPF}{1 - \text{haematocrit}}$$

RBF can be measured even more accurately by cannulating the renal artery and renal vein, sampling the PAH concentration in each and applying the Fick principle. However, this is far too invasive to be used routinely. In either case, using PAH always underestimates RBF, as only 90% of the RBF supplies the glomerulus – the remainder supplies the renal parenchyma, so cannot be secreted into the tubules.

Further reading

B. M. Koeppen, B. A. Stanton. *Renal Physiology: Mosby Physiology Monograph Series, 5th edition.* St Louis, Mosby, 2012.

C. Lote. *Principles of Renal Physiology, 5th edition.* Berlin, Springer, 2006.

M. A. Ferguson, S. S. Walkar. Established and emerging markers of kidney function. *Clin Chem* 2012; **58**(4): 680–9.

K. Karkouti. Transfusion and risk of acute kidney injury in cardiac surgery. *Br J Anaesth* 2012; **109**(Suppl. 1): i29–38.

E. M. Moore, R. Bellomo, A. D. Nichol. The meaning of acute kidney injury and its relevance to intensive care and anaesthesia. *Anaesth Intensive Care* 2012; **40**(6): 929–48.

J. Mårtensson, C.-R. Martling, M. Bell. Novel biomarkers of acute kidney injury and failure: clinical applicability. *Br J Anaesth* 2012; **109**(6): 843–50.

Chapter

68

Renal Filtration and Reabsorption

How does filtration occur in the kidney?

The basic filtration unit of the kidney is the renal corpuscle, consisting of a glomerulus surrounded by a Bowman's capsule. The high glomerular capillary hydrostatic pressure forces a fraction of the plasma (i.e. water and solutes) through the capillary wall and into the Bowman's space. This filtration barrier is composed of three layers:

- **Glomerular capillary endothelium**, a specialised endothelium with large fenestrations.
- **Glomerular basement membrane**, a layer of supportive basal lamina.
- **Podocytes**, the epithelial cells of a Bowman's capsule. These cells have foot-like projections that wrap around glomerular capillary endothelial cells, leaving slit-like openings between them.

It is important that filtration permits the passage of water and solutes, but that the capillary retains blood cells and proteins. This selectivity results from:

- **The effective pore size of the glomerular capillaries**. This is determined by the size of the capillary wall fenestrations and the spacing between podocyte foot processes:
  - *Particles below 7 kDa* are freely filtered into the Bowman's space.
  - *Particles above 70 kDa* (e.g. immunoglobulins – around 150 kDa) cannot pass between through the pores.
  - *Between 7 and 70 kDa*, partial filtration occurs.

  Albumin (67 kDa) is just small enough to fit through the pores, but filtration is prevented due to its negative charge (see below). Haemoglobin (Hb) is a 69.8-kDa protein, and so is just small enough to be filtered. Hb must therefore be sequestered within red blood cells to prevent filtration.

- **Particle charge**. Most plasma proteins are negatively charged, as their pK_a is less than physiological pH. As a result:
  - *Plasma proteins are retained*. When negatively charged plasma proteins approach the glomerular fenestrations, they are repelled by the negative charges of the glomerular basement membrane and podocyte foot processes.
  - *Small anions are filtered*. Small anions do not come into close enough contact with the glomerular membrane proteins to be repelled.

A final determinant of whether a particle is filtered is the extent of its binding to plasma proteins: acidic compounds bind to albumin, whilst basic compounds bind to α-1-glycoprotein. The extent of protein binding is an important determinant in the clearance of many drugs.

What happens to the filtrate in the renal tubules?

Filtration results in a tubular fluid that contains not only metabolic waste products, but also useful solutes such as electrolytes, glucose and amino acids. The nephron reabsorbs these essential components.

Most of the reabsorption occurs in the proximal convoluted tubule (PCT). Here, 67% of Na^+, K^+, Cl^- and water, 85% of HCO_3^- and (in normal subjects) 100% of glucose and amino acids are reabsorbed. Reabsorption takes place through active or passive processes:

- **Active reabsorption**. The reabsorption of most substances is active (i.e. requires energy), accounting for the high metabolic activity of the kidney. In the basolateral membrane of the tubular cells, Na^+/K^+-ATPase ion pumps actively extrude Na^+ ions from the tubular cells into the peritubular capillaries in exchange for K^+.

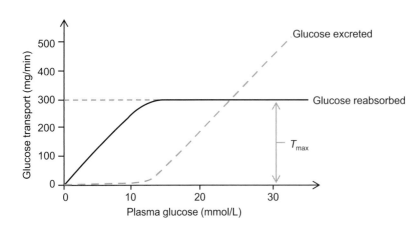

Figure 68.1 Reabsorption of glucose in the proximal convoluted tubule.

The resulting low intracellular Na^+ concentration is used to drive:

- *Co-transporters*: for example, the sodium–glucose-linked transporter (SGLT2) responsible for glucose reabsorption;
- *Counter-transporters*: for example, the Na^+/H^+ counter-transporter, which is involved in acid excretion.

- **Passive reabsorption**. Water is reabsorbed passively: the balance of Starling forces favours bulk reabsorption of water (see Chapter 36). Some of the dissolved electrolytes and small molecules such as urea are passively reabsorbed with water.

Clinical relevance: hyperglycaemia

The reabsorption capacity of the co-transporters in the PCT is limited. In the case of glucose, the SGLT2 transporters have a maximum reabsorption capacity T_{max} of approximately 300 mg/min. T_{max} is reached when filtrate glucose concentration is around 12 mmol/L.

This is relevant in diabetes mellitus: when plasma glucose concentration exceeds the ability of the kidney to reabsorb, glucose will appear in the urine (Figure 68.1).

Glomerular filtration rate (GFR) increases in pregnancy (see Chapter 82). As a result, there is an increased filtration of glucose into the renal tubules: T_{max} is exceeded at a lower plasma glucose concentration. Along with hormonal changes, this accounts for the increased incidence of glycosuria in pregnancy.

How else may substances be renally excreted?

The PCT also actively secretes waste products into the tubular filtrate. Secretion is an active, energy-consuming process in which substances are transported from the peritubular capillaries to the PCT. It allows more effective excretion of waste products than filtration alone. Of clinical importance, many drugs are cleared from the blood with the aid of active secretion through two different carriers:

- **The organic anion transporter**, which secretes a number endogenous and exogenous anionic substances, such as uric acid, penicillin, probenecid and aspirin. Because the same transporter is used for all substances and has a limited capacity for secretion, the presence of one substance affects the clearance of another. For example, probenecid is secreted by the anion transporter in preference to penicillin; co-administration therefore reduces the clearance of penicillin. This pharmacological interaction was exploited during World War II, when penicillin supplies were limited.
- **The organic cation transporter**, which secretes a number of important cationic substances, such as creatinine, catecholamines and morphine.

What is meant by the term 'clearance'?

The clearance of a given solute quantifies the capacity of the kidney to eliminate that solute from the blood, whether through filtration, reabsorption or secretion.

The concept develops from a simple conservation condition, in which

Amount (i.e. moles) of X cleared from plasma

= Amount of X in urine

As moles = volume × concentration:

Volume of plasma filtered × $[X]_{plasma}$

= Volume of urine excreted × $[X]_{urine}$

which rearranges to:

Volume of plasma filtered

$$= \frac{\text{Volume of urine excreted} \times [X]_{urine}}{[X]_{plasma}}$$

Therefore:

Key equation: clearance

$$\text{Clearance} = \frac{\dfrac{\text{Volume of urine excreted}}{\text{per unit time}} \times [X]_{urine}}{[X]_{plasma}}$$

What is GFR? How is it related to the Starling forces?

The GFR is the volume of fluid passing into the tubules from the glomerular capillaries per unit time. The typical GFR of a healthy adult is 125 mL/min. This means 180 L of fluid is filtered by the glomerulus per day. GFR is determined by the balance of Starling forces:

Key equation: Starling filtration equation applied to the kidney

$$GFR = K_f[(P_i - P_o) - (\pi_i - \pi_o)]$$

where P_i and P_o are the hydrostatic pressures inside and outside the glomerular capillary, respectively,

and π_i and π_o are the oncotic pressures inside and outside the glomerular capillary, respectively.[1]

- **The glomerular filtration coefficient** K_f reflects the ease with which fluid leaves the glomerular capillaries under the forces acting across the glomerular filtration barrier. It depends on pore size, which is essentially constant, and surface area of the glomerular capillaries, which can be altered a little through contraction and relaxation of the glomerular mesangial cells (see Chapter 67).
- **The balance of Starling filtration forces** across the filtration barrier (see Chapter 36). The unique arrangement of afferent and efferent arterioles results in a high glomerular capillary hydrostatic pressure (see Chapter 67). A typical value of P_i is 48 mmHg, whilst a typical value of P_o is 10 mmHg. This gives a driving hydrostatic pressure across the glomerular capillary of 38 mmHg.

Oncotic pressure is a measure of the number of osmotically active particles within a compartment. π_i is the result of the osmotic properties of plasma proteins and is typically 25 mmHg. In contrast, as essentially no protein is filtered, π_o is zero.

Overall:

$$GFR = K_f[(P_i - P_o) - (\pi_i - \pi_o)]$$
$$\Rightarrow GFR = K_f[(48 - 10) - (25 - 0)]$$
$$\Rightarrow GFR = K_f \times 13 \text{ mmHg}$$

That is, there is a net driving pressure of 13 mmHg that forces fluid from the glomerular capillaries to the Bowman's space and then on to the renal tubules. This driving pressure may be altered by changes in the glomerular hydrostatic pressure (e.g. decompensated systemic hypotension) or by changes to blood oncotic pressure (e.g. hypoalbuminaemia).

---

[1] In a normal glomerulus, the reflection coefficient σ, normally appearing as the coefficient before the osmotic pressure term, approaches 1, as proteins are almost perfectly excluded and are therefore ignored (see Chapter 36).

How is clearance used in the measurement of GFR?

GFR is an indicator of kidney function and is used clinically to assess the degree of renal failure. If a substance X is freely filtered at the glomerulus and not secreted or reabsorbed later in the tubule, then the rate at which the substance appears in the urine must be equal the rate of its filtration. GFR can therefore be indirectly measured using the clearance formula. A number of substances have been used for the estimation of GFR:

- **Inulin** (not to be confused with insulin) is a small, exogenous polysaccharide that is freely filtered at the glomerulus and not reabsorbed or secreted later along the tubule. Measurement of inulin clearance represents the 'gold standard' in GFR calculation, but is relatively invasive (requiring a continuous infusion of inulin) and is really only used in research where very accurate measurements of GFR are required.
- **Creatinine** is an endogenous molecule produced during skeletal muscle metabolism. Its clearance can be accurately measured using blood and 24-h urine samples. However, creatinine clearance is only an estimate of GFR:
  - The rate of creatinine production is dependent on skeletal muscle mass. This in turn is influenced by age, sex and race, amongst other factors. Numerous algorithms exist to try to compensate for these factors; for example, the Cockcroft–Gault formula compensates for age, sex and weight.
  - Creatinine is actively secreted into the PCT, accounting for 10–20% of excreted creatinine. This results in a slight overestimation of creatinine clearance and therefore an overestimation of GFR. Whilst this error is tolerable in normal patients, in those with advanced renal impairment, the error becomes proportionally much larger: filtration reduces with disease progression, but secretory mechanisms are left intact.
  - In clinical practice, it is not practical to collect 24-h urine samples to perform a formal creatinine clearance calculation. However, by measuring plasma creatinine alone, GFR may fall by as much as 50% (from 180 to 90 L/day) without being detected.

Many researchers have tried to identify an alternative biomarker with which to estimate GFR. Urea has previously been used, but is produced at an even more variable rate than creatinine, being dependent on dietary protein, catabolism and hormonal status. Urea is also reabsorbed in large quantities in the PCT and collecting ducts, making it a very inaccurate measure of GFR. Cystatin C is a small, endogenous molecule that is freely filtered at the glomerulus and then reabsorbed and almost totally metabolised by the tubular cells. In the future, a combination of creatinine and cystatin C may prove to be the best estimate of GFR.

Clinical relevance: renal replacement therapy

Renal failure may occur acutely or insidiously – there are a multitude of causes, and the pathogenesis is complex. The end result is a loss of the essential functions of the kidney, most notably failure of:

- Clearance of toxic substances, leading to uraemia;
- Electrolyte homeostasis, leading to life-threatening hyperkalaemia;
- Water excretion, leading to fluid overload;
- Acid excretion, leading to acidaemia.

Management of renal failure involves artificially performing the key functions of the kidney. Methods of renal replacement therapy (RRT) are:

- **Peritoneal dialysis**. Hyperosmolar dialysate solution is infused into the peritoneal cavity. 'Filtration' is achieved by using the peritoneum as a semipermeable membrane. Water is reabsorbed by making use of the osmolar gradient across the peritoneum. Diffusion along concentration gradients across the peritoneum allows clearance of toxic substances and correction of electrolyte abnormalities.
- **Intermittent haemodialysis and continuous haemofiltration**. Whilst conceptually simple, these methods are inherently complex, involving extracorporeal circuits and an artificial semipermeable membrane. 'Filtration' occurs within an artificial 'kidney', a cellulose or synthetic semipermeable membrane. Like the native kidney, this membrane selectively 'sieves' the blood, allowing small molecules (H_2O, electrolytes and waste products) to pass through, but retaining cells and large proteins in the blood. Depending on the type of RRT, simple diffusion, convection or a combination of the two may be utilised. Reabsorption is achieved by returning electrolyte-rich, pH-balanced fluid to the blood.

- **Renal transplant**. The best method of replacing the function of a failed native kidney is through transplantation of a donor kidney.

What is meant by the term 'filtration fraction'?

The filtration fraction is the fraction of the plasma that is filtered by the glomerulus. For example, the kidney receives a blood at a rate of 1000 mL/min. Assuming a haematocrit of 0.4, glomerular plasma flow is approximately 600 mL/min. We know that a healthy adult's GFR is 125 mL/min. Therefore, the filtration fraction is (125/600) × 100 ≈ 20%.

Further reading

D. C. Eaton, J. D. C. Eaton, J. Pooler. *Vander's Renal Physiology, 8th edition*. New York, McGraw-Hill Medical, 2013.

B. M. Koeppen, B. A. Stanton. *Renal Physiology: Mosby Physiology Monograph Series, 5th edition*. St Louis, Mosby, 2012.

C. Lote. *Principles of Renal Physiology, 5th edition*. Berlin, Springer, 2006.

G. Choi, C. D. Gomersall, Q. Tian, et al. Principles of antibacterial dosing in continuous renal replacement therapy. *Crit Care Med* 2009; 37(7): 2268–82.

N. A. Hall, A. J. Fox. Renal replacement therapies in critical care. *Continuing Educ Anaesth Crit Care Pain* 2006; 6(5): 197–202.

Renal Regulation of Water and Electrolyte Balance

How is water distributed in the body?

Water is the most abundant component of the human body. On average, 60% of the body is composed of water (this value varies with sex, body habitus and age). Body water is distributed between the two major body compartments: intracellular and extracellular. For the average 70-kg man:

- Total body water is 42 L (60% of 70 kg, where 1 kg of water has a volume of 1 L).
- Approximately two-thirds of body water is intracellular fluid (ICF); that is, 28 L.
- Approximately a third of body water is extracellular fluid (ECF); that is, 14 L. Of the ECF:
    - Approximately a fifth is intravascular fluid; that is, plasma volume is around 3 L.
    - A smaller proportion (around 1 L) is transcellular fluid, such as cerebrospinal fluid, ocular fluid, synovial fluid.
    - The remainder is interstitial fluid (around 10 L), the fluid that occupies the spaces between cells. It is within this fluid that capillaries and cells exchange nutrients and waste products.

How is the volume of water within different body compartments measured?

Body fluid compartments are typically measured using an indicator-dilution method. A known quantity of an indicator substance is administered, allowed to equilibrate across the body compartment of interest and its concentration measured. The key to this method is an understanding of the barriers between body compartments and selection of the correct indicator and its permeability properties, ensuring that it selectively accesses the relevant compartment:

- Calculation of plasma volume requires an indicator that, once infused into the circulation, cannot cross the capillary endothelium, such as radio-labelled albumin.
- Calculation of ECF volume requires an indicator that is able to cross the capillary endothelium but cannot gain access to the ICF by crossing the cells' phospholipid bilayer, such as thiosulphate.
- Calculation of total body water requires an indicator that can distribute across all body fluid compartments. The indicator must be able to cross both the capillary endothelium and the cells' phospholipid bilayer. Deuterated water (^2H_2O) is often used.
- The volumes of the ICF and interstitial fluid compartments cannot be directly measured. Instead, interstitial fluid volume can be calculated from the difference between ECF and plasma volumes. Likewise, ICF volume can be calculated from the difference of total body water and ECF volume.

How is plasma volume regulated?

The maintenance of intravascular volume is a problem familiar to anaesthetists:

- Too low a blood volume results in reduced venous return, reduced cardiac preload and therefore reduced cardiac output, systemic hypotension and organ ischaemia.
- Too high a blood volume is also potentially harmful: excessive preload stretches cardiac myocytes, which may precipitate left ventricular failure, and induces hypertension, which damages organs such as the kidneys, heart and retina.

The body cannot control the volume of ECF by moving water directly between compartments: there are no water pumps in the body. Na^+ is the major cation of the ECF; together with its conjugate anion, Na^+ accounts for over 90% of the body's osmotic activity. ECF volume is therefore regulated by controlling the movement of Na^+ and thus water. Extracellular Na^+ concentration is a balance of:

- **Na^+ intake** – dietary or intravenous;
- **Extra-renal Na^+ loss** – for example, sweating, faeces;
- **Renal Na^+ excretion**.

The kidney is essentially responsible for plasma Na^+ regulation, as it can significantly vary its Na^+ excretion. The kidney therefore regulates plasma volume and thus ECF volume:

- Net renal Na^+ loss = ECF volume reduction;
- Net renal Na^+ gain = ECF volume expansion.

What is osmolarity? How does it differ from molarity?

Osmolarity is a measure of the number of dissolved osmotically active particles per unit *volume* of a solution.

> **Key definitions: osmolarity and molarity**
>
> Osmolarity is defined as the number of osmoles per litre of solution, where osmoles denotes the number of moles of particles that are able to exert an osmotic pressure.
>
> In contrast, molarity is the number of moles of solute dissolved per litre of solution; that is, the concentration.

For example, 1 mol of sodium chloride dissolved in water completely dissociates into Na^+ and Cl^- ions, thereby yielding 2 Osmol of osmotically active particles. In comparison, 1 mol of glucose dissolves in water but cannot dissociate into ions, thus yielding only 1 Osmol of osmotically active particles.

Plasma osmolarity can be estimated at the bedside by summing the concentrations of the most common osmolytes:

> **Key equation: estimated plasma osmolarity**
>
> Plasma osmolarity = $2[Na^+] + 2[K^+] + [glucose] + [urea]$, where [X] (mmol/L) is the concentration of substance X.

In this estimate, the concentrations of Na^+ and K^+ are doubled to account for their conjugate anions (some of which may not be routinely measured in the laboratory).

What is osmolality? How does it differ from osmolarity?

Osmolality is a measure of the number of dissolved osmotically active particles per unit *mass* of a solution. The problem with using osmolarity results from changes in volume of solvent (water) with changes in temperature and with the introduction of solute. As solvent mass does not vary with temperature, osmolality is independent of temperature and the weight of the solute. Osmolality is measured in the laboratory by a method based on the depression of the freezing point of the solution.

> **Key definition: osmolality**
>
> Osmolality is defined as the number of osmoles per kilogram of solvent.

Osmolarity and osmolality are often used interchangeably, as numerically they are similar in normal patients. However, in certain situations, an osmolar gap exists – a difference between the measured osmolality and the calculated osmolarity:

> **Key equation: osmolar gap**
>
> Osmolar gap = osmolality – osmolarity

An osmolar gap indicates the presence of additional unmeasured osmotically active particles in the plasma that are not included in the estimation of osmolarity. Clinically important causes of a high osmolar gap include alcohol intoxication, hypertriglyceridaemia and methanol and ethylene glycol poisoning.

Why is it so important that plasma osmolarity is regulated?

Osmolarity must be tightly regulated, as it alters the fluid tonicity; tonicity refers to the response of intracellular water to the osmolarity of the surrounding ECF:

- If the ECF is isotonic, the cells stay the same size.
- If the ECF is hypertonic, the cells shrink due to the extracellular movement of water by osmosis.
- If the ECF is hypotonic, the cells swell due to the intracellular movement of water by osmosis.

> **Clinical relevance: hypotonicity**
>
> Infusion of sterile water into a peripheral vein acutely lowers the osmolarity of venous blood. The

circulating red blood cells (RBCs) find themselves surrounded by hypotonic solution. Water moves into the RBCs, causing them to swell and potentially haemolyse. An RBC can only accommodate a limited amount of extra water before haemolysis occurs. For this reason, infusions of 5% dextrose are used in place of sterile water:

- 5% dextrose is approximately isotonic (osmolarity of 278 mOsmol/L compared with plasma osmolarity of 285–295 mOsmol/L).
- Once the glucose is metabolised, it is as if free water has been infused, but without the acute drop in osmolarity.

Severe hyponatraemia is usually accompanied by a fall in plasma osmolarity, which results in generalised cell swelling. This is particularly dangerous in the brain, which is confined within the rigid structure of the skull. Cerebral oedema may result in raised intracranial pressure, seizures, altered consciousness and brainstem herniation.

How is plasma osmolarity controlled in the body?

Plasma osmolarity is controlled by means of a feedback loop. Like all feedback loops in the body, there are:

- **Sensors**. Osmoreceptors are located in the organum vasculosum of the lamina terminalis and subfornical organ within the hypothalamus.
- **Control centre**. The hypothalamus interprets the response from the osmoreceptors. Osmoreceptors are extremely sensitive: they can detect as little as a 1% change in plasma osmolarity. The normal set point of plasma osmolarity is 285–295 mOsmol/L.
- **Effectors**. The hypothalamus responds to a rise in plasma osmolarity in two ways:
  - *Stimulating thirst*: oral water intake is increased.
  - *Reducing water excretion by the kidney*: antidiuretic hormone (ADH; also known as arginine-vasopressin) is synthesised by the hypothalamus and transported to the posterior lobe of the pituitary gland through nerve axons, where it is stored in granules. In response to an increase in plasma osmolarity, the hypothalamus signals the posterior lobe of the pituitary to secrete ADH into the systemic

circulation. ADH acts at the collecting ducts of the kidney, increasing the reabsorption of free water and thus reducing plasma osmolarity.

Similarly, if plasma osmolarity were to fall, the hypothalamus reduces the sensation of thirst and inhibits the secretion of ADH, thereby increasing the amount of water excreted by the kidney.

What is the mechanism by which ADH acts at the kidney?

ADH regulates the water permeability of the collecting ducts in the kidney (Figure 69.1):

- Normally, the luminal wall of the collecting ducts is impermeable to water. Therefore, any renal filtrate that passes through the distal convoluted tubule (DCT) and into the collecting duct is destined for excretion as urine.
- ADH binds to V_2 receptors in the collecting ducts, which, through a cyclic AMP second messenger system, results in a water channel (aquaporin 2) being inserted in the luminal walls of the collecting ducts.
- This makes the collecting ducts permeable to water, which flows along an osmotic gradient, from an area of low osmolarity (the filtrate) to an area of high osmolarity (the renal medulla). A reduced volume of water is therefore excreted in the urine.
- The key to this process is the extremely high osmolarity of the renal medulla, generated by the loops of Henle (LOH) and its countercurrent mechanism, and through urea cycling.

How is the high osmolarity of the renal medulla generated?

As discussed in Chapter 67, the LOH is located in the renal medulla, where it connects the proximal convoluted tubule (PCT) to the DCT. It is composed of three functional parts:

- **The thin descending limb**, which is permeable to water but relatively impermeable to ions and urea;
- **The thin ascending limb**, which is permeable to ions and urea, but impermeable to water, potentially leading to a separation of ion and water movement;
- **The thick ascending limb**, which is also impermeable to water, but additionally moves

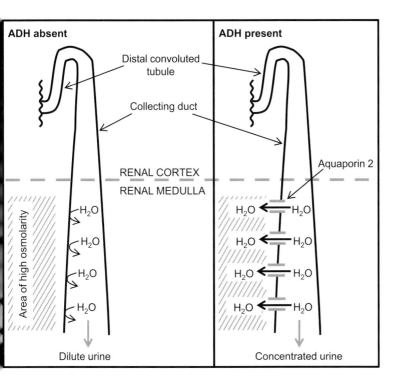

Figure 69.1 H_2O reabsorption at the collecting ducts.

ions via secondary active transport involving luminal $Na^+/K^+/2Cl^-$ co-transporters powered by secondary active transport from the basolateral Na^+/K^+-ATPase.

Figure 69.2 summarises alterations in the renal filtrate as it passes along the LOH:

- In the PCT, water is reabsorbed in conjunction with ions, amino acids and glucose. The osmolarity of the fluid entering the descending limb of the LOH is therefore roughly the same as plasma osmolarity; that is, 300 mOsmol/L (1).
- When the filtrate reaches the thick ascending limb of the LOH, the $Na^+/K^+/2Cl^-$ co-transporter moves Na^+, K^+ and Cl^- from the filtrate to the medullary interstitium (2). As the ascending limbs are impermeable to water:
  - The filtrate entering the DCT becomes hypo-osmolar.
  - The renal medullary interstitium becomes hyper-osmolar.
- Filtrate entering the descending limb of the LOH now passes by the hyper-osmolar medullary interstitium. Because the walls of the descending limb are water permeable, water moves down its osmotic gradient into the medullary interstitium.

As water leaves, the remaining filtrate becomes more concentrated; that is, the osmolarity increases (3).

- Filtrate moves along the LOH, until it reaches the thin ascending limb (4). Here, ions move out of the tubule into the interstitium down a concentration gradient. Ions continue to move into the interstitium in the thick ascending limb, but by secondary active transport (5).
- This countercurrent multiplier mechanism results in a medullary interstitial osmolar gradient, with the tip of the LOH having the highest osmolarity (1200 mOsmol/L) (6).

As the LOH is highly metabolically active, it requires a good blood supply. However, if blood vessels were to simply pass through the renal medulla, they would carry solutes away, washing away the osmotic gradient (Figure 69.3a). To avoid this problem, the LOH has a specialised blood supply. The vasa recta – arteriolar branches of the efferent arterioles – follow the LOH deep into the medulla, descending with the ascending limb of the LOH, turning a hairpin bend and ascending with the descending limb to form a 'countercurrent' flow of blood. The hairpin design of the vasa recta is important in the maintenance of the medullary osmolar gradient (Figure 69.3b):

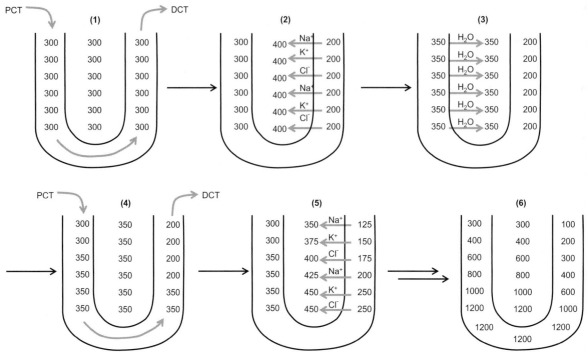

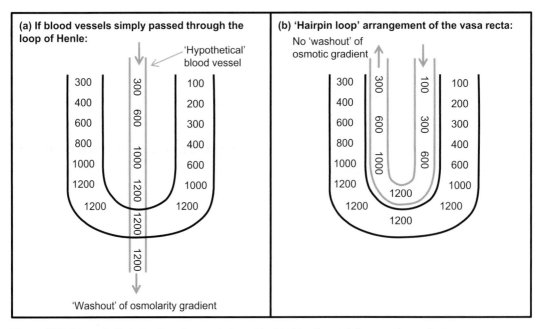

Figure 69.2 Generation of the medullary osmolar gradient.

Figure 69.3 Schematic illustrating how the vasa recta avoids disturbing the medullary osmolar gradient.

- As the vasa recta descend in the medulla, the electrolyte content and osmolarity of their blood equilibrates with that of the surrounding interstitium: ions diffuse into the vessel and water diffuses out.

- As the vasa recta ascend, their contents equilibrate with the surrounding interstitium: water diffuses into the vessel and solutes diffuse out.

- Blood flows sufficiently slowly in the vasa recta to allow near-complete equilibration between the blood and the medullary interstitium. The osmolarity of the blood leaving the vasa recta is near normal (around 320 mOsmol/L). Therefore, the interstitial medullary osmolar gradient is minimally disturbed.

Clinical relevance: clinical disorders of osmolarity

The hypothalamus is crucial to the regulation of plasma osmolarity through its roles in sensing plasma osmolarity and triggering the secretion of ADH. The hypothalamus may malfunction; for example, following a head injury. Two important clinical syndromes are:

- **Central diabetes insipidus** (DI), in which the posterior lobe of the pituitary gland fails to secrete adequate ADH. Without ADH, water cannot be reabsorbed at the collecting ducts. Clinically, DI is characterised by the production of large amounts of excessively dilute urine and signs of hypovolaemia. Biochemically, excessive water excretion leads to hypernatraemia, high plasma osmolarity and an inappropriately low urine osmolarity. Note: nephrogenic DI, which may be caused by lithium therapy, has identical clinical and biochemical features, but a different mechanism: the collecting ducts fail to respond to circulating ADH.
- **Syndrome of inappropriate ADH secretion**. Circulating ADH is in excess of that required to maintain normal plasma osmolarity. Excess ADH may be secreted by the posterior lobe of the pituitary gland or by an ectopic source, such as a small-cell lung carcinoma. Excessive ADH secretion results in additional water reabsorption at the collecting duct. The clinical features are those of hyponatraemia (headache, nausea, confusion, seizures, coma), sometimes associated with fluid overload. Biochemically, in addition to hyponatraemia and low plasma osmolarity, urine osmolarity is inappropriately high.

Urea also makes a significant contribution to the high osmolarity of the medullary interstitium. Urea is produced by the liver as the end product of nitrogen metabolism. It is freely filtered at the glomerulus and then reabsorbed along the tubule. The result is that around 40% of the filtered urea is cleared into the urine. The remaining urea provides around half of the osmolarity of the medullary interstitium.

How does the kidney regulate Na^+ excretion?

As discussed in Chapter 68, the kidney filters 180 L of Na^+-containing plasma per day, significantly more than the total volume of body water. Typical urine output is in the region of 1.5 L/day. Clearly, most of the Na^+ – and therefore water – is reabsorbed by the kidney.

Na^+ excretion is controlled in two ways:

- **Changes in glomerular filtration rate** (GFR). When plasma volume is high, GFR is increased. More Na^+ is then filtered at the glomerulus and delivered to the nephron, resulting in more Na^+ being excreted in the urine. Perhaps more importantly, when plasma volume is low, Na^+ is conserved through a reduced GFR.
- **Changes in Na^+ reabsorption**. This is the main mechanism in operation during euvolaemia. Na^+ is reabsorbed in two phases in the kidney (Figure 69.4):

  - *Bulk reabsorption in the PCT and LOH.* Around 60% of filtered Na^+ is reabsorbed in the PCT, driven by the basolateral Na^+/K^+-ATPase pump. This ion pump keeps the Na^+ concentration within the tubular cells low. Na^+ is reabsorbed from the tubular lumen by a variety of means: passive diffusion, co-transport with molecules such as glucose and counter-transport with H^+ (see Chapter 70). Approximately 30% of filtered Na^+ is reabsorbed in the LOH through the $Na^+/K^+/2Cl^-$ co-transporter (see above).
  - *Reabsorption in the DCT and collecting duct.* Around 90% of the filtered Na^+ has been reabsorbed by the time the filtrate reaches the DCT. The intracellular Na^+ concentration in the DCT and collecting duct cells is kept low as a result of the basolateral Na^+/K^+-ATPase. Na^+ transfer across the tubular cell luminal membrane is controlled by aldosterone through two mechanisms:

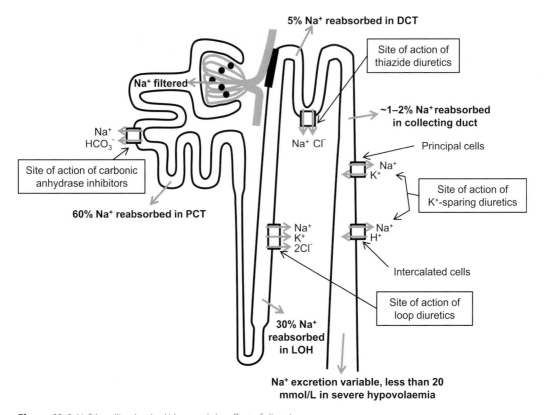

Figure 69.4 Na$^+$ handling by the kidney and the effect of diuretics.

- In the DCT, 5% of filtered Na$^+$ is reabsorbed through an Na$^+$/Cl$^-$ cotransporter in the luminal membrane. Aldosterone controls the number of transmembrane co-transporters.
- In the late DCT and collecting duct, aldosterone acts on two cell types to reabsorb Na$^+$ and water in exchange for the secretion of K$^+$ (principal cells) or H$^+$ (intercalated cells).

Summarise the physiological response to low plasma volume

Low-pressure mechanoreceptors monitor the degree of stretch within the cardiac atria and pulmonary vessels. Hypovolaemia results in reduced venous return and therefore reduced stimulation of the right atrial stretch receptors. Secretion of atrial natriuretic peptide (ANP) and brain natriuretic peptide (BNP) is reduced. Afferent nerve impulses relay information to the medulla oblongata and hypothalamus. In turn, thirst is stimulated and three 'hypovolaemia hormones' are released: noradrenaline, ADH and renin.

- Noradrenaline causes both afferent and efferent arterioles to vasoconstrict, reducing renal blood flow and therefore GFR. Na$^+$ excretion is consequently reduced.
- Renin is released in response to both sympathetic stimulation by the medulla oblongata and the reduced Na$^+$ content of the tubular filtrate, as detected by the juxtaglomerular apparatus. Renin leads to the production of both angiotensin II and aldosterone (see Chapter 68):
  - Angiotensin II acts at the PCT, where it increases Na$^+$ reabsorption, and at the afferent and efferent arterioles, where it causes vasoconstriction, thus reducing GFR.
  - Aldosterone acts on the DCT and collecting ducts, where it increases the reabsorption of Na$^+$ and water and the secretion of K$^+$ and H$^+$.
- ADH increases the permeability of the collecting duct to water, allowing the renal medullary

osmotic gradient to be used for the reabsorption of water.

In combination, these mechanisms result in the conservation of fluid through reductions in renal Na$^+$ excretion. The maximum possible concentration of urine is 1200 mOsmol/L; that is, the osmolarity at the inner renal medulla. The kidney must still excrete osmotically active waste products, accounting for around 600 mOsmol/day. Therefore, the minimum daily urine output is:

$$\frac{600 \text{ mOsmol}}{1200 \text{ mOsmol/L}} = 500 \text{ mL}$$

Around 500 mL/day of fluid is lost through sweating, faeces and respiration; these are termed 'insensible losses'. Therefore, to maintain euvolaemia, a minimum daily intake of 1000 mL water is required.

Clinical relevance: diuretics

A diuretic is a drug that increases the production of urine. Different classes of diuretics act at different sites within the kidney (Figure 69.4). Commonly used classes of diuretic include the following.

- **Osmotic diuretics** (e.g. mannitol) are osmotically active agents freely filtered at the glomerulus and not reabsorbed by the tubules. The increased osmolarity of the filtrate results in less water being reabsorbed, which increases the volume of urine produced.
- **Carbonic anhydrase (CA) inhibitors** (e.g. acetazolamide). CA is an enzyme located in the PCT. It is required for HCO_3^- reabsorption (see Chapter 70). Inhibition of CA increases renal HCO_3^- excretion.
- **Loop diuretics** (e.g. furosemide and bumetanide), which inhibit the Na$^+$/K$^+$/2Cl$^-$ co-transporter in the thick ascending limb of the LOH. Not only are Na$^+$, K$^+$ and Cl$^-$ not reabsorbed, but the countercurrent mechanism that generates the medullary osmolarity gradient is disrupted. Loop diuretics are therefore extremely effective.
- **Thiazide diuretics** (e.g. bendroflumethiazide). Thiazides act by blocking the Na$^+$/Cl$^-$ co-transporter in the early DCT.
- **Potassium-sparing diuretics** (e.g. spironolactone and amiloride). Spironolactone blocks aldosterone receptors in the DCT and collecting duct. It therefore exerts biochemical

effects opposite to those of aldosterone in the form of increased Na$^+$ excretion and reduced H$^+$ and K$^+$ excretion, hence the term 'potassium-sparing'. Amiloride blocks Na$^+$ channels in the DCT and collecting duct. The biochemical effects of amiloride are therefore similar to those of spironolactone.

ADH is involved in the regulation of both osmolarity and plasma volume. Which takes priority?

For absolute control of the volume and consistency of the plasma, osmolarity and volume should be regulated independently. However, the two regulatory mechanisms overlap:

- Even small changes in plasma osmolarity may be catastrophic owing to brain cell swelling in the closed compartment of the cranium. In contrast, small changes in plasma volume are relatively well tolerated owing to the high compliance of the venous circulation, which acts as a blood reservoir.
- The osmoreceptors in the hypothalamus are therefore sensitive to changes in osmolarity as small as 2–3%, whereas volume and baroreceptors require a 7–10% change in blood volume to trigger a response.
- Therefore, it is the osmolarity that is first conserved even if this disturbs the plasma volume; for example, intravenous infusion of hypertonic saline results in the secretion of ADH, which acts to conserve water to correct plasma osmolarity, despite an increase in volume.
- With larger volume losses (>7%), volume regulation takes priority owing to the potential for tissue ischaemia.

Summarise the physiological response to high plasma volume

The stretch receptors of the cardiac atria and pulmonary vessels respond to hypervolaemia by reducing their afferent output to the medulla oblongata. This reduces the release of the three hypovolaemia hormones. As a result, a greater amount of Na$^+$ and water is excreted in the urine. An expansion in plasma volume causes a relative dilution of plasma proteins – plasma oncotic pressure is reduced. This changes Starling's forces at the glomerular capillary, favouring an increase in filtration fraction.

In addition, ANP and BNP are released from the cardiac atria and ventricles, respectively, in response to stretch. ANP and BNP have a number of effects on the kidney, all of which increase Na^+ excretion:

- Afferent arteriolar vasodilatation with efferent arteriolar vasoconstriction. This increases glomerular capillary hydrostatic pressure, thus increasing GFR and Na^+ excretion.
- Relaxation of the glomerular mesangial cells, which increases the surface area for filtration, thus increasing GFR and Na^+ excretion.
- Inhibition of Na^+ channels in the DCT and collecting ducts, which directly inhibits Na^+ reabsorption.
- Inhibition of both renin secretion by the granular cells and aldosterone secretion by the adrenal glands.

How is plasma potassium concentration regulated?

K^+ is predominantly an intracellular ion:

- 98% of total body K^+ is found in the ICF, where the typical K^+ concentration is 150 mmol/L. As the major intracellular ion, K^+ is responsible for intracellular osmotic pressure.
- 2% of total body K^+ is found in the ECF, where normal K^+ concentration is 3.5–5.5 mmol/L.

Maintaining the large K^+ concentration difference between the ICF and ECF is very important, as it is responsible for the resting membrane potential (RMP; see Chapter 51).

Plasma K^+ concentration is a balance between K^+ intake, movement of K^+ between the intra- and extra-cellular spaces and K^+ excretion. The kidney is responsible for overall regulation of K^+ balance, but its mechanisms take time. Instead, rapid changes in plasma K^+ concentration are achieved by the movement of K^+ between the ICF and ECF.

- **K^+ intake.** A typical Western diet contains 70 mmol of K^+ per day (10 times more than is required), nearly all of which is absorbed in the gut. One might therefore expect a surge in plasma K^+ concentration following a meal. This is avoided through an important effect of insulin (released in response to ingested glucose), which stimulates

the activity of the basolateral Na^+/K^+-ATPase, thus increasing cellular K^+ uptake, which keeps the plasma K^+ concentration constant.

- **Movement between intra- and extra-cellular spaces**, through a number of mechanisms:
  - *Insulin* promotes intracellular movement of K^+ by increasing the activity of the Na^+/K^+-ATPase, as discussed above.
  - *Sympathetic stimulation.* α-adrenoceptor activation triggers K^+ release from cells. This mechanism is important in exercising muscle: local hyperkalaemia stimulates glycogenolysis and vasodilatation. $β_2$-adrenoceptor activation causes intracellular uptake of K^+. This is, in part, why hypokalaemia is commonly associated with the acute stress response and with the use of salbutamol.
  - *Extracellular pH.* In metabolic acidosis, much of the additional H^+ is buffered intracellularly. Intracellular acidosis impairs the basolateral Na^+/K^+-ATPase, leading to extracellular leak of K^+ ions, and thus hyperkalaemia (see Chapter 70). In metabolic alkalosis, the opposite occurs.
- **K^+ excretion by the kidney** (Figure 69.5). K^+ is freely filtered at the glomerulus. Almost all of the filtered K^+ is reabsorbed in the PCT (through diffusion) and LOH (through the $Na^+/K^+/2Cl^-$ co-transporter), irrespective of whether body K^+ is high or low. Instead, plasma K^+ is regulated through K^+ secretion in the DCT and collecting ducts:
  - *When plasma K^+ concentration is low*, the kidney tries to conserve as much K^+ as possible. Additional K^+ is reabsorbed in the DCT, probably through the H^+/K^+-ATPase. In total, up to 99% of K^+ is reabsorbed.
  - *When plasma K^+ concentration is high*, the adrenal cortex is directly stimulated to secrete aldosterone. As discussed above, aldosterone acts at the DCT and collecting ducts, where it reabsorbs Na^+ and water whilst secreting K^+ and H^+.

Clinical relevance: management of hyperkalaemia

Significant hyperkalaemia (plasma K^+ concentration >6 mmol/L) affects cells' RMP; membrane depolarisation may cause life-threatening cardiac

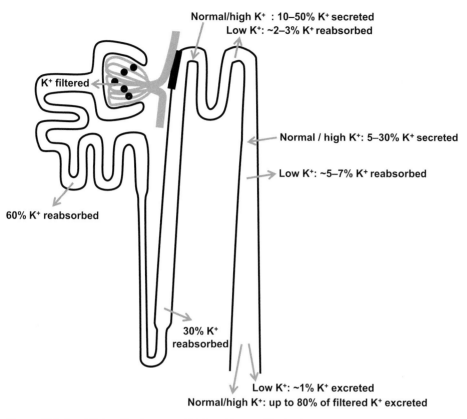

Normal/high K⁺ : 10–50% K⁺ secreted
Low K⁺: ~2–3% K⁺ reabsorbed

K⁺ filtered

Normal / high K⁺: 5–30% K⁺ secreted

Low K⁺: ~5–7% K⁺ reabsorbed

60% K⁺ reabsorbed

30% K⁺ reabsorbed

Low K⁺: ~1% K⁺ excreted
Normal/high K⁺: up to 80% of filtered K⁺ excreted

Figure 69.5 Renal K⁺ handling in states of high and low total body K⁺.

arrhythmias such as ventricular fibrillation. Classical electrocardiogram (ECG) changes include tall, tented T-waves and, later, widened QRS complexes. Hyperkalaemia is frequently the result of acute renal failure or severe metabolic acidosis, but can also be caused by drugs (e.g. spironolactone and suxamethonium), Addison's disease and cellular breakdown (haemolysis and rhabdomyolysis).

The clinical management of hyperkalaemia involves, in part, intracellular movement of plasma K⁺ through manipulation of the mechanisms described above:

- **Ca²⁺** (e.g. 10 mL of 10% calcium chloride solution) is given for cardioprotection; it stabilises the RMP as Ca²⁺ ions bind to the outer surface of the membrane. This creates a local high density of positive charge, leading to a relatively more negative intracellular voltage (see Chapter 51).
- **An insulin/dextrose infusion** reduces plasma K⁺ concentration by increasing cellular K⁺ uptake.
- **Salbutamol** promotes intracellular movement of K⁺ through its β_2-agonist activity.

- **A sodium bicarbonate infusion** may be useful in the context of hyperkalaemia and metabolic acidosis: by increasing the pH of ECF, sequestered intracellular H⁺ moves back into the ECF as K⁺ moves intracellularly.

The latter three management options merely move K⁺ between body compartments; they do not alter total body K⁺. In the longer term, K⁺ may need to be removed from the body. This can be achieved using calcium resonium (an ion-exchange resin) or by renal replacement therapy: haemodialysis or haemofiltration.

Clinical relevance: hypokalaemia

Like hyperkalaemia, significant hypokalaemia (K⁺ < 3 mmol/L) alters the RMP: hyperpolarisation makes the membrane more difficult to depolarise. Patients with hypokalaemia may therefore develop muscular weakness and myalgia; severe hypokalaemia may cause flaccid paralysis and respiratory failure. The classical ECG changes of hypokalaemia are flattened or inverted T-waves, increased PR interval, U-waves and ST-segment depression. The differential diagnosis of hypokalaemia is wide, including low dietary intake, diarrhoea, alkalosis and Conn's syndrome, an aldosterone-secreting tumour. As anaesthetists, we tend to become involved with severe hypokalaemia either because patients have developed severe weakness or because they need central venous replacement of K^+.

K^+ may be replaced enterally or intravenously; rapid replacement by the intravenous route risks ventricular tachyarrhythmias. A safe rate of peripheral venous K^+ replacement is 10 mmol/h, whilst central venous K^+ may be administered at up to 20 mmol/h, with appropriate monitoring. It is worth mentioning that half of patients with significant hypokalaemia also have significant hypomagnesaemia (the mechanisms of loss of both cations are similar). Hypokalaemia is often resistant to treatment in the presence of hypomagnesaemia, as Mg^{2+} is required for the Na^+/K^+-ATPase to function normally. Therefore, both electrolyte disturbances require treatment.

Further reading

M. A. Glasby, C. L.-H. Huang. *Applied Physiology for Surgery and Critical Care*. Oxford, Butterworth-Heinneman, 1995.

D. J. McLean, A. D. Shaw. Intravenous fluids: effects on renal outcomes. *Br J Anaesth* 2018; **120**(2): 397–402.

B. Taylor, D. J. Chambers, N. Patel, et al. Hypokalaemia: the dangers of a sweet tooth. *J Intensive Care Soc* 2012; **13**(4): 342–5.

M. Doherty, D. J. Buggy. Intraoperative fluids: how much is too much? *Br J Anaesth* 2012; **109**(1): 69–79.

J. P. Kokko, F. C. Rector Jr. Countercurrent multiplication system without active transport in inner medulla. *Kidney Int* 1972; **2**(4): 214–23.

Acid–Base Physiology

What is an acid?

The word 'acid' is derived from the Latin *acidus*, meaning sour. Early chemists defined an acid as a chemical substance whose aqueous solution tastes sour, changes the colour of litmus paper to red and reacts with certain metals to produce the flammable gas, hydrogen. Likewise, a base is a chemical substance whose aqueous solution tastes bitter, changes the colour of litmus paper to blue and reacts with acids to produce a salt.

What are the Brønsted–Lowry definitions of an acid and base?

Brønsted and Lowry independently recognised that acid–base reactions in aqueous solution involve the transfer of an H^+ from one molecule to another, and they suggested the following definitions:

- An acid is a proton donor.
- A base is a proton acceptor.

The generic reaction between an acid and base is:

$$HA + B \rightleftharpoons BH^+ + A^-$$

where HA is a Brønsted–Lowry acid (as it donates H^+), B is a Brønsted–Lowry base (as it accepts H^+), BH^+ is referred to as the conjugate acid and A^- is referred to as the conjugate base.

Acids may be classified as being either strong or weak:

- A strong acid is one that completely dissociates in solution.
- A weak acid is one that only partially dissociates in solution.

What is pH?

pH is a measure of the acidity of an aqueous solution. pH is the negative decadic logarithm of the H^+ ion concentration:

Key equation: pH

$$pH = -\log_{10}[H^+]$$

where $\log_{10}$ is the logarithm (base 10) and $[H^+]$ is the molar concentration of H^+ ions.

Note: pH is dimensionless; that is, it has no units.

Because the pH scale is logarithmic, a small change in pH represents a much larger change in $[H^+]$:

- The 'normal' body pH of 7.4 is equivalent to an H^+ concentration of 40 nmol/L.
- Acidaemia is defined as an arterial pH *below* 7.35.
- Alkalaemia is defined as an arterial pH *above* 7.45.
- A small reduction in pH from 7.4 to 7.0 represents more than a doubling of the H^+ concentration, from 40 to 100 nmol/L.

What is K_a?

K_a is the ionisation constant for H^+ from its acid in the equilibrium:

$$HA \underset{k_2}{\overset{k_1}{\rightleftharpoons}} H^+ + A^-$$

where k_1 is the rate constant for the forward reaction and k_2 is the rate constant for the backward reaction.

When the rate of the forward reaction equals the rate of the backward reaction, the reaction is said to be at equilibrium. The equilibrium constant K_a can then be written as:

$$K_a = \frac{k_1}{k_2} = \frac{[H^+][A^-]}{[HA]}$$

What is pK_a?

pK_a is defined as the negative decadic logarithm of the ionisation constant (K_a) of an acid. It equals the pH value at which equal concentrations of the acid and conjugate base forms of a substance are present.

Key equation: pK_a

$$pK_a = -\log_{10} K_a$$

---

pK_a is a measure of the strength of an acid. It is normally used to characterise weak acids.

From the equilibrium equation defining K_a above, it can be seen that:

- A high K_a represents greater dissociation of HA into H^+ and A^- and therefore a greater concentration of free H^+. A low pK_a therefore corresponds to increased acidity.
- A low K_a represents less dissociation of HA, resulting in a lower concentration of free H^+. A high pK_a therefore corresponds to reduced acidity.

Like pH, pK_a is a logarithmic scale. Therefore, a small reduction in pK_a represents a much larger increase in acidity.

The acidity of a substance in solution can be related to the pH in a more formal way. Rearranging the above equation:

$$[H^+] = K_a \frac{[HA]}{[A^-]}$$

As pH = $-\log_{10}[H^+]$:

$$pH = -\log_{10}\left(K_a \frac{[HA]}{[A^-]}\right)$$

Multiplying out the brackets:

$$pH = -\log_{10} K_a - \log_{10}\frac{[HA]}{[A^-]}$$

And as $pK_a = -\log_{10} K_a$:

Key equation: the Henderson–Hasselbalch equation

$$pH = pK_a + \log_{10}\frac{[A^-]}{[HA]}$$

or:

$$pH = pK_a + \log_{10}\frac{[\text{Conjugate base}]}{[\text{Acid}]}$$

Illustrate these principles of acid–base balance in the HCO_3^-/H_2CO_3 buffer system

The most important physiological buffering system is that of CO_2, H_2CO_3 and HCO_3^-, which follows the reaction:

$$CO_2 + H_2O \rightleftharpoons H_2CO_3 \rightleftharpoons H^+ + HCO_3^-$$

H_2CO_3 is the Brønsted–Lowry acid, water is the Brønsted–Lowry base, HCO_3^- is the conjugate base and H_3O^+ is the conjugate acid.

Applying the Henderson–Hasselbalch equation to the HCO_3^-/H_2CO_3 buffer system:

$$pH = pK_a + \log_{10}\frac{[HCO_3^-]}{[H_2CO_3]}$$

As the pK_a of the HCO_3^-/H_2CO_3 equilibrium is 6.1 and $[H_2CO_3]$ can be related to the solubility and partial pressure of CO_2 (P_aCO_2), this equation can be rewritten as:

$$pH = 6.1 + \log_{10}\frac{[HCO_3^-]}{0.23 \times P_aCO_2}$$

where 0.23 is a solubility factor. P_aCO_2 is measured in kilopascals.

Normal plasma pH can therefore be predicted by inserting the 'normal' plasma values of $[HCO_3^-]$ = 24 mmol/L and P_aCO_2 = 5.3 kPa:

$$pH = 6.1 + \log_{10}\frac{24}{0.23 \times 5.3} = 7.4$$

How are disorders of acid–base balance classified?

Acid–base disturbance is traditionally classified by pH disturbance (i.e. acidosis or alkalosis) and by aetiology (i.e. whether it is of respiratory or metabolic origin). Acids of respiratory origin – namely CO_2 – are known as volatile acids, as they may escape as a gas. Acids that are non-volatile (e.g. lactic acid) are known as fixed acids as they may not escape the system.

The four classes of acid–base disorders are:

- **Respiratory acidosis**, in which decreased $\dot{V}_A$ results in pH < 7.35 and P_aCO_2 > 6.0 kPa. Hypoventilation may be due to:

  - *Depression of the respiratory centre*; for example, due to opioids or obesity hypoventilation syndrome;

- *Nerve or muscle disorders*, such as Guillain–Barré syndrome and myasthenia gravis;
- *Chest wall disease*; for example, flail chest;
- *Airway disease*; for example, asthma and chronic obstructive pulmonary disease (COPD);
- *Lung parenchymal disease*; for example, acute respiratory distress syndrome (ARDS).

Of particular relevance to anaesthesia, hypercapnoeic acidosis may also occur due to:

- *Insufficient mechanical ventilation*, which may of course be intentional; for example, permissive hypercapnoea in patients with ARDS;
- *Increased CO_2 production* in malignant hyperpyrexia;
- *Exogenous CO_2 intake*; for example, re-breathing CO_2-containing exhaled gases or insufflation of CO_2 in laparoscopic surgery.

If a respiratory acidosis persists for a period of days, the kidneys increase HCO_3^- reabsorption; this is termed metabolic compensation. Raised plasma HCO_3^- concentration (>26 mmol/L) may be seen in patients with COPD, ARDS and obesity hypoventilation syndrome.

- **Metabolic acidosis**, in which there is an increase in fixed acid, which may be endogenous (e.g. lactic acid) or exogenous (e.g. salicylate). As the increased fixed acid is buffered by HCO_3^-, metabolic acidosis is characterised by low plasma HCO_3^- concentration (<22 mmol/L) and pH < 7.35. Identification of the cause of metabolic acidosis may be aided by the anion gap (see below). The respiratory system responds to a metabolic acidosis by rapidly increasing $\dot{V}_A$, thereby reducing P_aCO_2; this is referred to as respiratory compensation.
- **Respiratory alkalosis**, in which hyperventilation results in hypocapnoea ($P_aCO_2 < 4.7$ kPa) and alkalosis (pH > 7.45). Increased $\dot{V}_A$ may be the result of:

  - *Central causes*; for example, head injury, pain, anxiety, progesterone (in pregnancy) and drugs (such as salicylate overdose).
  - *Hypoxaemia*, in which afferent signals from peripheral chemoreceptors stimulate the respiratory centre. This may occur, for example, at high altitude.

  - *Activation of lung J-receptors*, as occurs in pulmonary embolus and pulmonary oedema.
  - *Excessive mechanical ventilation*.

- **Metabolic alkalosis** – the least common of the main acid–base disorders – in which plasma HCO_3^- exceeds 26 mmol/L in the absence of a primary respiratory acidosis. The more common causes of metabolic alkalosis are:

  - *Gain of exogenous alkali*; for example, an infusion of sodium bicarbonate and massive transfusion, where citrate is metabolised to HCO_3^-;
  - *Loss of endogenous acid*; for example, from the stomach through severe vomiting or nasogastric drainage or from the kidney through the use of diuretics.

What is the base excess?

Acid–base imbalance is often of mixed aetiology. One of the failings of the Henderson–Hasselbalch approach is that, when an acidosis or alkalosis is of mixed metabolic and respiratory origin, it is difficult to quantify each component.

The base excess (BE) is defined as the amount of acid or base that must be added to titrate the blood sample to pH 7.40, when P_aCO_2 has been corrected to 5.3 kPa and the temperature of blood is 37°C. Therefore:

- Blood that is already at pH 7.40 and has a P_aCO_2 of 5.3 kPa will have a BE of 0.
- In metabolic acidosis, BE will be negative.
- In metabolic alkalosis, BE will be positive.
- Normal BE is considered to be –2 to +2 mEq/L.

BE is useful when identifying the cause of a metabolic acidosis. For example, a patient with pneumonia has the following blood gas results: pH 7.2, BE –8 mEq/L and lactate 3 mmol/L. A BE of –8 mEq/L represents a significant metabolic acidosis. As lactate is only 3 mmol/L, there must be another source of acid present to account for the remaining 5 mEq/L. Given the history, this may be the result of acute kidney injury with failed excretion of fixed acids.

What is the anion gap?

The anion gap is the apparent difference between the total concentration of measured cations and the total concentration of measured anions. In practice, only the most common cations and anions are measured by the blood gas machine, giving the formula:

Key equation: anion gap

$$\text{Anion gap} = \text{sum of cation concentrations}$$
$$-\text{sum of anion concentrations}$$
$$= ([Na^+] + [K^+]) - ([Cl^-] + [HCO_3^-])$$

The normal anion gap is 10–20 mEq/L, which represents unmeasured anions such as sulphates, phosphates and plasma proteins. The anion gap is used clinically to identify the cause of a metabolic acidosis. A raised anion-gap metabolic acidosis may be the result of:

- **Increased endogenous anions**; for example:
  - *Lactic acid*, produced during anaerobic metabolism;
  - *Fixed acids*, which accumulate in acute kidney injury;
  - *Ketoacids*, whose production is increased by diabetic ketoacidosis.
- **Increased exogenous anions**; for example:
  - *Salicylate*;
  - *Ethanol*;
  - *Methanol*;
  - *Ethylene glycol*.

A normal anion-gap metabolic acidosis, which occurs much less commonly, may be caused by chronic gastrointestinal HCO_3^- loss or renal tubular acidosis.

Albumin is the major unmeasured anion. Hypo-albuminaemia, which is common in critically ill patients, is therefore associated with a reduced anion gap. It is important to note that a metabolic acidosis may be missed in a hypoalbuminaemic critical care patient, as the anion gap may be normal.

How is body pH regulated?

pH homeostasis is very important, as the effects of acidaemia and alkalaemia on the body are potentially very serious. Body pH is normally[1] maintained between 7.35 and 7.45 through three mechanisms. As acidosis is much more frequently

encountered than alkalosis, these mechanisms are primarily concerned with limiting the harmful effects of acidosis:

- **Buffering**. A buffer is a substance that responds rapidly to oppose the change in pH when an acid or base is added to the plasma, according to Le Chatelier's principle. Buffers are salts of weak acids or bases, and they work by releasing or absorbing H^+ in response to the addition of a stronger base or acid, respectively. Buffer systems can be classified as:
  - *Extracellular buffers*:
    - The H_2CO_3/ HCO_3^- buffer system is the most important extracellular buffer owing to the abundance of HCO_3^- in plasma and to the fact that CO_2 (in equilibrium with H_2CO_3) may be eliminated by the lungs (see below). The pK_a of the H_2CO_3/HCO_3^- system is 6.1; therefore, at pH 7.4, HCO_3^- is a good buffer of acids but not alkalis.
    - Haemoglobin (Hb). The histidine side chains of Hb act as a buffer by binding H^+ ions. Deoxyhaemoglobin is better able to bind H^+ than oxyhaemoglobin (see the Haldane effect, Chapter 9).
  - *Intracellular buffers*:
    - The phosphate buffer system ($H_2PO_4^-$/ HPO_4^{2-}). The concentration of phosphate is low in extracellular fluid, making it a less important buffer. Phosphate is, however, an important buffer of both intracellular fluid and urine, where the phosphate concentration is higher.
    - Proteins. Amino acid side chains can buffer both acids (amine side chains) and alkalis (carboxyl side chains). Whilst plasma proteins play only a minor role in buffering, intracellular proteins are present at higher concentrations, making them important intracellular buffers.

- **Respiratory regulation**. The respiratory system responds within minutes to correct pH disturbances. The P_aCO_2 is inversely related to $\dot{V}_A$ (see Chapter 11). In turn, pH is related to P_aCO_2. Therefore:
  - An increase in $\dot{V}_A$ results in an increase in blood pH.

---

[1] In pregnancy, a mild physiological alkalosis is expected (see Chapter 82).

- A reduction in $\dot{V}_A$ results in a decrease in blood pH.

The respiratory centre responds rapidly to a pH disturbance, increasing or decreasing $\dot{V}_A$ in response to acidaemia or alkalaemia, respectively:

- Metabolic acidosis is sensed by the carotid bodies (see Chapter 22), which stimulate the respiratory centre; $\dot{V}_A$ increases in proportion to the degree of acidosis. The increase in $\dot{V}_A$ is predominantly due to an increase in V_T with little increase in respiratory rate; this breathing pattern is called 'Kussmaul breathing' and is commonly seen in diabetic ketoacidosis.
- Hypercapnoea is sensed by both the peripheral and central chemoreceptors (see Chapter 22), which stimulate an increase in $\dot{V}_A$. Hypercapnoea is a potent stimulus: the combined effects of acidosis and hypercapnoea generate a twofold greater increase in $\dot{V}_A$ than acidosis alone.
- Alkalaemia reduces stimulation of the carotid bodies and thus causes a limited reduction in $\dot{V}_A$. However this compensation is limited, as ventilation must continue to maintain P_AO_2.

- **Renal regulation.** The kidneys correct pH disturbances over a period of days through three mechanisms:

- *Excretion of fixed acids*; for example, phosphoric, sulphuric and keto acids. Renal filtration and excretion constitutes the only means of excreting fixed acids.
- *Controlled reabsorption of filtered HCO_3^-.* HCO_3^- is freely filtered at the glomerulus. Around 80% of filtered HCO_3^- is reabsorbed in the proximal convoluted tubule (PCT), irrespective of changes in plasma pH. The mechanism of reabsorption is as follows (Figure 70.1):

  ▪ HCO_3^- cannot directly cross the apical membrane of the tubules.
  ▪ Instead, H^+ is secreted into the tubular lumen (1), where it combines with HCO_3^-, resulting in CO_2 (2). This reaction is catalysed by the brush border enzyme carbonic anhydrase (CA). H^+ is secreted into the PCT lumen by secondary active transport using an Na^+/H^+-antiporter and the Na^+ gradient generated by the basolateral Na^+/K^+-ATPase.
  ▪ As CO_2 is lipid soluble, it diffuses along its concentration gradient across the apical membrane of the tubule and into the PCT cell (3).

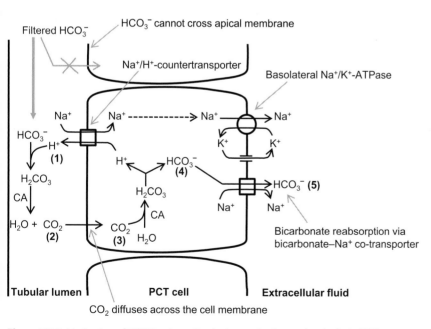

Figure 70.1 Mechanism of HCO_3^- reabsorption in the proximal convoluted tubule (PCT).

- In the PCT cell, the reverse reaction occurs: CA catalyses the reaction between CO_2 and water, producing H^+ and HCO_3^- (4). H^+ is secreted back into the tubular lumen through the Na^+/H^+-antiporter and HCO_3^- moves into the blood through a sodium bicarbonate co-transporter (5). Overall, HCO_3^- is reabsorbed from the renal filtrate.

In the distal convoluted tubule and collecting ducts, the type A intercalated cells and principal cells control the reabsorption of the remaining tubular HCO_3^-. The mechanism for HCO_3^- reabsorption is similar to the PCT, relying on H^+ secretion into the tubular lumen. Under normal conditions, nearly all of the filtered HCO_3^- is reabsorbed. Alkalaemia leads to less HCO_3^- being reabsorbed; more HCO_3^- appears in the urine, resulting in a higher urinary pH.

- *Ammoniagenesis.* In response to acidosis, the liver shifts from turning ammonium (NH_4^+) ions and HCO_3^- into urea to producing glutamine. Glutamine travels in the blood to the cells of the PCT, where NH_4^+ and HCO_3^- are reproduced. NH_4^+ is secreted into the tubular lumen in exchange for Na^+ (again, the process is driven by the basolateral Na^+/K^+-ATPase) and HCO_3^- is moved into the blood in exchange for Cl^-. This generation of HCO_3^- is beneficial in the correction of the acidosis, but the kidney must now excrete the NH_4^+:

  - In the thick ascending limb of the LOH, NH_4^+ is reabsorbed via the $Na^+/K^+/2Cl^-$ transporter (NH_4^+ passes through the K^+ site).
  - In the medullary interstitium, NH_4^+ loses an H^+ to become NH_3.
  - The membrane of the medullary collecting duct is permeable to NH_3; therefore, NH_3 diffuses into the collecting duct.
  - In continued acidosis, H^+ ions are present in high concentration within the tubular fluid and thus bind to NH_3 to reform NH_4^+. The collecting duct membrane is impermeable to NH_4^+ and thus it is excreted.

Overall, one H^+ ion is excreted into the renal filtrate per molecule of glutamine metabolised. The capacity of this system to excrete H^+ is very high, even when the tubular filtrate is already very acidic.

What are the main systemic consequences of acid–base disturbance?

At a molecular level, pH affects:

- **Enzyme function** – outside a narrow range of pH, enzymes may become denatured and their function impaired.
- **The ionisation of molecules** – this may alter their ability to cross cell membranes or affect their shape and function.
- **Ion channel function** – a pH disturbance may alter the permeability of neuronal membrane ion channels, which in turn affects the resting membrane potential (RMP) and action potential.

The clinical effects of acid–base disturbance can be considered system by system:

- **Cardiovascular system.** It is difficult to separate the effects of acidosis from the effects of hypercapnoea on the heart and vasculature. In general:
  - *Sympathetic response.* Hypercapnoea stimulates catecholaminergic release from the adrenal medulla.
  - *Effect on cardiac output.* Acidosis causes direct myocardial depression, manifesting as a decrease in stroke volume. However, in mild acidosis, these effects are offset by catecholaminergic release from the adrenal medulla. Below pH 7.0, the negative inotropy associated with acidosis outweighs the positively inotropic effects of adrenaline. In addition, parasympathetic outflow increases, which counteracts the effects of catecholamines on heart rate, resulting in bradycardia. As a result of these two effects, cardiac output falls.
  - *Cardiac arrhythmias,* including ventricular ectopic beats and atrial fibrillation, are common in acidosis, whether metabolic or respiratory in origin. This is a consequence of increased circulating adrenaline and electrolyte disturbance (see below).

– *Vascular tone.* The effects of acidosis and hypercapnoea on the vasculature is complex: whilst acidosis per se causes arteriolar vasoconstriction, hypercapnoea causes many vascular beds to vasodilate (thus accounting for the bounding pulse found in hypercapnoeic patients), such as in skin and the cerebral arterioles.

Alkalosis increases myocardial contractility by increasing the responsiveness of the myocardium to circulating catecholamines; therefore, myocardial O_2 demand increases. However, alkalosis also reduces myocardial O_2 delivery through vasoconstriction of the coronary circulation and by shifting the oxyhaemoglobin dissociation curve to the left, thus impairing offloading of O_2 to the myocardium.

- **Respiratory system.** As discussed above, the main effect of acidosis on the respiratory system is an increase in alveolar ventilation ($\dot{V}_A$). The respiratory centre in the medulla oblongata is stimulated by the carotid bodies in response to decreased plasma pH and by the central chemoreceptors in response to hypercapnoea (see Chapter 22).

  Additional effects of acid–base disturbance on the respiratory system are:

  – *The oxyhaemoglobin dissociation curve* is shifted to the right by acidosis and to the left by alkalosis (see Chapter 8).
  – *Airway resistance.* The effect of acidosis on airway calibre is complex. Hypercapnoea causes bronchodilatation through a direct effect of CO_2 on the bronchial smooth muscle. But hypercapnoea also triggers an increase in parasympathetic outflow to the bronchi, indirectly causing bronchoconstriction. In otherwise-healthy hypercapnoeic patients, indirect bronchoconstriction outweighs direct bronchodilatation, resulting in an increase in airway resistance and consequently an increase in the work of breathing.

- **Electrolyte changes.** Acidosis is commonly associated with hyperkalaemia, which may precipitate cardiac arrhythmias. Plasma K^+ increases by 0.6 mmol/L for every 0.1-unit decrease in plasma pH. It was previously thought that H^+ underwent intracellular buffering through exchange with intracellular K^+, but it is now thought that acidosis impairs the Na^+/K^+-ATPase, resulting in net leak of K^+ into the extracellular fluid. Despite the high plasma K^+ concentration, total body K^+ stores are frequently depleted. Thus, the treatment of acidosis may result in hypokalaemia if K^+ is not simultaneously replaced.

  Plasma calcium occurs in two forms: biologically active, ionised Ca^{2+} and protein-bound, unionised Ca^{2+} (see Chapter 81). In acidosis, H^+ ions compete for the same binding sites as Ca^{2+} on albumin, displacing Ca^{2+} and thus increasing the fraction of ionised Ca^{2+}. Conversely, alkalosis reduces the fraction of ionised Ca^{2+}. As ionised Ca^{2+} is the biologically active form, alkalosis results in an effective hypocalcaemia. Hypocalcaemia increases the Na^+ permeability of the neuronal cell membrane, making the RMP more unstable. Paraesthesias (spontaneous depolarisation of sensory receptors) and tetany (spontaneous depolarisation of motor neurons) may therefore occur.

- **Central nervous system** (CNS). Whilst H^+ cannot cross the blood–brain barrier owing to its charge, the high lipid solubility of CO_2 allows it to diffuse into the brain. As discussed in Chapter 49, hypercapnoea causes vasodilatation of the cerebral vasculature. Cerebral blood flow (CBF) is therefore directly proportional to P_aCO_2, between the limits of 3.5 and 8.0 kPa. Patients with respiratory acidosis may therefore experience headaches (due to the increased CBF), confusion and impaired consciousness, extensor plantar responses and asterixis (CO_2 flapping tremor).

  Respiratory alkalosis may precipitate seizures. Hypocapnoea induces an alkalosis within the CNS. In a similar way to the peripheral nerves, the RMP of the brain's neurons becomes more unstable, which results in neuronal excitation and spontaneous depolarisation.

- **Bones.** Chronic metabolic acidosis leads to bone decalcification as bone phosphate is mobilised to buffer H^+ ions. In chronic renal failure, this contributes to the development of renal osteodystrophy.

How does pH change with temperature?

Consider the dissociation equilibrium of pure water:

$$H_2O \rightleftharpoons H^+ + OH^-$$

The pH of pure water is temperature dependent: a decrease in temperature shifts the equilibrium to the left, thus reducing the concentration of free H^+, which consequently increases the pH of water.

Likewise, the pH of blood is temperature dependent. Blood pH increases by 0.015 for every 1°C decrease in temperature. In addition, as temperature decreases, the blood solubility of CO_2 increases and therefore P_aCO_2 falls.

Arterial blood gas analysers operate at 37°C. As long as the patient's temperature is near to 37°C, the pH measured by blood gas analysis will roughly correlate with the patient's actual blood pH. However, in a hypothermic patient, the pH measured at 37°C may be significantly lower than the patient's actual blood pH and the measured P_aCO_2 will be higher than the actual P_aCO_2. The pH and P_aCO_2 can be mathematically corrected to determine their actual values at the patient's temperature. For example, a patient whose temperature is 27°C may have blood gas analysis (measured at 37°C) demonstrating normal pH and P_aCO_2; that is, 7.4 and 5.3 kPa, respectively. However, when mathematically corrected to 27°C, these values are significantly different: pH is 7.55 and P_aCO_2 is 3.3 kPa.

Clinical relevance: hypothermic cardiopulmonary bypass

Clinically, the temperature dependence of pH is important in the context of hypothermic cardiopulmonary bypass, when the patient's P_aCO_2 and thus pH are controlled by the perfusionist:

- **The pH-stat method** involves adding CO_2 to blood in the bypass circuit in order that the patient's pH and P_aCO_2 are maintained at nominally normal values when corrected to the patient's body temperature. It has been suggested that this practice counteracts the leftward shift in the oxyhaemoglobin dissociation curve that occurs with hypothermia, thereby improving O_2 delivery. However, increased P_aCO_2 causes cerebral vasodilatation, which in turn increases CBF and abolishes cerebral autoregulation. This increase in CBF may possibly increase the embolic load, thus increasing the

risk of post-operative cognitive dysfunction and stroke.
- **The alpha-stat method** involves permitting the alkaline drift that occurs with hypothermia, instead targeting nominally normal pH and P_aCO_2 when measured at 37°C and accepting that the patient's actual blood pH will be >7.45. This method is thought to maintain cerebral autoregulation and electrochemical neutrality at a cellular level, thus maintaining the function of cellular enzymes.

Despite many studies, it remains unclear whether pH-stat or alpha-stat is the better technique in hypothermic cardiopulmonary bypass and deep hypothermic circulatory arrest.

What is the Stewart approach to acid–base physiology?

The traditional Henderson–Hasselbalch approach outlined above is well established and can easily be applied to most clinical situations. However, the traditional approach often fails to explain the complex acid–base abnormalities that occur in critical care patients.

The Stewart approach was developed in the 1980s. Though academically sound, the new acid–base theory was often considered too complex for routine clinical use. The Stewart approach has recently seen a resurgence of interest amongst intensive care physicians since the publication of simplified versions of the Stewart theory, most notably by Story et al. in 2004 (see Further reading). A full explanation is beyond the scope of this book, but a brief account is given below.

There are three independent variables when considering acid–base balance:

- P_aCO_2, which is determined by the balance of CO_2 production through cellular metabolic processes and CO_2 elimination by alveolar ventilation.
- **Strong ions**, electrolytes such as Na^+, K^+ and Cl^-, which are always fully dissociated from their counterions. In plasma, strong cations outnumber strong anions – the difference is called the strong ion difference.
- **Weak acids**, which are only partially dissociated in solution. Weak acids are mainly plasma proteins, of which albumin is the major contingent.

Key equations: Stewart–Fencl–Story approach

The simplified Stewart model involves two equations:

$$BDE_{NaCl} = [Na^+] - [Cl^-] - 38 \qquad (1)$$

where BDE_{NaCl} (mEq/L) is the base deficit excess for Na^+/Cl^-/free water.

$$BDE_{Alb} = 0.25 \times (42 - [albumin]) \qquad (2)$$

where BDE_{Alb} (mEq/L) is the base deficit excess for albumin (in units of grams per litre).

The BDE_{NaCl} is the Stewart equivalent of BE in Henderson–Hasselbalch theory:

- $BDE_{NaCl} > 0$ implies alkalaemia.
- $BDE_{NaCl} < 0$ implies acidaemia.

The greater the BDE_{NaCl}, the greater the extent of the acid–base disturbance.

As albumin is negatively charged, hypoalbuminaemia causes a metabolic alkalosis, the extent of which is quantified by BDE_{Alb}.

These simple equations agree with the original, complex Stewart equations surprisingly well. Crucially, the Stewart model can be used to explain the complex acid–base disturbances that occur in critical care.

Clinical example: complex acid–base disturbance in a critical care patient

A patient is admitted to intensive care following a laparotomy for bowel perforation. Over the next day, the patient developed severe sepsis. Several days of mechanical ventilation later, arterial blood gas analysis demonstrated: pH 7.45, P_aO_2 12.1 kPa, P_aCO_2 5.0 kPa, HCO_3^- 26 mmol/L, Na^+ 147 mmol/L, Cl^- 115 mmol/L, albumin 12 g/L.

Using the Henderson–Hasselbalch approach, one might think there was no acid–base abnormality: the pH and HCO_3^- are just within the normal range. However, using the Stewart–Fencl–Story approach:

- $BDE_{NaCl} = 147 - 115 - 38 = -6 \text{ mEq/L}.$
- $BDE_{Alb} = 0.25 \times (42 - 12) = 7.5 \text{ mEq/L}.$

This approach demonstrates a concomitant hyperchloraemic metabolic acidosis and an alkalosis due to severe hypoalbuminaemia.

Further reading

T. Post, B. Rose. *Clinical Physiology of Acid–Base and Electrolyte Disorders, 5th edition.* New York, McGraw-Hill, 2001.

K. A. A. Aziz, A. Meduoye. Is pH-stat or alpha-stat the best technique to follow in patients undergoing deep hypothermic circulatory arrest? *Interact Cardiovasc Thorac Surg* 2010; **10**(2): 271–82.

C. G. Morris, J. Low. Metabolic acidosis in the critically ill: part 1. Classification and pathophysiology. *Anaesthesia* 2008; **63**(3): 294–301.

C. G. Morris, J. Low. Metabolic acidosis in the critically ill: part 2. Causes and treatment. *Anaesthesia* 2008; **63**(4): 396–411.

A. Badr, P. Nightingale. An alternative approach to acid–base abnormalities in critically ill patients. *Continuing Educ Anaesth Crit Care Pain* 2007; 7(4): 107–11.

D. A. Story, H. Morimatsu, R. Bellomo. Strong ions, weak acids and base excess: a simplified Fencl–Stewart approach to clinical acid–base disorders. *Br J Anaesth* 2004; **92**(1): 54–60.

Micturition

How is urine stored and excreted from the body?

The bladder is a hollow, muscular organ situated in the pelvis. Its role is the storage and voiding of urine. Urine is produced in the kidneys, enters the bladder through the ureters and exits via the urethra.

Important aspects of lower urinary tract anatomy are:

- **Urothelium** lines the inner wall of the ureters, bladder and urethra, providing a highly impermeable barrier to ion, solute and water flux. This is the same type of epithelium that lines the renal collecting duct and renal pelvis (see Chapter 67).
- **The detrusor muscle** is the smooth muscle of the bladder wall and is arranged in spiral, longitudinal and circular bundles. The detrusor muscle exhibits an unusually high compliance – as the bladder fills, the detrusor muscle relaxes and stretches, resulting in only a small increase in intravesical pressure. This is known as viscoelasticity. The detrusor is innervated by both the sympathetic (via the hypogastric nerve) and parasympathetic (via the pelvic splanchnic nerves) nervous systems and is therefore under involuntary control.
- **The internal urethral sphincter** (IUS) surrounds the urethra at its junction with the bladder. The IUS is an extension of the detrusor smooth muscle and is under control of the sympathetic nervous system.
- **The external urethral sphincter** (EUS) is a portion of striated muscle that surrounds the urethra distal to the internal sphincter (females) or distal to the prostate (males). Because the EUS consists of striated muscle, it is under voluntary control via the pudendal nerve.

What is urinary continence? How is it achieved?

Urinary continence is the ability to store urine without leakage until the bladder can be emptied at an appropriate time. Biomechanically, urine will not leak from the bladder so long as the outlet resistance exceeds intravesical pressure. Overall control of urinary continence is directed by two pontine centres: the storage centre and the micturition centre.

During the storage phase of micturition, the pontine storage centre increases sympathetic nervous system outflow, causing:

- **Relaxation of the detrusor muscle** through stimulation of β_3-adrenoreceptors in the fundus and body of the bladder;
- **Tonic contraction of the IUS** through stimulation of α_1-adrenergic receptors at the bladder neck.

The coordinated relaxation of the bladder and contraction of the IUS allows the bladder to fill without leakage of urine.

What happens to intravesical pressure as the bladder fills?

As the bladder fills and its radius increases, bladder wall tension increases due to the law of LaPlace (see Chapter 20). Bladder wall compliance is relatively high at low urine volumes; above 400 mL capacity, the compliance of the bladder wall decreases substantially. When intravesical pressure rises above 10 cmH$_2$O (around 200 mL stored urine):

- **Stretch receptors in the bladder wall are activated.** Afferent signals are relayed to the lumbar spinal cord via the hypogastric nerve, where two reflexes are triggered:
  - *The micturition reflex* triggers firing of parasympathetic cholinergic neurons (originating from the S2–S4 segments of the spinal cord), resulting in a transient contraction of the detrusor muscle. The micturition reflex is self-regenerative; that is, detrusor contraction results in further bladder wall stretch receptor activation, which triggers further detrusor contraction.

- *The guarding reflex* is a reflex contraction of the EUS during these transient detrusor contractions that prevents urinary leakage.

- **Sensation of bladder fullness**: the afferent signals produced by the stretch receptors are interpreted by higher brain centres as a sensation of bladder fullness. As the bladder fills, the micturition reflex occurs more frequently and the detrusor contracts more powerfully:

  - The first desire to void occurs when the bladder contains around 200 mL of urine.
  - The bladder feels 'uncomfortably full' at around 350–400 mL.
  - When the bladder reaches 700 mL capacity, pain ensues.

- **Involuntary micturition**: once the micturition reflex is powerful enough, it causes reflex opening of the EUS (unless higher centres inhibit this) and micturition (voiding) occurs. This is the situation for babies and infants, before full maturation of the pontine micturition centre has developed.

- **Voluntary micturition**:

  - *If voiding is not desired* or is inconvenient, the frontal cortex instructs the pontine control centres to increase sympathetic outflow and decrease parasympathetic outflow, which relaxes the detrusor and contracts the IUS, preventing leakage of urine. As the micturition reflex becomes more powerful, the pontine control centres also initiate tonic contraction of the EUS to counteract the increasing intravesical pressure. Higher centres can also prevent voiding when the micturition reflex is becoming more powerful by voluntary tonic contraction of the EUS.
  - *When it is convenient to urinate*, abdominal muscles contract to increase the pressure within the bladder, thus stretching the bladder walls. The pontine micturition centre simultaneously triggers a micturition reflex and inhibits the EUS so that urination can occur.

Clinical relevance: spinal cord injury and neurogenic bladder

Sympathetic and parasympathetic nervous system input to the bladder and IUS are essential for urinary continence and complete bladder emptying. In the event of a complete spinal cord injury above the sacral level, these autonomic pathways are disrupted:

- **Acute phase of spinal shock**: in the period of weeks immediately following spinal cord injury, there is flaccid paralysis and loss of reflexes below the level of the injury. The bladder loses both its sympathetic and parasympathetic inputs – the bladder becomes paralysed (atonic) and conscious awareness of a full bladder is lost. In contrast, the activity of the EUS is markedly increased. The result is acute urinary retention, with 'overflow' urinary incontinence occurring when the bladder is very full (high intravesical pressure overcoming bladder outlet resistance). A urinary catheter is used for bladder management to prevent acute kidney injury, which historically was the leading cause of death following acute spinal cord injury.
- **Hyperreflexia and spasticity**: following the period of spinal shock, the patient develops abnormally strong reflexes and spasticity. The detrusor is commonly hyperreflexic, developing powerful reflex contractions in response to bladder wall stretch. The result is that the bladder fills and empties spontaneously, a condition known as automatic bladder. Bladder emptying is often incomplete due to non-sustained detrusor contractions and reflex contraction of the EUS (called detrusor–sphincter dyssynergia), which increases the risk of urinary tract infections.

Clinical relevance: post-operative urinary retention

Post-operative urinary retention (POUR) is the inability to void urine following surgery in the presence of a full bladder, complicating approximately 15% of surgical episodes. While there is no standard definition of POUR, it usually includes:

- **Clinical criteria**, such as the sensation of a full bladder, suprapubic pain and palpable bladder;
- **Evidence of a full bladder**, such as an ultrasound scan estimating a bladder volume of >500 mL or a post-catheterisation residual volume of >500 mL urine.

Risk factors for POUR include:

- **Patient factors**: previous history of lower urinary tract symptoms.
- **Type of surgery**: anorectal and inguinal hernia surgery.

- **Intraoperative intravenous fluid** exceeding 750 mL increases the risk of POUR.
- **Neuraxial blockade**: spinal anaesthesia, particularly if combined with intrathecal opioids, significantly increases the risk of POUR compared to general anaesthesia. This is hardly surprising – during spinal anaesthesia, signals from the autonomic nervous system to the detrusor are abolished, resulting in a situation similar to that following spinal cord injury. The risk of POUR is reduced by using lower-dose or shorter-acting (e.g. prilocaine) intrathecal local anaesthetics.
- **Analgesia**: opioid use increases the risk of POUR by 1.5 times.

Catheterisation, usually when the bladder volume has exceeded 600 mL, is the standard treatment for POUR in order to alleviate patient discomfort and to prevent complications (e.g. kidney injury and urinary tract infection).

Further reading

C. Tai, J. R. Roppolo, W. C. de Groat. Spinal reflex control of micturition after spinal cord injury. *Restor Neurol Neurosci* 2006; **24**(2): 69–78.

G. Baldini, H. Bagry, A. Aprikian, F. Carli. Postoperative urinary retention: anesthetic and perioperative considerations. *Anaesthesiology* 2009; **110**(5): 1139–57.

Chapter

72

Haemostasis

What is haemostasis?

'Haemostasis' is a collective term for the mechanisms that stop blood loss. Macroscopically, the most obvious haemostatic mechanism is the conversion of liquid blood to a solid gel – a process called coagulation. The process of clot formation is known as thrombosis.

Haemostasis can be life-saving: when blood vessels have been damaged, it is important that haemostasis occurs rapidly to prevent excessive blood loss. However, it is equally important that the haemostatic response is controlled and localised to the area of vessel damage. Widespread coagulation could prevent blood flow completely, damage red blood cells (RBCs) through microangiopathic haemolytic anaemia or lead to paradoxical bleeding due to depletion of clotting factors through disseminated intravascular coagulation (DIC). Therefore, the mechanisms that promote and inhibit haemostasis are finely balanced.

The three main components involved in haemostasis are:

- Platelets;
- Endothelium;
- Coagulation proteins.

All three must be intact for haemostasis to be effective.

How does the vascular endothelium prevent haemostasis?

The endothelium is extremely important in the balance between haemostasis and anti-haemostasis. Its normal function is to prevent haemostasis and promote blood flow, but when damaged, it rapidly initiates a haemostatic response. The endothelium prevents haemostasis by:

- **Inhibition of platelet adhesion** through the secretion of nitric oxide (NO) and prostacyclin

(PCI_2). The endothelium also produces the enzyme adenosine diphosphatase, which degrades ADP, an essential compound for platelet activation.

- **Anticoagulant effects** result from two endothelial membrane-bound proteins:
  - *Heparan sulphate*, which has a similar structure to heparin, activates the plasma protein antithrombin III, which in turn inactivates thrombin (also known as factor IIa) and factor Xa.
  - *Thrombomodulin* has two roles: it directly binds thrombin, effectively removing thrombin from the circulation. The thrombin–thrombomodulin complex also activates protein C. Together with a cofactor (protein S), activated protein C is a potent anticoagulant, inactivating factor Va and VIIIa.

- **Fibrinolytic effects** – endothelial cells also secrete the enzyme tissue plasminogen activator (t-PA). This potent enzyme cleaves the proenzyme plasminogen to form plasmin. Plasmin degrades fibrin clots from the endothelial cell surface in a process called fibrinolysis (see p. 348).

Outline the steps involved in haemostasis

Clot formation has three key steps:

- Vasoconstriction;
- Platelet aggregation;
- Coagulation.

When a vessel is disrupted, platelets must aggregate and plug the hole. To prevent the platelet plug being washed away as it is being formed, the vessel first vasoconstricts, resulting in decreased blood flow – this also has the effect of minimising blood loss.

The plasma coagulation proteins then trigger a fibrin mesh to form around the platelet plug, resulting in a stable clot.

How is haemostasis initiated?

When a vessel is damaged, plasma becomes exposed to a number of substances:

- **von Willebrand factor** (vWF). Endothelial cells are the main site of the synthesis and storage of vWF. Normally, a limited amount of vWF is secreted into the vessel lumen, where it binds to factor VIII, protecting the clotting factor from degradation. A damaged vessel releases a large amount of vWF from its endothelial cells; vWF then binds platelets to subendothelial collagen fibres.
- **Collagen fibres**. Vessel damage exposes subendothelial collagen fibres. Platelets bind to collagen (through a bridging vWF molecule) and become activated.
- **Tissue factor** (TF) is expressed by subendothelial cells, such as smooth muscle cells, but not normally by endothelial cells, unless they become damaged. TF activates plasma coagulation proteins (through the extrinsic pathway), culminating in the production of thrombin.

Describe the steps involved in platelet activation and aggregation

Platelets are disc-shaped (hence the name) anuclear cell fragments. They have a short lifespan in the circulation, typically of 7 days. Blood vessel damage exposes TF, collagen and vWF. Passing platelets are activated by collagen and vWF, and also by thrombin itself, produced by TF activation of the coagulation cascade. When platelets are activated, they change shape from disc-like to stellate and release a number of molecules from storage granules (Figure 72.1):

- Serotonin (5-HT);
- Thromboxane A_2;
- ADP;
- Platelet activating factor (PAF);
- vWF;
- Fibrinogen;
- Thrombin;
- Ca^{2+} ions;
- Platelet-derived growth factor (PDGF).

The key steps of platelet aggregation are:

- Serotonin and thromboxane A_2 are potent vasoconstrictors that reduce blood flow at the site of injury.
- Platelets are attracted to the site of injury. Initially, platelets are activated by and bind to subendothelial collagen (via vWF); the exposed collagen becomes coated in a layer of platelets. The next cohort of platelets cannot make contact with collagen. Instead, they are activated by the ADP molecules released from the first cohort of platelets. Binding of ADP causes the platelets to change shape and release more chemicals from storage granules.
- Activated platelets exhibit a glycoprotein Ilb/IIIa receptor on their surface. Fibrinogen and vWF 'glue' platelets together through this receptor (Figure 72.1). More and more platelets become activated and bind to the site of injury, forming a soft platelet plug.
- The soft platelet plug formed is often not enough to achieve haemostasis – the plug must be reinforced to make a strong clot. Conveniently, the strands of fibrinogen that are interwoven in the soft platelet plug are converted to fibrin (a strong insoluble protein) by thrombin, the end point of the coagulation cascade.

Describe the steps of the coagulation cascade

The coagulation cascade is a complex biochemical pathway involving a number of plasma proteins, culminating in the formation of thrombin. The coagulation cascade is an example of a biological amplification system: starting from a small number of activated molecules, the sequential activation of circulating coagulation proteins results in a magnified response.

Classically, the coagulation cascade is initiated by one of two distinct pathways: intrinsic or extrinsic (Figure 72.2). The two pathways converge on a final common pathway, resulting in thrombin formation. These classical pathways explain the mechanism of coagulation *in vitro* and reflect the laboratory clotting screen. However, there are a number of flaws with the classical model that have more recently led to the development of a cell-based coagulation model, which is thought to better reflect the mechanism of *in vivo* coagulation.

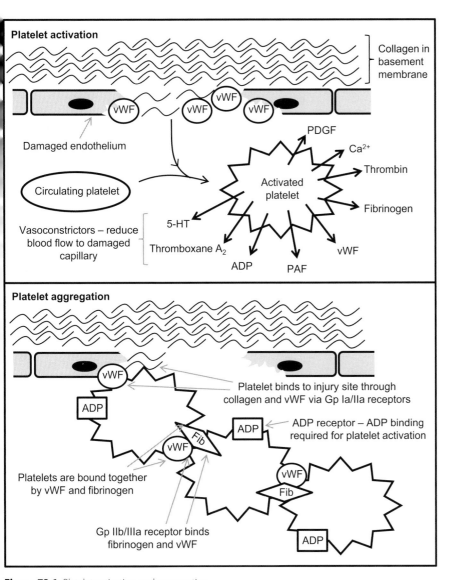

Figure 72.1 Platelet activation and aggregation.

Clinical relevance: antiplatelet drugs

Antiplatelet drugs are commonly prescribed for patients at risk of arterial thrombosis, such as those with myocardial infarction or stroke. Antiplatelet drugs act through different mechanisms, each targeting a different part of the platelet activation and aggregation mechanism:

- **Cyclo-oxygenase (COX) inhibitors**; for example, aspirin. Thromboxane A_2 is a potent platelet activator and vasoconstrictor produced from platelet membrane phospholipid, a process that

is catalysed by the enzyme COX. At the same time, endothelial cells produce PGI_2, a platelet inhibitor also catalysed by COX. The balance between thromboxane A_2 and PGI_2 determines whether a clot is formed. Aspirin is a non-specific, irreversible inhibitor of COX that prevents platelets from producing thromboxane A_2 and endothelial cells from producing PGI_2. However, as platelets contain no nucleus, COX remains inhibited for the entirety of their lifespan (approximately 7 days). Conversely, endothelial

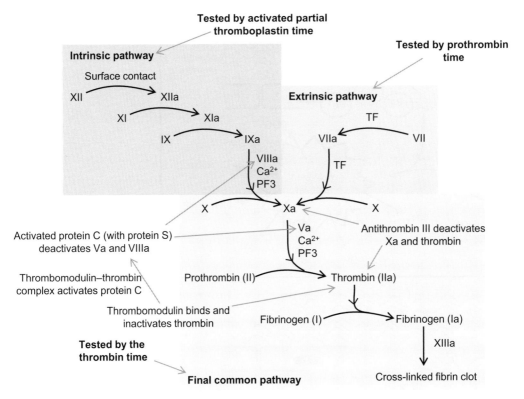

Figure 72.2 The classical coagulation cascade. Roman numerals represent unactivated clotting factors; 'a' denotes activated clotting factors (PF3 = platelet factor 3).

cells may produce new COX within hours. The result is a net increase in platelet inhibition.

- **ADP receptor antagonists**; for example, clopidogrel, ticagrelor and prasugrel. This class of drug specifically blocks the platelet ADP receptor, which prevents further platelet activation and inhibits the expression of the glycoprotein IIb/IIIa complex, thus inhibiting platelet aggregation.
- **Glycoprotein IIb/IIIa inhibitors**; for example, tirofiban and abciximab. Platelet aggregation is inhibited by preventing platelets from binding to fibrinogen.
- **Phosphodiesterase inhibitors**; for example, dipyridamole, which acts through a number of possible mechanisms. One mechanism is the inhibition of the platelet phosphodiesterase enzyme, whose usual role is to break down cyclic AMP (cAMP). Increased platelet cAMP inhibits ADP release, resulting in impaired platelet aggregation and reduced thromboxane A_2 synthesis.

Key features are:
- **Extrinsic pathway**. The extrinsic pathway is so called because it is activated by TF, which is not normally found within the lumen of intact blood vessels. Blood vessel disruption exposes circulating clotting factors to subendothelial TF: any factor VII passing the site of injury is activated to factor VIIa. Factor VIIa activates factor X, the clotting factor at the start of the final common pathway (Figure 72.2).
- **Intrinsic pathway**. The intrinsic pathway is so called because it was recognised that initiation of coagulation did not always require TF, especially *in vitro*; plasma can clot without the addition of any extrinsic material. It has since been found that the intrinsic pathway is activated by contact with negatively charged substances such as subendothelial collagen *in vivo* or glass *in vitro*. The intrinsic pathway involves a number of clotting factors, culminating in the activation of factor X at the start of the final common pathway

(Figure 72.2). Whilst the intrinsic pathway is now thought to have only a minor haemostatic role *in vivo*, an understanding of it remains important for the interpretation of laboratory coagulation studies and the diagnosis of specific clotting factor deficiencies.

- **Final common pathway**. Along with a number of cofactors (factor V, Ca^{2+} and platelet factor 3, PF3), factor Xa (produced by either the intrinsic or extrinsic pathway) converts prothrombin (factor II) to thrombin (factor IIa). Thrombin then acts on the fibrinogen mesh within the platelet plug, hydrolysing the soluble fibrinogen to produce insoluble fibrin strands. In addition, thrombin has other key roles:

  - *Activation of factor XIII*. Factor XIIIa forms covalent crossbridges between fibrin strands in the platelet plug, forming a stable clot.
  - *Generation of a positive-feedback loop*. Thrombin activates factors V and VIII, which feed into the coagulation cascade to produce more thrombin.
  - *Activation of protein C*. Thrombin forms a complex with thrombomodulin (an endothelial cell membrane protein). The plasma glycoprotein protein C is activated by the thrombin–thrombomodulin complex, producing activated protein C. Activated protein C is an important inhibitor of coagulation, as it deactivates factors Va and VIIIa.

Clinical relevance: haemophilia and von Willebrand disease

Haemophilia A is an X-linked autosomal recessive disease that results in a deficiency of factor VIII. Following vessel injury, a soft platelet plug forms, but fibrin cannot be produced to reinforce the platelet plug. As a consequence, patients with haemophilia bleed for a much longer time than patients with normal coagulation. Bleeds into joints may cause permanent disability, and intracerebral bleeds are frequently fatal.

Management is either prophylactic or by treatment of bleeding episodes when they occur: infusions of human or recombinant factor VIII are used in severe haemophilia. Alternatively, patients with mild haemophilia may use desmopressin (DDAVP, a synthetic form of antidiuretic hormone) to boost the body's own production of factor VIII.

von Willebrand disease is the most common hereditary coagulation disorder: patients have either deficient or defective vWF. vWF normally has two roles:

- Forming a bridge between platelets and subendothelial collagen;
- Binding to clotting factor VIII, thus protecting it from degradation.

Therefore, if vWF is reduced or ineffective, both formation of the platelet plug and coagulation are affected. von Willebrand disease has a wide disease spectrum, but fortunately most cases are mild – patients present with nosebleeds, easy bruising and bleeding following dental extraction.

Treatment for mild bleeding is usually unnecessary. Like haemophilia A, DDAVP can be used to boost the body's own factor VIII and vWF production and is commonly used prior to surgery or dental extraction. In severe bleeding, a factor VIII concentrate rich in vWF can be given intravenously.

What is the cell-based model of coagulation?

Whilst the classical coagulation cascade accurately reflects *in vitro* laboratory coagulation tests, it does not adequately explain *in vivo* haemostasis. The cell-based model of coagulation is thought to better represent the *in vivo* mechanism of coagulation (Figure 72.3). Of particular interest, several of the proteins traditionally included in the intrinsic pathway (e.g. factor XII and prekallikrein) have been shown to make little *in vivo* contribution to coagulation and are not included in the cell-based coagulation model:

- **Initiation phase**. Coagulation is triggered by vessel damage, which exposes plasma to TF. The initiation phase of coagulation takes place on a TF-bearing endothelial cell. Any nearby factors V and VII become activated. These activated factors go on to activate other nearby clotting factors. This culminates in the formation of a small amount of thrombin. In addition, passing platelets are activated by TF and vWF and by the small amount of thrombin that has been formed.
- **Amplification phase**. The amplification phase involves the further activation of clotting factors and platelets in preparation for the large-scale generation of thrombin.

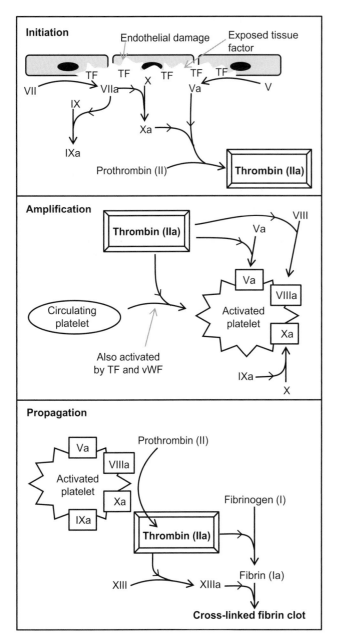

Figure 72.3 Cell-based coagulation model.

- **Propagation phase**. The propagation phase occurs on the surface of an activated platelet loaded with activated clotting factors. With all of its cofactors in place, the activated platelet can catalyse the formation of large amounts of thrombin.

The cell-based coagulation model has thrombin at its centre. Thrombin is involved in its own generation and regulation through feedback loops, as well as the conversion of fibrinogen to a cross-linked fibrin polymer.

What are the main laboratory tests of clotting?

The main laboratory tests of clotting are:

- **Prothrombin time** (PT), a test of the extrinsic pathway. The test involves adding TF to a sample of plasma and measuring the time of clot formation. The international normalised ratio (INR) is the ratio of a patient's PT compared with the average PT of a control sample. PT mainly assesses clotting factor VII of the extrinsic pathway, along with clotting factors II, X and fibrinogen of the final common pathway. PT is prolonged by:

- *Decreased hepatic synthesis* of the vitamin K-dependent clotting factors: II, VII, IX and X. This may be the result of warfarin therapy (vitamin K antagonism), vitamin K deficiency (e.g. fat malabsorption) or liver disease.
- *DIC* due to the consumption of clotting factors.

- **Activated partial thromboplastin time** (APTT), a test of the intrinsic pathway. The test involves adding phospholipid and an activator (e.g. silica) to a plasma sample and measuring the time taken to clot. APTT mainly assesses clotting factors VIII, IX, XI and XII of the intrinsic pathway and clotting factors II, X and fibrinogen of the common pathway. APTT is prolonged by:

- *Unfractionated heparin therapy* through activation of antithrombin III (which inactivates factors Xa and thrombin). Low-molecular-weight heparins are too small to activate antithrombin III effectively, instead inactivating factor Xa directly. APTT is then usually not prolonged.
- *Haemophilia* (factor VIII deficiency), Christmas disease (factor IX deficiency) and von Willebrand disease (vWF deficiency).
- *DIC* due to the consumption of clotting factors.

In addition, there are other less commonly used tests that may be indicated in certain circumstances:

- **Thrombin time** (TT), a test of the final common pathway. Thrombin is added to plasma and the clotting time is measured. TT tests the interaction between thrombin and fibrinogen and is prolonged in fibrinogen deficiency (e.g. due to DIC).
- **Bleeding time**. A standard incision is made and time to stop bleeding is measured; that is, the time it takes for an effective platelet plug to form. Bleeding time is therefore a test of platelet

function. This test is rarely performed, as it does not help to predict surgical bleeding.

Clinical relevance: oral anticoagulants

Oral anticoagulant therapy is most commonly used in the following clinical situations:

- **Atrial fibrillation** to prevent systemic embolisation; for example, ischaemic stroke;
- **Deep vein thrombosis** and pulmonary embolus, including following lower limb arthroplasty;
- **Metallic heart valves** to prevent systemic embolisation.

Until relatively recently, only one oral anticoagulant was in common usage: warfarin. Warfarin is a coumarin derivative that acts by inhibiting vitamin K synthesis and thereby reduces the production of the vitamin K-dependent clotting factors II, VII, IX and X and proteins C and S. Warfarin is 99% protein bound, which means that it can easily be displaced by other highly protein-bound drugs, leading to an increased anticoagulant effect. Warfarin is also metabolised by the liver cytochrome P450 enzymes; variations in anticoagulant effect are due to genetic differences in P450 activity, as well as foods and drugs that are co-metabolised by P450. Warfarin must therefore be closely monitored through blood sampling and testing of the PT (or INR). Despite this, there are a few remaining advantages of warfarin therapy. Its easy reversibility means that, in the event of a life-threatening bleed (e.g. intracranial haematoma), the anticoagulant effects of warfarin can be rapidly reversed by administering vitamin K and a pre-calculated dose of prothrombin complex concentrate. It is also thought to be safer in severe renal impairment. Warfarin is the only oral anticoagulant licenced for metallic heart valves.

Direct oral anticoagulants (DOACs) have become widely used for both short- and long-term anticoagulation. DOACs are preferred because of their favourable pharmacokinetics with fixed dosing, decreased drug–drug interactions and lack of monitoring requirements. DOACs in current use are:

- **Direct thrombin inhibitors**, such as dabigatran;
- **Direct factor Xa inhibitors**, such as rivaroxaban, apixaban and edoxaban.

The downside of DOACs has traditionally been their reversibility in the event of a life-threatening bleed when compared to that of warfarin. DOACs are associated with less intracranial bleeding than is warfarin, although they may have a higher incidence of gastrointestinal bleeding. The anticoagulant effects of

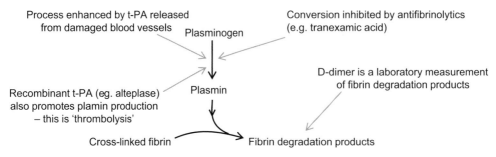

Figure 72.4 Fibrinolysis.

dabigatran may be reversed by haemodialysis and a specific monoclonal antibody, idarucizumab, which is now available for emergency use in most UK hospitals.[1] DOACs are not currently licenced for mechanical heart valves due to a higher incidence of thrombotic events when compared with warfarin.

What is thromboelastography?

Thromboelastography is a near-patient method of testing the whole haemostatic process. It assesses platelet function, coagulation and fibrinolysis in a single test. Not only is thromboelastography quicker to perform than laboratory-based tests, it is also thought to better represent *in vivo* haemostasis.

A sample of whole blood is added to a slowly rotating cuvette – the low-shear environment mimics sluggish venous flow. A plastic pin attached to a torsion wire is lowered into the cuvette. As the blood clots, fibrin strands form between the cuvette and the pin and the torsion of the wire changes. The speed and strength of clot formation are calculated from the change in torsion of the wire, resulting in a cigar-shaped graph.

Gross abnormalities of haemostasis can be quickly assessed from the shape of the thromboelastogram, or a more detailed analysis of haemostasis can be made by analysing various parameters.

What is the fibrinolysis pathway?

Fibrinolysis is a physiological mechanism in which the fibrin within blood clots is slowly dissolved. It is a normal part of wound healing and is an important

mechanism to keep small vessels patent. The fibrinolysis pathway is shown in Figure 72.4.

Key points are:

- Plasminogen is a β-globulin, a proenzyme synthesised by the liver.
- Plasminogen becomes interwoven into the fibrin clot as it is formed.
- Plasminogen is converted to plasmin, a serum protease. The main physiological activator of plasminogen is t-PA, expressed by the endothelial cells: it helps to keep the endothelial cell surface free of fibrin deposits and therefore small vessels patent.
- Fibrin is cleaved by plasmin, producing fibrin degradation products (FDPs). One of these FDPs is called the D-dimer, a cleavage product of cross-linked fibrin. D-dimer concentration is a laboratory test commonly used to aid the diagnosis of venous thromboembolic disease (for example, pulmonary embolus, PE).
- Fibrinolysis is a much slower process than coagulation. The time lag between clot formation and clot dissolution allows healing to take place.

The fibrinolysis pathway can be manipulated as required:

- **Thrombolysis.** In life-threatening thrombosis (e.g. ST-elevation myocardial infarction, acute ischaemic stroke, massive PE), thrombolytic drugs may be used to dissolve the thrombus. These drugs (e.g. alteplase, streptokinase) all promote the conversion of plasminogen to plasmin, thus increasing fibrinolysis.
- **Inhibition of fibrinolysis.** Antifibrinolytic drugs (e.g. tranexamic acid) inhibit the activation of plasminogen. It may be advantageous to inhibit fibrinolysis (e.g. following haemorrhage), thus

---

[1] Andexanet alfa is a reversal agent for rivaroxaban and apixaban that was approved in 2018 by the Food and Drug Administration and will soon enter clinical practice.

promoting haemostasis. Tranexamic acid is commonly used in trauma, orthopaedic, spinal and cardiac surgery and for the treatment of menorrhagia.

Further reading

J. W. Eikelboom, S. Kozek-Langenecker, A. Exadaktylos, et al. Emergency care of patients receiving non-vitamin K antagonist oral anticoagulants. *Br J Anaesth* 2018; **120**(4): 645–56.

J. W. Simmons, M. F. Powell. Acute traumatic coagulopathy: pathophysiology and resuscitation. *Br J Anaesth* 2017; **119**(Suppl. 3): ii31–43.

G. Ramalingam, N. Jones, M. Besser. Platelets for anaesthetists – part 1: physiology and pathology. *BJA Education* 2016; **16**(4): 134–9.

E. Ortmann, M. W. Besser, A. A. Klein. Antifibrinolytic agents in current anaesthetic practice. *Br J Anaesth* 2013; **111**(4): 549–63.

A. N. G. Curry, J. M. T. Pierce. Conventional and nearpatient tests of coagulation. *Continuing Educ Anaesth Crit Care Pain* 2007; **7**(2): 45–50.

B. T. Colvin. Physiology of haemostasis. *Vox Sanguinis* 2004; **87**(Suppl. 1): S43–6.

M. Hoffman. Remodelling the blood coagulation cascade. *J Thromb Thrombolysis* 2003; **16**(1–2): 17–20.

Chapter 73

Transfusion

What are red blood cell antigens?

As discussed in Chapter 8, red blood cells (RBCs) can be thought of as 'bags of haemoglobin' (Hb). However, the composition of the 'bag' itself differs between patients. The RBCs have surface antigens that act as markers, identifying the RBC to the immune system. RBC surface antigens may be polypeptides, polysaccharides or glycoproteins. Which specific antigens are expressed is determined genetically. There are at least 30 different RBC antigen systems, the most important of which are:

- The ABO blood group system;
- The Rhesus (Rh) blood group system.

Minor blood group systems include Kell, MNS, Lewis, P and Duffy.

Describe the ABO system

As well as being the first RBC antigen system discovered, the ABO blood system remains the most important for blood transfusion. The ABO blood groups are carbohydrate-based antigens. All patients' RBCs have a disaccharide 'core' antigen, called the H antigen. Patients then fall into one of four blood groups:

- **Group O.** These patients' RBCs only express the H antigen; 'O' signifies that no other sugars are added.
- **Group A.** An additional carbohydrate group (N-acetylgalactosamine) is bound to the H antigen, making a trisaccharide: the A antigen.
- **Group B.** A different carbohydrate group (D-galactose) is bound to the H antigen, making a different trisaccharide: the B antigen.
- **Group AB.** These patients' RBCs express both A and B antigens.

In the UK, the most common blood groups are O (44%) and A (42%). Group B makes up 10%, while group AB is found in only 4% of patients.

What is the Rh system?

The Rh blood group is the second most important in transfusion medicine. It is named after the Rhesus monkey, the animal whose blood was used in the discovery of the Rh system. There are 50 different Rh antigens discovered to date, of which the most important are: D, C, c, E and e. By far the most important Rh antigen is D – this is the antigen that is present when patients are referred to as being Rhesus positive, Rh factor positive or RhD positive.

The RhD antigen is a large (30-kDa) cell membrane protein that is thought to be a subunit of an ammonia transport protein. As with other blood group systems, the presence or absence of the RhD antigen on a patient's RBCs is genetically determined – around 85% of the UK population are RhD positive.

Why does the immune system develop antibodies to RBC antigens?

The immune system develops antibodies to fragments of foreign material presented by antigen-presenting cells (see Chapter 75). Patients may develop antibodies to non-self RBC antigens for two reasons:

- Exposure to foreign RBCs, such as following a blood transfusion or placental abruption.
- Exposure to environmental antigens (food, bacteria, etc.) that happen to have a chemical structure similar to that of a non-self RBC antigen results in the production of antibodies that also cross-react with non-self RBCs.

The two main blood groups exemplify this:

- **ABO blood group system.** At birth, antibodies to non-self ABO antigens are not present: they appear in the plasma from around 6 months of age. Antibody development is thought to be an immune response to environmental antigens that have a similar chemical structure to the ABO antigens. As a result, antibodies are raised to non-self antigens:

- *Blood group O*: develop anti-A and anti-B antibodies;
- *Blood group A*: develop anti-B antibodies only;
- *Blood group B*: develop anti-A antibodies only;
- *Blood group AB*: do not develop anti-A or anti-B antibodies.

The anti-A and anti-B antibodies produced are immunoglobulin M (IgM). This is important as IgM is unable to cross the placenta – if it could, every foetus of a different ABO blood group to the mother would have its RBCs attacked by the maternal immune system.

- **Rh blood group system.** In contrast to the ABO blood group system, the 15% of the population who are genetically RhD antigen negative do not naturally develop RhD antibodies. Anti-RhD antibodies are only acquired on exposure to foreign RBCs carrying the RhD antigen. Clinically, this may occur due to:

  - *Incompatible blood transfusion.* Transfusion of RhD-positive blood into an RhD-negative patient will trigger anti-RhD antibody production.
  - *Foetal–maternal haemorrhage.* If the blood of an RhD-positive foetus and RhD-negative mother mix (e.g. following childbirth, abortion, trauma or placental abruption), the maternal immune system will be exposed to RhD antigen and will develop anti-RhD antibodies.

Unfortunately, RhD antibodies are usually IgG and are therefore able to cross the placenta.

Clinical relevance: Rh disease

Rh disease affects RhD-negative mothers with RhD-positive offspring. When an RhD-negative mother is exposed to RhD-positive foetal blood (e.g. following trauma), her immune system produces anti-RhD IgG. Maternal anti-RhD IgG is then able to cross the placenta and attack the RBCs of an RhD-positive foetus, either for the same or a subsequent pregnancy. The foetus develops a severe anaemia *in utero* and, if the foetus survives to birth, Rh disease (haemolytic disease of the newborn).

RhD-negative mothers are given anti-RhD immunoglobulin once or twice during pregnancy and at delivery in an attempt to prevent maternal

---

sensitisation to RhD. The parenteral anti-RhD IgG binds any foetal RBCs that pass into the maternal circulation.

What is meant by the terms 'allogenic' and 'autologous' blood transfusion?

Allogenic blood transfusion is where donor blood – usually packed RBCs – is given intravenously to a recipient. In contrast, autologous blood transfusion is where blood is taken from a patient and reinfused back into the same patient when required (e.g. intraoperative cell salvage, preoperative autologous blood donation, acute normovolaemic haemodilution).

What is meant by the term 'haemolytic transfusion reaction'?

Early allogenic blood transfusions were fraught with complications: many patients died after receiving incompatible blood. It was not until the ABO blood group system was discovered that the reasons for these deaths became clear.

A haemolytic transfusion reaction will occur if the recipient's plasma contains antibodies that are reactive against the donor's RBC antigens. The recipient's antibodies coat the donor RBCs: the antibody–antigen complex activates complement, leading to haemolysis of donor RBCs. Haemolytic transfusion reactions are of two types:

- **Immediate haemolytic transfusion reaction.** ABO incompatibility causes rapid intravascular haemolysis, with the severity depending on the antibody titre. Urticaria, flushing, chest pain, dyspnoea, jaundice, tachycardia, shock, haemoglobinuria and disseminated intravascular coagulation may occur. Transfusion of RhD-incompatible blood tends to result in extravascular haemolysis, which is usually less severe than intravascular haemolysis.
- **Delayed haemolytic transfusion reaction.** Minor RhD antigens and the minor blood group systems may cause a delayed haemolytic transfusion reaction, occurring 7–21 days following transfusion. Delayed transfusion reactions are difficult to prevent. Following a prior exposure to a blood antigen, patients develop a low titre of antibody – too low for laboratory detection. When incompatible blood is transfused, a secondary

immune response occurs: it takes time for new IgG antibodies to be produced, leading to a delay before haemolysis is evident.

What is meant by the terms 'universal donor' and 'universal recipient'?

There are two groups of patients of particular importance in transfusion medicine – the universal donor and the universal recipient:

- **The universal donor** is a blood group O, RhD-negative patient. This is because:

  - Group O RBCs only express the core H antigen, so are safe for donation to recipients with anti-A or anti-B antibodies.
  - RhD-negative RBCs are safe to transfuse in recipients with anti-RhD antibodies.

  In an emergency situation where there is insufficient time to establish the blood type of the recipient (e.g. trauma, ruptured aortic aneurysm, obstetric haemorrhage), it is considered safe to transfuse with O negative blood. However, there may still be minor blood group antigen–antibody incompatibility reactions; a full crossmatch is required to ensure blood is fully compatible.

- **The universal recipient** is more of academic than clinical interest. Blood group AB, RhD-positive patients can receive donor blood irrespective of its ABO and Rh status:

  - Their plasma has neither anti-A nor anti-B antibodies, because their RBCs contain both antigens.
  - Similarly, their plasma does not contain anti-RhD antibodies, because their RBCs express the RhD antigen.

  It is important to note that the minor blood group antigens are not necessarily compatible; a crossmatch is still required.

What is a 'crossmatch'?

Crossmatch is a compatibility test between donor and recipient blood. There are two types:

- **Major crossmatch**. The recipient's serum is mixed with donor RBCs – this is a test of compatibility between the recipient's antibodies and donor antigens. If donor RBCs clump together, the blood is incompatible.
- **Minor crossmatch**. The recipient's RBCs are mixed with the donor's plasma. Minor crossmatch

is no longer routinely performed because RBCs are now transfused as packed cells and thus contain an insignificant amount of donor plasma.

How are blood products stored?

The three main blood products are packed RBCs, fresh frozen plasma (FFP) and platelets:

- **Packed RBCs**. Donated whole blood is spun in a centrifuge and the plasma removed. The RBCs are resuspended in the minimum amount of fluid, resulting in a haematocrit of >75%. Citrate, adenine and glucose are added and the mixture stored at 4° C, resulting in a shelf life of 42 days. During storage:

  - Some RBCs become spherical, reducing their lifespan.
  - K^+ concentration rises to 30 mmol/L by 28 days' storage.
  - ATP and 2,3-diphosphoglycerate (2,3-DPG) levels fall. Following transfusion, it takes 24 h for 2,3-DPG concentrations to return to normal. Transfused blood therefore has a higher O_2-binding affinity than native blood and thus O_2 offloading to the tissues is impaired (see Chapter 8). Whether this is clinically significant is a matter of debate.

- **FFP**. As the name suggests, the plasma removed from whole blood during the process of producing packed RBCs is cooled to –30°C within 8 h of donation. FFP has a shelf life of 1 year. FFP is used to replace coagulation factors and should be blood-type matched to ensure compatibility. Other FFP-derived blood products are:

  - *Cryoprecipitate*: FFP is frozen to –70°C then thawed and centrifuged and the precipitate collected. Cryoprecipitate is rich in factors VIII, XIII, fibrinogen and von Willebrand factor and is used in clotting factor deficiencies and hypofibrinogenaemia.
  - *Freeze-dried factor VIII concentrate*, which also contains a small amount of fibrinogen, is used to replace factor VIII in patients with haemophilia A.
  - *Freeze-dried factor IX concentrate*, which also contains a small amount of factors II, VII and X, is used to replace factor IX in patients with factor IX deficiency (Christmas disease).

- **Platelet concentrate**. Platelets are either pooled from the whole blood of multiple donors or collected from one donor by a process called apheresis. Platelet concentrates are ultraviolet irradiated to reduce the risk of transmission of infectious diseases. Platelets are stored at room temperature as they quickly become nonfunctional at 4°C, and so only have a short shelf life (5 days). Platelets can be transfused without crossmatch, but the platelet count rises more if they are ABO-type specific.

What are the other serious complications of blood transfusion?

Complications of transfusion range from mild to fatal reactions. Transfusion complications can be classified as immunological and non-immunological:

- **Immunological complications**. In addition to immediate and delayed haemolytic transfusion reaction, the immune system is responsible for other transfusion complications:

  - *Non-haemolytic febrile reactions*. Recipient antibodies react with antigens on the small number of donor leukocytes contained within donor blood. The antibody–antigen complex activates complement and cytokines are released. Febrile reactions were previously common, but have become much rarer since the introduction of universal leukodepletion. Febrile reactions are usually mild, but it is important to note that fever is also an early symptom of the life-threatening immediate haemolytic transfusion reaction.

  - *Allergic reactions*. Foreign protein in the donor blood cross-reacts with recipient IgE. Allergic reactions are usually mild, causing urticaria and pruritus.

  - *Transfusion-related acute lung injury* (TRALI), the most common cause of death following blood transfusion. TRALI is thought to occur through both immune and non-immune mechanisms. In immune TRALI, antibodies within the donor blood attack the recipient's tissues. Non-immune TRALI is thought to be due to neutrophil activation following release of reactive lipid products from the donor RBC membranes. Whatever the mechanism, TRALI causes a spectrum of lung disease indistinguishable from acute respiratory distress syndrome.

  - *Graft-versus-host disease*. In immunocompromised patients, T-lymphocytes within the donor blood launch an immune response against the recipient's tissues. Following the introduction of universal leukodepletion, this has become a rare but very serious complication of blood transfusion. Certain high-risk immunocompromised patients therefore require irradiated blood.

- **Non-immunological complications**. These are divided into infective and non-infective types:

  - *Septicaemia*. Bacterial contamination of blood products can lead to septicaemia. Platelets are at a particular risk because they are stored at room temperature, which allows bacteria to replicate.

  - *Infectious disease transmission*; for example, hepatitis B, hepatitis C, HIV, cytomegalovirus, malaria and prion disease. Donors are screened for blood-borne infectious diseases both by questionnaire and serology. Rarely, disease transmission may occur in the early stages of an infection when the donor is infectious but has not developed antibodies: serological screening tests are therefore negative. No serological tests for prion disease exist; screening is based on questionnaire alone, but the risk of transmission has been reduced following leukodepletion.

  - *Transfusion-associated circulatory overload* (TACO). Rapid transfusion can lead to left ventricular failure in susceptible patients (those with heart or renal failure, the elderly, those with hypoalbuminaemia). Transfusions in these patients are often accompanied by the administration of furosemide. The resulting dyspnoea may be confused with TRALI.

  - *Iron overload*. The body does not have a disposal mechanism for excess iron; only the absorption of iron is regulated. Haemosiderosis (iron overload) can occur in patients who require frequent blood transfusions, such as those with thalassaemia or sickle cell disease. Excess iron deposits in the liver, heart and endocrine organs, resulting in organ damage.

What is cell salvage?

Cell salvage is a method of autologous blood transfusion: a patient's own blood is collected, processed, stored and retransfused. It is an important method of reducing the requirement for allogenic transfusion, with all its associated risks. Cell salvage is usually performed intraoperatively, where spilt blood is collected from the surgical field. This blood is then processed and returned to the patient. The steps involved in the processing of blood depend on the particular cell salvage equipment – for example, RBCs may be centrifuged, washed and resuspended in saline. Cell salvage has some obvious advantages, but also has some disadvantages:

- **Advantages**:
  - Cell salvage is more cost-effective than autologous transfusion.
  - It does not have the infective and immune risks of autologous transfusion.
  - Cell salvage is accepted by some Jehovah's Witnesses.

- **Disadvantages**:
  - Electrolyte abnormalities may occur, particularly in massive transfusion.
  - Clotting factors are lost when blood is processed; a dilutional coagulopathy may occur.
  - In obstetric haemorrhage, there is a risk of precipitating an amniotic fluid embolus, as amniotic fluid mixed with the salvaged RBCs may not be completely removed by the washing process and subsequently be reinfused. However, cell salvage is now considered safe if used in combination with a leukocyte depletion filter.
  - In cancer surgery, there is a risk that malignant cells suctioned along with spilt blood from the surgical site may not be completely removed by the washing process and be reinfused. Again, a number of studies have shown that the use of a leukocyte depletion filter reduces this risk significantly.

What is massive transfusion? What additional complications occur?

Massive transfusion is the transfusion of a greater volume of stored blood than a patient's circulating volume in a 24-h period or transfusion of more than half a patient's circulating volume in a 4-h period (note: there are many other similar definitions).

Massive transfusion carries all the risks of a single-unit transfusion outlined above, but also has additional risks:

- **Hypothermia**. Transfusion of multiple units of refrigerated packed cells leads to a fall in core body temperature through conduction. Hypothermia is associated with coagulopathy, cardiac arrhythmias, reduced tissue oxygenation (as the oxyhaemoglobin dissociation curve is shifted to the left) and a worse overall outcome. The risk of hypothermia can be reduced by warming all transfused blood and fluids, as well as active warming of the patient; for example, by using a forced-air warmer.

- **Dilutional coagulopathy**. Multiple transfusions of packed RBCs along with crystalloid administration leads to dilution of plasma constituents. Of particular importance are clotting factors and platelets because haemostasis will become impossible, leading to further haemorrhage and a requirement for more blood products. Aggressive and pre-emptive replacement of clotting factors and platelets with FFP, cryoprecipitate and platelet concentrate is required.

- **Hypocalcaemia**. Packed cells contain only a small amount of the anticoagulant citrate; FFP and platelet concentrate contain much higher citrate concentrations. The role of citrate is the chelation of Ca^{2+}, preventing the coagulation of stored blood products. In massive transfusion, there is sufficient intravascular citrate to cause a severe hypocalcaemia. Without Ca^{2+} replacement, this can lead to hypotension and electrocardiogram changes (bradycardia, flat ST segments, prolonged QT interval). Hypocalcaemia should be treated with 10 mL of 10% calcium chloride.

- **Hyperkalaemia**. As discussed above, when RBCs are stored, K^+ seeps out of the erythrocytes. When blood is transfused, K^+ tends to diffuse back into the RBCs, but this process is hindered if the patient is acidotic or hypothermic, leading to hyperkalaemia.

- **Acidosis**. A unit of packed RBCs has a lower pH (around 6.8) than plasma, mainly as a result of lactate accumulation due to the anaerobic metabolism of erythrocytes during storage. Massive transfusion may therefore worsen acidosis, though the additional lactate is usually rapidly cleared by the liver.

Is there any alternative to using blood for oxygen carriage?

There are a number of alternative O_2-carrying solutions (blood substitutes) currently undergoing clinical trials, which can be classified as:

- **Hb-based O_2 carriers.** Pure Hb from RBCs cannot be used as it causes renal tubular damage. Instead, Hb must be cross-linked, polymerised or encapsulated.
- **Perfluorocarbon-based O_2 carriers.** These man-made chemicals are able to dissolve significant quantities of gases, including O_2 and CO_2. However, perfluorocarbons are hydrophobic and therefore must be prepared as an emulsion to mix with blood. They do not have the same complex dissociation kinetics as Hb.

There are some potential advantages to using blood substitutes over human blood:

- Blood transfusion is expensive and associated with a number of immune and non-immune complications (see above).
- Human blood can only be stored for 30 days and must be refrigerated. Blood substitutes have a much greater shelf life and can be stored at ambient temperature, which makes them an attractive prospect in military trauma medicine.
- Alternative O_2-carrying solutions are likely to be acceptable to Jehovah's Witnesses.

Further reading

J. Overfield, M. M. Dawson, D. Hamer. *Transfusion Science, 2nd edition.* Banbury, Scion, 2007.

S. V. Thakrar, B. Clevenger, S. Mallett. Patient blood management and perioperative anaemia. *BJA Education* 2017; **17**(1): 28–34.

A. A. Klein, P. Arnold. R. M. Bingham, et al. AAGBI guidelines: the use of blood components and their alternatives. *Anaesthesia* 2016; **71**(7): 829–42.

D. Orlov, K. Karkouti. The pathophysiology and consequences of red blood cell storage. *Anaesthesia* 2015; **70**(Suppl. 1): 29–37.

J. P. Cata, H. Wang, V. Gottumukkala, et al. Inflammatory response, immunosuppression, and cancer recurrence after perioperative blood transfusions. *Br J Anaesth* 2013; **110**(5): 690–701.

Anaemia and Polycythaemia

What steps are involved in red blood cell production?

Erythropoiesis, the production of red blood cells (RBCs), occurs within the bone marrow. Erythrocytes differentiate through several cell types during their development:

- The starting point is the common pluripotent haemopoietic stem cell. This stem cell differentiates into myeloid progenitor stem cells dedicated to erythropoiesis, first called burst-forming unit erythroid (BFU-E) cells, before becoming colony-forming unit erythroid (CFU-E) cells.
- CFU-E cells then pass through a series of erythroblast phases in the bone marrow. Erythroblasts require both vitamin B_{12} and folate for their DNA synthesis.
- Erythroblasts synthesise haemoglobin (Hb) from the early stages of their maturation. Globin chains are produced in the cytoplasm, whilst the haem moiety, which requires iron, is synthesised in the mitochondria.
- The penultimate cell type is the reticulocyte. By this stage of maturation, the cell has lost its nucleus. However, Hb continues to be synthesised by the residual ribosomal RNA within the cytoplasm.
- At 1–2 days following their release into the circulation, reticulocytes lose their RNA (and therefore their ability to synthesise Hb) and become mature erythrocytes.

Erythropoiesis is controlled by the hormone erythropoietin (EPO). EPO is a glycoprotein secreted mainly by the kidney in response to hypoxaemia.[1] EPO increases erythropoiesis by stimulating the differentiation of BFU-E and CFU-E progenitor cells. A negative-feedback loop is therefore created: hypoxaemia stimulates EPO production, which increases RBC production, which increases O_2-carrying capacity, counteracting the initial hypoxaemia.

Why do patients become anaemic?

Anaemia is defined as an Hb concentration below the expected value when gender, pregnancy and altitude have been taken into account. The World Health Organization defines anaemia as Hb < 130 g/L in men and Hb < 120 g/L in non-pregnant women. The prevalence of anaemia in the surgical population has been found to be as high as 60%.

Anaemia occurs when RBC loss exceeds RBC production. There are many causes of anaemia, which may be classified as follows.

- **Insufficient RBC production.** Examples include:
  - *Iron-deficiency anaemia.* Deficient haem synthesis results in a reduced number of microcytic and hypochromic RBCs.
  - *Folic acid and vitamin B_{12} deficiency.* RBCs produced are megaloblastic.
  - *End-stage renal disease.* Insufficient EPO is produced by the kidneys; RBCs are normocytic.
  - *Anaemia of chronic disease.* This is now thought to result from cytokine-mediated (especially interleukin-6) hepatic synthesis of a protein hormone called hepcidin. Hepcidin blunts the response of the erythropoietic progenitor cells to EPO and reduces the gastrointestinal (GI) absorption of iron (see later).
- **RBC haemolysis.** RBCs are haemolysed either intravascularly or (more commonly) extravascularly within the spleen. Examples include:

---

[1] Note that around 10% of the EPO originates from the liver; this EPO is especially important in end-stage renal failure.

  – *Inherited abnormalities of RBCs*; for example, hereditary spherocytosis. Abnormally shaped RBCs are taken out of circulation by the spleen, reducing their lifespan.

  – *Inherited abnormalities of Hb*; for example, sickle cell disease. The spleen haemolyses sickle-shaped cells, significantly reducing the average RBC lifespan.

  – *RBC enzyme deficiencies*; for example, glucose-6-phosphate dehydrogenase deficiency causes some Hb in the ferrous state (Fe^{2+}) to be oxidised to the ferric state (Fe^{3+}), forming MetHb (see Chapter 8). RBCs containing MetHb are haemolysed by the spleen.

  – *Transfusion reactions*; transfusion of ABO-incompatible blood leads to an antibody-mediated intravascular haemolysis reaction (see Chapter 73).

  – *Autoimmune haemolytic anaemia*; RBCs are haemolysed by autoimmune attack.

  – *Mechanical trauma to RBCs*; for example, cardiopulmonary bypass and valvular dysfunction may result in traumatic haemolysis.

● **Bleeding**. This may be acute (e.g. postpartum haemorrhage) or chronic (e.g. colonic carcinoma, menstruation). In critical care patients, repeated arterial blood sampling is a major contributor to anaemia.

What are the adverse consequences of anaemia?

In itself, mild anaemia has few consequences. However, the disease underlying the anaemia may be very significant, such as colonic carcinoma. Therefore, it is important to investigate and establish the cause of anaemia where possible.

Patients with acute blood loss exhibit the signs of hypovolaemia: tachycardia, hypotension and oliguria. Patients with chronic anaemia develop signs and symptoms dependent on its severity:

● Those with mild anaemia may develop general malaise and dyspnoea on exertion.

● In severe anaemia, reduced O_2-carrying capacity necessitates an increase in cardiac output; patients may experience palpitations.

● Those with pre-existing coronary artery disease or peripheral arterial disease may experience angina or claudication, respectively; high-output heart failure may develop.

> **Clinical relevance: patient blood management**
>
> Perioperative anaemia and blood transfusion are both independent risk factors for poor post-operative outcomes. Patient blood management is a multidisciplinary approach that aims to reduce unnecessary perioperative blood transfusions through:
>
> ● *Preoperative optimisation of red cell mass*: for example, through use of intravenous iron therapy in iron-deficiency anaemia (the most common cause of preoperative anaemia).
>
> ● *The minimisation of intraoperative blood loss*, which may include minimally invasive surgical techniques, the use of topical haemostatic agents, the use of antifibrinolytic drugs (tranexamic acid) and cell salvage. Where blood products are required, these should be guided using thromboelastography.
>
> ● *The management of post-operative anaemia*: the National Institute for Health and Care Excellence (NICE) recommends a transfusion trigger of 70 g/L, or 80 g/L in patients with cardiovascular disease. A 'single-unit' transfusion strategy is recommended in stable patients without active bleeding.

How is iron handled in the body?

Iron is an extremely important element in all living organisms. In humans, iron is primarily involved in:

● **O_2 transport and storage** – Hb and myoglobin.

● **Catalysis of biological reactions** – the cytochrome class of enzymes, catalase and peroxidase all have iron atoms at their active site.

Total body iron is typically 3–5 g. The majority of iron in the body is found within Hb (60–70%), with a further 5–10% incorporated within myoglobin and iron-containing enzymes. The rest (20–30%) is found in the liver, where it is stored as ferritin and its degradation product, haemosiderin. Key features of iron absorption are:

● A typical Western diet contains 15 mg of iron per day, but usually only 1–2 mg of this is absorbed. However, iron absorption can double in pregnancy and iron deficiency.

● There are two forms of dietary iron, both of which are absorbed in the duodenum:

  – *Haem groups* can be directly absorbed by the enterocytes through a haem transport protein. Once inside the enterocytes, iron is released.

  – *Dietary iron salts* are found in both oxidation states: ferrous (Fe^{2+}) and ferric (Fe^{3+}).

Enterocytes can only absorb iron in the ferrous state; this is why iron supplements are ferrous rather than ferric (e.g. ferrous fumarate). Fe^{3+} salts precipitate when the environmental pH is greater than pH 3 (i.e. the duodenum) and therefore cannot be absorbed.

- The low-pH environment of chyme entering the duodenum facilitates the enzymatic reduction of iron from Fe^{3+} to Fe^{2+}, thus allowing duodenal absorption. Drugs that reduce the acidity of the stomach (e.g. proton-pump inhibitors) significantly decrease duodenal ferrous iron, leading to iron deficiency.

How does the body control iron homeostasis?

Iron homeostasis is tightly regulated. Unusually, the body does not have a mechanism for iron excretion, so control of the body's iron content is solely through regulation of iron absorption. This is why iron overload can be a major problem in patients requiring regular blood transfusions.

When body iron stores are low, more iron is transported across the enterocyte basolateral membrane. Conversely, when iron stores are plentiful, iron absorption is inhibited. Traditionally, it was thought that the GI mucosal cells somehow inherently regulated iron absorption; this is 'mucosal block theory'. Recently, our understanding of the iron absorption mechanism has progressed: it is regulated by a liver protein hormone called hepcidin. Hepcidin binds to and inhibits ferroportin, the enterocyte basolateral membrane iron channel:

- **When hepcidin levels are high**, Fe^{2+} cannot be transported out of the enterocyte. Iron is therefore stored within the enterocyte's cytoplasmic ferritin before being excreted from the body as the mucosal cell sloughs.
- **When hepcidin levels are low**, Fe^{2+} is allowed to pass into the circulation through the enterocyte basolateral ferroportin channels.

Once within the plasma, Fe^{2+} is oxidised to Fe^{3+} and bound to the plasma transport protein transferrin. Transferrin transports Fe^{3+} within the circulation to where it is needed, such as the bone marrow. Excess iron is stored by the intracellular protein ferritin.

Conservation of iron within the body is extremely important: iron absorption is as little as 1 mg/day, yet erythropoiesis requires 20 mg of iron per day. At the end of the erythrocyte lifespan, iron is liberated from Hb and carried by transferrin to the bone marrow, where it is recycled.

Hepcidin deficiency is implicated in hereditary haemochromatosis, a genetic condition of iron overload: hepcidin levels are inappropriately low, resulting in an excess of total body iron. Exactly how hepatocytes regulate hepcidin production and what goes wrong in haemochromatosis are not yet established.

What is polycythaemia?

Polycythaemia is a persistently increased ratio of RBCs to plasma (i.e. haematocrit) – above 0.51 in men and 0.48 in women. Polycythaemia is classified as:

- **Primary polycythaemia**, where an abnormality in the bone marrow results in the inappropriate production of an increased number of RBCs. For example, polycythaemia rubra vera (PRV) is a myeloproliferative condition in which the bone marrow undergoes excessive erythropoiesis.
- **Secondary polycythaemia**, where increased erythropoiesis is due to increased EPO secretion. EPO is usually secreted in response to chronic hypoxaemia (e.g. high altitude, smoking, chronic respiratory disease, congenital heart disease), but is occasionally due to an EPO-secreting tumour.

Patients with primary polycythaemia are at greatly increased risk of thrombosis, both arterial and venous. This is due to:

- **Hyperviscosity**. Increased haematocrit results in increased blood viscosity, which, according to the Hagen–Poiseuille equation, increases resistance to blood flow. The resultant reduction in venous blood flow predisposes to venous thrombosis. Cardiac work is also increased.
- **Hypercoagulability**. The coagulation cascade is abnormal in patients with PRV – they are at greater risk of thrombotic disease, even when their haematocrit is normalised by venesection.
- **Thrombocytosis**. Some patients with PRV also have excessive platelet production, increasing their risk of arterial thrombosis.

Patients with secondary polycythaemia also have increased blood viscosity, but seem not to have an increased risk of thrombosis.

Clinical relevance: anaesthesia for patients with PRV

Patients with primary polycythaemia are at increased risk of perioperative arterial and venous thromboses, including stroke, pulmonary embolus, myocardial infarction and hepatic and portal venous thrombosis. Paradoxically, these patients are also at greater risk of haemorrhage as platelet function is often abnormal.

The management of patients with PRV differs for elective and emergency surgery. Before elective surgery, patients' Hb concentration should be reduced to 'normal' levels by phlebotomy or drugs such as hydroxyurea. Prior to urgent surgery, Hb concentration can be normalised by venesection: replacing whole blood with the same volume of crystalloid. The potential for abnormal coagulation and platelet function means that neuraxial blockade is relatively contraindicated.

Further reading

A. V. Hoffbrand, P. A. H. Moss. *Hoffbrand's Essential Haematology, 7th edition*. Hoboken, Wiley-Blackwell, 2015.

S. V. Thakrar, B. Clevenger, S. Mallett. Patient blood management and perioperative anaemia. *BJA Education* 2017; **17**(1): 28–34.

A. Shander, M. Javidroozi, S. Ozawa, et al. What is really dangerous: anaemia or transfusion? *Br J Anaesth* 2011; **107**(Suppl. 1): i47–59.

G. Papanikolaou, K. Pantopoulos. Iron metabolism and toxicity. *Toxicol Appl Pharmacol* 2005; **202**(2): 199–211.

Immune System

What is an antigen? How does an antigen differ from a hapten and an allergen?

An antigen is a substance that stimulates the immune system, resulting in an immune response. Antigens are either proteins or polysaccharides. The immune system produces antibodies that specifically bind to the antigen.

A hapten is a small molecule that may also stimulate the immune system, but only when attached to a larger carrier protein. The immune system produces antibodies to the hapten–carrier complex; these antibodies can also bind to the hapten (when not attached to a carrier protein).

An allergen is an environmental antigen that produces a vigorous immune response, even though the allergen is usually harmless.

What are the differences between the innate and adaptive immune systems?

The role of the immune system is to defend the body against microorganisms, abnormal host cells, toxins and other foreign material. The two main parts of the immune system are the innate and adaptive immune systems.

- **Innate immune system**. Key features are:
  - *Immediate line of defence.*
  - *Rapid but non-specific response* to a potential threat. No previous exposure to an invading microorganism is required.
  - *Composed of several parts*:
    - Anatomical/biochemical – including skin, mucociliary escalator of the respiratory tract, low gastric pH, peristalsis and biliary secretions of the gastrointestinal tract. Lysozyme secretion in saliva and tears

causes bacterial cell wall lysis. Transferrin secretion in mucosa creates a low-iron environment, thus inhibiting bacterial replication.
    - Inflammation.
    - Complement system.
    - Cellular components – neutrophils, macrophages, natural killer (NK) cells, mast cells, basophils and eosinophils.
    - Acute-phase proteins; for example, C-reactive protein, α_1-antitrypsin.

- **Adaptive immune system**. Key features are:
  - *Slower response, but specific* to the invading microorganism. The adaptive immune response is slower than the innate immune system, but has the advantage of 'memory' – a much quicker response occurs if the same microorganism invades for a second time.
  - *Involvement of both cellular and humoral elements*:
    - Cytotoxic T cells are responsible for cell-mediated immunity – defence against intracellular pathogens and abnormal host cells.
    - B cells and T helper cells are responsible for antibody-mediated (humoral) immunity – defence against pathogens within body fluids.

Which cells are involved in the innate immune response?

The innate immune response involves different types of white blood cells (leukocytes):

- **Neutrophils** account for 60% of all leukocytes. They are involved in the phagocytosis (engulfing and ingestion) of bacteria and fungi. A neutrophil can phagocytose around 5–20 bacteria before it dies.

- **Monocytes** migrate from blood into tissues, where they become macrophages. Macrophages phagocytose microorganisms and cellular debris. A macrophage may phagocytose up to 100 bacteria before it dies.
- **Eosinophils** are involved in the killing of multicellular microorganisms, such as helminths and parasites. Eosinophils (along with mast cells) are also important in the pathogenesis of allergic reactions and asthma (serum eosinophil count increases in both conditions).
- **Basophils** are the least common of the leukocytes. Basophils seem to act like circulating mast cells: they have granules that contain inflammatory mediators, including histamine and heparin. Basophils are involved in allergic reactions and defence against parasites.
- **NK cells** are classed as lymphocytes, but in contrast to the other lymphocytes (B and T cells), NK cells are non-specific in their immune function. NK cells are extremely important: they destroy tumour cells and cells infected with viruses. They are also thought to be involved in the suppression of a pregnant mother's immune system to prevent immune attack of the foetus.

What is inflammation?

Inflammation is a non-specific response triggered by either microorganism invasion or tissue injury. First described over 2000 years ago, the symptoms of inflammation are redness, heat, swelling and pain. Inflammation is characterised by the following processes:

- **Vasodilatation**, which increases blood flow to the site of injury/infection, thus explaining the redness and heat associated with inflammation.
- **Increased vascular permeability**, which allows plasma proteins to leak from the vessels to the site of injury/infection. The leak of plasma to the interstitial space accounts for the oedema associated with inflammation.
- **Migration of phagocytes**, which kill invading microorganisms and remove debris in preparation for tissue healing.

Inflammation can be initiated by a number of insults. The mechanisms of initiation are complex and not fully understood. A simplified sequence of events is:

- **Recognition of tissue damage**. The two most common causes of tissue damage are trauma and infection. The body recognises these threats in different ways:
  - *Trauma*. Mechanical damage causes blood vessel disruption and local mast cell degranulation. Blood vessel disruption activates platelets and the coagulation cascade (see Chapter 72), whilst mast cells release histamine and other inflammatory mediators.
  - *Infection*. Tissue macrophages recognise the presence of microorganisms. In addition to phagocytosing the microorganisms, macrophages release proinflammatory cytokines including interleukins-1 and -6, and tumour necrosis factor-α (IL-1, IL-6 and TNF-α, respectively) that trigger local mast cells to degranulate, releasing more proinflammatory cytokines.
- **Local inflammatory response**. Irrespective of the mechanism of initiation, inflammation follows a stereotypical series of events:
  - *Local arterioles vasodilate in response to histamine*. This increases blood flow to the area of injury, thus delivering the necessary quantities of leukocytes and plasma proteins.
  - *Post-capillary venules increase their permeability*. These venules already have very thin walls with little muscle or connective tissue. The vessels swell in response to proinflammatory cytokines, mainly TNF-α and histamine, allowing gaps to develop between endothelial cells. Large volumes of plasma, including large molecules such as complement, coagulation proteins and, later on in the inflammatory process, antibodies, pass into the interstitial space. Complement acts in two main ways (see below): by triggering further degranulation of mast cells and through opsonisation (coating) of microorganisms to facilitate their phagocytosis.
  - *Recruitment of cellular components*. The increased permeability of the post-capillary venules is not in itself a sufficient signal to induce leukocytes to migrate into the interstitial space. Capillaries' endothelial cells need a way of signalling to passing leukocytes, informing them of a pathogen threat. In response to inflammatory mediators, endothelial cells express cell surface adhesion

molecules that slow down circulating neutrophils and macrophages, allowing them to pass between the endothelial cells in a process known as 'transmigration'. The leukocytes are then guided towards the site of injury/infection by attractant molecules called chemotactic molecules.

- **Systemic inflammatory response.** Proinflammatory cytokines are usually concentrated at the site of injury/infection. However, in severe inflammation or in cases where a microorganism escapes from the site of invasion, proinflammatory cytokines are released into the systemic circulation, causing:
  - *Pyrexia* which augments phagocytosis and impairs bacterial multiplication.
  - *Release of neutrophils from the bone marrow.*
  - *Release of acute-phase proteins from the liver*: plasma C-reactive protein concentration correlates with the degree of inflammation.

What are eicosanoids and kinins? How are these involved in inflammation?

- **Eicosanoids** are a family of signalling molecules whose main role is that of a proinflammatory cytokine. Eicosanoids are all derived from arachidonic acid and are subclassified into prostaglandins, prostacyclins, thromboxanes and leukotrienes. One of the enzymes involved in the synthesis of prostaglandins, prostacyclins and thromboxanes is cyclo-oxygenase (COX; also termed prostaglandin-endoperoxide synthase). The COX-1 and COX-2 enzymes are important targets for the clinical management of inflammation.
- **Kinins** are poorly understood. During acute inflammation, bradykinin is produced through cleavage of inactive precursors. Like histamine, bradykinin causes arteriolar vasodilatation and increases the permeability of post-capillary venules. Bradykinin is also implicated in the sensitisation of peripheral pain fibres.

Clinical relevance: systemic inflammatory response syndrome

Following severe tissue damage or infection, inflammation can spiral out of control when proinflammatory

---

cytokines are released into the systemic circulation. Systemic inflammatory response syndrome (SIRS) results from this cytokine storm and is defined by two or more of the following signs:

- Pyrexia $> 38°C$ (or $< 36°C$);
- Heart rate > 90 bpm;
- Respiratory rate > 20 breaths/min;
- White cell count $> 12 \times 10^9$/L or $< 4 \times 10^9$/L.

The same stereotyped processes that usually only occur local to the site of tissue damage now spread to the whole body, resulting in:

- **Generalised vasodilatation and leaky post-capillary venules.** This leads to systemic hypotension and intravascular fluid depletion, respectively.
- **Neutrophil migration** into organs distant to the site of infection/injury.
- **A pro-coagulant state**, resulting in microvascular thrombosis.
- **Myocardial depression**, probably due to delayed Ca^{2+} uptake and release by the sarcoplasmic reticulum.
- **Mitochondrial dysfunction**, resulting in a failure of oxidative phosphorylation.

As many of these complications result in reduced O_2 delivery to the tissues, it is no surprise that patients with SIRS may go on to develop multiple organ dysfunction. Organ dysfunction is usually a combination of macro- and micro-vascular ischaemia. The lung is the most common organ to malfunction in response to systemic inflammation, leading to acute respiratory distress syndrome. Note: SIRS is most commonly triggered by severe infection (especially Gram-negative infection), but is also triggered by non-infective aetiology, such as acute pancreatitis and severe trauma.

What are the roles of complement?

The complement system is a collection of 25 plasma proteins. Although it is considered part of the innate immune system, the complement system also contributes to the adaptive immune system, as it 'complements' the activity of antibodies. The complement system may be activated in two ways:

- **Coming into contact with a particular type of bacterial cell wall** – this is called the alternative pathway.
- **Exposure to an antibody–antigen complex** – this is called the classical pathway.

Once activated, complement has a number of roles:

- **Bacterial cell lysis.** Many activated complement proteins come together to form a 'membrane attack complex'. This complex kills bacteria by punching holes in their cell membranes. Water diffuses along its osmotic gradient through these holes, causing the bacteria to swell and burst.

- **Opsonisation.** Fragments of complement protein coat the microorganisms and then act as binding sites for neutrophils and macrophages, making phagocytosis more efficient.

- **Chemotaxis.** After leukocytes migrate into the tissues from the circulation, bits of complement act as homing beacons, guiding leukocytes towards the site of infection.

- **Triggering local mast cells to degranulate,** releasing vasoactive mediators such as histamine, thus augmenting inflammation.

What is lymphoid tissue? How is the thymus involved in lymphocyte maturation?

Lymphoid tissue is a collective term for tissues that:

- **Produce lymphocytes** – bone marrow;
- **Process lymphocytes** – thymus;
- **Store lymphocytes** – lymph nodes, spleen, tonsils, appendix, gut-associated lymphoid tissue (Peyer's patches).

The bone marrow produces naïve B and T lymphocytes from common lymphoid progenitor stem cells. B cells mature in the bone marrow, whilst T cells leave the bone marrow and migrate to the thymus, where they mature.

The importance of the thymus is obvious when it is absent: DiGeorge syndrome is a genetic disorder that results in a midline congenital defect, which usually includes thymic aplasia. Children born without a thymus suffer from severe immunodeficiency.

The thymus is very important in T-cell maturation as its epithelial cells are able to synthesise and express all of the proteins found elsewhere in the body. Each T cell has a receptor (the T-cell receptor, TCR) whose protein sequence is essentially generated at random. Each TCR is therefore able to bind a different antigen. In the thymus, the T cells undergo processing; any T cell that interacts strongly with a host protein is eliminated through apoptosis. This process results in the death of almost all immature T cells (around 98%). Despite only 2% of immature T cells surviving

to full maturation, there are still an estimated 100 million different T cells, each with a unique TCR.

Like T cells, immature B cells are tested for reactivity against self-antigens in the bone marrow before being released into the circulation. Any B-cell receptor (BCR; which is actually a cell surface-bound antibody molecule) that reacts strongly with self-antigens is prevented from maturing further and is eliminated through apoptosis. All remaining B cells complete their maturation in the bone marrow before being released into the circulation. Once in the circulation, they are taken up by lymphoid tissue, where they are stored.

What are antibodies? How are they produced?

An antibody, exemplified by immunoglobulins (Ig), is a 'Y'-shaped protein produced by the adaptive immune system. Antibodies are produced in response to pathogen invasion and are specific to the invading pathogen; that is, they bind to specific parts of the pathogen. The functions of antibodies are:

- **Opsonisation.** Antibodies label pathogens, making them easier for leukocytes to identify. The F_c region forming the tail of the antibody points away from the pathogen (see below) and acts as a binding site for leukocytes, thus facilitating phagocytosis.

- **Agglutination.** Antibodies all have more than one binding site. Binding more than one pathogen causes pathogens to clump together, making them bigger targets for leukocytes.

- **Inactivation of the pathogen.** The antigenic part of the microorganism may be important to its function; binding of an antibody may render the microorganism harmless. Alternatively, the antibody may bind a toxin produced by the pathogen, making it innocuous.

- **Activation of complement.** As discussed above, when antibodies bind to an antigen (e.g. a microorganism), the complement cascade is activated through the classical pathway. Complement aids phagocytosis through chemotaxis and opsonisation, promotes inflammation through mast cell degranulation and directly attacks the pathogen by forming a membrane attack complex.

When a pathogen invades, the adaptive immune system responds in a well-defined series of steps (Figure 75.1). These result in the mass production of a highly specific antibody:

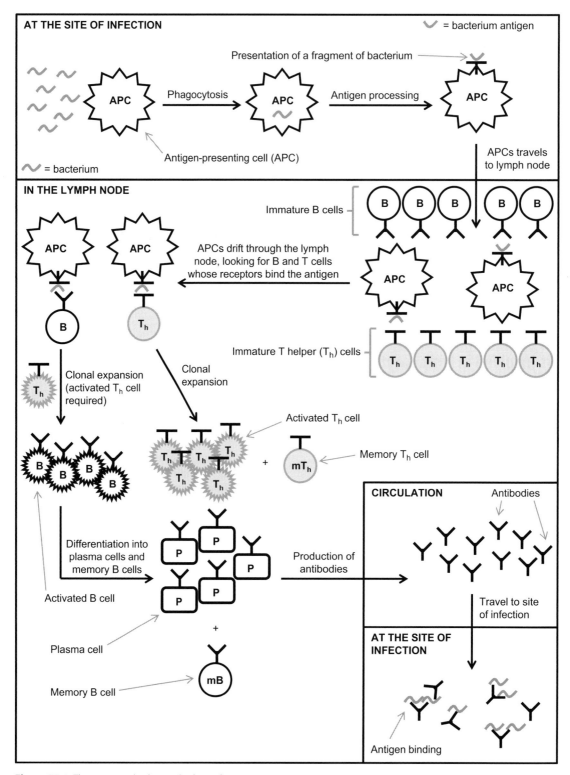

Figure 75.1 The steps involved in antibody production.

- Macrophages and dendritic cells (similar to macrophages) are collectively known as antigen-presenting cells (APCs).
- When APCs phagocytose pathogens, they take small parts of the microorganism (antigens) and express them on their cell surface. The antigens are displayed on the cell membrane by a large protein called major histocompatibility complex (MHC) class II. The APCs then travel from the site of infection to nearby lymphoid tissue, often a lymph node.
- The lymph nodes contain a huge number of B cells and T helper cells, each with uniquely different BCRs and TCRs. The APCs wander through the lymph node, presenting their cell surface antigen to every B and T helper cell that passes. Eventually, the APCs find B and T helper cells whose receptors are an exact match for the APC antigen.
- Antibodies are produced as a result of the interaction of B and T helper cells with APCs (Figure 75.1):
  - *T helper cells* become activated when their TCR matches the APC antigen. Activated T helper cells become blast cells that undergo rapid proliferation, resulting in a clone of identical T helper cells, all with TCRs specific to the same antigen. A small proportion of activated T helper cells become memory T helper cells – these cells lie dormant, ready to be rapidly reactivated if the same pathogen invades again. T helper cells are also called $CD4^+$ T cells, as it is the T cell $CD4^+$ receptor that interacts with the APC MHC class II molecule.
  - *B cells* are also activated when their membrane surface Ig (the BCR) binds to a matching APC antigen, but this activation process (usually) requires help from the corresponding T helper cell. This is effectively a safety mechanism built into the design of the immune system – in order for a B cell to become activated, the APC antigen must make two exact matches: one with a T helper cell and one with a B cell. Activated B cells then rapidly divide to produce a clone of daughter cells, all with identical membrane-bound Ig. The daughter B cells differentiate into either plasma cells (the majority) or memory cells.

  - *Plasma cells* are antibody production factories. The rate of antibody production is astonishing: each plasma cell can produce 2000 antibody molecules per second. They are so committed to antibody synthesis that they do so to the detriment of protein synthesis for normal cellular function and thus only survive for around a week.
  - *Memory cells* are dormant plasma cells that are ready to be reactivated if the same pathogen were to invade again.

What is the difference between the primary and secondary immune response?

The steps outlined above constitute the primary immune response. The whole process from pathogen invasion to antibody production takes around 5 days. The main Ig produced by the plasma cells is IgM, with some IgG produced later. Most of the plasma cells and T helper cells die within the next 5 days, after the pathogen has been destroyed.

If the same pathogen were to invade again, the immune response would be much faster and more vigorous; this is the secondary immune response. APCs transport antigen to the lymph nodes as before, but this time memory T helper cells and memory B cells formed during the clonal expansions of the primary immune response are activated. These memory cells are primed to divide rapidly and can produce antibodies within hours of infection. In contrast to the primary immune response, IgG is the main Ig produced by the secondary immune response, with IgM making up the minority. The secondary immune response is so rapid that pathogens can be killed before they make the host ill – this is called active immunity, where a person is immune from a particular infection as a result of a previous exposure.

What is the difference between active and passive immunisation?

Immunisation is the process whereby a person is made immune or resistant to an infectious disease:

- **Active immunisation**. An inactive portion of a virus or bacterium is given to the patient, usually through injection (vaccination). The patient's immune system produces antibodies to the antigen, during which memory B and T helper cells are produced. If the individual were subsequently exposed to the active pathogen, a rapid secondary immune response would occur, making the pathogen effectively harmless. Active immunisation requires the patient to be immunocompetent; that is, able to mount an immune response to the vaccine.

- **Passive immunity**. Preformed antibodies are given to a patient. Two important uses of passive immunisation are:

  - *Physiological*. Antibodies (IgG) are transferred across the placenta from mother to foetus in order to protect the foetus from pathogens at a time when its immune system is immature and unable to mount an immune response. After birth, antibodies (IgA) are also transferred to the infant through breast milk.

  - *Clinical*. Recombinant antibodies can be given parenterally to a patient to neutralise a pathogen or toxin. Examples include varicella zoster Ig, which is given to at-risk pregnant patients to prevent foetal infection, and tetanus Ig, which is given to neutralise the tetanus toxin in severe tetanus infection.

What is cell-mediated immunity? How are T cells involved?

Some pathogens, particularly some viruses, parasites, yeasts and certain bacteria (e.g. *Mycobacterium tuberculosis*), hide in the body's own cells, where they grow, manipulate the cells' protein synthesis and replicate.

All of the body's cells are programmed to take samples of intracellular protein, process them and display them on the cell membrane. These small portions of intracellular proteins are displayed on the cell membrane MHC class I molecules. When the host cell is infected, this intracellular protein sampling continues; foreign protein is amongst the protein displayed on the cell membrane. Cytotoxic T cells patrol the body, checking that none of the body's cells display foreign material. Cytotoxic T cells are also known as CD8$^+$ T cells, as it is the T-cell CD8$^+$ receptor that interacts with the MHC class I molecule. As discussed above, during their development, cytotoxic T cells are only allowed to leave the thymus if their TCR does not bind to any proteins normally found in host cells.

Therefore, any host cell that displays a protein that binds to the cytotoxic T cell's receptor is likely to be infected. When this happens, the cytotoxic T cell becomes activated (Figure 75.2):

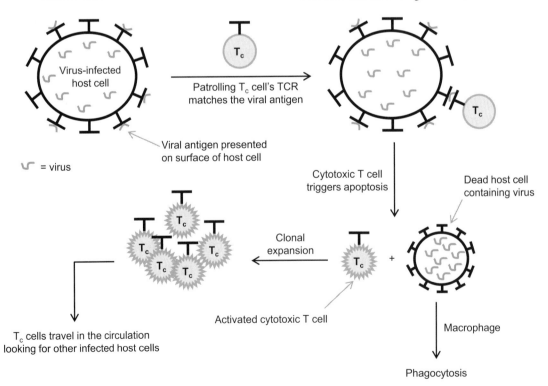

Figure 75.2 Cell-mediated immunity (T_C = cytotoxic T cell).

- The cytotoxic T cell induces apoptosis in the host cell. The pathogen remains within the cell as it undergoes apoptosis. Tissue macrophages then ingest the dead host cell, killing the intracellular pathogen.
- The cytotoxic T cell rapidly divides, producing a large number of clonal daughter cells, each with an identical TCR. These daughter cells travel in the circulation, looking for other infected cells.

This is known as cell-mediated immunity, an immune response that does not involve antibodies or complement. Importantly, it is not just intracellular infections that result in foreign protein being displayed on the cell membrane. Malignant cells also display abnormal proteins on their cell membranes. Cytotoxic T cells are involved in inducing the apoptosis of these abnormal host cells.

What is the basic structure of immunoglobulin? What are the different types?

An antibody is a large 'Y'-shaped protein consisting of two identical heavy chains and two identical light chains, linked by disulphide bridges (Figure 75.3). Antibodies have two regions:

- **The variable region,** F_{ab} – the area that recognises and binds antigen. Every antibody has a different F_{ab}.
- **The constant region,** F_c – the area that binds to other parts of the immune system, such as phagocytes and complement. Each different type of Ig (i.e. IgG, IgM, etc.) has an identical F_c.

There are five types of Ig – all types of Ig contain the same basic 'Y' structure, but some aggregate into polymers:

- **IgM** is the largest Ig, consisting of an aggregate of five 'Y' Ig subunits. This is the first type of antibody produced in the primary immune response and is particularly good at binding large antigens.
- **IgG** is most abundant Ig. IgG is composed of a single 'Y' Ig and is the only Ig that can cross the placenta.
- **IgA** is a dimer of 'Y' Ig. It is found in the mucosa (respiratory tract, gut, etc.), saliva, tears and breast milk.
- **IgE** is a monomer Ig found on the surface of mast cells. When an antigen binds to IgE, the mast cell

is triggered to degranulate. This is the mechanism of type 1 hypersensitivity (see below). IgE is normally present in the plasma in low concentration, but this may be increased with atopy (e.g. in asthma), parasitic infections and hypersensitivity reactions.
- **IgD** is a monomer Ig, usually attached alongside IgM to the cell membrane of naïve B cells (cells not yet activated by antigen). The physiological purpose of IgD is a bit of a mystery – IgD disappears once the B cell is activated, when it becomes entirely covered with IgM.

How can immunodeficiency be classified?

Immunodeficiency is a disorder in which the immune system is impaired or absent. The complications of immunodeficiency depend on which component of the immune system is affected, but generally include opportunistic infection and an increased incidence of certain malignancies. Immunodeficiency may be classified as:

- **Primary immunodeficiency** due to a defect of immune system development. Various parts of the immune system may be dysfunctional:
  - *T-cell dysfunction*: for example, DiGeorge syndrome, in which thymic aplasia results in failure of T-cell maturation, as described above;
  - *Combined B- and T-cell dysfunction*: for example, severe combined immunodeficiency;
  - *B-cell dysfunction*: for example, X-linked agammaglobulinaemia, in which genetically defective B cells fail to synthesise antibodies;
  - *Complement deficiency*: in which the absence of single complement proteins leads to infection or an autoimmune disease.
- **Secondary immunodeficiency.** Causes include:
  - *Iatrogenic*: most commonly due to steroids, chemotherapy agents, radiotherapy and specific immunosuppressive drugs to prevent transplant rejection;
  - *Ageing and malnutrition*: which is associated with a general reduction in immune function;
  - *Specific diseases*: cancer (especially those affecting the immune cells; e.g. leukaemia and myeloma) and acquired immunodeficiency syndrome (AIDS).

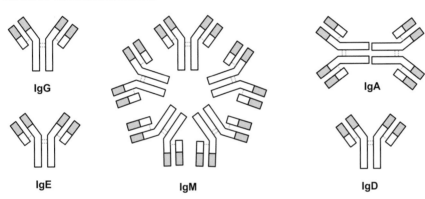

Figure 75.3 Structure and types of immunoglobulin.

TYPES OF IMMUNOGLOBULIN:

IgG

IgE

IgM

IgA

IgD

What is hypersensitivity? What types are there?

Hypersensitivity is an exaggerated or inappropriate immune response that causes discomfort, tissue damage or even death. Hypersensitivity is classified as:

- **Type I or immediate hypersensitivity**. This occurs in asthma, allergic rhinitis (hay fever) and the feared anaphylaxis. This is an allergic reaction that occurs following re-exposure to an allergen. On first exposure to the allergen, T helper and B cells interact as usual, producing IgE specific to the allergen. IgE travels in the circulation and coats the surface of mast cells. On subsequent exposure, the allergen binds to the specific IgE on mast cells, causing rapid degranulation and release of inflammatory mediators: histamine, leukotrienes and prostaglandins. The clinical

effects depend on the location of the mast cells and the route of entry of the allergen:

- *Asthma*: inhaled allergens bind to mast cell IgE within the bronchial smooth muscle, causing degranulation. Release of histamine and leukotrienes triggers bronchospasm.
- *Allergic rhinitis*: allergens (e.g. grass pollen) bind to mast cell IgE in the mucosa of the nasopharynx. Mast cell degranulation releases histamine, causing itchy eyes and inflammation of nasal mucosa with an increased secretion of mucus.
- *Anaphylaxis*: allergens that reach the systemic circulation cause widespread mast cell degranulation, resulting in a potentially life-threatening vasodilatation, bronchospasm and fluid extravasation. Anaphylaxis is especially

severe when the allergen is injected directly into the circulation, which is why it occurs most commonly in association with anaesthesia.

- **Type II or cytotoxic hypersensitivity.** Antibodies produced by the immune system bind to antigens on the surface of the body's own cells. The antibody–antigen complex triggers complement, which initiates inflammation and facilitates phagocytosis by macrophages. Examples of type II hypersensitivity reactions include:

  - *Idiopathic thrombocytopaenic purpura.* IgG antibodies coat platelets and their precursor megakaryocytes, resulting in phagocytosis by splenic and hepatic macrophages. The result is a very low platelet count.
  - *Goodpasture's disease.* IgG binds to type IV collagen in the basement membrane of the renal glomerulus and pulmonary alveolus, causing acute kidney injury and pulmonary haemorrhage, respectively.

- **Type III hypersensitivity or immune complex disease.** Sometimes when antibodies (usually IgG) bind antigens, there are insufficient antibody–antigen complexes to activate complement, particularly when the amount of antibody is small. The antibody–antigen complexes float around in the circulation and get lodged in small blood vessels, joints and glomeruli, where they cause inflammation. Examples include:

  - *Systemic lupus erythematosus*, in which antinuclear antibodies complex with nuclear antigens, causing skin, glomerulus and joint inflammation.
  - *Farmer's lung*, a hypersensitivity pneumonitis in which inhaled mould spores trigger antibody production. The resulting antibody–antigen complexes deposit in the lungs, causing inflammation.

- **Type IV or delayed-type hypersensitivity.** Some allergens trigger a type of hypersensitivity that involves T cells, not antibodies. The response is much slower, taking 2–3 days to develop. T helper cells recognise an antigen presented by an APC. The activated T helper cells divide and secrete cytokines, initiating inflammation. Cell damage is caused by the macrophages that become activated in response to these cytokines. Examples include:

  - *Tuberculosis*, the classic delayed-type hypersensitivity. Activated macrophages fuse to form giant cells around the tuberculosis antigen, the centre of which may become necrotic – this is known as a caseating granuloma. The importance of T helper cells is seen when they are absent: patients with AIDS are very susceptible to intracellular pathogens such as *M. tuberculosis*.
  - *Contact dermatitis*, where contact with certain allergens (e.g. nickel) causes a delayed skin reaction.

Clinical relevance: immune consequences of anaesthesia and surgery

The immune system is affected in the perioperative period in a number of ways:

- **Disruption of physicochemical barriers**, allowing easier access for pathogens. The most obvious route of pathogen entry is the site of surgery where the skin or mucosa has been breached. In addition, endotracheal intubation and breathing dry air inhibits ciliary function in the tracheobronchial tree, predisposing to pneumonia.
- **Exposure to allergens.** The UK 6th National Audit Project found the incidence of anaphylaxis during general anaesthesia to be 1/10,000; 4% of cases were fatal. The most common precipitants of anaphylaxis in the perioperative period were:

  - *Muscle relaxants*, most notably suxamethonium, accounting for 33% of cases;
  - *Antibiotics*, most notably penicillins and teicoplanin, accounting for 47% of cases;
  - *Antiseptics*, including chlorhexidine-impregnated central lines, accounting for 9% of cases;
  - *More rarely*: latex. colloids, blood products, amide local anaesthetics (esters have a very low incidence of allergy) and induction agents.

- **Depression of the immune system.** Various parts of the immune system may be suppressed in the perioperative period:

  - *The stress response to surgery* depresses lymphocyte function and phagocytosis.
  - *Opioids* impair macrophage, neutrophil and NK cell function, lymphocyte proliferation and cytokine release. NK cells are particularly

important in cancer surgery as they kill the stray tumour cells that evade the surgeon. Recently, small retrospective clinical trials have suggested that regional anaesthesia is associated with improved survival in cancer surgery; for example, using paravertebral blocks instead of systemic opioids in breast surgery.

- *Anaesthetic agents*: volatile anaesthetics have been shown to reduce NK cell function. In contrast, the use of propofol has no effect on NK cell activity. Recently, the use of total intravenous anaesthesia in cancer surgery has been shown to significantly reduce cancer recurrence in a large retrospective trial (see Further reading).
- *Transfusion-related immunomodulation* (TRIM), where allogenic blood transfusion causes a temporary depression of the immune system. TRIM may sometimes be useful; for example, improved graft survival has been demonstrated when patients undergoing kidney transplantation had a preoperative blood transfusion.
- *Perioperative hypothermia* depresses both innate and adaptive immune systems, which may reduce survival in cancer surgery.

Further reading

K. Murphy, C. Weaver. *Janeway's Immunobiology, 9th edition*. New York, Garland Science, 2016.

T. Cook, N. Harper. Anaesthesia, surgery and life-threatening allergic reactions – report and findings of the Royal College of Anaesthetists' 6th National Audit Project: perioperative anaphylaxis, 2018; www.nationalauditprojects.org.uk/NAP6Report#pt.

T. J. Wigmore, K. Mohammed, S. Jhanji. Long-term survival for patients undergoing volatile versus IV anesthesia for cancer surgery: a retrospective analysis. *Anesthesiology* 2016; **124**(1): 69–79.

Á. Heaney, D. J. Buggy. Can anaesthetic and analgesic techniques affect cancer recurrence or metastasis? *Br J Anaesth* 2012; **109**(Suppl. 1): i17–28.

S. Gando. Microvascular thrombosis and multiple organ dysfunction syndrome. *Crit Care Med* 2010; **38**(Suppl. 2): S35–42.

G. L. Snyder, S. Greenburg. Effect of anaesthetic technique and other perioperative factors on cancer recurrence. *Br J Anaesth* 2010; **105**(2): 106–15.

C. Snowden, E. Kirkman. The pathogenesis of sepsis. *Continuing Educ Anaesth Crit Care Pain* 2002; **2**(1): 11–14.

76

Plasma Constituents

What are the components of blood?

The constituents of blood are:

- **Plasma** (55%), consisting of:

  - *Water*;
  - *Electrolytes*;
  - *Dissolved gases* (O_2, CO_2);
  - *Plasma proteins*;
  - *Other dissolved substances*, including hormones, glucose, amino acids, coagulation proteins, lactic acid and urea.

- **Cellular components** (45%), consisting of:

  - *Erythrocytes*;
  - *Leucocytes*;
  - *Platelets*.

Classify the different plasma proteins

The plasma contains over 500 different proteins. The total plasma protein concentration is 60–85 g/dL. Plasma proteins are traditionally classified into:

- **Albumin**, making up 60% of plasma proteins;
- **Globulins**, making up 35% of total plasma protein, subclassified as α-, β- and γ-globulins;
- **Fibrinogen**, making up 4% of total plasma protein.

Most plasma proteins, with the major exception of γ-globulin, are synthesised in the liver. The most important type of γ-globulin is Ig, which is produced by plasma cells.

Alternatively, plasma proteins can be classified according to function:

- **Transport proteins**; for example:

  - *Transferrin* transports iron;
  - *Ceruloplasmin* transports copper;
  - *Lipoproteins* transport lipids;
  - *Thyroxine-binding globulin* transports the thyroid hormone thyroxine;
  - *α_1-acid glycoprotein* transports basic and neutrally charged drugs.

- **Enzyme inhibitors**; for example, α_1-antitrypsin is a protease inhibitor.
- **Coagulation and anticoagulation**; for example, fibrinogen, protein C and antithrombin III.
- **Endocrine**; for example, antidiuretic hormone and angiotensin II.
- **Immunological**; for example, IgG and IgM.
- **Mixed function**; for example, albumin has major roles in both transport and colloid oncotic pressure.

What are the functions of albumin?

Albumin has many roles:

- **Colloid oncotic pressure**. Albumin is responsible for around 80% of the intravascular oncotic pressure. The development of peripheral oedema mainly depends on the oncotic gradient between the intravascular and interstitial spaces (see Chapter 36). At a molecular weight of 67 kDa, albumin is normally too large to pass between the capillary fenestrations. However, if the capillaries become leaky, two patients with the same serum albumin may have very different degrees of peripheral oedema. Thus:

  - A malnourished elderly patient with a serum albumin of 20 g/dL and normal capillaries will have minimal peripheral oedema.
  - A patient with severe sepsis, a serum albumin of 20 g/dL and leaky capillaries will have significant peripheral oedema.

- **Transport of endogenous substances and drugs**. Albumin has a number of organic and inorganic binding sites through which it transports a variety of substances: unconjugated bilirubin, bile salts, electrolytes and free fatty acids. Albumin also binds and transports some important drugs: warfarin, digoxin, non-steroidal anti-inflammatory drugs (NSAIDs) and thiopentone. This is clinically important, as many of these drugs compete with each other for the same binding site, leading to an increased fraction of free drug and potentially toxic effects. Thus, if a patient who already takes warfarin is given an NSAID, some warfarin will be displaced from albumin, thus increasing the unbound fraction: prothrombin time and international normalised ratio will increase.

- **Free radical scavenging.** Sulphydryl groups within albumin act as free radical scavengers.

- **Acid–base balance.** Albumin is negatively charged, contributing significantly to the anion gap – the unmeasured anions within the plasma.

  In hypoalbuminaemia, the anion gap is therefore reduced. Albumin also contributes to acid–base balance: hypoalbuminaemia results in a mild metabolic alkalosis. This is why albumin concentration is included in the Stewart method of acid–base analysis (see Chapter 70).

- **Plasma Ca^{2+} handling.** The negative charge of albumin also sequesters Ca^{2+} ions in the plasma, reducing the amount of free Ca^{2+}.

Further reading

C. A. Burtis, E. R. Ashwood, D. E. Bruns. *Tietz Textbook of Clinical Chemistry and Molecular Diagnostics*, 5th edition. Philadelphia, Saunders, 2012.

Metabolism

Metabolism refers to the whole range of biochemical reactions that occur within living organisms. Metabolism broadly encompasses anabolism (the building up of larger molecules from smaller ones) and catabolism (their breaking down into smaller entities with the extraction of energy).

What is meant by the term 'cellular respiration'?

Cellular respiration is the series of catabolic processes by which carbohydrates, fats and proteins are broken down to yield ATP through a series of redox reactions, ultimately using O_2 as the oxidising agent. As O_2 is too reactive to be used directly, this process employs a series of intermediate electron carriers, including nicotinamide adenine dinucleotide (NAD^+) and flavin adenine dinucleotide (FAD).

How are carbohydrates, fats and proteins metabolised to adenosine triphosphate?

Details of the metabolic processes involved are complex, but an overview remains useful for clinical practice. Catabolism involves a number of processes:

- **Glycolysis**, the process by which glucose is converted to pyruvate, which then enters the citric acid cycle. Glycolysis takes place in the cytoplasm and can occur in either aerobic or anaerobic conditions.
- **Lipolysis**, the process by which free fatty acids are oxidised to acetyl-CoA, which then enters the citric acid cycle.
- **Protein catabolism**, a process of oxidative deamination in which amino acids have their amino groups removed to form keto acids. The keto acids may then enter the citric acid cycle or be converted to glucose or fatty acids. The amino groups are converted to urea by the urea cycle.

- **The citric acid cycle**, in which acetyl-CoA and other metabolites are broken down through a series of redox reactions within the inner mitochondrial matrix. The resulting NADH, $FADH_2$ and H^+ are then processed by the electron transport chain.
- **The electron transport chain**, located within the inner mitochondrial matrix, is the final step of aerobic metabolism. NADH and $FADH_2$ transfer electrons to O_2, releasing energy that is used to pump H^+ across the inner mitochondrial membrane. The resulting electrochemical gradient is used to generate ATP.

Describe the important steps of the glycolytic pathway

Glycolysis (also called the Embden–Meyerhof pathway) is the metabolic pathway through which glucose is converted into pyruvate, with the generation of two ATP and two NADH molecules (Figure 77.1). Key features of the glycolysis pathway are:

- Glycolysis occurs in the cytoplasm.
- The first step is the phosphorylation of glucose, resulting in glucose-6-phosphate – the 'active' form of glucose. One ATP molecule is consumed and converted to ADP in this process. This reaction is catalysed by the enzymes glucokinase (in the liver) or hexokinase (in the other tissues).[1] Phosphorylation of glucose maintains the low cytoplasmic concentration of glucose. This thereby maintains the concentration gradient for glucose diffusion from the extracellular to the intracellular space.

---

[1]   Glucose-6-phosphate is also obtained from the breakdown of the storage molecule glycogen by the enzyme glycogen phosphorylase (see p. 380).

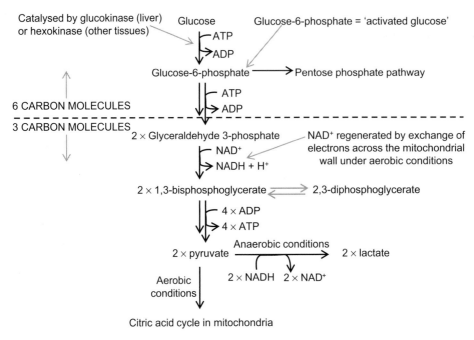

Figure 77.1 The glycolytic pathway (simplified).

- Glucose-6-phosphate (a six-carbon molecule) is broken down to two molecules of pyruvate (a three-carbon molecule) through a series of seven intermediates. During this process, a further molecule of ATP is consumed to form ADP, and then four molecules of ATP are produced from ADP.
- The overall glycolysis reaction is

$$C_6H_{12}O_6 + NAD^+ + 2ADP + 2P_i \rightarrow 2C_3H_4O_3$$
$$+ 2H^+ + 2ATP + 2H_2O + 2NADH$$

- It is important to note that O_2 is not consumed and CO_2 is not produced. Glycolysis can therefore occur under both aerobic and anaerobic conditions.
- NAD^+ is required for glycolysis. This is where aerobic and anaerobic conditions differ:
  - *Under aerobic conditions*: NADH produced during glycolysis exchanges electrons with NAD^+ or FAD across the mitochondrial wall, which regenerates NAD^+, thus allowing glycolysis to continue. Pyruvate then passes into the mitochondrion, where it enters the citric acid cycle.

  - *Under anaerobic conditions*: the electron transport chain is not active, so there are no NAD^+ or FAD molecules within the mitochondrion with which to exchange electrons. Glycolysis can only continue if NAD^+ is regenerated through a different reaction: the production of lactic acid. Pyruvate is reduced to lactate by NADH in a reaction catalysed by the enzyme lactate dehydrogenase. This regenerates NAD^+ in order that glycolysis can continue:

  Pyruvate + NADH $\rightarrow$ Lactate + NAD^+

Lactate has a number of fates:

- If the PO_2 is restored, it can be oxidised back to pyruvate and enter the citric acid cycle.
- Lactate can leave the cell cytoplasm and travel in the circulation to the liver, where it can be either oxidised back to pyruvate or converted to glucose through a process called gluconeogenesis. This is known as the Cori cycle.
- In organisms without a liver (e.g. yeast), lactate is converted to ethanol to regenerate NAD^+ in a process called fermentation.

- An important intermediate in the glycolytic pathway is 1,3-bisphosphoglycerate (1,3-BPG). 1,3-BPG isomerises to 2,3-diphosphoglycerate (2,3-DPG), a molecule that binds strongly to deoxyhaemoglobin. Under conditions of low PO_2, the rate of glycolysis becomes increased, as the enzyme phosphofructokinase involved in glycolysis is O_2 sensitive. This results in increased 2,3-DPG levels, which aids the offloading of O_2 from haemoglobin (Hb) (see Chapter 8).

Clinical relevance: lactic acidosis

Lactic acidosis usually results from either regionally or globally reduced O_2 delivery, such as in limb ischaemia, mesenteric ischaemia, cardiac arrest and severe shock (septic, cardiogenic, etc.). However, it is important to remember that lactic acidosis may occur for other reasons, including:

- **Reduced clearance of plasma lactate**. This may occur in hepatic or renal dysfunction. Metformin (a biguanide) reduces hepatic gluconeogenesis. As lactate is used by the liver as a substrate for gluconeogenesis, metformin reduces hepatic lactate uptake, thus exacerbating a lactic acidosis.
- **Cytotoxic hypoxia**. The electron transport chain can be poisoned by substances such as cyanide. Cells are then no longer able to utilise O_2 for aerobic respiration and are reliant on glycolysis for ATP production.

Treatment of lactic acidosis is focused on diagnosis and correction of the underlying cause; this may involve surgery or organ support (by O_2 administration, fluid or inotropic support, haemofiltration, etc.). Rarely, administration of sodium bicarbonate may be indicated if there is cardiovascular compromise as a result of profound acidosis or severe hyperkalaemia accompanying the acidosis.

What are the important steps of the citric acid cycle?

The citric acid cycle (also known as the Krebs cycle and the tricarboxylic acid cycle) takes place in the inner mitochondrial matrix. It involves a complex cycle of metabolic intermediates, producing CO_2, ATP and electron donors (NADH and $FADH_2$) that are then utilised in the electron transport chain (Figure 77.2). Whilst O_2 is not consumed in the citric acid cycle, the cycle nevertheless ceases to operate under anaerobic conditions corresponding to a mitochondrial $PO_2 < 0.4$ kPa. This is because the electron transport chain, which is dependent upon O_2, is needed to regenerate NAD^+ and FAD for use in the citric acid cycle.

The main substance consumed by the citric acid cycle is acetyl-CoA. Acetyl-CoA is a two-carbon molecule (the acetyl part) attached to the carrier coenzyme A (CoA or CoA-SH, derived from vitamin B). Acetyl-CoA is produced either from:

- **Pyruvate**, according to the reaction:

$$Pyruvate\ (3) + CoA - SH + NAD^+ \rightarrow$$
$$Acetyl - CoA\ (2) + CO_2 + NADH$$

(numbers in parentheses refer to number of carbon atoms in the molecule); or
- **β-oxidation of fatty acids** – see below.

However, other substances (e.g. keto acids formed from the deamination of amino acids) can enter the citric acid cycle at different points.

The citric acid cycle is a complex system of eight molecular intermediates, enzymes and coenzymes. Key features of the citric acid cycle are:

- Acetyl-CoA (2) reacts with oxaloacetate (4) to form citrate (6). Citrate is considered the starting point of the cycle (hence the name) and is traditionally drawn at the 12 o'clock position.
- Citrate (6) (through an intermediate) decarboxylates to give α-ketoglutarate (5), NADH and CO_2.
- α-ketoglutarate (5) decarboxylates when it reacts with CoA to give succinyl-CoA (4), NADH and CO_2.
- The four-carbon succinyl-CoA undergoes a series of reactions and isomerisations, passing through a number of intermediate states before regenerating oxaloacetate (4). No CO_2 is produced during these changes – the carbon number of the molecules is unchanged. However, the process does produce a molecule each of ATP, NADH and $FADH_2$.
- The NADH, $FADH_2$ and H^+ produced in the citric acid cycle are used in the electron transport chain to produce ATP.
- The overall reaction for each acetyl group entering the citric acid cycle is:

$$Acetyl - CoA + 3NAD^+ + FAD + ADP + P_i +$$
$$2H_2O \rightarrow CoA - SH + 3NADH + FADH_2 + 3H^+$$
$$+ ATP + 2CO_2$$

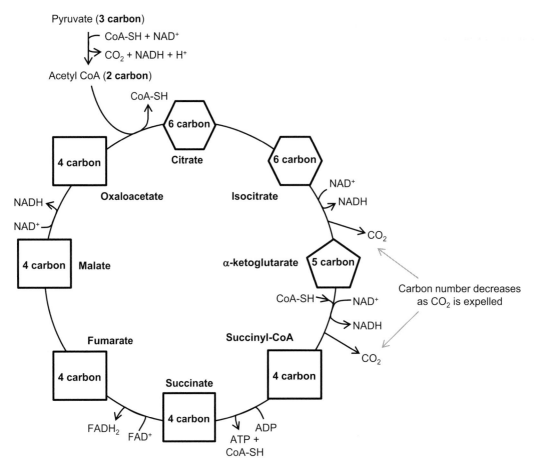

Figure 77.2 The citric acid cycle (simplified).

Describe the key steps of the electron transport chain

The electron transport chain is the final step of carbohydrate, fat and protein catabolism. The electron transport chain consists of five protein complexes on the inner surface of the inner mitochondrial membrane that use the electron donors NADH and $FADH_2$ to produce ATP (Figure 77.3).

Key features of the electron transport chain are:

- Electrons are transferred from NADH to Complex I and from $FADH_2$ to Complex II.
- Coenzyme Q (also called ubiquinone) is involved in facilitating electron transfer from Complexes I and II to Complex III.
- Cytochrome c is involved in electron transfer between Complexes III and IV.

- Complex IV (also called cytochrome c oxidase) transfers the collected electrons to O_2, forming water. Complex IV is the part of the electron transport chain that is affected by cyanide poisoning: cyanide binds to the Complex IV haem group, preventing it from binding O_2.
- As electrons are transferred along the electron transport chain and as electrons are combined with O_2, the energy released is used to pump H^+ from the inner mitochondrial matrix to the intermembrane space. This generates an electrochemical gradient between the intermembrane space and the inner mitochondrial matrix.
- The final stage in the electron transport chain is ATP synthesis. Complex V (also known as ATP synthase) is a pore in the inner mitochondrial

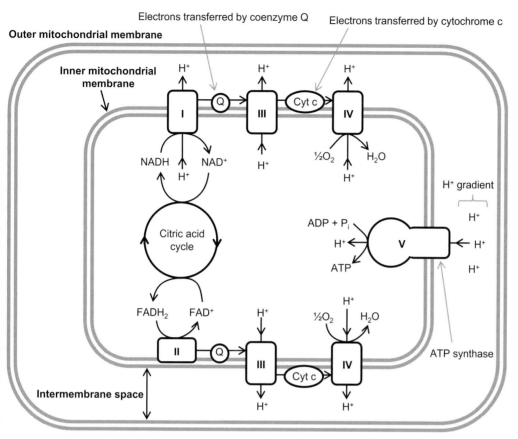

Figure 77.3 The electron transport chain (simplified).

matrix through which the intermembrane H$^+$ ions pass, generating ATP in the process. This final step of the electron transport chain is known as oxidative phosphorylation.

Oxidative phosphorylation is usually coupled; that is, H$^+$ movement across the inner mitochondrial membrane is used to generate ATP. In brown adipose tissue, pores can be opened that allow H$^+$ ions to travel down their electrochemical gradient from the intermembrane space to the inner mitochondrial matrix without passing through Complex V. This is called uncoupling, where oxidation and phosphorylation are no longer strictly matched. The energy released during H$^+$ movement generates heat instead of ATP. This is an important mechanism for thermogenesis in neonates. Overall at the electron transport chain:

- NADH generates three ATP molecules.
- FADH$_2$ generates one ATP molecule.

How much ATP is generated from a molecule of glucose during aerobic and anaerobic metabolism?

- **Anaerobic metabolism = 2 × ATP:**

    - Metabolism of glucose involves glycolysis only.
    - Two molecules of ATP are generated.
    - Two molecules of NADH are also generated, but cannot be utilised under anaerobic conditions.

- **Aerobic metabolism = 36 × ATP:**

    - Through glycolysis, one glucose molecule results in 2 × ATP, 2 × pyruvate and 2 × NADH.
    - As each pyruvate is converted to acetyl-CoA, one NADH molecule is generated.
    - In the citric acid cycle, each acetyl-CoA generates 3 × NADH, 1 × FADH$_2$ and 1 × ATP.

- Overall, one molecule of glucose thus produces $4 \times$ ATP, $10 \times$ NADH and $2 \times$ FADH$_2$.
- In the electron transport chain, each NADH produces $3 \times$ ATP and each FADH$_2$ produces $1 \times$ ATP. In total, one molecule of glucose produces $36 \times$ ATP.

How are fats metabolised?

Fats are a useful source of energy, as they produce more than twice the amount of ATP than equivalent masses of carbohydrate or protein.

Free fatty acids are catabolised by the cells in a process called β-oxidation. β-oxidation takes place in the mitochondrial matrix and involves removing successive two-carbon units from the fatty acid, with each event producing one molecule of acetyl-CoA (Figure 77.4). Acetyl-CoA then enters the citric acid cycle, as described above.

Key features of fat catabolism are:

- Free fatty acids are stored as triglyceride: three fatty acids esterified with glycerol. When needed, triglycerides are hydrolysed by lipases to regenerate free fatty acids and glycerol. Glycerol can also be metabolised: in the liver, glycerol is transformed into glucose through a process called gluconeogenesis. The newly formed glucose enters the circulation, where it is taken up by cells and used to produce ATP.
- Short- and medium-chain fatty acids are small enough to directly enter the mitochondria. Long-chain fatty acids have to be bound to a carrier – the carnitine shuttle – in order to cross the mitochondrial membrane.

Clinical relevance: ketone bodies

When carbohydrates are scarce (as occurs during starvation) or unable to enter the cell (as occurs in diabetic ketoacidosis), fat metabolism becomes the main source of energy, and so β-oxidation results in a high mitochondrial acetyl-CoA concentration. When acetyl-CoA concentration is high, ketone bodies (acetone, acetoacetic acid and β-hydroxybutyric acid) are spontaneously formed by condensation of two molecules of acetyl-CoA. Ketone bodies are a normal finding during starvation, but are pathological in diabetic ketoacidosis.

Ketone bodies can be utilised by the liver, heart and brain:

- The liver converts ketone bodies back into acetyl-CoA, which then enter the citric acid cycle.
- The heart usually favours fatty acids as its main energy source, but can also use ketone bodies in times of starvation.
- The brain does not normally metabolise fatty acids; it is usually entirely dependent on glucose for its ATP. In times of starvation, the brain can adapt to using ketone bodies as its energy source. During prolonged starvation, up to 70% of the brain's metabolic demands can be provided by ketone bodies.

Red blood cells (RBCs) do not have mitochondria, so they are entirely dependent on glycolysis for their metabolism and are unable to utilise ketone bodies.

How are proteins catabolised?

Proteins are the basic building blocks of the body's structures; the body therefore treats them differently to the other energy sources. Proteins are only used for energy production if amino acids are plentiful or in times of starvation. Protein catabolism is an inefficient process: 1.75 g of protein is required to produce the same energy as 1 g of carbohydrate.

Proteins are first broken down into their constituent amino acids. To be of any use, amino acids must first have their amino groups removed through oxidative deamination or transamination:

- **Oxidative deamination**. This takes place in the liver and is catalysed by deaminase enzymes. The amino group is removed, producing a keto acid and ammonia (NH$_3$). The keto acid enters the citric acid cycle, where it may be used for energy, transformed into glucose (gluconeogenesis) or used to synthesise another amino acid or a fatty acid. NH$_3$ is a toxic substance; it is converted to nontoxic urea through a process called the urea cycle (or ornithine cycle). Conversion of NH$_3$ to urea is an energy-consuming process, requiring three ATP molecules per urea molecule formed. Unlike other amino acids, glutamate can also be deaminated in the kidney and its NH$_3$ immediately excreted into the urine. This is important, as it means NH$_3$ can be excreted without the need for the energy-consuming urea cycle.
- **Transamination**. The amino group of an amino acid is transferred, through catalysis by

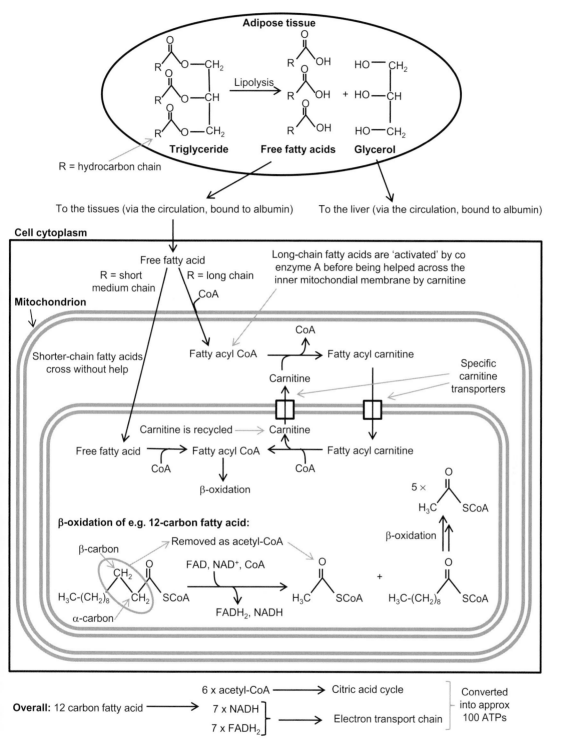

Figure 77.4 β-oxidation (simplified) (SCoA = thiocoenzyme A).

aminotransferases, to a keto acid or another amino acid to form a new amino acid. There are nine essential amino acids: phenylalanine, valine, threonine, tryptophan, isoleucine, methionine, leucine, lysine and histidine. These amino acids cannot be synthesised by transamination and must be supplied from the diet.

How are carbohydrates, fats and proteins stored in the body?

Humans eat sporadically, with gaps in between meals. At the same time, constant ATP production is required to maintain cellular processes. Therefore, the storage and gradual release of nutrients is of great importance:

- **Glycogen**. Carbohydrates are stored as glycogen, a polymer of glucose analogous to the plant glucose-storage molecule, starch. Glycogen is found in the liver and muscles:

  - The liver contains approximately 100 g of glycogen, which can be released as glucose into the circulation for use by other organs. Liver glycogen is only sufficient to maintain plasma glucose concentration for around 24 h, after which gluconeogenesis becomes the dominant mechanism (see below).
  - The muscle glycogen store contains around 200 g of glucose, but its glucose cannot be released back into the circulation. Muscle glycogen can only be used for metabolic processes within the muscle.

  Following a carbohydrate-based meal, the hormone insulin facilitates the production of glycogen in a process called glycogenesis. Glucose-6-phosphate, the active form of glucose, is joined together in chains. This process is catalysed by the enzyme glycogen synthase: increased insulin concentration upregulates this enzyme's activity (Figure 77.5).

  When plasma glucose levels fall, the liver glycogen store liberates glucose, thus returning the plasma glucose concentration to normal. This process is called glycogenolysis and is stimulated by the hormones glucagon and adrenaline. Growth hormone causes glycogenolysis in skeletal muscle.

- **Triglyceride**. The body's main energy storage form is triglyceride, mainly found within adipose cells. Triglycerides are either absorbed from the diet or synthesised from carbohydrate or protein precursors:

  - Dietary triglyceride is packaged by enterocytes into chylomicrons (see Chapter 64). Chylomicrons circulate in the plasma, offloading exogenous triglycerides to the tissues. Any excess triglyceride is taken up by adipose tissue for storage.
  - Hepatocytes synthesise triglyceride in an anabolic process called lipogenesis. After a meal, insulin levels are high. Once the liver glycogen store is full, any excess carbohydrates or amino acids are converted to fatty acids and glycerol, which are esterified to give triglyceride. This newly formed triglyceride is packaged as very-low-density lipoprotein (VLDL) in the liver. VLDL is released into the circulation, where it distributes endogenous triglyceride to the tissues.

- **Protein**. Although protein is primarily a structural material, the muscles provide a store of amino acids that can be catabolised at times of starvation.

What is gluconeogenesis?

Gluconeogenesis, as the name suggests, is an energy-consuming anabolic process in which glucose is synthesised from non-carbohydrate precursors. Gluconeogenesis mainly occurs in the liver, with a minor contribution by the kidney. It is one of two mechanisms that prevent plasma glucose concentration from falling too low, the other being glycogenolysis. It may seem odd that the liver synthesises glucose by an energy-consuming process so that the newly formed glucose can be catabolised by other tissues. However, some tissues are predominantly (brain) or entirely (RBCs) dependent on glucose as their source of energy.

Gluconeogenesis is another complex metabolic pathway. Its key features are:

- Molecules used as substrates for gluconeogenesis include lactate, pyruvate, glycerol, amino acids and all the intermediates of the citric acid cycle.
- The gluconeogenesis pathway is a separate biochemical pathway – it is not simply the reverse of glycolysis.
- Gluconeogenesis starts from oxaloacetate, a four-carbon intermediate of the citric acid cycle.
- Gluconeogenesis is controlled by the hormone glucagon, released when plasma glucose concentration is low (see below).

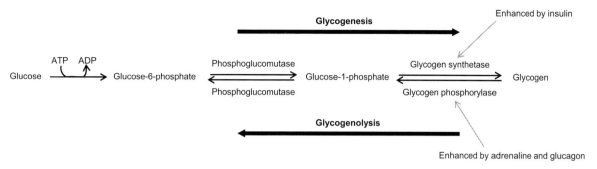

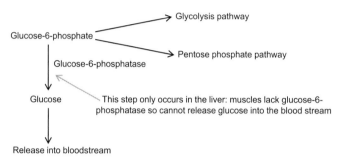

Fates of glucose-6-phosphate regenerated by glycogenolysis:

Figure 77.5 Glycogenesis and glycogenolysis (simplified).

- The biguanide metformin works by inhibiting gluconeogenesis.

What is the pentose phosphate pathway?

The pentose phosphate pathway (PPP; also called the hexose monophosphate shunt) is an anabolic carbohydrate pathway with two functions:

- **To produce pentose sugars** for nucleic acid synthesis;
- **To produce NADPH** for intracellular reduction reactions (i.e. the reverse of oxidation).

Key features are:

- The PPP starts with the active form of glucose, glucose-6-phosphate.
- Whether glucose-6-phosphate proceeds along the glycolytic pathway or the PPP depends on the activity of the enzyme that catalyses the first step of the PPP: glucose-6-phosphate dehydrogenase (G6PD). G6PD is controlled by the cellular concentration of $NADP^+$, becoming more active if $NADP^+$ levels are high.

- The PPP accounts for approximately 60% of the NADPH required by the cells, which is used to reduce glutathione. Glutathione is an antioxidant used to prevent cellular damage from reactive oxygen species (see Chapter 24). It is also important in RBCs, where it helps maintain Hb in its ferrous (Fe^{2+}) state. Patients with G6PD deficiency cannot utilise the PPP, which leads to a loss of reducing power, predisposing the patient to MetHb (Fe^{3+}) formation (see Chapter 8).

Summarise the effects of insulin and glucagon

Resting plasma glucose concentration is usually tightly controlled – it is maintained between 3.5 and 5.5 mmol/L by the balance of two hormones:

- **Insulin**, which acts to reduce plasma glucose concentration;
- **Glucagon**, which acts to increase plasma glucose concentration.

Insulin is the body's main anabolic hormone. Insulin is a peptide hormone produced in the β-cells of the islets of Langerhans in the pancreas:

- **Proinsulin**. This is an insulin precursor consisting of an A- and B-chain joined together by two disulphide bridges and a C-peptide.
- **Insulin**. This is formed when the C-peptide of proinsulin is cleaved by endopeptidases. Insulin and free C-peptide are packaged together in vesicles, awaiting a physiological trigger for release.
- **Exocytosis**. The primary trigger for insulin vesicles to undergo exocytosis is an increase in plasma glucose concentration.
- **Plasma insulin secretion** occurs in two phases. Initially, a rise in plasma glucose concentration stimulates a rapid increase in plasma insulin concentration as vesicles empty their contents filled with preformed insulin. When all of the vesicles have emptied, the β-islet cells release insulin as it is synthesised.
- **The sympathetic nervous system** inhibits the release of insulin from the β-islet cells by direct innervation through α_2-adrenoceptor action. However, adrenaline, which is released in response to sympathetic nervous activity at the adrenal medulla, causes an increase in insulin secretion through β_2-adrenoceptor activation. This is important during exercise: muscles require insulin for glucose uptake through the GLUT-4 glucose transporter (see below).

Insulin has three main physiological effects:

- **Facilitation of glucose uptake**. The cell membrane glucose transporter GLUT-4 requires insulin to facilitate cellular glucose uptake. GLUT-4 transporters are present in adipose tissue, skeletal muscle and the heart. Note: the cells of the brain and liver have GLUT-1 and GLUT-2 glucose transporters, respectively, which are not insulin dependent.
- **Storage of metabolic substrates**. Increased plasma insulin concentration promotes substrate storage:
  - *Hepatic glycogenesis*;
  - *Fatty acid synthesis* in the liver;
  - *Increased esterification of fatty acids* (to synthesise triglyceride) in adipose tissue.
- **Inhibition of endogenous glucose production**. Insulin inhibits the breakdown of stored substrates (i.e. lipolysis and glycogenolysis) and gluconeogenesis.

Insulin also promotes the cellular uptake of amino acids and K^+:

- Increased amino acid uptake promotes protein synthesis.
- The physiological role of increased K^+ uptake is a feedforward response to prevent hyperkalaemia following a meal – the presence of increased glucose suggests feeding and the likelihood of increased K^+. The mechanism can be manipulated in hyperkalaemic patients: plasma K^+ concentration can be reduced through the use of an insulin and dextrose infusion.

Clinical relevance: diabetic ketoacidosis

In type 1 diabetes, there is an absolute lack of endogenous insulin due to autoimmune attack of the β-cells in the islets of Langerhans. Patients are treated with exogenous insulin.

When exogenous insulin is insufficient (e.g. due to an acute illness or patient noncompliance with treatment), plasma glucose concentration increases due to:

- Reduced glucose uptake into cells;
- Increased hepatic glycogenolysis;
- Increased gluconeogenesis.

In addition, low insulin plasma concentration results in lipolysis and β-oxidation. As discussed above, when the acetyl-CoA concentration in the liver is high, ketone bodies are synthesised. Hyperglycaemia and ketone body formation result in adverse effects:

- **Osmotic diuresis**. Hyperglycaemia results in an osmotic diuresis, which can cause significant hypovolaemia and renal electrolyte loss. In particular, significant hypokalaemia may occur.
- **Acidosis**. Synthesis of ketone bodies may result in significant acidaemia. The respiratory centre is stimulated by the carotid bodies, resulting in an increased V_T, known as 'Kussmaul respiration'. In addition, acidosis may be exacerbated by lactic acid production in significantly hypovolaemic patients.

The paradox in diabetic ketoacidosis is that, despite a high plasma glucose concentration, most of the body's cells are deficient in glucose, as the insulin-dependent glucose transporter GLUT-4 is inactive.

Glucagon is a peptide hormone produced by the α-cells of the islets of Langerhans. Unlike the β-islet cells, α-islet cells have no glucose sensing apparatus, and therefore:

- **Secretion of glucagon is stimulated by** a hypoglycaemia-induced increase in autonomic nervous system activity. In addition, glucagon is secreted in response to an increase in circulating adrenaline.
- **Glucagon release is inhibited by**:
  - *Insulin*;
  - *Somatostatin*;
  - *Increased plasma free fatty acid and ketone body concentrations.*

Glucagon acts to increase plasma glucose concentration by:
- **Promoting gluconeogenesis**;
- **Promoting glycogenolysis**;
- **Inhibiting glycolysis in the liver** – intermediates of the glycolysis pathway are instead used as substrates for gluconeogenesis.

Glucagon is especially important during starvation. Maintenance of a normal plasma glucose concentration is important, as the brain is very dependent on glucose for its metabolism (see Chapter 78).

What is meant by the term 'basal metabolic rate'?

Basal metabolic rate (BMR) is the amount of energy a patient consumes per unit time in a state of mental and physical rest in a comfortable environment, 12 h after a meal. BMR is corrected for age and surface area. Normal BMR for an adult is approximately $200 \text{ kJ m}^{-2} \text{ h}^{-1}$, or $40 \text{ kcal m}^{-2} \text{ h}^{-1}$. The body's metabolic rate is increased by:

- **Exercise.**
- **Raised catecholamine levels**, including stress.
- **Hyperthyroidism** – thyroid hormones play a major role in the basal control of metabolic rate.
- **Pregnancy and lactation** – BMR increases by 20% in pregnancy as a consequence of foetal and placental metabolism, as well as the growth of the uterus and breasts. In the postnatal period, the metabolic processes involved in the production of breast milk cause an increased BMR; breastfeeding is promoted as a means of postnatal weight loss.
- **High and low environmental temperature** – pyrexia causes an increase in BMR.

- **A recent meal** – BMR is raised for the 6 h following a large meal, mostly due to oxidative deamination of amino acids in the liver.
- **Children** – BMR is increased in children owing to the metabolic needs of growth and thermoregulation; neonates have a BMR approximately twice that of adults (see Chapter 84).

BMR is reduced by:
- **Hypothyroidism.**
- **Starvation.** BMR is reduced to preserve body fat and protein stores.
- **Advancing age.** BMR declines by approximately 2% per decade.

It was previously thought that BMR was lower in females than males. However, taking lean body mass into account, there is no BMR difference between the sexes.

Clinical relevance: the metabolic equivalent

The metabolic equivalent (MET) of a task is a method of expressing the energy cost of a particular physical activity. Exercise is graded against multiples of BMR:

- 1 MET equals in a state of rest, awake, fasted for >12 h.
- 3 MET equals walking at moderate pace on the flat.
- 4 MET equals climbing two flights of stairs without stopping.
- 8 MET equals jogging.
- 10 MET equals strenuous exercise.

METs can be used in the preoperative anaesthetic assessment to grade physiological reserve. A functional capacity of less than 4 MET represents poor physiological fitness, associated with a higher risk of perioperative cardiac events (see Chapter 43).

Further reading

R. L. Miesfeld, M. M. McEvoy. *Biochemistry*. New York, W. W. Norton & Company, 2017.

D. Voet, J. G. Voet. *Biochemistry, 4th edition*. Hoboken, John Wiley & Sons, 2011.

Taskforce for the European Society of Cardiology. Guidelines for pre-operative cardiac risk assessment and perioperative cardiac management for non-cardiac surgery. *Eur Heart J* 2009; **30**(22): 2769–812.

F. C. Luft. Lactic acidosis – update for critical care clinicians, *J Am Soc Nephrol* 2001; **12**(Suppl.): S15–19.

Starvation

Describe the changes that occur during starvation

Starvation is defined as the failure to ingest or absorb sufficient dietary calories to sustain normal body function, resulting in behavioural, physical and metabolic changes.

During starvation, the body must survive partially or totally on endogenous stores. As starvation progresses, the balance of the hormones insulin and glucagon alters: insulin concentration decreases to very low levels, whilst glucagon concentration increases. This, in turn, is responsible for the major metabolic changes that occur during starvation.

Describe the biochemical changes of starvation

During periods of starvation, the body's main concern is maintaining plasma glucose concentration; some tissues, particularly the brain and red blood cells, are dependent on glucose for their metabolism.

- **During the first 24–48 h**, a reduction in plasma glucose concentration causes a fall in plasma insulin concentration and a rise in glucagon concentration:

  - *Glycogenolysis in the liver* is promoted by glucagon, releasing glucose into the circulation. The liver glycogen store is exhausted after 48 h.
  - *Lipolysis* is promoted by high glucagon concentration and low insulin concentration, resulting in the liberation of free fatty acids and glycerol from stored triglyceride.
  - *β-oxidation of fatty acids* is promoted by low plasma insulin concentration. Most of the energy produced in the early stages of starvation comes from β-oxidation.

    This process leads to high acetyl-CoA concentration within the mitochondria, resulting in the formation of ketone bodies.

- **Over the next few days:**

  - *Gluconeogenesis increases*: the substrates for gluconeogenesis are glycerol, lactate and amino acids.
  - *Plasma insulin concentration becomes very low*, which increases ketone body synthesis.

- **Over the next few weeks:**

  - *Gluconeogenesis gradually declines* as tissues adapt to metabolise ketone bodies. Plasma ketone concentration rises as high as 7 mmol/L.
  - *Basal metabolic rate (BMR) decreases*.

The brain still requires 100–120 g of glucose per day, and gluconeogenesis is the only means of supplying this demand. Whilst glycerol released during lipolysis remains the main substrate for gluconeogenesis, amino acids are increasingly used; high glucagon concentration stimulates the release of amino acids from skeletal muscle.

What other changes occur during starvation?

Along with biochemical changes, starvation induces behavioural changes:

- Initially, energy is conserved through a reduction in unnecessary movement.
- In severe starvation, all but life-saving movement ceases.

There are also some additional physiological changes: the activity of the sympathetic nervous system is reduced in severe starvation, leading to difficulty with temperature and blood pressure control.

What is the usual mode of death in starvation?

Total fat stores vary between patients, but a typical 70-kg man has enough triglyceride to survive around

40–60 days of starvation. After triglyceride stores have been exhausted, the amino acids within skeletal muscle are liberated and used for gluconeogenesis. However, once half the muscle mass has been catabolised, there is insufficient respiratory muscle remaining to adequately clear respiratory secretions and pneumonia ensues.

Clinical relevance: enhanced recovery

Traditionally in major surgery, to protect against aspiration pneumonia on induction of anaesthesia, patients are starved preoperatively for at least 6 h and often significantly longer. The metabolic consequences of major surgery are complex (see Chapter 79), including insulin resistance, hyperglycaemia and protein catabolism, all of which worsen outcome.

The enhanced recovery programme is a structured approach to managing the perioperative period in patients undergoing major surgery. Factors such as neuraxial blockade and early mobilisation are incorporated into a protocol-based perioperative care bundle that has been shown to reduce the length of hospital stay and post-operative complications. One of the factors included in the enhanced recovery bundle is preoperative carbohydrate loading. Allowing patients to drink carbohydrate-based drinks up to 2 h preoperatively is associated with less insulin resistance and a reduced loss of muscle mass without increasing the risk of aspiration. Glucose is said to have a protein-sparing effect that is thought to be due to the effects of insulin preventing protein catabolism.

What is refeeding syndrome?

Refeeding syndrome is the severe metabolic disturbance that can occur following reinstitution of nutrition to patients who have been starved or severely malnourished. It was first reported amongst survivors of Japanese concentration camps in World War II.

Patients at risk of refeeding syndrome include those who have been starved for 5 days or longer; refeeding syndrome may therefore be encountered in emergency surgical and critical care patients. The onset of refeeding syndrome is usually within a few days of reinstitution of food, causing:

- *Hypophosphataemia*;
- *Hypokalaemia*;
- *Hypomagnesaemia*;
- *Increased extracellular fluid*.

During starvation, plasma insulin concentration falls to very low levels. When feeding is re-established and plasma glucose concentration rises, there is a massive increase in insulin secreton by the pancreatic β-islet cells. The high insulin concentration promotes cellular glucose, Mg^{2+}, phosphate and K^+ uptake, causing the plasma concentrations of these substances to fall dramatically. In addition, there is excessive Na^+ and water retention (the mechanism for which is unknown), which may precipitate left ventricular failure. Reintroduction of carbohydrate increases the respiratory quotient: the respiratory system, already potentially weak from respiratory muscle catabolism, must increase $\dot{V}_A$ to compensate for the increased production of CO_2 when carbohydrates are metabolised.

Management of refeeding syndrome is by slow institution of feeding with aggressive correction of electrolytes.

Clinical relevance: anorexia nervosa

Anorexia nervosa is a psychiatric disorder characterised by strict, psychologically driven weight loss through dietary restriction, excessive exercise and purging (self-induced vomiting and laxative use). Anorexia has significant physiological sequelae with implications for anaesthesia:

- **Respiratory**. Purging may result in a metabolic alkalosis. The respiratory centre may partially compensate through bradypnoea.
- **Cardiovascular**. Anorexic patients are typically hypotensive and bradycardic as a result of decreased sympathetic outflow. The baseline electrocardiogram may demonstrate abnormalities as a result of electrolyte disturbances; perioperative arrhythmias are common. Myocardial contractility may be impaired; excessive fluid administration may precipitate overt cardiac failure.
- **Gastrointestinal**. Repeated vomiting results in salivary gland hyperplasia, dental caries, oesophageal strictures and Mallory–Weiss tears. Gastric emptying times are prolonged; all anorexic patients should be considered to have a 'full stomach', warranting rapid sequence induction. Refeeding syndrome is almost universal.
- **Renal**. Significant electrolyte disturbances (especially K^+, Mg^{2+}, Ca^{2+} and Cl^-) may occur in

those who abuse diuretics and laxatives. Glomerular filtration is often impaired.

- **Thermoregulation**. Decreased subcutaneous fat and an inadequate shivering mechanism predispose anorexic patients to perioperative hypothermia. In addition to the usual warming methods, the ambient theatre temperature may need to be increased.
- **Positioning**. The lack of subcutaneous fat predisposes anorexic patients to peripheral nerve injuries – careful positioning and padding are required.
- **Pharmacological**. A decrease in plasma protein concentration results in a greater fraction of unbound drug – doses need to be adjusted for this, as well as for the patient's weight. In addition, drug clearance may be reduced due to reduced BMR and renal function. Hypokalaemia and hypocalcaemia may prolong the duration of neuromuscular blockade.

Further reading

W. J. Fawcett, O. Ljungqvist. Starvation, carbohydrate loading, and outcome after major surgery. *BJA Education* 2017; **17**(9): 312–16.

C. Jones, S. A. Badger, R. Hannon. The role of carbohydrate drinks in pre-operative nutrition for elective colorectal surgery. *Ann R Coll Surg Engl* 2011; **93**(7): 504–7.

A. M. Denner, S. A. Townley. Anorexia nervosa: perioperative implications. *Continuing Educ Anaesth Crit Care Pain* 2009; **9**(2): 61–4.

M. D. Kraft, I. F. Btaiche, G. S. Sacks. Review of the refeeding syndrome. *Nutr Clin Pract* 2005; **20**(6): 625–33.

Stress Response

What is the stress response?

The stress response is a complex neuroendocrine response to physiological stress. The most commonly encountered stressors are trauma, burns, surgery and critical illness; the magnitude of the neuroendocrine response is directly related to the magnitude of the stressor. In addition to its metabolic effects, the stress response leads to activation of the immunological and haematological systems.

The stress response, often referred to as the 'fight or flight' response, was once a useful survival strategy. However, in the context of modern surgery, many of the physiological changes that accompany the stress response adversely affect surgical outcomes and extend hospital stay.

How is the stress response initiated? What are its effects on the endocrine system?

The hypothalamus coordinates the stress response through the secretion of pituitary hormones and the activation of the sympathetic nervous system. It is stimulated to do so through two mechanisms:

- *Relay of autonomic and sensory afferent nervous impulses* from the area of injury to the hypothalamus.
- *Local activation of inflammation* in the area of injury with cytokine release, complement activation, leukocyte attraction, platelet activation and initiation of the coagulation cascade. Cytokines such as interleukin-6, interferons and tumour necrosis factor spill over into the systemic circulation, triggering the hypothalamus to activate the stress response.

Once activated, the hypothalamus:

- **Increases sympathetic nervous outflow**, resulting in:
  - *Systemic release of adrenaline* from the adrenal medulla;

  - *Systemic release of noradrenaline* from postganglionic sympathetic nerve terminals, resulting in some spillover of noradrenaline into the systemic circulation;
  - *Renin release* by the kidney, which increases aldosterone secretion from the adrenal cortex (through the production and action of angiotensin II);
  - *Glucagon release* from the α-cells of the islets of Langerhans;
  - *Reduced insulin secretion* from the β-cells of the islets of Langerhans (see Chapter 77).

- **Signals the pituitary to release**:
  - *Adrenocorticotropic hormone*, which stimulates cortisol release from the adrenal cortex. Cortisol is known as the 'stress hormone' owing to the multitude of effects it mediates in response to physiological stress. The mineralocorticoid effects of aldosterone and cortisol result in excess Na$^+$ and water reabsorption.
  - *Growth hormone* (GH).
  - *Antidiuretic hormone* (ADH). Increased ADH results in reabsorption of water at the renal collecting duct.

The secretion of the other pituitary hormones is not altered by the stress response.

What are the metabolic effects of the hormonal changes?

The stress response has effects on all of the major metabolic substrates:

- **Carbohydrate.** Hyperglycaemia occurs in proportion to the severity of trauma due to:
  - *Low insulin concentration*;
  - *High glucagon concentration*;
  - *The anti-insulin effects* of catecholamines, cortisol and, to a lesser extent, GH.

- **Protein**. Protein metabolism has two phases:
  - *Initially*, protein anabolism is inhibited.
  - *After 12–14 h*, skeletal muscle is catabolised: amino acids are required for use as substrates for gluconeogenesis and for the synthesis of acute-phase proteins.

The extent of protein catabolism is proportional to the severity of the trauma. This is referred to as negative nitrogen balance, where the amount of nitrogen excreted from the body is greater than that ingested. The hormones involved are:

- *Cortisol*, which promotes protein breakdown and gluconeogenesis;
- *GH*, which has greater anabolic than catabolic effects on body protein and thus may limit skeletal muscle breakdown.
- **Fat**. Lipolysis and ketogenesis are promoted by:
  - *High glucagon concentration*;
  - *Low insulin concentration*;
  - *Increased catecholamine, cortisol and GH concentrations*.

What are the adverse consequences of the stress response?

The stress response has many adverse consequences:

- **Cardiovascular**. Increased levels of catecholamines and angiotensin II result in peripheral vasoconstriction, hypertension and tachycardia, all of which increase myocardial work, with the potential to precipitate myocardial ischaemia in susceptible patients.
- **Hyperglycaemia**. Raised plasma glucose is associated with poor wound healing and wound infection. In critical illness, hyperglycaemia is associated with increased mortality, increased risk of nosocomial infection, requirement for renal replacement therapy and critical illness polyneuropathy. The plasma glucose concentration at which insulin therapy should be started is controversial: tight glucose control (e.g. plasma glucose 4.4–6.1 mmol/L) may reduce these adverse complications, but it carries an increased risk of iatrogenic hypoglycaemia.
- **Protein catabolism**. Negative nitrogen balance is a major consequence of the stress response. Loss of skeletal muscle mass can be significant (up to 0.5 kg/day) following major surgery. Generalised

loss of skeletal muscle makes patients feel weak and contributes to post-operative immobility, thus increasing venous thromboembolism risk. Loss of respiratory muscle predisposes patients to post-operative respiratory failure. In the severely malnourished, cardiac muscle mass may be lost, predisposing to arrhythmias. Unfortunately, no strategy has ever successfully prevented stress-related protein catabolism. However, protein catabolism does appear to be reduced by preoperative carbohydrate loading and perioperative low-dose glucose infusion.

- **Electrolyte disturbance**. A consequence of increased mineralocorticoid activity (due to aldosterone and cortisol) is increased Na^+ and water reabsorption and increased K^+ excretion. Hypokalaemia is very common in hospitalised patients, particularly after major surgery and in critical illness. Hypokalaemia may result in muscle weakness, arrhythmias and ileus.
- **Fluid overload**. Excess ADH and mineralocorticoid activity, along with intravenous fluid administration, can result in fluid overload, precipitating left ventricular failure in susceptible patients and contributing to wound breakdown and anastomotic leak.
- **Thromboembolism**. The stress response produces a pro-coagulant state, increasing the risk of deep-vein thrombosis and pulmonary embolus.
- **Immunological**. Cortisol, released as part of the stress response, has significant effects on T cells. Cortisol stimulates the division of $CD8^+$ cytotoxic T cells, which in turn suppresses the division of $CD4^+$ T helper cells. Overall, the effect on T helper cells results in the body being more susceptible to invading pathogens. Cortisol also decreases inflammation by decreasing capillary permeability, prostaglandin synthesis (through inhibition of the enzyme phospholipase), cytokine release and leukocyte migration.

How may anaesthetists reduce the stress response to surgery?

Looking through the list of adverse consequences of the stress response, it is likely to be advantageous if the stress response to surgery could be reduced or eliminated completely. As discussed above, the stress response is initiated by afferent sensory and auto-nomic neural input to the hypothalamus and by cytokine release. Methods to reduce the stress response include:

- **Epidural and spinal anaesthesia**. This is the most studied and most successful method of reducing the stress response. Preoperative neuraxial blockade prevents initiation of the stress response by afferent neural input, but does not influence cytokine release. Lumbar epidurals are more effective than thoracic epidurals at attenuating the stress response, as the lumbar autonomic nerves are less reliably blocked by thoracic epidurals. Neuraxial blockade also improves post-operative pain, reduces thromboembolic risk (especially in lower limb surgery) and reduces post-operative ileus.

- **Systemic opioids**. Opioids are well known to suppress the hypothalamic–pituitary–adrenal axis. High-dose fentanyl has been shown to abolish the stress response to abdominal and pelvic surgery, but increases the need for post-operative ventilation.

- **General anaesthetic agents**. Etomidate is an inhibitor of 11-β-hydroxylase in the adrenal cortex: an induction dose of etomidate reduces aldosterone and cortisol synthesis for up to 8 h (see Chapter 81). Other general anaesthetic agents appear to have minimal influence on the stress response.

- **Intraoperative warming**. Maintaining normothermia intraoperatively has been shown to reduce the magnitude of the stress response.

- **Surgical technique**. Surgeons also have a role to play in reducing the stress response to surgery. Laparoscopic and other minimally invasive surgical techniques are associated with reduced cytokine release compared with the equivalent open procedures.

Further reading

F. Fant, E. Tina, D. Sandblom, et al. Thoracic epidural analgesia inhibits the neuro-hormonal but not the acute inflammatory stress response after radical retropubic prostatectomy. *Br J Anaesth* 2013; **110**(5): 747–57.

M. Mikura, I. Yamaoka, M. Doi, et al. Glucose infusion suppresses surgery-induced muscle protein breakdown by inhibiting ubiquitin–proteasome pathway in rats. *Anaesthesiology* 2009; **110**(1): 81–8.

D. Burton, G. Nicholson, G. Flail. Endocrine and metabolic response to surgery. *Continuing Educ Anaesth Crit Care Pain* 2004; **4**(5): 144–7.

J. P. Desborough. The stress response to trauma and surgery. *Br J Anaesth* 2000; **85**(1): 109–17.

Hypothalamus and Pituitary

What is a hormone?

A hormone is a substance released by a cell, gland or organ into the blood, allowing it to exert its signalling effects on tissues elsewhere in the body.

What types of hormone exist?

Hormones are classified on the basis of their chemical structure:

- **Peptide hormones**, the most common type, may be subclassified as:

  - *Short peptide chains*; for example, thyrotropin-releasing hormone (TRH), antidiuretic hormone (ADH), adrenocorticotrophic hormone (ACTH) and insulin;
  - *Longer protein chains*; for example, growth hormone (GH) and prolactin (PRL);
  - *Glycopeptides*: a protein chain with carbohydrate groups attached; for example, luteinising hormone (LH), follicle-stimulating hormone (FSH) and thyroid-stimulating hormone (TSH).

  In general, peptide hormones are stored in granules and are released into the circulation by exocytosis. Once they reach their target tissue, peptide hormones exert their effects by binding to cell surface receptors.

- **Lipid- and phospholipid-derived hormones**, of which there are two main subtypes:

  - *Steroid hormones*; for example, aldosterone, testosterone, oestrogen and cortisol;
  - *Eicosanoids*; for example, prostaglandins, thromboxanes and leukotrienes.

  The steroid hormones are all derived from cholesterol, whilst the eicosanoids are derived from the phospholipid bilayer of cell membranes. Both types of lipid-derived hormone are synthesised as required and immediately released

into the circulation; neither is stored. The high lipid solubility of steroid hormones allows them to diffuse across target cell membranes, where they exert their effects by binding to cytosolic receptors. The steroid hormone–receptor complex then travels to the cell nucleus, where it influences gene transcription. The eicosanoids have a wide range of functions in the body and their mechanisms of action are complex.

- **Monoamine derivatives**; that is, hormones derived from a single amino acid. For example:

  - *Catecholamines* are synthesised from phenylalanine or tyrosine.
  - *Serotonin* is derived from tryptophan.
  - *Thyroxine* is derived from tyrosine.

  The monoamine-derived hormones behave very differently:

  - Catecholamines and serotonin are stored in granules prior to release, whilst thyroxine is incorporated within thyroglobulin (see Chapter 81).
  - Catecholamines and serotonin exert their effects at the target tissue through cell membrane receptors, whilst thyroxine binds to receptors at the cell nucleus.

What are the functions of the hypothalamus?

The hypothalamus is located below the thalamus, making up the ventral part of the diencephalon. Though relatively small, the hypothalamus exerts control over a large number of body functions, acting as the link between brain, autonomic nervous system and endocrine system. The functions of the hypothalamus may be classified as:

- **Autonomic.** The hypothalamus receives inputs from the limbic system and relays them to the medulla oblongata. Thus, emotional stress (e.g. fear) triggers a sympathetic nervous system response.

- **Thermoregulation**. The hypothalamus integrates signals from peripheral and central (hypothalamic) thermoreceptors and controls the balance of activities of the two hypothalamic centres: the heat loss centre and the heat gain centre (see Chapter 89).
- **Regulation of hunger**. Food intake is controlled through the relative activities of the hypothalamic feeding and satiety centres. These centres are influenced by hypothalamic glucose concentration, gastrointestinal hormones (cholecystokinin and glucagon) and leptin (a hormone released from adipose tissue).
- **Regulation of body water**. As discussed in Chapter 69, the hypothalamus regulates body water through two mechanisms:
    - *The thirst centre* controls water intake.
    - *Osmoreceptors* control renal water excretion, in conjunction with ADH secretion by the pituitary gland.
- **Control of sleep–wake cycles**. Stimulation of the anterior hypothalamus leads to sleep, whilst stimulation of the posterior hypothalamus causes wakefulness. Circadian rhythms are thought to originate in the hypothalamus.
- **Control of pituitary function**. The hypothalamus exerts control over the pituitary gland through two mechanisms:
    - *The anterior lobe* is controlled by the secretion of hypothalamic hormones into the long portal vein.
    - *The posterior lobe* is controlled by direct neural connections from the hypothalamus.
- **Behaviour**. The hypothalamus contains 'punishment' and 'reward' centres, which moderate behaviour.
- **Regulation of sexual function**. The hypothalamus controls the pulsatile release of gonadotropins and the surge of gonadotropins that leads to ovulation.

Describe the anatomy of the pituitary gland

The pituitary gland is a pea-sized gland located in the sella turcica, a depression in the sphenoid bone at the base of the skull. The pituitary gland is situated directly below the hypothalamus, to which it is connected by the pituitary stalk. The pituitary gland is almost entirely covered superiorly by a fold of dura mater called the diaphragma sella; a gap allows the pituitary stalk to pass through.

The pituitary gland lies close to some key structures:

- *Superiorly*, the pituitary stalk, optic chiasm and third ventricle;
- *Laterally*, the cavernous sinus, which contains cranial nerves III, IV, VI, V_1 and V_2, and the internal carotid artery (ICA).

The pituitary gland itself comprises two main lobes, anterior (larger) and posterior, which are separated by a small pars intermedia. These lobes have different embryological origins:

- **The anterior lobe**, or adenohypophysis, develops from a depression of oral ectoderm in the embryo's pharynx, known as Rathke's pouch.
- **The posterior lobe**, or neurohypophysis, develops from a downgrowth of neural ectoderm from the hypothalamus. The posterior lobe never separates from the hypothalamus; the downgrowth persists as the pituitary stalk.
- **The pars intermedia** is a very thin layer of cells located between the anterior and posterior lobes that also develops from Rathke's pouch. It is often considered to be part of the anterior lobe and is not well developed in humans.

Describe the blood supply to the pituitary gland

The blood supply to the pituitary gland is complex.

- **The anterior lobe** receives blood from:
    - *The superior hypophyseal artery*, a branch of the ICA.
    - *The long portal veins*, which supply the anterior lobe with the majority of its blood. A portal vein connects two capillary networks. The long portal veins connect the capillary network of the lower hypothalamus and pituitary stalk to the capillary network of the anterior lobe. Thus, hormones released by the neurosecretory cells of the hypothalamus are delivered directly to the anterior lobe.
    - *The short portal veins*, which transport some capillary blood from the posterior lobe to the capillary networks of the anterior lobe.

- **The posterior lobe** receives blood from the inferior hypophyseal artery, a branch of the ICA.

Venous blood from both anterior and posterior lobes drains into the cavernous sinuses.

Which hormones does the hypothalamus secrete?

The hypothalamus secretes six hormones into the long portal vein, which exert control over the anterior lobe of the pituitary gland:

- *TRH*, which stimulates the release of TSH;
- *Gonadotropin-releasing hormone* (GnRH), which causes the release of FSH and LH;
- *Corticotropin-releasing hormone* (CRH), which triggers the secretion of ACTH;
- *GH-releasing hormone* (GHRH), which stimulates the release of GH;
- *Somatostatin*, which inhibits GH release and also moderately inhibits TSH release;
- *Dopamine*, which inhibits the release of PRL.

What is meant by the term 'hypothalamic–pituitary axis'?

The hypothalamic–pituitary axis refers to the set of complex endocrine interactions between the hypothalamus, the anterior lobe of the pituitary gland and the target organ. Hormone secretion by the hypothalamus and anterior lobe is controlled by two negative-feedback loops (Figure 80.1):

- **Short-loop feedback** – hormones secreted by the anterior lobe inhibit the release of their respective hypothalamic hormones.
- **Long-loop feedback** – the peripheral endocrine glands secrete hormones in response to anterior lobe hormones (e.g. cortisol is secreted by the adrenal cortex in response to ACTH). The resulting peripheral hormones then inhibit further secretion of both pituitary and hypothalamic hormones.

Which hormones are secreted by the anterior lobe?

The anterior lobe secretes six hormones, classified as:

- **Directly acting hormones** – PRL and GH. These hormones exert their effects through PRL and GH receptors at their target tissues.

- **Stimulating hormones** – TSH, FSH, LH and ACTH. These hormones act at their respective endocrine glands, stimulating them to release thyroid hormones, oestrogen, testosterone and cortisol, respectively. Their endocrine axes are named:
  - The hypothalamic–pituitary–thyroid axis;
  - The hypothalamic–pituitary–gonadal axis;
  - The hypothalamic–pituitary–adrenal axis.

Taking each anterior lobe hormone in turn:

- **TSH** is a glycoprotein hormone that acts on the thyroid gland, promoting the synthesis and release of the biologically active thyroid hormone T_3 and its precursor T_4. TSH release is promoted by hypothalamic TRH release and inhibited by negative feedback from circulating T_3.
- **LH** is a glycoprotein hormone. In females, a rapid increase in LH stimulates ovulation; following ovulation, LH promotes the development of the corpus luteum. In males, LH stimulates the synthesis and secretion of testosterone by Leydig cells.
- **FSH** is also a glycoprotein hormone. In females, FSH promotes oestrogen synthesis and the development of ovarian follicles. In males, FSH aids sperm maturation. FSH and LH are collectively known as gonadotropins. FSH and LH secretion is promoted by the pulsatile release of hypothalamic GnRH and is inhibited by negative feedback from circulating testosterone or oestrogen.
- **ACTH** is a small peptide hormone that exerts its effects on the adrenal gland. In response to ACTH, cortisol is released from the zona fasiculata. ACTH release is promoted by CRH release from the hypothalamus and is inhibited by feedback from circulating cortisol. Of interest, ACTH is degraded over time to produce α-melanocyte-stimulating hormone (α-MSH), which accounts for the pigmentation of skin that occurs in Addison's disease when ACTH levels are high.
- **GH** is a protein hormone that has anabolic effects on tissues throughout the body. GH has two types of effect:
  - *Direct effects.* GH stimulates lipolysis through its action on adipose cell GH receptors, thus increasing the concentration of circulating fatty acids.

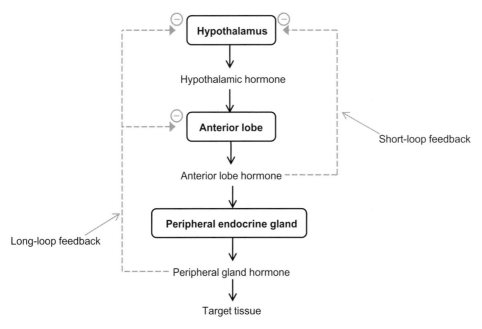

Figure 80.1 Feedback loops and the hypothalamic–pituitary axis.

– *Indirect effects.* The majority of GH effects are mediated through insulin-like growth factor 1 (IGF-1), a hormone secreted by the liver in response to circulating GH. IGF-1 promotes cell growth and development.

GH is released from the pituitary gland in a pulsatile fashion, particularly at night. Regulation of pituitary GH secretion is complex: GH secretion is promoted by the release of hypothalamic GHRH, but is inhibited by hypothalamic secretion of somatostatin. In addition, GH secretion is part of a negative-feedback loop in which IGF-1 inhibits pituitary secretion of GH. Overall, plasma GH concentration is usually very low, but it is increased at times of physiological stress, hypoglycaemia and exercise.

- **PRL** is a protein hormone that has an important role in lactation, where it promotes breast development during pregnancy and induces milk production following delivery. Regulation of PRL release is different from that of the other anterior lobe hormones: there is no hypothalamic stimulating hormone. Instead, the hypothalamus controls PRL secretion through tonic dopamine release, which in turn inhibits pituitary PRL release. In the context of breastfeeding, PRL secretion is stimulated by suckling. PRL concentration also rises following sexual intercourse and as part of the stress response; PRL concentration is raised following an epileptic seizure. Tumours may also increase prolactin concentration both as a direct result of increased secretion (adenomas) and from compression of the pituitary stalk, which prevents dopamine from travelling to the anterior pituitary.

In addition, the pars intermedia secretes a seventh hormone: α-MSH. Increased α-MSH secretion is responsible for the skin pigmentation of pregnancy and in Addison's disease.

Which hormones are released by the posterior lobe?

The posterior lobe of the pituitary gland releases two hormones: ADH and oxytocin. It is important to note that these hormones are not synthesised in the posterior lobe. Instead, the two hormones are synthesised in the hypothalamus, packaged into tiny vesicles, transported to the posterior lobe through nerve axons and stored in granules within the nerve terminals. Following an action potential from the hypothalamus, the storage granules are released into the systemic circulation.

The two posterior lobe hormones are:

- **ADH**, a small peptide hormone with two main physiological effects:

– *Antidiuretic effects*: ADH acts in the kidney, where it causes the insertion of water channels (aquaporins) and urea transporters (UT-A1) into the cell membrane of collecting duct cells, thus increasing water reabsorption (see Chapter 69). ADH is primarily secreted in response to increased plasma osmolarity. Again, there is a negative-feedback loop, in that ADH secretion increases water reabsorption by the kidney. This decreases plasma osmolarity, which in turn decreases ADH secretion.

– *Vasoconstriction*, hence the alternative name for ADH: vasopressin. At normal concentrations, ADH seems to contribute little to the resting tone of arterioles. In high concentrations, ADH acts as a powerful vasoconstrictor. In hypovolaemic shock, the dramatic increase in ADH secretion is an important compensatory mechanism for restoring systemic blood pressure.

ADH is also secreted in times of physiological stress; ADH secretion is inhibited by alcohol, leading to a diuresis.

- **Oxytocin**, a small peptide hormone that is structurally very similar to ADH. The best-known effects of oxytocin are:

  – *Contraction of uterine smooth muscle during labour*. Oxytocin is released by the posterior lobe in response to stretching of the cervix by the foetal head.

  – *The let-down reflex in lactation*. Oxytocin is secreted in response to suckling, where it stimulates contraction of myoepithelial cells in the mammary glands, which squeeze newly produced milk into the duct system.

  – *Psychological*. Oxytocin is involved in pair bonding, particularly between mother and child following birth. Studies suggest it is also important for generating trust between adults and it has therefore earned the nickname 'cuddle hormone'.

Clinical relevance: pituitary adenoma

Tumours of the anterior lobe of the pituitary gland are usually benign. However, they still have significant clinical consequences, presenting in four ways:

- **Hormone hypersecretion**. Functional pituitary tumours (i.e. those that secrete hormones) tend to become apparent at a smaller size owing to the clinical effects of hormone hypersecretion. For example, PRL hypersecretion causes galactorrhoea.
- **Hormone hyposecretion**. Larger pituitary tumours tend to be non-secreting. These large tumours encroach on the surrounding normal pituitary cells with the potential to cause hypothyroidism, adrenocortical insufficiency or infertility.
- **Mass effect**. Larger pituitary tumours compress important structures surrounding the pituitary gland: the optic chiasm (which classically results in a bitemporal hemianopia), cranial nerves (which result in cranial nerve palsy) and the third ventricle (which may cause an obstructive hydrocephalus).
- **Incidental finding**. Many pituitary adenomas are now identified when the brain undergoes computed tomography or magnetic resonance imaging for another reason.

Patients with pituitary adenomas may present the anaesthetist with a number of problems:

- **Nature of surgery**. Pituitary debulking surgery is commonly carried out via the trans-sphenoidal route, which has implications for the anaesthetist, such as shared airway and the requirements of minimal haemodynamic instability and a smooth extubation.
- **Co-morbidities**. Cushing's disease results from an ACTH-secreting adenoma. It is associated with hypertension and diabetes mellitus. Acromegaly (a GH-secreting adenoma) is also associated with hypertension and diabetes, as well as cardiomyopathy and sleep apnoea.
- **Implications for the airway**. A combination of macrognathia, macroglossia and upper airway soft tissue expansion can potentially make acromegalic patients difficult to intubate.

Further reading

P. E. Molina. *Endocrine Physiology, 5th edition*. New York, McGraw-Hill, 2018.

R. Menon, P. G. Murphy, A. M. Lindley. Anaesthesia and pituitary disease. *Continuing Educ Anaesth Crit Care Pain* 2011; **11**(4): 133–7.

M. Lim, D. Williams, N. Maartens. Anaesthesia for pituitary surgery, *J Clin Neurosci* 2006; **13**(4): 413–18.

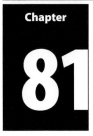

Chapter

81

Thyroid, Parathyroid and Adrenal

The thyroid gland

Which hormones are synthesised by the thyroid gland?

The thyroid gland is located in the anterior neck and consists of two lobes connected by an isthmus. It secretes two hormones:

- **Triiodothyronine** (T_3), the strongly biologically active thyroid hormone. T_3 comprises only 10% of the hormones released by the thyroid gland. In the circulation, T_3 is very highly protein bound (99.7%), mainly to albumin, and has a short half-life (24 h). Only the unbound fraction of T_3 is able to diffuse into the tissues to exert its effects.
- **Thyroxine** (T_4), a weakly biologically active hormone, is the main hormone synthesised by the thyroid gland (90%). T_4 is also very highly protein bound, but mainly to a specific carrier protein: thyroxine-binding globulin. At 7 days, the half-life of T_4 is much longer than that of T_3. Around half of the weakly active T_4 is converted to the active form, T_3, in the peripheral tissues. The other half is converted to an inactive hormone called reverse T_3. Bound T_3 and T_4 provide a large reservoir of thyroid hormone, which delays the onset of symptoms in hypothyroidism.

What are the physiological effects of triiodothyronine?

T_3 is able to diffuse across cell membranes to reach the cell nucleus, where it regulates gene transcription. T_3 therefore has physiological effects on most tissue types in the body, with the exception of the spleen and the thyroid gland itself. The main physiological effects of T_3 are perhaps best illustrated when T_3 concentration is either abnormally high or low, as occurs in hyperthyroidism and hypothyroidism, respectively:

- **Metabolism**. T_3 affects the activity of a wide range of metabolic processes, such as lipolysis and gluconeogenesis. Hyperthyroidism results in an increase in basal metabolic rate (BMR) and an increased availability of metabolic substrates, such as free fatty acids and glucose. In hypothyroidism, the opposite occurs.
- **Growth and development**. Hypothyroidism in childhood causes growth retardation. T_3 is especially important in the development of the central nervous system (CNS), where it stimulates neuronal myelination and nerve axon growth.
- **Respiratory system**. In hyperthyroidism, O_2 consumption and CO_2 production are increased due to the increase in BMR. In turn, $\dot{V}_E$ increases.
- **Cardiovascular system**. In hyperthyroidism, T_3 increases the number of β-adrenergic receptors in the heart. The result is an increase in heart rate (HR) and myocardial contractility, leading to an increase in cardiac output.
- **CNS**. T_3 has an important effect on mood: in hypothyroidism, depression and psychosis may occur, whilst hyperthyroidism is associated with anxiety.
- **Musculoskeletal system**. In hyperthyroidism, T_3 induces protein catabolism, which predominantly affects proximal muscles, resulting in proximal myopathy.

How are triiodothyronine and thyroxine synthesised?

The thyroid gland is made up of multiple follicles: spheres of follicular cells surrounding a core of thyroglobulin, a large protein containing many tyrosine residues. T_3 and T_4 are synthesised as follows (Figure 81.1):

- **Iodide (I^-) uptake**. I^- is actively transported from the circulation to the follicular cells through a Na^+/I^- co-transporter. As a result of this secondary active transport, 25% of the body's I^- is

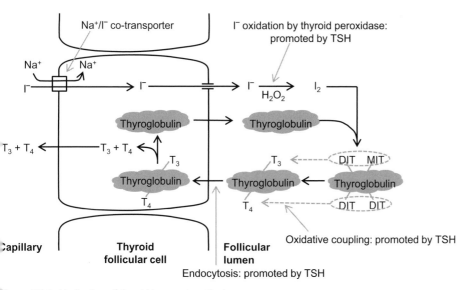

Figure 81.1 Mechanism of thyroid hormone synthesis.

stored within the thyroid. The uptake of I^- is stimulated by thyroid-stimulating hormone (TSH). I^- diffuses through the follicular cell and into the follicular lumen.

- **I^- oxidation.** As I^- is relatively inert, it must be oxidised to the more reactive iodine (I_2) by thyroid peroxidase involving hydrogen peroxide (H_2O_2), a reaction that is promoted by TSH.

  I_2 reaction with tyrosine. Once synthesised, I_2 reacts with the tyrosine residues of the surrounding thyroglobulin protein. Tyrosine may be iodinated at one or two positions, resulting in mono-iodotyrosine (MIT) or di-iodotyrosine (DIT), respectively.

- **Oxidative coupling.** Two of the iodinated tyrosine molecules are then coupled together. If two DIT molecules join, the resulting compound is T_4; if MIT is coupled to DIT, the result is T_3. This oxidative coupling of tyrosine residues is promoted by TSH.

The end result of this process is small T_3 and T_4 molecules dispersed throughout the large thyroglobulin protein.[1] It is estimated that the thyroid gland contains a sufficient store of T_3 and T_4 to meet the body's requirements for 1–3 months. In response to TSH, droplets of thyroglobulin are endocytosed by

the follicular cells. Within the follicular cell, T_3 and T_4 are separated from thyroglobulin and released into the circulation.

How is the plasma concentration of thyroid hormones regulated?

TSH has multiple roles in both the synthesis and release of thyroid hormones. TSH is released by the anterior lobe of the pituitary gland in response to hypothalamic secretion of thyrotropin-releasing hormone (TRH; see Chapter 80). In turn, TRH release is controlled through a negative-feedback loop: T_3, the biologically active thyroid hormone, inhibits the release of TRH at the hypothalamus. T_3 is highly protein bound; only the unbound fraction is able to inhibit the hypothalamus.

Disturbances in the hypothalamic–pituitary–thyroid axis usually result from thyroid gland dysfunction:

- **Hypothyroidism** most commonly results from Hashimoto's thyroiditis, an autoimmune disease of the thyroid gland in which antibodies are directed against thyroid peroxidase or thyroglobulin. The result is a reduction in T_3 and T_4 secretion. In response, the hypothalamus and anterior lobe of the pituitary gland increase their secretion of TRH and TSH, respectively; a high measured TSH normally implies hypothyroidism.

- **Hyperthyroidism** is most commonly due to Graves' disease, an autoimmune condition that

---

This is why thyroglobulin is often called a colloid; that is, a substance dispersed within another substance.

results in increased synthesis and secretion of T_3 and T_4. The hypothalamus and anterior lobe of the pituitary gland respond by decreasing their secretion of TRH and TSH. A low measured TSH normally implies hyperthyroidism.

What is Graves' disease?

Graves' disease is an autoimmune disease: autoantibodies stimulate TSH receptors in the thyroid gland, causing excessive synthesis and release of T_3 and T_4. The clinical effects of Graves' disease can be divided into:

- **Those due to hyperthyroidism.** Symptoms include palpitations, heat intolerance, weight loss despite increased appetite, fine tremor, diarrhoea and excessive sweating. Clinical signs include sinus tachycardia, atrial fibrillation, lid lag and a smooth, diffusely enlarged thyroid gland (a 'goitre').
- **Those caused by the autoantibodies.** Graves' eye disease is caused by the same TSH receptor autoantibodies that also target fibroblasts in the extraocular muscles. The resulting inflammation causes exophthalmos (upper lid retraction), proptosis (bulging eyes) and conjunctivitis.

What are the management options in Graves' disease?

There are three treatment options in hyperthyroidism:

- **Anti-thyroid drugs.** Carbimazole and propylthiouracil mainly act by inhibiting the thyroid peroxidase-catalysed oxidation of I^- to I_2. Without I_2, the iodination of tyrosine cannot occur.
- **Radioiodine.** As discussed above, I^- is actively concentrated in the thyroid gland. Likewise, radioactive iodine (^{131}I) is also actively taken up by the thyroid gland, where the β-radiation emitted causes damage and necrosis of thyroid tissue.
- **Surgery.** Total thyroidectomy is a permanent solution to hyperthyroidism, but carries additional risks: recurrent laryngeal nerve injury, parathyroid gland damage and post-operative haematoma, which may cause airway obstruction.

All of the above options (usually) render the patient hypothyroid: T_4 replacement is therefore required. None of the above options have any effect on Graves' eye disease. As it is mediated by autoantibodies,

severe Graves' eye disease may be treated with corticosteroids or by surgical debulking.

Clinical relevance: anaesthesia for thyroid surgery

There are many indications for thyroid surgery: thyroid malignancy, hyperthyroidism and goitre with associated complications, such as tracheal compression. Anaesthesia for thyroid surgery may be particularly challenging owing to the proximity of the thyroid gland to the trachea.

Prior to thyroid surgery, the patient should be rendered euthyroid by one of the medical methods above. In addition to the usual clinical assessments of the airway, a computed tomography scan of the neck may be used to assess the size and position of any goitre. It is also important to identify compression or invasion of the structures surrounding the thyroid gland: the trachea (resulting in stridor), superior vena cava (obstruction), sympathetic chain (Horner's syndrome) and recurrent laryngeal nerve (hoarse voice).

Induction of anaesthesia may require a gaseous or awake fibre-optic technique if the trachea is compressed or the anatomy significantly distorted. Occasionally, the only airway option is a tracheostomy performed under local anaesthesia. Intraoperative electrophysiological testing of the recurrent laryngeal nerve may preclude the use of muscle relaxants following induction – a remifentanil infusion is therefore commonly used.

A number of serious post-operative complications may occur:

- **Haemorrhage,** which can cause tracheal compression and rapid airway obstruction. Any suspicion of developing airway obstruction warrants an urgent surgical review and removal of the surgical clips – a clip remover should be kept at the patient's bedside.
- **Recurrent laryngeal nerve palsy,** which may be due to surgical retraction or transection and may be unilateral or bilateral. Bilateral recurrent laryngeal nerve palsy results in complete adduction of the vocal cords and therefore complete airway obstruction. Immediate reintubation is required and a tracheostomy may be necessary.
- **Severe hypocalcaemia** – the parathyroid glands may be inadvertently damaged or excised during thyroid surgery, resulting in hypocalcaemia. The signs and symptoms of hypocalcaemia are discussed below. Of note: severe hypocalcaemia may result in laryngospasm.
- **Tracheomalacia,** characterised by flaccid tracheal cartilage that collapses on inspiration, resulting in airway obstruction. Patients who

have long-standing or very large goitres are at much greater risk of tracheomalacia. Prior to extubation, it is useful to deflate the endotracheal tube cuff to check for air leak.

Regulation of calcium homeostasis

What are the physiological functions of calcium?

Ca^{2+} has numerous biological roles, the most important of which are:

- **Structural** – calcium phosphate gives bone its rigidity.
- **Haemostasis** – Ca^{2+} is an essential cofactor in the coagulation cascade. Blood samples are prevented from clotting through the addition of EDTA or citrate, which irreversibly binds Ca^{2+} (see Chapter 72).
- **Resting membrane potential** (RMP) – extracellular Ca^{2+} concentration affects the cell membrane Na^+ permeability, which in turn affects the RMP of excitable cells. Hypocalcaemia acts to depolarise the cell membrane towards the threshold potential. Thus, nerves may undergo spontaneous depolarisation, resulting in tetany (see Chapter 52). Clinical signs of hypocalcaemia include Trousseau's sign (carpal spasm following inflation of a blood pressure cuff) and Chvostek's sign (inducing facial spasm when tapping over the zygoma).
- **Neurotransmitter release** – Ca^{2+} influx into the terminal bouton triggers the exocytosis of vesicles filled with neurotransmitter into the synaptic cleft (see Chapter 53).
- **Excitation–contraction coupling** – Ca^{2+} influx into skeletal, cardiac or smooth muscle is essential for the binding of myosin to actin (see Chapters 54, 56 and 57).
- **Cell signalling** – Ca^{2+} is an important second messenger. For example, G proteins that act via inositol triphosphate use Ca^{2+} as the intracellular messenger.

What proportion of body calcium is located in the plasma?

The proportion of body Ca^{2+} located in the plasma is actually very low:

- The mass of Ca^{2+} in an adult is approximately 1 kg.
- Almost all Ca^{2+} is located in bone (99%). This Ca^{2+} cannot be rapidly mobilised. The remaining 1% is located in teeth and soft tissues.
- Only 0.1% of body Ca^{2+} is located in the extracellular fluid (ECF) and only a third of this is located in the plasma.

The normal range of plasma Ca^{2+} is 2.2–2.6 mmol/L. Only around 45% of plasma Ca^{2+} is in the biologically active ionised form. The remaining 55% is either protein bound or associated with various anions, such as HCO_3^-, citrate and phosphate. It is important to note that whilst the total amount of plasma Ca^{2+} falls when albumin is low, the ionised portion of Ca^{2+} remains the same. Plasma Ca^{2+} can be mathematically corrected for hypoalbuminaemia[2] or, alternatively, ionised Ca^{2+} can be measured by arterial blood gas analysis. The normal range for ionised Ca^{2+} is 1.1–1.4 mmol/L.

How is plasma calcium concentration regulated?

Logically, plasma Ca^{2+} concentration may be altered by:

- An increase or decrease in intestinal absorption of dietary Ca^{2+};
- An increase or decrease in renal excretion of Ca^{2+} salts;
- Movement of Ca^{2+} between body compartments.

Three hormones are involved in Ca^{2+} homeostasis. Parathyroid hormone (PTH) and vitamin D act to increase plasma Ca^{2+} concentration, whilst calcitonin acts to decrease plasma Ca^{2+} concentration:

- **PTH** is a protein hormone secreted by the parathyroid glands. There are usually four parathyroid glands, located on the posterior surface of the thyroid gland. Plasma Ca^{2+} concentration is sensed by parathyroid Ca^{2+}-sensing receptors (CaSRs). Low plasma Ca^{2+} triggers PTH secretion, which acts at:
  - *The kidney.* Here, it increases Ca^{2+} reabsorption and decreases phosphate reabsorption.

---

[2] Corrected Ca^{2+} = measured Ca^{2+} + 0.02 × (40 – serum albumin), where Ca^{2+} is measured in mmol/L and albumin in g/L. Therefore, each 1-g/L decrease in serum albumin decreases plasma Ca^{2+} by 0.02 mmol/L.

- – *Bone*. Here, it increases the activity of osteoclast cells (the cells that resorb bone), releasing stored Ca^{2+}.
- – *The intestine*. This is an indirect effect: PTH upregulates the renal enzyme 1-α-hydroxylase, which is responsible for activating vitamin D (see below). Vitamin D increases the intestinal absorption of dietary Ca^{2+} and phosphate.

- **Vitamin D**, a steroid hormone. Vitamin D must go through a series of modifications before it can exert its effects (Figure 81.2):
  - – *In the skin*: cholecalciferol (vitamin D_3) is synthesised through the effects of sunlight on 7-dehydrocholesterol in the skin. Cholecalciferol also originates in the diet; vitamin D is not a vitamin in the strictest sense: individuals who have adequate exposure to sunlight do not require dietary supplementation.
  - – *In the liver*: vitamin D_3 is 25-hydroxylated by the enzyme 25-hydroxylase, resulting in calcidiol (25-hydroxy vitamin D_3).
  - – *In the kidney*: calcidiol is 1-α-hydroxylated to give calcitriol (1,25-dihydroxy vitamin D_3),

the biologically active form of vitamin D. The enzyme that catalyses this process is 1-α-hydroxylase, which is upregulated by PTH.

Vitamin D increases plasma Ca^{2+} concentration through its actions on:

- – *The intestine*, where the absorption of dietary Ca^{2+} and phosphate is increased.
- – *The kidney*, where Ca^{2+} and phosphate reabsorption is increased.

In addition, vitamin D acts on the bone, where it increases bone calcification.

It is important to note that, under normal circumstances, the rate-determining step in the synthesis of calcitriol is 1-α-hydroxylation. PTH controls the activity of the enzyme involved in this step; PTH therefore directly controls the plasma concentration of calcitriol.

- **Calcitonin** is a peptide hormone secreted by the parafollicular C cells of the thyroid gland. Calcitonin has a minor role in Ca^{2+} homeostasis in humans, only being secreted when plasma Ca^{2+} rises above 2.4 mmol/L. Calcitonin decreases plasma Ca^{2+} concentration through its actions on:
  - – *The intestine*, where it decreases the absorption of dietary Ca^{2+} and phosphate;
  - – *The kidney*, where it decreases the reabsorption of Ca^{2+} and phosphate and decreases the activity of the enzyme 1-α-hydroxylase, thereby decreasing the effects of vitamin D.
  - – *Bone*, where osteoclast activity is decreased, thereby decreasing bone resorption.

Other hormones such as gonadal steroids (increase bone density), glucocorticoids (decrease bone density) and growth hormone (increase bone density) also affect Ca^{2+} homeostasis.

In summary:

- **Low plasma ionised Ca^{2+} concentration:**
  - – Increases parathyroid PTH secretion, which, in turn, increases the rate of vitamin D activation.
  - – The combined effects of vitamin D and PTH increase intestinal absorption and renal reabsorption of Ca^{2+}. The effect on bone is negligible, as the increase in bone resorption by PTH is cancelled out by the bone calcification effect of vitamin D.

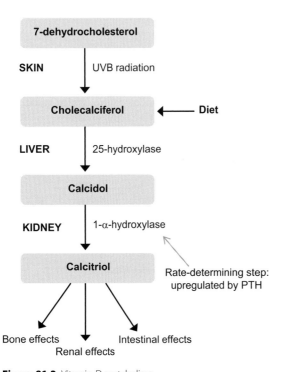

Figure 81.2 Vitamin D metabolism.

- **High plasma ionised Ca^{2+} concentration**:
  - Decreases PTH secretion and, in turn, decreases the rate of activation of vitamin D. In addition, the parafollicular C cells release calcitonin.
  - The combined effect of reduced PTH, reduced vitamin D and increased calcitonin results in a decrease in intestinal Ca^{2+} absorption and renal Ca^{2+} reabsorption.

Clinical relevance: kidney and liver dysfunction

As discussed above, 25-hydroxylation of vitamin D occurs in the liver and 1-α-hydroxylation occurs in the kidney.

In chronic kidney disease (CKD), 1-α-hydroxylation of calcidiol is impaired – activated vitamin D cannot be synthesised. Without vitamin D, renal excretion of Ca^{2+} exceeds intestinal absorption, resulting in hypocalcaemia. PTH secretion increases as the parathyroid glands attempt to normalise plasma ionised Ca^{2+} concentration. This is referred to as secondary hyperparathyroidism. PTH causes extensive demineralisation of the bones as Ca^{2+} is redistributed to the ECF, resulting in renal osteodystrophy. Patients with CKD are treated with a pre-activated form of vitamin D, alfacalcidol, thereby bypassing the renal 1-α-hydroxylation mechanism.

The aetiology of bone disease in cirrhosis patients is more complex than in CKD; for example, alcoholism is associated with a dietary Ca^{2+} deficiency and haemochromatosis is complicated by gonadal failure, which is associated with osteoporosis. Severe liver dysfunction may also cause impaired 25-hydroxylation of cholecalciferol: activated vitamin D levels are low, which contributes to bone disease.

Clinical relevance: hyperparathyroidism

Other than surgery, hyperparathyroidism may also be treated using the 'calcimimetic', cinacalcet. Cinacalcet increases the sensitivity of the CaSR, resulting in decreased PTH secretion. It has been used in primary, secondary and tertiary hyperparathyroidism.

The adrenal glands

Describe the anatomy of the adrenal glands

The adrenal glands are triangular organs closely related to the superior poles of the kidneys at the level of the T12 vertebral body. Each adrenal gland is surrounded by a protective fat pad and renal fascia. The adrenal gland consists of two distinct parts that differ in their embryological origins:

- **The (outer) adrenal cortex** makes up 70% of the adrenal glands' weight. The adrenal cortex is derived from mesoderm and is composed of three layers:[3]
  - *Zona glomerulosa*, the outermost layer, is the main site of aldosterone production.
  - *Zona fasciculata*, the middle layer, is the main site of glucocorticoid synthesis.
  - *Zona reticularis*, the inner layer, produces androgens. The main androgens produced are dehydroepiandrosterone and androstenedione. These are weak androgens that are converted to testosterone by the peripheral tissues.
- **The (inner) adrenal medulla** is innervated by T5–T9 pre-ganglionic sympathetic neurons; the adrenal medulla can be considered to be a modified sympathetic ganglion. Sympathetic nervous system activity stimulates the chromaffin cells to release granules containing adrenaline (approximately 80%) and noradrenaline (approximately 20%).

Discuss the physiology of aldosterone

Aldosterone is a steroid hormone produced by the zona glomerulosa. It accounts for 95% of the mineralocorticoid activity in the body, with cortisol contributing much of the remainder. It therefore promotes Na^+ and water reabsorption, along with K^+ and H^+ excretion. Aldosterone therefore plays an important role in the regulation of blood volume and consequently blood pressure.

There are four main triggers to aldosterone secretion:

- **Angiotensin II** is the most important factor in aldosterone release. The renin–angiotensin–aldosterone axis is a complex feedback loop that helps regulate blood volume. As discussed in Chapter 67, the main trigger for renin release is a reduction in renal blood flow (RBF). Renin converts angiotensinogen to angiotensin I.

---

[3] A mnemonic for remembering the order of these layers is: GFR – glomerulosa, fasiculata, reticularis. A mnemonic for remembering the hormones secreted by each layer is: ACTH – aldosterone, cortisol, 'testosterone' hormones.

Angiotensin I is converted to angiotensin II by angiotensin-converting enzyme in the lungs. Angiotensin II then triggers aldosterone release, amongst other effects. Aldosterone increases plasma volume, thereby restoring RBF.

- **Hyperkalaemia** directly stimulates aldosterone secretion from the adrenal cortex. Similarly, hypokalaemia decreases aldosterone secretion.
- **Plasma acidosis** directly stimulates aldosterone release, which in turn promotes renal H^+ secretion.
- **Adrenocorticotropic hormone** (ACTH), whose main role is stimulating the release of cortisol (see p. 402), plays a minor role in aldosterone secretion.

What are the functions of cortisol?

Cortisol is a steroid hormone secreted mainly by the zona fasiculata. It is the main glucocorticoid of the body; corticosterone, which has a closely related chemical structure, has a minor role. Cortisol is important in the physiological response to stress and has actions throughout the body, the most important of which are:

- **Metabolic**, essentially the opposite to those of insulin:
  - *Mobilisation of amino acids* from skeletal muscle for use as substrates for gluconeogenesis.
  - *Stimulation of lipolysis*, which releases free fatty acids and glycerol. Glycerol is used as a substrate for gluconeogenesis.
  - *Peripheral glucose utilisation is decreased*, thus increasing plasma glucose concentration.
  - *Stimulation of gluconeogenesis*, which further increases plasma glucose concentration.
- **Cardiovascular**. Cortisol is essential for normal cardiovascular function. Cortisol increases the sensitivity of the vasculature to the effects of catecholamines – without cortisol, widespread vasodilatation occurs. The mineralocorticoid effects of cortisol result in an increase in plasma volume.

In chronic excess (e.g. in Cushing's disease), cortisol has additional effects:

- Osteoporosis;
- Anti-inflammatory and immunosuppressive effects;
- Effects on the CNS, such as psychosis and memory loss;
- Peptic ulceration.

How is cortisol secretion regulated?

Cortisol secretion is controlled by a negative-feedback loop involving the hypothalamus and pituitary gland:

- Corticotropin-releasing hormone (CRH) is released by the hypothalamus. Normally, CRH is released in a diurnal pattern, with peak release in the early morning. CRH release is increased under conditions of physiological stress, such as pain, infection and following surgery.
- ACTH is released from the anterior lobe of the pituitary gland in response to CRH.
- Cortisol is released from the zona fasiculata in response to ACTH. Some 90% of plasma cortisol is bound to cortisol-binding protein and albumin. Only 10% of plasma cortisol is unbound and therefore biologically active.
- The unbound fraction of cortisol inhibits CRH release from the hypothalamus and ACTH release from the anterior lobe of the pituitary gland.

Clinical relevance: etomidate

Etomidate is an intravenous anaesthetic induction agent with a reputation for cardiovascular stability. However, the use of etomidate has diminished since a study demonstrated an increased mortality rate when a continuous infusion of etomidate was used for the sedation of critically ill trauma patients.

The synthesis of steroid hormones is complex, involving many intermediate compounds. The final step in the biosynthesis of cortisol is hydroxylation of 11-deoxycortisol by the enzyme 11-β-hydroxylase. This enzyme is reversibly inhibited by etomidate. Etomidate therefore suppresses cortisol synthesis, which, at a times of physiological stress (e.g. the perioperative period and severe sepsis), has the potential for adrenocortical insufficiency.

Despite the theoretical risk of adrenocortical suppression, a single dose of etomidate for the rapid sequence induction of a critically ill patient has not been shown to increase mortality.

How are catecholamines synthesised in the adrenal medulla?

Structurally, catecholamines consist of catechol (a benzene ring with two hydroxyl groups) with an amine side chain. Catecholamines are derived from the amino acid tyrosine (Figure 81.3):

- Tyrosine is acquired from the diet or through the hydroxylation of phenylalanine in the liver.

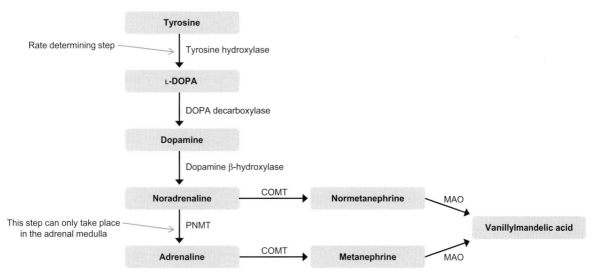

Figure 81.3 Catecholaminergic synthetic pathway.

- Tyrosine is taken up into the cytoplasm of chromaffin cells, where it is converted to L-3,4-dihydroxyphenylalanine (L-DOPA). This is the rate-determining step of catecholamine synthesis.
- L-DOPA is converted into dopamine.
- Dopamine is converted into noradrenaline.
- Noradrenaline is converted into adrenaline by the enzyme phenylethanolamine N-methyl transferase (PNMT). This enzyme is only present in the chromaffin cells of the adrenal medulla. Therefore, whilst noradrenaline may be synthesised elsewhere (e.g. sympathetic nerve terminals), adrenaline can only be synthesised within the adrenal medulla.
- Noradrenaline and adrenaline are then packaged into granules, which also contain ATP, chromogranin A and opioid peptides such as metenkephalin.

How is catecholamine secretion controlled?

Whilst the hormones of the adrenal cortex are controlled by negative-feedback loops, the catecholamines of the adrenal medulla are secreted in response to sympathetic nervous system activity; there is no negative-feedback control of catecholamine secretion.

Secretion of catecholamines takes place as follows:
- In response to various stimuli (exercise, trauma, pain, hypovolaemia, hypoglycaemia, hypothermia and anxiety), action potentials are generated in the pre-ganglionic sympathetic nerves that terminate on the chromaffin cells of the adrenal medulla.
- Like other pre-ganglionic sympathetic neurons (see Chapter 59), acetylcholine (ACh) is released from the terminal bouton.
- ACh activates nicotinic receptors on the chromaffin cell membrane, increasing cell membrane Na^+ and K^+ permeability, which results in net depolarisation.
- Membrane depolarisation opens voltage-gated Ca^{2+} channels; the influx of Ca^{2+} into the chromaffin cells triggers exocytosis of the catecholamine-containing granules, releasing adrenaline and noradrenaline into the circulation.

It is important to note that catecholamine release from the adrenal medulla does not take place in isolation – it is part of a wider sympathetic nervous response that includes extensive noradrenaline release at sympathetic nerve terminals.

What are the physiological effects of adrenaline and noradrenaline?

The most important physiological effects of adrenaline are:
- **Metabolic.** Adrenaline stimulates glycogenolysis, which in turn increases plasma glucose concentration. Free fatty acids are liberated from adipose tissue and amino acids are released from skeletal muscle.

- **Heart**. Adrenaline has positive chronotropic and positive inotropic effects on the heart, increasing HR and myocardial contractility, respectively, through stimulation of β_1-adrenergic receptors.
- **Vasculature**. Adrenaline causes peripheral vasoconstriction, except in skeletal muscle capillary beds, where it causes vasodilatation.
- **Lungs**. Adrenaline relaxes bronchial smooth muscle through β_2-adrenergic receptors, resulting in bronchodilatation.

Noradrenaline causes peripheral vasoconstriction through the activation of α_1-adrenoceptors, with baroreceptor-mediated reflex bradycardia. Noradrenaline promotes gluconeogenesis and lipolysis. In addition, noradrenaline plays an important role in the normal functioning of the CNS.

How are catecholamines metabolised?

The plasma half-life of catecholamines is very short: both noradrenaline and adrenaline have plasma half-lives of around 2 min. Noradrenaline and adrenaline are both sequentially metabolised by catechol-O-methyltransferase (COMT) and monoamine oxidase (MAO), two enzymes distributed widely throughout the body. Metanephrine is an intermediate in this process, with vanillylmandelic acid produced after both enzymes have exerted their effects. Phaeochromocytoma, a tumour of chromaffin cells associated with excessive secretion of catecholamines, may be diagnosed through raised plasma metanephrine concentrations.

Further reading

P. E. Molina. *Endocrine Physiology, 5th edition*. New York, McGraw-Hill, 2018.

D. E. Kerr, T. Wenham, J. Newell-Price. Endocrine problems in the critically ill 2: endocrine emergencies. *BJA Education* 2017; **17**(11): 377–82.

T. Miller, B. Gibbison, G. M. Russell. Hypothalamic–pituitary–adrenal function during health, major surgery, and critical illness. *BJA Education* 2017; **17**(1): 16–21.

D. S. Ross. Radioiodine therapy for hyperthyroidism. *N Engl J Med* 2011; **364**(6): 542–50.

S. Malhotra, V. Sodhi. Anaesthesia for thyroid and parathyroid surgery. *Continuing Educ Anaesth Crit Care Pain* 2007; 7(2): 55–8.

Maternal Physiology during Pregnancy

How does endocrine function alter during pregnancy?

It comes as no surprise that there are major endocrine changes during pregnancy. These endocrine changes are the driving force for many of the other physiological and anatomical changes associated with pregnancy.

The main hormones involved are:

- **β-human chorionic gonadotropin** (β-hCG), a glycoprotein hormone with a structure similar to that of luteinising hormone, follicle-stimulating hormone and thyroid-stimulating hormone (TSH). It is secreted by the placenta shortly after implantation of the embryo and can be detected in the maternal circulation from the second week of pregnancy. β-hCG levels rise rapidly, doubling every 2 days until a peak is reached at 10 weeks' gestation. Its main role is to prolong the life of the corpus luteum:

    - In the second half of the menstrual cycle, the corpus luteum secretes progesterone and a small amount of oestrogen.
    - After 14 days, in the absence of an implanted embryo, progesterone secretion stops and the corpus luteum degenerates into the corpus albicans. The decline in progesterone triggers sloughing of the uterine lining (the endometrium).
    - If an embryo implants in the endometrium (or fallopian tube in the case of an ectopic pregnancy), the syncytiotrophoblast cells of the newly formed placenta produce progressively increasing amounts of β-hCG, which stimulates the corpus luteum to continue secreting progesterone. This prevents sloughing of the endometrium, which would cause miscarriage.

    - After 10 weeks' gestation, the placenta slowly takes over oestrogen and progesterone synthesis from the corpus luteum. β-hCG concentration then falls and the corpus luteum degenerates.

    β-hCG is also thought to be involved in suppressing the maternal immune response, protecting the placenta and embryo from immune destruction.

- **Human placental lactogen** (hPL), a polypeptide hormone whose structure is similar to that of growth hormone. Like β-hCG, hPL is secreted by the syncytiotrophoblast cells of the placenta. Throughout pregnancy, hPL concentration increases in proportion to foetal and placental growth, peaking near term. Its function is to ensure adequate provision of nutrients for the growing foetus through manipulation of maternal metabolism:

    - *Increased maternal lipolysis* increases the availability of free fatty acids.
    - *Decreased maternal peripheral insulin sensitivity* results in decreased peripheral utilisation of glucose and thus increased maternal plasma glucose concentration. It is important that the foetus has access to ample glucose, as this is its primary source of energy. hPL is implicated in the development of gestational diabetes.
    - *Stimulation of breast growth and development.* As the name suggests, hPL mimics the action of prolactin (PRL); whilst it has a much weaker effect than PRL, the high concentration of hPL is thought to be partly responsible for breast development during pregnancy.

- **Progesterone**, a steroid hormone often referred to as the 'pregnancy hormone', reflecting its many important roles. Progesterone is secreted by the corpus luteum in early pregnancy and by the placenta in the second and third trimesters. The main functions of progesterone are:

- *Preparing the endometrium for implantation* and promoting growth of the endometrium following implantation;
- *Uterine muscle relaxation*, suppressing myometrial contractions and preventing miscarriage;
- *Formation of a cervical mucus plug*, thus protecting the developing foetus from ascending infection;
- *Development of milk glands* in preparation for lactation.

In addition, progesterone is responsible for many of the other physiological changes associated with pregnancy, which are discussed in more detail below.

- **Oestrogen**. Three oestrogens are synthesised by the placenta: oestradiol, oestrone and oestriol. Each oestrogen comes from a different precursor, and the amount of each oestrogen produced is proportional to the amount of each precursor delivered to the placenta. The main oestrogen produced in pregnancy is oestriol, whose main role is to increase uteroplacental blood flow (in contrast, oestradiol dominates the menstrual cycle). Importantly, oestriol is produced from a foetal adrenal precursor called dehydroepiandrosterone sulphate. Consequently, uteroplacental blood flow is under the control of the growing foetus. Other roles of oestrogens include:

  - *Stimulation of uterine growth*;
  - *Sensitisation of the myometrium to oxytocin* in preparation for labour.

In addition, oestriol is responsible for the increased risk of thromboembolic disease associated with pregnancy.

Other pregnancy-related endocrine changes include:

- **Thyroid hormones**. In pregnancy, oestriol stimulates the liver to synthesise additional thyroxine-binding globulin. Therefore, one might expect unbound triiodothyronine (T_3) and thyroxine (T_4) concentrations to decrease. However, thyrotropin-releasing hormone secretion increases as a result of the negative-feedback loop, which increases TSH secretion by

the pituitary. Increased TSH stimulates the thyroid to secrete additional T_3 and T_4, bringing the free fractions of thyroid hormones back to normal.

- **PRL**. Oestrogen stimulates a dramatic increase in the pituitary secretion of PRL, whose role is the preparation of the breasts for lactation. The pituitary gland doubles in size to accommodate the number of extra lactotrophs required. Because of the increased metabolic demands of the enlarged pituitary gland, it becomes vulnerable to ischaemia. Pituitary infarction can occur if the patient suffers prolonged hypotension, as may result from post-partum haemorrhage – this is known as Sheehan's syndrome.
- **Parathyroid hormone** (PTH). Ca^{2+} is transferred across the placenta to meet the requirements of the growing foetus. As maternal absorption of dietary Ca^{2+} cannot meet this placental loss, one might expect maternal ionised Ca^{2+} concentration to fall. However, the maternal parathyroid glands sense the fall in plasma Ca^{2+} and respond by increasing secretion of PTH. PTH increases plasma Ca^{2+} concentration by increasing bone resorption, renal tubular Ca^{2+} reabsorption and activation of vitamin D. Of clinical significance, pregnant patients at high thromboembolic risk, such as those with prosthetic heart valves, may be treated with low-molecular-weight heparin (LMWH). LMWH has the undesirable effect of worsening the PTH-related reduction in bone mineral density, potentially leading to osteopenia.

Which other physiological changes of pregnancy are of interest to anaesthetists?

This is best answered using a system-by-system approach:

Respiratory system. Changes to the respiratory system begin by as early as 4 weeks' gestation, but the most significant changes occur from 20 weeks' gestation:

- **Airway**. Pregnancy-related capillary engorgement causes oedema of the oropharyngeal mucosa and larynx. In pre-eclampsia, the change in capillary dynamics can significantly worsen airway oedema.

- **Minute ventilation**. From early pregnancy, progesterone stimulates the respiratory centre in the medulla:

  – $\dot{V}_E$ *increases* by 50% at term: the increase in V_T is substantially greater (40%) than that of respiratory rate (10%). $\dot{V}_E$ increases further in labour due to pain.

  – *Anatomical dead space increases* due to bronchodilatation; that is, progesterone-induced smooth muscle relaxation.

  – *A mild reduction in* P_aCO_2 (typically 4.3 kPa) due to progesterone-induced maternal hyperventilation. This mild respiratory alkalosis triggers a compensatory renal HCO_3^- loss (typical plasma HCO_3^- concentration is 20 mmol/L), which usually corrects the pH disturbance.

  This is of clinical significance when anaesthetising a pregnant patient: special attention should be paid to $\dot{V}_E$. One should aim for a P_aCO_2 of ~4.3 kPa, which represents a normal value for pregnancy:

  – The foetus cannot correct a pH disturbance by respiratory or renal compensation. Therefore, maternal respiratory acidosis can cause foetal acidosis.

  – Likewise, maternal alkalosis should be avoided: the oxyhaemoglobin dissociation curve is shifted to the left, reducing O_2 transfer to the foetus with the potential for foetal hypoxia.

- **Lung volumes**. The gravid uterus causes an upwards displacement of the diaphragm and flaring of the lower ribs: the anterior–posterior diameter of the ribs increases by 2–3 cm. Diaphragmatic contraction is not restricted, but lung volumes are affected:

  – *Functional residual capacity (FRC) is reduced* by 20% when standing and by a further 30% in the supine position. The reduction in FRC is mainly due to a reduction in residual volume.

  – *Vital capacity remains unchanged.*

- **O_2 consumption**. The O_2 requirements of the growing foetus result in a 20% increase in O_2 consumption at term. O_2 consumption is further increased during labour due to uterine contractions.

- **Respiratory compliance**. Lung compliance is unaffected by pregnancy, but thoracic wall compliance is reduced by 20%. This is another consequence of the upward displacement of the diaphragm.

Clinical relevance: general anaesthesia and pregnancy

Beyond 12 weeks' gestation, the risk of gastro-oesophageal reflux increases. The higher risk of aspiration pneumonitis on induction of anaesthesia necessitates a rapid sequence induction and antacids. However, general anaesthesia in obstetric patients has additional difficulties:

- The incidence of difficult airway in the obstetric population is around 1 in 250, eight times higher than the general population. Difficult airway may be due to:

  – *Airway oedema*, as discussed above.
  – *Increased mucosal vascularity*. Repeated attempts at laryngoscopy may result in laceration and bleeding. In pre-eclampsia, coagulopathy only worsens the situation.
  – *Weight gain*. Large breasts and short neck make laryngoscopy more challenging.
  – *Poorly applied cricoid pressure.*

- The combination of increased O_2 consumption and decreased FRC (the main O_2 store) means that obstetric patients desaturate quickly.

As always, preparation is the key to success:

- Good head, neck and shoulder position can be achieved with standard pillows or with a specially designed elevation pillow.
- Adequate pre-oxygenation over at least 3 min is essential; the time pressure of an emergency caesarean section makes it all too easy to cut corners here!
- Most important is an experienced assistant with a range of ready-prepared airway equipment.

Cardiovascular system. Pregnancy causes major changes to cardiovascular physiology, increasing the demands on the heart considerably. Myocardial workload is further increased in labour, with the early post-partum period being particularly high risk. Cardiac disease is the leading indirect cause of death in pregnant patients (MBRRACE-UK triennium 2013–15 report: published 2017). The major cardiovascular changes in pregnancy are:

- **Blood volume**. Total blood volume increases gradually throughout pregnancy, by around 40% for a singleton pregnancy and even more for a multiple pregnancy:
  - *Red cell mass increases* by 20–30% due to an increase in erythropoietin secretion. Plasma volume increases by 45% due to oestrogenic stimulation of the renin–angiotensin–aldosterone system. The discrepancy between the increases in red cell mass and plasma volume results in the physiological anaemia of pregnancy. Haemoglobin (Hb) concentration falls from a typical pre-pregnancy concentration of 150 g/L to around 120 g/L at term; haematocrit falls to around 0.35.
  - *Each uterine contraction squeezes 300–500 mL of blood* from the uterus to the systemic circulation during labour.
  - *Blood loss* at delivery is typically 300 mL for vaginal delivery and 500 mL for caesarean section. The mother is protected from the impact of this haemorrhage by 'autotransfusion', in which around 500 mL of blood is returned to the systemic circulation during uterine involution.

- **Cardiac output** (CO). The increase in CO starts in early pregnancy, from the fourth week of gestation. CO increases by up to 50% by the third trimester. The factors involved are:
  - *A reduction in afterload.* Systemic vascular resistance (SVR) falls by 20% due to progesterone-induced vasodilatation. As a result, systolic blood pressure falls by 5% and diastolic blood pressure falls by 10%.
  - *Increased heart rate* (HR). In response to decreased blood pressure, there is a reflex increase in HR of 25% over the course of the pregnancy.
  - *An increase in preload.* Increased circulating blood volume results in an increase in cardiac preload. As a result, stroke volume (SV) increases by 30%. Much of the increase in SV occurs during the first trimester.
  - *Myocardial contractility is unchanged* by pregnancy.

During labour, CO is increased further (25–50%) in response to catecholamine secretion. In addition, CO increases by an additional 20–30%

during uterine contractions. Epidural analgesia reduces the secretion of catecholamines in response to pain, which can lessen the impact of labour on the heart. Following delivery, the autotransfusion of 500 mL of uterine blood to the venous system increases cardiac preload, resulting in a 60–80% increase in CO. This is a moment of great danger to parturients at risk of cardiac failure.

- **Aortocaval compression**. From 20 weeks' gestation, the enlarging uterus can compress the inferior vena cava (IVC) and the descending aorta when the parturient is supine. This has serious implications:
  - *Reduced maternal venous return.* Reduced cardiac preload causes a fall in CO, leading to a feeling of nausea, pallor, hypotension or cardiovascular collapse when supine. Symptoms and signs resolve in the lateral position, where IVC compression is relieved.
  - *Reduced placental blood flow.* Blood flow to the placenta is not autoregulated; instead, blood flow is directly proportional to perfusion pressure (see Chapter 83). IVC compression by the gravid uterus reduces CO, which impairs placental perfusion. In addition, compression of the descending aorta further reduces uteroplacental blood flow. Impaired placental blood flow may result in inadequate foetal gas exchange, sometimes with fatal consequences.

Most non-anaesthetised parturients are able to compensate, at least partially, for aortocaval compression through two mechanisms:
  - *Sympathetic outflow increases,* which in turn increases SVR and HR.
  - *Some blood bypasses the compressed IVC,* returning from the lower limbs to the heart through collateral pathways: the azygos, paravertebral and epidural veins.

General anaesthesia and neuraxial blockade abolish the sympathetic response to aortocaval compression; severe hypotension or even cardiac arrest may develop rapidly when the patient is supine. It is therefore very important that the parturient is never supine and that the uterus is always displaced from the great vessels. Aortocaval compression is usually relieved by a lateral tilt (on the operating table or with a wedge), but relief can only be guaranteed in the full lateral position. Lateral tilt with a wedge is especially important to remember during cardiopulmonary resuscitation of pregnant patients.

Gastrointestinal (GI) system. The changes in GI physiology are of particular importance to the anaesthetist. There is a significantly increased risk of gastro-oesophageal reflux in pregnancy due to:

- **Decreased lower oesophageal sphincter (LOS) tone.** Progesterone-induced smooth muscle relaxation decreases the tone of the LOS, leading to sphincter incompetence.

- **Mechanical changes at the gastro-oesophageal junction.** The gravid uterus displaces the stomach and diaphragm upwards, reducing the acute angle of the oesophagus as it passes through the diaphragm.

- **Increased intra-gastric pressure.** In the third trimester, the gravid uterus increases gastric pressure. This further reduces the lower oesophageal barrier pressure.

- **Delayed gastric emptying.** Gastric emptying is unaffected by pregnancy. However, in labour, there is a significant delay in gastric emptying, which may be further worsened by opioids.

- **Gastric pH.** The hormone gastrin is secreted by the placenta from the 15th week of gestation. Compared with non-pregnant patients, gastric volume is increased and gastric pH decreased; aspiration causes a greater degree of lung injury.

Gastro-oesophageal reflux commonly causes heartburn in pregnancy, but its main anaesthetic implication is an increased risk of Mendelson's syndrome (see Chapter 63), a pneumonitis resulting from pulmonary aspiration of acidic gastric contents under general anaesthesia. Rapid sequence induction and non-particulate antacids are indicated for general anaesthesia in pregnant patients beyond the first trimester; the exact gestational week is a matter of controversy.

Haematological physiology. In addition to the physiological anaemia of pregnancy described above, there are other important pregnancy-induced haematological changes:

- **White cell count** (WCC) is elevated in pregnancy due to an increase in neutrophils and monocytes. The normal range of WCC in pregnancy is not universally accepted, but is often taken as $6000-16,000/mm^3$ from the 12th gestational week. WCC may increase to as much as $30,000/mm^3$ during labour.

- **Platelet count** falls gradually throughout pregnancy; at term, the lower limit of a normal platelet count is $115 \times 10^9/L$. The decreased platelet count is due to both haemodilution (a relatively increased plasma volume) and shorter platelet lifespan.

- **Hypercoagulable state.** Pregnant patients are at significantly increased risk of venous thromboembolism due to:

    - An increase in fibrinogen and clotting factors VII, X and XII;
    - Decreased fibrinolysis.

- **Renal physiology.** Pregnancy induces both anatomical and physiological changes to the kidneys and ureters:

    - *Dilatation of the ureters and renal pelvis* as a result of both mechanical obstruction by the gravid uterus and progesterone-induced smooth muscle dilatation. These changes make urinary tract infection and pyelonephritis more common in pregnancy.
    - *Increased glomerular filtration rate* (GFR). Renal blood flow increases by 50%, reflecting the increase in CO. GFR is increased by a similar amount; pregnant patients have lower serum creatinine and urea concentrations.
    - *Uric acid levels.* In early pregnancy, increased GFR results in a lower uric acid concentration. In the third trimester, uric acid concentration steadily increases above the pre-pregnancy level due to increased tubular reabsorption of uric acid. Hyperuricaemia in pregnancy is associated with pre-eclampsia and has been suggested (controversially) to correlate with its severity.
    - *Glycosuria.* Tubular reabsorption of glucose cannot keep pace with the increase in GFR. The result is glucose passing into the urine, making urinary dipstick testing an unreliable test for diabetes mellitus in pregnancy.
    - *Proteinuria.* In a similar way to glucose, tubular protein reabsorption mechanisms are insufficient to match the 50% increase in GFR. Proteinuria is therefore more common in

pregnancy; the upper limit of the normal range is generally taken as 300 mg of protein in a 24-h urine collection (compared with 150 mg per 24-h period in the non-pregnant state). Pre-eclampsia causes a pathological increase in proteinuria.

Central nervous system (CNS). The endocrine changes of pregnancy have a significant effect on the CNS. The minimum alveolar concentration (MAC) of volatile anaesthetics needed to prevent movement in 50% of subjects in response to surgical stimulus is reduced by 30–40%. This is thought to be due to:

- **Progesterone.** This is known to have sedative effects and reduce the MAC of volatile anaesthetic agents in both male and female animal models.
- **β-endorphins.** These are secreted by the placenta throughout pregnancy, but especially in labour. Their exact role is unknown, but β-endorphins are thought to be analgesic in labour, to contribute to the reduction in MAC and possibly to increase neural sensitivity to local anaesthetics, which partially explains why lower doses of local anaesthetic are required for regional anaesthesia in pregnancy.

Pregnancy also causes changes to the epidural and subarachnoid spaces:

- **Epidural pressure is increased** to around +1 cmH$_2$O, compared with –1 cmH$_2$O in the non-pregnant state.

  The higher epidural pressure is due to engorgement of the epidural veins secondary to mechanical compression of the IVC by the gravid uterus. In the first stage of labour, epidural pressure increases to +4–10 cmH$_2$O. Bearing down in the second stage of labour can increase epidural pressure to +60 cmH$_2$O. Epidural vein engorgement means accidental venous cannulation is more common when introducing an epidural catheter.

- **Cerebrospinal fluid pressure is unchanged** from its pre-pregnancy value. However, cerebrospinal

fluid pressure undergoes a significant increase in the second stage of labour, up to 70 cmH$_2$O.

Hepatic physiology. Levels of the hepatic enzymes glutamyltransferase, alanine aminotransferase and lactic acid dehydrogenase are slightly elevated, and some clinical signs usually associated with chronic liver disease (e.g. palmar erythema, spider naevi) may occur normally in pregnancy. Alkaline phosphatase (ALP) levels are also increased; ALP originates from both the liver and the placenta. Hepatic protein production does not keep pace with the increase in plasma volume, leading to decreased plasma protein concentration. Thus:

- **Albumin concentration decreases throughout pregnancy,** from around 35 g/L to 25 g/L.
- **Plasma cholinesterase concentration decreases** by 25% due to both decreased hepatic synthesis and increased plasma volume. This is of particular interest to anaesthetists, as suxamethonium is metabolised by plasma cholinesterase; decreased enzyme activity leads to prolonged suxamethonium action.

Musculoskeletal. Ligaments become increasingly lax as pregnancy progresses due to placental secretion of the hormone relaxin. During general anaesthesia, it is important to pay close attention to positioning in order to minimise the risk of post-operative back and joint problems.

Further reading

D. Katz, Y. Beilin. Disorders of coagulation in pregnancy. *Br J Anaesth* 2015; **115**(Suppl. 2): ii75–88.

A. T. Dennis, C. B. Solnordal. Acute pulmonary oedema in pregnant women. *Anaesthesia* 2012; **67**(6): 646–59.

E. Reitman, P. Flood. Anaesthetic considerations for nonobstetric surgery during pregnancy. *Br J Anaesth* 2011; **107**(Suppl. 1): 172–8.

B. H. Heidemann, J. H. McClure. Changes in maternal physiology during pregnancy. *Continuing Educ Anaesth Crit Care Pain* 2003; **3**(3): 65–8.

83

Foetal Physiology

What are the functions of the placenta?

The placenta has the following functions:

- Exchange of nutrients between the foetal and maternal circulations;
- Endocrine;
- Immunological.

How does the anatomy of the placenta relate to these functions?

- **Exchange of nutrients**. The placenta is an unusual organ because it is derived from the tissues of two different organisms: endometrial cells (known as decidual cells in pregnancy) from the mother and trophoblastic cells from the foetus. The foetus is entirely reliant on exchange with the maternal circulation for nutrition (supply of O_2, glucose, amino acids, etc.) and excretion (elimination of CO_2, urea, creatinine, uric acid, etc.). Key features of placental development are:

  - The foetal cells form a ball of cells – the blastocyst – which implants within the endometrium.
  - The placenta develops from trophoblast cells, derived within the outer cell layer of the blastocyst.
  - The trophoblastic cells develop into two layers, which together form the chorion. The outer chorionic layer consists of syncytiotrophoblast cells, whilst the inner layer is made up of cytotrophoblast cells.
  - The chorion invades the maternal decidua, releasing enzymes that produce cavities within the decidua. When the maternal spiral arteries (which supply the decidua) are invaded, their blood fills these cavities.
  - Projections called chorionic villi form an extensive network of finger-like chorionic

projections into the blood-filled cavities and then become vascularised.

  - When the foetal heart becomes active at 5 weeks' gestation, foetal blood supplies the placenta through the two umbilical arteries. The umbilical arteries give rise to chorionic arteries, which branch over the foetal surface of the placenta until the capillaries of the chorionic villi are reached. The capillaries of the chorionic villi converge and return blood to the foetus through a single umbilical vein.

The foetal and maternal blood are thus separated only by the foetal endothelium and two (syncytiotrophoblastic and cytotrophoblastic) chorionic cell layers. Nevertheless, there is normally no mixing of maternal and foetal blood. The placenta grows to match the increasing nutritional demands of the developing foetus. As a result, at term, uterine blood flow has increased 10-fold over its pre-gestational value to 750 mL/min, with placental blood flow accounting for approximately 85% of this flow.

- **Endocrine function**. The placenta is an important endocrine organ during pregnancy, producing both peptide and steroid hormones. Hormone production takes place in syncytiotrophoblast cells. The hormones produced are:

  - *β-human chorionic gonadotropin*;
  - *Human placental lactogen*;
  - *Oestrogen*;
  - *Progesterone*.

The roles of these four hormones in pregnancy is more fully discussed in Chapter 82.

Clinical relevance: pre-eclampsia

Pre-eclampsia is a potentially life-threatening complication of pregnancy characterised by hypertension and proteinuria in the third trimester. Pre-eclampsia has many associated complications including: eclampsia, HELLP (**H**aemolysis, **E**levated **L**iver enzymes and **L**ow **P**latelet count) syndrome, liver rupture and cerebral haemorrhage.

The exact pathogenesis of pre-eclampsia is not yet fully established. A possible sequence of events is:

- There is dysfunction of the spiral arteries that constitute the sole blood supply of the placenta. It is not clear whether this is due to foetal (e.g. inadequate trophoblast invasion) or maternal factors.
- The syncytial cells of the chorion – the endocrine cells of the placenta – produce a number of substances in response to hypoxia. These include cytokines, eicosanoids and the soluble vascular endothelial growth factor receptor 1. There is also an increased rate of apoptosis of syncytiotrophoblast cells.
- These released placental factors cause a systemic inflammatory response in the mother, resulting in widespread endothelial dysfunction and subsequent organ dysfunction.

The only definitive treatment of pre-eclampsia is delivery of the placenta; the risks of pre-eclampsia to the mother must be balanced against the early delivery of the foetus.

- **Immunological function**. The foetus is genetically distinct from the mother and would accordingly be expected to provoke a maternal immune response. However, this rarely occurs, and this immune tolerance is attributed to the placenta:
  - After implantation, trophoblast cells lose many of their cell surface major histocompatibility complex molecules, making them less immunogenic. The trophoblast cells cover themselves in a coat of mucoprotein, further disguising them from the maternal immune system.
  - The chorionic cells act as an immunological barrier, preventing maternal T cells and antibodies from reaching the foetal circulation.
  - Progesterone and α-fetoprotein produced by the yolk sac at implantation act as maternal immunosuppressive agents, specifically damping down cellular immunity. However, this also decreases the ability of the mother to launch effective cell-mediated reactions in

defence against certain microorganisms, such as *Listeria monocytogenes*.

The chorion also acts as a barrier to prevent bacteria and viruses infecting the foetus. However, some bacteria (e.g. *Listeria*) and many viruses (including rubella, parvovirus B19 and HIV) manage to cross into the foetal circulation. The foetal immune system is not fully developed until 6 months after birth. *In utero*, the foetus relies on maternal antibodies to fight infections: syncytiotrophoblasts have immunoglobulin G (IgG) receptors, allowing IgG, but not other forms of immunoglobulin, to cross the placenta by endocytosis.

Clinical relevance: placental antibody transfer

The foetus requires maternal IgG as a defence against infections. However, allowing the placental transfer of IgG also has negative consequences:

- **Haemolytic disease of the newborn**. Rhesus (RhD) antigen-negative mothers previously exposed to the RhD antigen (e.g. through blood transfusion or previous foetomaternal haemorrhage) produce anti-RhD IgG. When pregnant with an RhD-positive foetus, maternal anti-RhD IgG crosses the placenta and attacks foetal erythrocytes, resulting in haemolysis.
- **Transient neonatal myasthenia**. Myasthenia gravis is an autoimmune condition in which the immune system produces IgG against the acetylcholine receptors of the neuromuscular junction, causing fatigable muscular weakness (see Chapter 53). Placental transfer of these antibodies causes some neonates to have temporary muscle weakness, resulting in respiratory distress, a weak cry and poor feeding.
- **Congenital heart block**. Placental transfer of anti-Ro IgG antibodies from mothers with systemic lupus erythematosus can cause congenital heart block and neonatal lupus erythematosus.

What are the different mechanisms by which substances cross the placenta?

Substances may cross the placenta through different mechanisms:

- **Simple diffusion** of gases, particularly O_2 and CO_2.

- **Facilitated diffusion**. Glucose crosses the placenta through facilitated transport by the insulin-independent glucose transport proteins GLUT-1 and GLUT-3. Glucose transfer is proportional to maternal glucose concentration and is increased in diabetic mothers with poor glycaemic control, with a consequent high average foetal plasma glucose concentration.
- **Active transport**. Amino acids are transferred across the placenta by Na^+-dependent active transport. Many amino acids are metabolised in the placenta. For example, serine is converted to glycine before being released into the foetal circulation.
- **Transcytosis**. IgGs are endocytosed by syncytiotrophoblast cells, transferred across the placenta in a vesicle and exocytosed into the foetal circulation.
- **Bulk flow**. In a similar way to other capillary systems in the body, water passes between the cells of the placenta along its osmotic gradient. Any small molecules dissolved in the water are also transported by solvent drag.

Clinical relevance: placental drug transport

Transfer of drugs across the placenta depends on:

- **Concentration gradient**. Rates of diffusion are proportional to concentration gradient.
- **Molecular size**. Drugs with smaller molecular weights (<500 Da) cross the placenta more easily.
- **Charge**. Neutral molecules cross much more readily than charged molecules. The degree of ionisation of a drug may change with pH.
- **Lipid solubility**. Highly lipid-soluble drugs readily diffuse across the lipid-rich placenta.
- **Protein binding**. Highly protein-bound drugs show less diffusion across the placenta compared with drugs with lower protein binding. Maternal hypoalbuminaemia or acidosis may significantly alter drug protein binding and therefore placental drug transfer.

Any drug given to the mother has the potential to reach the foetus. Some drugs (e.g. thalidomide) have serious adverse effects on the growing foetus, whilst others (e.g. amoxicillin) are considered safe. Of interest to the anaesthetist are the following:

- Glycopyrrolate (a charged quaternary NH_4^+ salt) cannot cross the placenta, whilst atropine (an uncharged tertiary amine) crosses easily.

- Muscle relaxants are charged molecules, so they do not cross the placenta.
- The intravenous anaesthetic agents thiopentone, ketamine and propofol are highly lipophilic and are readily transferred across the placenta. However, redistribution in the foetus is rapid, so the residual effects are negligible following delivery.
- Opioids are lipophilic, so they diffuse readily across the placenta. Of particular note is pethidine, which is metabolised by the foetus to norpethidine. Norpethidine is less lipid soluble than pethidine, so it is less able to diffuse back to the maternal circulation. Foetal accumulation occurs, risking respiratory depression and poor feeding in the immediate neonatal period.
- Placental transfer of local anaesthetics is greatest for those with lower protein binding (e.g. lignocaine). Toxic levels in the foetus occur with high maternal local anaesthetic plasma concentrations – if the mother has symptoms and signs of local anaesthetic toxicity, so will the foetus. In addition, an acidaemic foetus may also develop local anaesthetic toxicity by a mechanism called 'ion trapping'. Low foetal pH causes ionisation of any local anaesthetic that crosses the placenta – the local anaesthetic is then unable to diffuse back to the maternal circulation.

What are the factors involved in foetal oxygen delivery?

Foetal oxygenation is determined by:

- **Delivery of O_2 to the placenta**. Placental O_2 delivery is a product of placental blood flow and maternal blood O_2 content, which in turn depends on maternal P_aO_2 and maternal haemoglobin (Hb) concentration.
- **Transfer of O_2 across the placenta**. In addition to the large surface area of the placenta, a number of factors aid the transfer of O_2 from maternal Hb (HbA) to foetal Hb (HbF):
  - *A large O_2 pressure gradient across the placenta*. The P_aO_2 of intervillous blood is around 6.7 kPa, compared with the foetal umbilical arterial P_aO_2 of 2.7 kPa.
  - *HbF has a higher O_2-binding affinity than maternal HbA*. The HbF oxyhaemoglobin

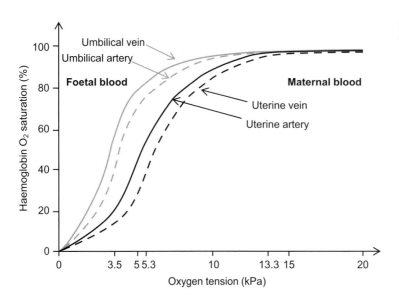

Figure 83.1 Oxyhaemoglobin dissociation curves for HbA and HbF.

dissociation curve is therefore positioned to the left of the HbA curve (Figure 83.1). This difference is primarily due to 2,3-diphosphoglycerate (2,3-DPG) binding: the placenta actively produces 2,3-DPG, which binds avidly to β-globin chains of HbA, but cannot bind to the γ-globin chains of HbF. 2,3-DPG shifts the oxyhaemoglobin dissociation curve of maternal HbA to the right, offloading additional O_2 to HbF.

- *The double Bohr effect.* CO_2 diffuses down its concentration gradient from the foetus (typical umbilical artery P_aCO_2 of 6.7 kPa) to the mother (typical intervillous P_aCO_2 of 4.9 kPa).

  - As foetal P_aCO_2 decreases, the HbF oxyhaemoglobin dissociation curve shifts to the left, further increasing HbF O_2-binding affinity – this is the Bohr effect (see Chapter 8).
  - As CO_2 crosses the placenta, the intervillous P_aCO_2 increases. The HbA oxyhaemoglobin dissociation curve shifts to the right, offloading even more O_2 – this is the double Bohr effect.

- **Foetal O_2-carrying capacity.** The foetus has a higher Hb concentration than adults (around 18 g/dL at birth), which increases the foetal O_2-carrying capacity.

What is the double Haldane effect?

The Haldane effect is the increased ability of deoxy-haemoglobin to carry CO_2 (see Chapter 9). The Haldane effect is particularly relevant at the placenta:

- As O_2 is offloaded from maternal oxyhaemoglobin, the resulting deoxyhaemoglobin is better able to carry the CO_2 transferred across the placenta from foetus to mother.
- Likewise on the foetal side of the placenta, binding of O_2 facilitates the release of CO_2 from HbF.

Together, these effects are termed the double Haldane effect.

What happens to foetal oxygenation during labour?

As discussed above, the foetus is entirely dependent on the placenta for its blood supply. The spiral arteries directly supply the placenta; these arise from the radial arteries, which pass through the myometrium. Importantly, uterine blood flow to the placenta is not autoregulated: blood flow is pressure dependent. Consequently, in labour, when myometrial contractions compress the radial arteries, placental blood flow is temporarily reduced, resulting in mild foetal hypoxaemia. The foetus can accommodate a degree of hypoxaemia without consequence. The severe hypoxaemia that causes foetal distress usually results from other pathology:

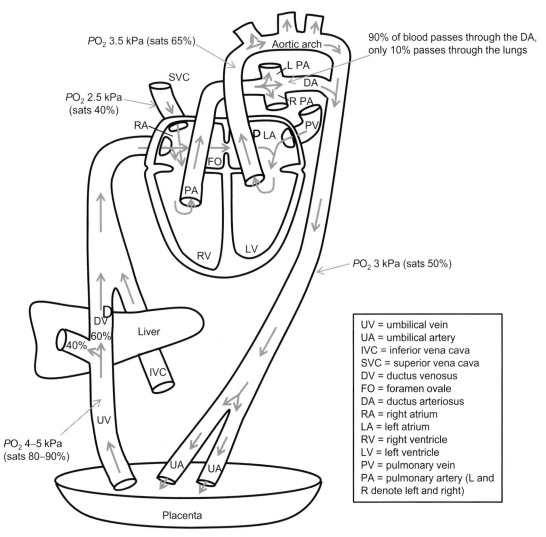

PO$_2$ 3.5 kPa (sats 65%)

Aortic arch

90% of blood passes through the DA, only 10% passes through the lungs

SVC

L PA

PO$_2$ 2.5 kPa (sats 40%)

DA

R PA

RA

PV

LA

FO

PA

PO$_2$ 3 kPa (sats 50%)

RV

LV

DV

60%

Liver

40%

IVC

UV

PO$_2$ 4–5 kPa (sats 80–90%)

UA   UA

Placenta

UV = umbilical vein
UA = umbilical artery
IVC = inferior vena cava
SVC = superior vena cava
DV = ductus venosus
FO = foramen ovale
DA = ductus arteriosus
RA = right atrium
LA = left atrium
RV = right ventricle
LV = left ventricle
PV = pulmonary vein
PA = pulmonary artery (L and R denote left and right)

Figure 83.2 Schematic of the foetal circulation.

- **Maternal factors** – hypotension; for example, as a result of sepsis or aortocaval compression;
- **Foetal factors** – for example, malpresentation;
- **Placental factors** – for example, placenta praevia, placental abruption;
- **Umbilical cord factors** – for example, entanglement around the foetus, true knots.

How does the foetal circulation differ from the adult circulation?

The foetal circulation is shown in Figure 83.2.

The foetal circulation differs from the adult circulation in the following respects:

- The presence of the umbilical vessels;
- Two vascular shunts: the ductus venosus and ductus arteriosus;
- A defect in the atrial septum, the foramen ovale.

As a result, patterns of foetal blood flow differ from those of an adult:

- Blood in the umbilical vein flowing from the placenta is oxygenated. The umbilical vein *PO*$_2$ is 4.0–5.0 kPa, equivalent to Hb O_2 saturations of around 80–90%.[1]

---

[1] Note: the HbF oxyhaemoglobin dissociation curve is shifted to the left in relation to HbA, so S_aO_2 is higher for a given O_2 tension.

- Of the blood flowing from the placenta, 40% enters the foetal liver, whilst 60% bypasses the liver and flows into the inferior vena cava (IVC) through the ductus venosus.
- Blood from the IVC flows into the right atrium (RA). A flap of tissue called the Eustachian valve directs the flow of the freshly oxygenated blood from the ductus venosus through the foramen ovale and into the left atrium (LA). From here, blood flows into the left ventricle (LV) and then into the ascending aorta (P_aO_2 of around 3.5 kPa, equivalent to saturations of 65%). The ascending aorta supplies the upper half of the body, including the heart and brain, the organs most in need of fully oxygenated blood.
- Deoxygenated blood (PO_2 of around 2.5 kPa, equivalent to saturations of 40%) from the superior vena cava, the coronary sinus and the remaining blood from the IVC (the blood returning from the lower limbs) flows through the RA and into the right ventricle (RV). When the RV contracts, blood is ejected into the pulmonary artery. However, only 10% of this blood enters the pulmonary circulation – pulmonary vascular resistance (PVR) is high owing to the effects of hypoxic pulmonary vasoconstriction (HPV) (see Chapter 23). Instead, the majority of blood flows through the lower-resistance ductus arteriosus to the descending aorta, which perfuses the lower half of the body. In this way, the least oxygenated blood flows back to the placenta for re-oxygenation.

The foetal heart shows many differences from the adult heart:

- The LV pumps half of the venous return to the upper half of the body, whilst the RV pumps the remaining blood to the lower half of the body. Unlike the adult heart, both ventricles pump blood into high-pressure systems – the foetal RV and LV are therefore of similar sizes and wall thicknesses.
- The foetal myocardium is immature, with a high proportion of non-contractile protein. It cannot increase its wall tension in response to increased preload, in contrast to the adult heart. The stroke volume (SV) is therefore fixed: cardiac output (CO) is consequently dependent on heart rate (HR; remember CO = SV × HR). The normal foetal HR at term is 110–160 bpm.

- The foetal HR is under autonomic control:
  - *The parasympathetic nervous system* is responsible for the normal baseline variability in HR.
  - *The sympathetic nervous system* is responsible for the accelerations in HR seen with foetal activity.

Clinical relevance: labour and foetal cardiovascular reflexes

During labour, foetal HR may be measured by cardiotocography (CTG). The CTG records the baseline foetal HR and the response to uterine contractions.

During uterine contractions, maternal spiral arteries are compressed, resulting in a transient fall in O_2 delivery to the placenta. A healthy foetus may exhibit an early deceleration on the CTG trace – a parasympathetic-mediated fall in HR shortly after the onset of a uterine contraction due to mild hypoxaemia or compression of the foetal head.

A late deceleration is more sinister. In response to severe foetal hypoxaemia, the peripheral chemoreceptors trigger peripheral vasoconstriction to redirect blood to vital organs. The resulting hypertension stimulates the baroreceptor reflex, resulting in a bradycardia. The deceleration in HR is late relative to the onset of uterine contractions because of the time taken in this two-step reflex response.

What are the physiological changes that occur at birth?

In utero, the foetus is dependent on the placenta for gas exchange and nutrition. Following birth, the neonate must fend for itself, with its lungs as the newly established gas-exchange organ and a circulation of adult configuration. Key changes are as follows:

- **Respiratory system:**
  - The newly delivered neonate is bombarded with tactile, thermal, visual and auditory stimuli.
  - Along with sensory stimulation, the falling P_aO_2, rising P_aCO_2 and falling pH stimulate both central and peripheral chemoreceptors, triggering the neonate to take its first breath.
  - The first breath requires a large amount of inspiratory work; the lungs are entirely fluid filled and poorly compliant, though some of the fluid is squeezed out of the lungs as a result of thoracic compression during labour.

– As O_2 enters the alveoli, PVR rapidly falls as HPV is reversed, permitting pulmonary blood flow.

- **Cardiovascular system**: the circulation changes from foetal to adult configurations.

  – Immediately following birth, the umbilical arteries vasoconstrict in response to mechanical stimulation and exposure to cold air. Delaying the clamping of the umbilical arteries for 40–60 s allows additional venous return from the placenta to the foetus. The removal of the low-resistance placenta from the arterial and venous circulations results in an increase in systemic vascular resistance and a reduction in right atrial venous return, respectively. Reduced blood flow through the ductus venosus results in its closure within 1–3 h.

  – Following the first breath, PVR decreases and blood flows into the lungs. Left atrial blood flow increases; when left atrial pressure exceeds right atrial pressure, a flap-like valve closes the foramen ovale.

  – Physiological closure of the ductus arteriosus occurs over the next 10 h through a number of mechanisms:

    - Following birth, the higher P_aO_2 stimulates vasoconstriction of the ductus arteriosus (the mechanism for this is not known). There is a higher incidence of failed ductus arteriosus closure in neonates with significant hypoxaemia and those born at altitude.

    - Vasodilatory prostaglandins are produced in foetal life by the ductus arteriosus. Following birth, prostaglandin production is reduced.

  - Bradykinin released from the lungs following the first breath is also implicated in ductus arteriosus closure.

Clinical relevance: transitional circulation

The physiological changes that follow birth are not irreversible. In certain circumstances they may be reversed, resulting in a transitional circulation that often has disastrous consequences for the neonate. The main causes for reversion to a transitional circulation are hypoxia, hypercapnoea, acidosis and hypothermia.

For example, in hypoxaemic neonates, HPV results in high PVR. Right atrial pressure is increased whilst left atrial pressure is reduced, resulting in the foramen ovale reopening. Hypoxaemia also prevents closure of the ductus arteriosus. The right-to-left shunting of blood through a patent foramen ovale and the patent ductus arteriosus exacerbates hypoxaemia and acidosis, further increasing PVR: a vicious cycle ensues.

Treatment aims to reverse hypoxaemia using specific therapies like exogenous surfactant (for infant respiratory distress syndrome) and general supportive therapies: O_2 administration, continuous positive airway pressure and mechanical ventilation. PVR may be reduced using inhaled nitric oxide as a pulmonary arterial vasodilator.

Further reading

S. Blackburn. *Maternal, Fetal, and Neonatal Physiology, 5th edition*. Philadelphia, Saunders, 2017.

S. Guller. Role of the syncytium in placenta-mediated complications of preeclampsia. *Thromb Res* 2009; **124**(4): 389–92.

P. J. Murphy. The fetal circulation. *Continuing Educ Anaesth Crit Care Pain* 2005; **5**(4): 107–12.

Chapter

84

Paediatric Physiology

Children are not simply 'small adults'. The anatomical and physiological differences between children and adults have a significant impact on their anaesthetic management.

Childhood is classified into the following age groups.

- *Neonate*: the first 28 days of life (or, more precisely, a baby under 44 weeks in terms of post-conceptual age);
- *Infant*: 28 days to 1 year;
- *Child*: 1–12 years;
- *Adolescent*: 13–17 years.

Describe the main anatomical and physiological differences between children and adults

The differences between children and adults are most evident below the age of 1 year. System by system, key features are as follows.

- **Airway.**

  - *Relatively large head with a prominent occiput*; relatively short neck and large tongue. Optimal head position is 'neutral' rather than the 'sniffing the morning air' position of the adult.
  - *Neonates and infants are obligate nasal breathers*. Nasal obstruction with secretions or nasogastric tubes can significantly impact breathing. This risk diminishes beyond the age of 4 months.
  - *Large 'U'-shaped epiglottis*. A straight-bladed laryngoscope may be required.
  - *A more cephalad larynx*. The larynx is at vertebral level C3 in the neonate and C4 in the child, compared with C5 or C6 in adults.
  - *A short trachea* (as little as 4 cm). This increases the risk of accidental endobronchial intubation. Intubation of the left main

bronchus is as likely as the right, as the angle at the carina is similar. This is in contrast to the situation in the adult, where the left bronchus takes a more acute angle than the right, making the right bronchus more susceptible to endobronchial intubation. The endotracheal tube (ETT) should be positioned at least 1 cm above the carina and should be fixed to the maxilla (otherwise accidental endobronchial intubation may occur with intraoperative head and jaw movement).

  - *The narrowest part of the trachea is the cricoid ring* in prepubescent children. The mucosa here is loosely bound, pseudostratified ciliated epithelium that, following airway trauma, is very prone to developing oedema.

Clinical relevance: choice of ETT in children

In young children, the trachea is very narrow. Even a small amount of oedema will have a significant impact on the radius of the trachea and therefore the resistance to airflow: the Hagen–Poiseuille equation indicates that resistance to flow is inversely proportional to the fourth power of the radius (see Chapter 21).

Traditionally, smaller versions of the adult high-pressure, low-volume cuff ETTs were used in children. Pressure on the tracheal mucosa caused oedema, which had the potential to cause airway obstruction following extubation. Therefore, uncuffed ETTs were used for children below the age of 10, whose tracheas were the narrowest, with the ETT size calculated using the following formula: (age/4) + 4. When inserted, a correctly sized, uncuffed ETT should not feel tight and there should be an air leak when positive pressure is applied. However, getting the right-sized ETT for a particular patient sometimes required multiple changes of ETT in order to find one that was not too tight and did not have a large air leak.

More recently, ETTs designed for use in children have been developed with low-pressure, high-volume cuffs. Cuffed ETTs are sized using the following formula: (age/4) + 3.5 (i.e. half a size smaller than an uncuffed ETT). The use of a cuffed ETT means that the large air leaks (and resultant suboptimal ventilation) associated with uncuffed ETTs are avoided. However, the reduced internal diameter of a cuffed ETT inevitably leads to greater airways resistance, meaning that a spontaneous breathing technique may not be possible.

- **Respiratory physiology.** Children (especially neonates and infants) have limited respiratory reserve.

  - *High O_2 consumption.* Arguably the most important feature of paediatric physiology is a high basal metabolic rate (BMR), resulting in increased O_2 consumption in relation to body mass: a neonate has an O_2 consumption double that of an adult: 6 mL kg^{-1} min^{-1} versus 3 mL kg^{-1} min^{-1}.

  - *Increased alveolar ventilation.* As a result of their high BMR, CO_2 production in children is increased. P_aCO_2 remains within the normal range due to increased $\dot{V}_A$.

  - *Increased respiratory rate* (RR). V_T is 6–8 mL/kg; that is, similar to adults. The increased $\dot{V}_A$ is achieved by increasing RR rather than V_T.

  - *The diaphragm is the main muscle of inspiration.* Ribs are soft and aligned horizontally; the 'bucket-handle' mechanism of the thoracic cage does not occur. V_T is fairly static; high intrapleural pressure results in intercostal recession rather than lung expansion, especially in neonates and infants. An acute abdomen or gas insufflation of the stomach splints the diaphragm, impairing ventilation.

  - *Reduced functional residual capacity* (FRC). Their soft ribs mean that chest wall compliance is increased in children. The elastic recoil of the lung is only slightly less than that of an adult. Overall, FRC (the point at which inward lung elastic forces match the outward elastic recoil of the chest wall) is reduced. As FRC is the O_2 reservoir of the lung, rapid desaturation may occur during periods of apnoea, such as following induction of anaesthesia. FRC is further reduced during general anaesthesia: the physiological mechanisms that maintain FRC (partial adduction of the vocal cords during expiration and inspiratory muscle tone) are abolished.

  - *Closing capacity (CC) exceeds FRC.* The increase in chest wall compliance and lower lung volumes mean that small airways collapse easily: CC exceeds FRC in neonates, leading to a significant $\dot{V}/\dot{Q}$ mismatch.

  - *The muscles of respiration are easily fatigued.* The work of breathing is higher due to lower lung volumes, excessive chest wall compliance and the inadequacy of the bucket-handle mechanism. The diaphragm and intercostal muscles fatigue easily due to a lack of type I muscle fibres.

- **Cardiovascular physiology.** The cardiovascular differences between children and adults are most stark in neonates, becoming more adult-like with age.

  - *Cardiac index* (i.e. cardiac output (CO) corrected for body surface area) is increased by 30–60% in neonates. The high CO is required to increase O_2-carrying capacity so that the high metabolic demands of the neonate are met.

  - *The Frank–Starling response is limited.* The neonatal myocardium has a lower proportion of contractile proteins. The ventricles generate less tension during contraction and cannot increase their tension in response to increased preload. The end result is a relatively fixed stroke volume; CO is largely heart rate (HR) dependent. As a result, bradycardia is poorly tolerated: a neonatal HR of <60 bpm is an indication for cardiopulmonary resuscitation.

  - *HR decreases with age,* from a typical value of 120 bpm in neonates to 75 bpm in adults.

  - *Sinus arrhythmia,* the variation of HR with breathing, which, despite its name, is not pathological. It is thought to be due to suppression of vagal tone on inspiration leading to an increase in HR, and vice versa on expiration. It is often seen on the electrocardiogram of children below teenage years as a sinusoidal variation in R–R interval. In adults, sinus arrhythmia may be preserved in athletes who have a higher vagal tone.

419

- – *Blood pressure increases with age*, from typical systolic values of 70 mmHg in neonates to 120 mmHg in adults.
- – *Autonomic nervous system reflexes*. The parasympathetic nervous system and baroreceptor reflexes are mature in neonates, but the sympathetic nervous system is relatively immature. The neonatal response to stress (e.g. hypoxia) is therefore predominantly parasympathetic, resulting in bradycardia. Bradycardia associated with hypoxia should be initially treated with O_2 and ventilation rather than atropine!

- **Central nervous system**. Key features are:
  - – *Intracranial pressure* (ICP). Neonates and infants have a large anterior fontanelle. Raised ICP can be partially compensated for by expansion of the fontanelle and separation of the cranial sutures; palpation of the fontanelle can be used to assess ICP.
  - – *The blood–brain barrier* (BBB) is immature and incomplete in neonates. Bilirubin and drugs (e.g. opioids and barbiturates) cross the BBB more easily. This explains the increased sensitivity of neonates to respiratory depressants.
  - – *Spinal cord*. The spinal cord ends at the level of L3 in neonates and L2/3 at 1 year of age. The adult level of L1/2 is reached at around the age of 8. Incomplete myelination of nerves results in better penetration of local anaesthetic; doses may be reduced slightly. The immaturity of the sympathetic nervous system means that central neuraxial blockade is well tolerated, with hypotension being uncommon.

- **Renal physiology**. The neonatal kidneys are immature. Renal function gradually reaches adult levels by 2 years of age:
  - – Glomerular filtration rate in infants is around half that of the adult (65 mL/min compared with 120 mL/min).
  - – Tubular function is immature and concentrating ability is reduced, especially in the first week of life; a dehydrated infant has a limited ability to conserve water.
  - – Preterm neonates are unable to significantly increase their Na^+ excretion if excessive volumes of crystalloid are administered.

- **Haematology**.
  - – At birth, foetal haemoglobin (HbF) predominates. By 3 months of age, 95% of Hb is adult HbA.
  - – During foetal life, the HbF concentration is high (around 180 g/L) to maximise O_2 carriage. In the days following birth, Hb concentration rises by 10–20 g/L as fluid loss results in haemoconcentration. Over the first 3 months of life, Hb concentration falls to 100 g/L, before it rises slowly to adult levels by puberty.
  - – During foetal life, vitamin K (a fat-soluble vitamin) barely crosses the placenta. Neonates are relatively vitamin K deficient, leading to impaired hepatic synthesis of clotting factors II, VII, IX and X, with the potential for bleeding exemplified by haemorrhagic disease of the newborn. Breast milk is low in vitamin K; this is why neonates are routinely given prophylactic vitamin K shortly after birth.
  - – Blood volume is approximately 90 mL/kg in the neonate and 80 mL/kg at 6 months. By 1 year of age, blood volume reaches the adult value of 70 mL/kg.

- **Hepatic physiology**. The neonatal liver has impaired enzymatic function:
  - – The function of glucuronosyltransferase, which catalyses the glucuronidation of bilirubin, is especially poor. Plasma unconjugated bilirubin increases and crosses the immature BBB, predisposing to kernicterus.
  - – Drugs that undergo hepatic metabolism by phase 1 and 2 reactions have prolonged action, such as barbiturates and opioids.

The liver reaches normal adult function by three months.

- **Metabolic**.
  - – Neonatal BMR is double that of an adult (50 kcal/kg per day versus 25 kcal/kg per day), resulting in increased O_2 consumption and CO_2 production. This is due to the metabolic demands of growth and thermoregulation. Neonatal BMR is higher than foetal BMR; the neonate must expend energy to achieve gas exchange (up to 25% of BMR), a process that

was performed passively by the placenta in foetal life.

– Neonates are prone to hypoglycaemia due to their high BMR coupled with both low liver glycogen stores and immature gluconeogenesis enzymes. Neonates should therefore not be fasted excessively prior to surgery, and most centres would commence an intravenous glucose infusion.

- **Thermoregulation.** Neonates and infants are prone to heat loss due to:

  – A large surface area-to-body weight ratio;
  – Minimal insulating subcutaneous tissue;
  – Poorly developed shivering and vasoconstriction mechanisms.

Neonates and infants have an additional method of heat production: non-shivering thermogenesis (see Chapter 77). Under the influence of the sympathetic nervous system, brown adipose tissue oxidises free fatty acids for heat generation instead of ATP production. This process is referred to as the uncoupling of oxidative phosphorylation. O_2 consumption is significantly increased.

   Hypothermia in neonates is associated with acidosis, respiratory depression and decreased CO. Under general anaesthesia, the main mechanism of heat loss is radiation. In addition to the usual measures to prevent heat loss (forced-air warming blankets, heat and moisture exchangers, etc.), ambient theatre temperature should be increased for younger children.

- **Fluid compartments.**

  – Neonatal total body water is 75% of body weight, compared with 60% in an adult. Premature neonates have an even higher proportion of body water: up to 85%.
  – Extracellular fluid is 40% of total body weight in the neonate, compared with 20% of total body weight in an adult.
  – When nil-by-mouth, dehydration occurs more rapidly in neonates than in adults owing to:

    ▪ Increased evaporative losses due to the neonate's high surface area-to-body weight ratio.
    ▪ Increased respiratory loss of water vapour due to higher $\dot{V}_E$.
    ▪ Impaired ability to concentrate urine.

Clinical relevance: pharmacokinetic differences between children and adults

The differences between a child's and an adult's handling of drugs is most pronounced below the age of 6 months. Important features are:

- **Increased volume of distribution of water-soluble drugs.** Young children have higher proportions of extracellular and total body water. Water-soluble drugs (e.g. suxamethonium) therefore have a higher volume of distribution and require a higher per-kilogram loading dose. An exception is the non-depolarising muscle relaxants. These drugs are also water soluble, but the amount of acetylcholine released at a young child's neuromuscular junction is reduced; overall, the dose of drug required is about the same.
- **Reduced body fat.** Muscle and fat contribute a smaller proportion of body weight in very young children; drugs that normally redistribute to fat (e.g. thiopentone) will therefore have prolonged effects.
- **Immature renal and hepatic function.** This is relevant in neonates, where drug metabolism and elimination may be impaired, prolonging drug action.
- **Reduced protein binding.** As a result of reduced plasma protein concentration, the fraction of unbound drug may be higher in children than in adults. This is particularly important for drugs that are highly protein bound, such as barbiturates, phenytoin, bupivacaine and diazepam.
- **Inhalational anaesthetics.** Minimum alveolar concentration is the same at birth as in adulthood, but is 50% higher in infants, gradually decreasing throughout childhood to reach adult values by adolescence. Gaseous induction and emergence from anaesthesia are quicker in children; this is due to a smaller FRC, a greater cerebral blood flow and a greater $\dot{V}_A$.

Further reading

N. A. Chambers, A. Ramgolam, D. Sommerfield, et al. Cuffed vs. uncuffed tracheal tubes in children: a randomised controlled trial comparing leak, tidal volume and complications. *Anaesthesia* 2018; **73**(2): 160–8.

S. Bell, D. Monkhouse. Age-related pharmacology. *Anaesth Intensive Care Med* 2005; **6**(3): 89–92.

Chapter 85

Physiology of Ageing

What makes surgery and anaesthesia in older people higher risk?

Ageing involves processes not only of physical but also of psychological and social change. Increasing numbers of elderly people are undergoing elective and emergency surgery, with post-operative complications being more common in the older population. It is important to understand the normal changes that occur with advancing age so that anaesthetic techniques can be modified and to allow early identification of anaesthetic and surgical complications.

Whilst the chronological age of a patient is easily measured (i.e. years), a patient's functional age is both more important and more difficult to measure. Ageing is associated with a decline in the physiological reserve of every organ system. The mechanism of this decline is either loss of cells from an organ or reduced function of the remaining cells. The decline in organ function often begins early in adult life, but is often not clinically evident until almost all of the organ reserve is lost. Organ failure occurs either when organ function declines to a level that can no longer support life or when a disease state requires an increase in organ function that cannot be met due to insufficient reserve.

Older patients often have chronic diseases that may impact the development or progression of an acute illness. The polypharmacy that commonly accompanies chronic illness may also influence the medical and anaesthetic management of an acute illness.

Describe the physiological and anatomical changes of interest to anaesthetists

The physiological and anatomical changes associated with ageing can be classified according to organ system:

- **Respiratory system:**
  - *Airway.* The elderly are often edentulous, making bag–valve–mask ventilation more difficult, but intubation easier.
  - *Upper airway collapse.* The upper airway becomes more prone to collapse, particularly at night: partial obstruction (snoring) and arterial hypoxaemia are common. Decreased upper airway tone can be problematic during recovery from anaesthesia, with airway obstruction being more common.
  - *The thoracic cage.* With advancing age:
    - The thoracic cage becomes more rigid due to calcification of the coastal cartilages, leading to reduced thoracic wall compliance.
    - Vertebral column deformity leads to kyphosis, which adversely affects lung mechanics.
    - The diaphragm and intercostal muscles atrophy. At times of high respiratory workload, this makes the elderly more susceptible to respiratory muscle fatigue.
  - *Degeneration of the elastic fibres of the alveolar septae,* leading to:
    - Loss of support for alveoli and small airways, resulting in airway collapse in expiration (i.e. an increased closing capacity, CC). This is a major cause of $\dot{V}/\dot{Q}$ mismatch and hypoxaemia in the elderly (see Chapter 15).
    - Increased lung compliance, which partially offsets the reduced thoracic wall compliance. Overall, the combined respiratory compliance is lower in older patients; that is, the gradient of the pressure–volume curve is reduced (Figure 85.1).

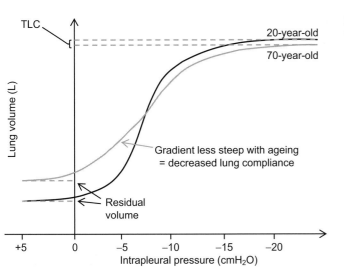

Figure 85.1 The change in lung compliance with age (TLC = total lung capacity).

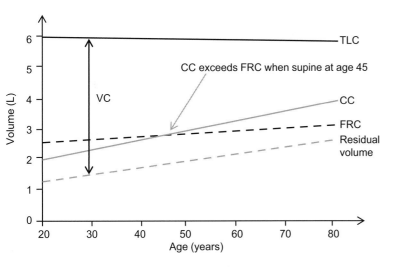

Figure 85.2 The change in lung volume with age (VC = vital capacity).

- An increase in residual volume and functional residual capacity (FRC) (Figure 85.2). FRC occurs at the point where the inward elastic forces match the outward spring of the thoracic cage. Reduced lung elastic recoil means that FRC occurs at increased lung volume. The anterior–posterior diameter of the lung increases as a consequence of the higher resting lung volume. This results in flattening of the hemi-diaphragms, putting

them at a mechanical disadvantage; the energy expended during inspiration increases.

- *Alveolar–arterial (A–a) O$_2$ gradient increases with age. This is in part due to $\dot{V}/\dot{Q}$ mismatch associated with increased CC, but is also due to:*

  - Reduced diffusing capacity of the alveoli due to both reduced alveolar surface area and increased alveolar–capillary membrane thickness;

- Hypoxic pulmonary vasoconstriction being less active, which further exacerbates $\dot{V}/\dot{Q}$ mismatch.

- **Cardiovascular system:**

  - *Arteries stiffen with age*, leading to systolic hypertension. This has two effects:

    - The walls of the aorta normally distend to accommodate the blood ejected from the left ventricle (LV). With ageing, the LV must generate a greater pressure to eject the stroke volume into a stiff aorta.
    - Normally, ejection of blood into the aorta causes a pressure wave that passes along the aorta and is reflected back towards the heart. The reflected wave reaches the heart after ejection of blood is complete and is responsible for the bump after the dicrotic notch in the arterial waveform. In the elderly, stiffened arteries cause an increase in the speed of the pressure wave. The reflected wave consequently reaches the heart in late systole, which further increases the pressure against which the ventricle must pump.

  - *Left ventricular hypertrophy.* As a consequence of the increase in afterload, the LV undergoes hypertrophy. Ventricular hypertrophy increases the stiffness of the LV, which impairs diastolic relaxation (see Chapter 30). This diastolic dysfunction worsens with age. The heart becomes progressively more dependent on atrial contraction for ventricular filling. This is why development of atrial fibrillation (AF) can so easily result in LV failure in the elderly.

  - *Veins stiffen with age.* Normally, veins act as a reservoir of blood to buffer changes in venous pressure, maintaining a constant right ventricular preload. With increasing age the veins stiffen, reducing their compliance and impairing the buffering mechanism. This is why the elderly are more likely to become hypotensive with mild hypovolaemia.

  - *Decreased response to β-adrenergic stimulation with ageing*, causing:

    - Reduced responsiveness of heart rate (HR) to catecholamines during exercise, resulting in a reduced maximum HR. Resting HR is unchanged.

  - The baroreceptors are less able to rapidly reflexively modify HR in response to changes in blood pressure, predisposing the elderly to postural hypotension.

  - *Cardiac output (CO) falls with age* at a rate of approximately 1% per year. This is due to reduced contractility of the LV as a result of both the reduced response to β-adrenergic stimuli and reduced myocyte function with advancing age.

  - *Conduction system abnormalities.* There is an increased tendency to supraventricular arrhythmias, particularly atrial and ventricular ectopic beats, and AF. This is thought to be due to fibrosis of the atria and sinoatrial node, as well as a large reduction in the number of pacemaker cells.

  - *Cardiac valve degeneration.* Calcification of the aortic valve is more common in older patients, leading to aortic sclerosis and aortic stenosis.

- **Central nervous system:**

  - *Loss of brain cells.* A generalised loss of cells leads to a reduced brain weight and the appearance of cerebral atrophy on computed tomography scan. The remaining neurons compensate by forming longer dendrites and making more connections to other neurons. Loss of dopaminergic neurons results in Parkinson's disease, whilst loss of cholinergic neurons in the hypothalamus is implicated in the development of dementia. The reduction in cell number results in a lower cerebral metabolic O_2 demand; cerebral blood flow is reduced by 10–20% as a result of the lower metabolic demand.

  - *Sensory impairment is common.* Deafness is very common in older people, and visual impairment affects around a third of the elderly population.

  - *Cognitive impairment becomes more common* with advancing age, affecting 20% of patients aged over 80.

- **Renal physiology:**

  - *Decrease in glomerular filtration rate.* Young adults have a significant reserve in renal function. From the age of 30 years, there is a progressive loss of glomeruli and reduced

renal plasma flow, resulting in a lower creatinine clearance.
- *Obstructive nephropathy* is common in elderly men due to prostatism.
- **Hepatic physiology**:
  - *Reduced liver size and hepatic blood flow* with advancing age. This results in reduced hepatic drug clearance.
  - *Decreased synthesis of plasma proteins* with advancing age. Of note, albumin concentration decreases and plasma cholinesterase levels are reduced.
- **Endocrine system**: diabetes mellitus is common in the elderly. There is an increase in peripheral insulin resistance and impaired insulin secretion in response to hyperglycaemia.
- **Locomotor and skin**:
  - The elderly tend to have reduced subcutaneous tissue, thin skin and fragile veins; achieving venous access can be difficult. Infusions of fluids or drugs can extravasate, especially if introduced under pressure. Pressure sores are more common, and additional care must be taken with patient positioning and padding of pressure points.
  - There is a generalised loss of muscle mass with advancing age, known as sarcopenia; 6 kg of muscle is lost by 80 years of age. This is thought to be due to loss of motor neurons, resulting in decreased levels of Ca^{2+} within the sarcoplasm.
  - Arthritis and bony deformities are very common in older people. This may lead to difficulty with mobility and positioning, potentially making regional anaesthesia more difficult. Larger-calibre spinal needles may be required to pass through calcified ligaments. Fortunately, post-dural puncture headache is far less common in the elderly.
- **Thermoregulation** is impaired with advancing age:
  - The elderly are at risk of hypothermia due to a reduction in heat production: basal metabolic rate decreases by 1% per year, and there is a reduction in the peripheral vasoconstrictor response to cold exposure.
  - Older patients are especially at risk of intraoperative hypothermia. Post-operative

shivering is the normal mechanism of returning to normothermia. The elderly may lack the muscle bulk to shiver effectively or may have insufficient cardiopulmonary reserve to meet the increased O_2 demand of shivering. Prevention of perioperative hypothermia in the elderly is crucial.
  - The elderly are also at risk of hyperthermia due to impairment of sweating.
- **Body compartments**:
  - *A reduced blood volume and a higher proportion of body fat* can lead to changes in the volume of distribution.
  - *Plasma protein concentration is reduced*, resulting in decreased drug protein binding, an increase in the free drug fraction and thus a higher free drug concentration.

What are the causes of ageing?

There are a number of theories of ageing. Ageing is thought to be:
- Caused by cell damage occurring throughout life; or
- Genetically pre-programmed.

Some of the more well-recognised theories of ageing are:
- **Telomere theory**. Telomeres are non-coding structures at the ends of chromosomes. During replication, DNA polymerase discards the three most distal base pairs, thus shortening the DNA sequence – the presence of a distal telomere segment therefore protects the coding section of DNA from shortening, which would result in the loss of genetic material. With ageing, the telomere is degraded and coding genetic information is lost. In response to DNA damage, cells undergo apoptosis.
- **Free radical theory**. Reactive O_2 species are highly reactive free radicals formed normally as part of metabolism. Free radicals cause oxidative stress, which results in ageing of cells.
- **Somatic mutation theory**. Cellular division can result in random mutations, producing inefficient cells. These cells accumulate with age, causing progressive organ dysfunction.

Clinical relevance: pharmacology and ageing

The physiological changes that occur with age have a number of pharmacological implications for the anaesthetist:

- **Altered drug pharmacokinetics**:
  - *Higher peak plasma concentration of drug* due to the lower volume of distribution.
  - *Prolonged terminal half-life of some drugs* due to sequestration of lipophilic drugs in the increased body fat and the reduced hepatic and renal clearance. Of particular note is that the effects of benzodiazepines given at induction of anaesthesia may persist into the post-operative period.
- **Vasopressors**. The reduced cardiac response to β-agonists means that mixed α- and β-agonists (e.g. ephedrine) become less effective with advancing age. Pure α-agonists (e.g. phenylephrine) are as effective in the elderly as in young people.
- **Intravenous induction agents**. The altered pharmacokinetics in the elderly leads to higher free drug plasma concentrations of the intravenous induction agents. The dose of induction agent therefore needs to be reduced. The reduced CO prolongs the arm–brain circulation time, so intravenous induction drugs must be injected slowly to avoid inadvertent overdose and the associated hypotension.
- **Inhalational agents**. Minimum alveolar concentration of inhalational anaesthetics is reduced by up to 30% in the elderly. The duration of inhalational induction may be prolonged due to the reduced alveolar diffusion and increased $\dot{V}/\dot{Q}$ mismatch that occur with advancing age.
- **Neuromuscular blockade**. The dose of non-depolarising muscle relaxants is unchanged in the elderly. The time taken to reach intubating conditions is increased due to reduced CO. The duration of neuromuscular blockade may be prolonged in the elderly depending on the mechanism of drug metabolism:
  - *Atracurium* has the same duration of action. Its metabolism is independent of renal and liver function as atracurium is metabolised by plasma esterases and through Hofmann elimination.
  - *Mivacurium and suxamethonium* have prolonged effects; these drugs are metabolised through the action of plasma cholinesterases, which are reduced in the elderly. The prolonged action of suxamethonium is clinically insignificant.
  - *Aminosteroid muscle relaxants* may have prolonged action in the elderly as their metabolism relies on both hepatic metabolism and renal excretion.

Further reading

G. Rai, A. Abdulla. *The Biology of Ageing and Its Clinical Implication: A Practical Handbook*. Boca Raton, CRC Press, 2012.

G. D. K. Matthews, C. L. H. Huang, L. Sun, et al. Translational musculoskeletal science: sarcopenia the next clinical target after osteoporosis? *Ann N Y Acad Sci* 2011; **1237**: 95–105.

J. F. Karp, J. W. Shega, N. E. Morone, et al. Advances in understanding the mechanisms and management of persistent pain in older adults. *Br J Anaesth* 2008; **101**(1): 110–20.

D. Murray, C. Dodds. Perioperative care of the elderly. *Continuing Educ Anaesth Crit Care Pain* 2004; **4**(6): 193–6.

Physiology of Obesity

What is the definition of obesity?

The World Health Organization classifies obesity based in the patient's body mass index (BMI); their weight (in kilograms) divided by the square of their height (in metres):

• <18.5	Underweight
• 18.5–24.9	Healthy weight
• 25.0–29.9	Overweight
• 30.0–34.9	Obesity class I (formerly known simply as 'obesity')
• 35.0–39.9	Obesity class II (formerly known as 'morbid obesity' if associated with an obesity-related comorbidity)
• >40.0	Obesity class III (formerly known as 'morbid obesity')

What are the physiological consequences of obesity of relevance to anaesthetists?

There is increasing evidence that obesity stimulates the innate immune system to increase production of the proinflammatory mediators tumour necrosis factor-α (TNF-α) and interleukin-6 (IL-6). The resulting state of low-grade inflammation is thought to be at least partially responsible for many of the pathophysiological changes associated with obesity.

System by system, the key features are:

- **Respiratory**:
  - *Airway*: increased prevalence of upper airway collapse (see Chapter 6) and difficult laryngoscopy. Correct patient head positioning before induction is crucial: a head-elevating laryngoscopy pillow may be required.
  - *Lung volume*: reduced functional residual capacity (FRC) due to weight of chest wall; closing capacity may exceed FRC, causing atelectasis and ventilation–perfusion ($\dot{V}/\dot{Q}$) mismatch; decreased thoracic compliance, leading to an increased work of breathing (see Chapter 21).
  - *Gas exchange*: increased O_2 consumption and CO_2 production due to the increased tissue mass – minute ventilation, $\dot{V}_E$, must increase to maintain normocapnoea.
  - *Obstructive sleep apnoea* (OSA): obesity increases the risk of OSA, which manifests as repeated cycles of overnight hypoxaemia and hypercapnoea (see Chapter 6).
  - *Asthma*: obese patients are twice as likely to develop asthma as the non-obese population. The cause is unclear, but may be related to the chronic inflammation associated with obesity or decreased airway calibre as a result of reduced lung volumes.

Overall: obese patients have the potential for rapid desaturation at induction of anaesthesia due to increased O_2 consumption combined with decreased FRC. Pre-oxygenation prior to induction of anaesthesia is of great importance and is perhaps best achieved using high-flow nasal oxygen therapy (see Chapter 6).

- **Cardiovascular** system changes occur as a result of adaptation to excess body mass and increased metabolic demands:
  - *Left-sided circulation*: excess body mass requires an increase in intravascular volume and cardiac output (mainly due to an increase in stroke volume, SV). Systemic hypertension is common in obesity and, together with the increased SV, results in left ventricular

hypertrophy and an increase in left ventricular work.
- *Coronary disease*: increased incidence of ischaemic heart disease due to systemic hypertension, dyslipidaemia and diabetes mellitus. It is important to note that symptoms of significant coronary artery stenosis may be masked by physical inactivity.
- *Right-sided circulation*: the changes in the respiratory system outlined above stimulate hypoxic pulmonary vasoconstriction, which leads to pulmonary hypertension and increased right ventricular work. This can lead to right ventricular hypertrophy and failure (cor pulmonale).
- *Venous system*: increased risk of venous thromboembolism. Intermittent calf compressors should be used intra- and post-operatively until the patient is adequately mobile.
- **Gastrointestinal**:
  - *Gastroesophageal reflux* is common due to lower oesophageal incompetence and increased intragastric pressure. General anaesthesia is associated with an increased aspiration risk.
  - *Hepatobiliary*: increased prevalence of gallstone disease and non-alcoholic steatohepatitis.
- **Endocrine**: the state of low-grade chronic inflammation promotes insulin resistance and the development of type 2 diabetes mellitus and hyperlipidaemia.
- **Musculoskeletal**: there is an increased prevalence of osteoarthritis (OA) and gout in the obese. As one would expect, there is a definite association between OA in weight-bearing joints and obesity. Interestingly, there is also an increased prevalence of OA in non-weight-bearing joints (e.g. those of the hand) in obese individuals, suggesting that the mechanism for the development of OA is not purely biomechanical, and possibly the low-grade state of inflammation plays a role.
- **Morphological**:
  - *Practical aspects*: obesity increases the difficulty of a number of practical procedures, including venous access, regional anaesthesia and surgical access. Limb tourniquets may not adequately fit.

- *Monitoring*: an upper arm non-invasive blood pressure cuff may have a poor fit and thus be unreliable. Instead, either the blood pressure cuff may be positioned at the forearm or calf or an invasive arterial line may be required.
- *Positioning and lifting* of an unconscious patient is more difficult, requiring a greater number of staff. Special equipment may be required, such as an intubation positioning aid, a hover mattress, a bariatric operating table and/or a bariatric bed.

What is the role of leptin in the control of appetite?

The control of appetite is complex, involving a number of hormones. Leptin and cholecystokinin are known to suppress appetite, whilst a number of agents stimulate appetite: ghrelin (a peptide hormone produced in the gut), insulin and the neurotransmitters dopamine and serotonin.

Leptin is a peptide hormone secreted by adipose cells that acts at the hypothalamus to inhibit hunger. Leptin is involved in a negative-feedback loop that aims to maintain body fat stores – the greater the number of adipose cells present, the greater the secretion of leptin, which acts to inhibits appetite. However, leptin levels are paradoxically high in obese patients: the hypothalamus becomes resistant to circulating leptin and fails to produce a feeling of satiety.

Clinical relevance: pharmacokinetics and obesity

In obese patients, the pharmacokinetics of many drugs are altered as a result of increased body lipid, reduced lean body mass (LBM) and decreased total body water.

- **Absorption**: gastric emptying may be increased or decreased; subcutaneous absorption is decreased due to poor blood supply; intravenous access may be challenging to achieve; the intramuscular route may fail if needles are too short.
- **Distribution**: there is an increased volume of distribution (V_d) for fat-soluble drugs such as midazolam, fentanyl, propofol and thiopentone. For these agents, ideal body weight (IBW) or LBM should be used instead of total body weight (TBW) when calculating bolus drug doses. For hydrophilic drugs, such as non-depolarising muscle relaxants, V_d is relatively unchanged –

LBM should be used when dosing. Exceptions are suxamethonium, which should be dosed on TBW, and remifentanil, whose pharmacokinetics are similar in obese and lean patients.

- **Metabolism**: hepatic clearance may be affected (may be increased or decreased) by fatty liver infiltration.
- **Elimination** may be affected by obesity-related co-morbidity, such as nephropathy secondary to diabetes or hypertension. Volatile anaesthetics show a similar time to recovery in obese and non-obese patients, with desflurane (least lipophilic) having only a minor advantage over isoflurane (most lipophilic).

Clinical relevance: obesity and target controlled infusions

Total intravenous anaesthesia (TIVA) is challenging in morbidly obese patients. TIVA is most commonly delivered using target controlled infusion pumps programmed with either the Marsh (propofol), Schnider (propofol) or Minto (remifentanil) pharmacokinetic models. However, there is controversy over which pharmacokinetic model to use in the morbidly obese and which weight to input:

- V_d **and rate constants** of all models were derived from normal-weight subjects – the pharmacokinetic models are therefore not formally validated in the morbidly obese.
- **The Marsh model** uses TBW to calculate the induction dose and maintenance infusion rates of propofol. However, in the morbidly obese, an induction bolus of propofol based on TBW is likely to represent a significant overdose and result in unwanted cardiovascular side effects. To prevent overdosing, pump manufacturers limit the input weight to the Marsh model at 150 kg. Anaesthetists may choose instead to use a modified input weight (e.g. Servin's formula:

input weight = IBW + 0.4 × (TBW – IBW)). This modification accurately predicts plasma propofol concentration in the early part of an anaesthetic, but increasingly underdoses patients after 40 min, risking accidental awareness.

- **The Schnider model** uses the inputs of age, height and TBW and calculates LBM[1] for use in its algorithm. The LBM calculation is accurate up to a BMI of 42 kg/m² in males and 37 kg/m² in females, but when patients exceed this BMI, the calculated LBM paradoxically decreases. As the Schnider model uses LBM to correct the rate constant for drug elimination from the central compartment, the clinical effect of this error is a higher maintenance infusion and anaesthetic overdose.
- **The Minto model** also uses the same LBM formula as the Schnider model and therefore suffers from inaccuracies at high BMI. The clinical effect here, however, is an underdosing of remifentanil during the maintenance infusion.

Despite the flaws of the above pharmacokinetic models in the morbidly obese, TIVA can still be used safely in this patient group. Arguably, the best strategy is to use the Schnider and Minto models titrated to surgical depth of anaesthesia using processed electroencephalogram monitoring.

Further reading

L. E. C. De Baerdemaeker, E. P. Mortier, M. M. R. F. Struys. Pharmacokinetics in obese patients. *Continuing Educ Anaesth Crit Care Pain* 2004; **4**(5): 152–5.

S. Lotia, M. C. Bellamy. Anaesthesia and morbid obesity. *Contuing Educ Anaesth Crit Care Pain* 2008; **8**(5): 151–6.

J. Ingrande, H. J. M. Lemmens. Dose adjustment of anaesthetics in the morbidly obese. *Br J Anaesth* 2010; **105**(Suppl. 1): i16–23.

A. R. Absalom, V. Mani, T. De Smet, M. M. R. F. Struys. Pharmacokinetic models for propofol – defining and illuminating the devil in the detail. *Br J Anaesth* 2009; **103**(1): 26–37.

---

[1] Using the formulae $LBM_{men} = 1.1 \times TBW - 128 \times (TBW/height\ (in\ cm))^2$; $LBM_{women} = 1.07 \times TBW - 148 \times (TBW/height\ (in\ cm))^2$.

Chapter

87

Altitude

High altitude has no consensus definition. It is most commonly defined as corresponding to >2500 m above sea level, where most individuals begin to show physiological adaptations. Long-term habitation at high altitude is possible – 100 million people live at altitudes >2500 m. Extreme altitude is defined as >6000 m – Mount Everest is 8848 m high. Humans are able to adapt their physiology to survive for short periods of time at extreme altitude, but long-term habitation is impossible.

What are the problems associated with high altitude?

High altitude presents a number of problems to the body, classified as:

- **Reduced barometric pressure** (P_B): during ascent, the P_B decreases exponentially.
- **Temperature**: the environmental temperature falls by 1°C for every 150 m elevation above sea level.
- **Reduced relative humidity**: this results in increased evaporative losses from the skin and respiratory tract.
- **Increased solar radiation**: due to reduced cloud cover.

How is alveolar oxygen tension P_AO_2 affected by altitude?

P_AO_2 is calculated using the alveolar gas equation (AGE) (see Chapter 18):

$$P_AO_2 = [F_iO_2 \times (P_B - P_{SVPwater})] - \frac{P_aCO_2}{R}$$

As the height above sea level increases, P_B decreases exponentially, but the inspired fractional oxygen concentration *remains the same* (21%); P_AO_2 will also therefore decrease. In turn:

- As alveolar gas is in equilibrium with the arterial gas, P_aO_2 will fall.
- A fall in P_aO_2 results in lower haemoglobin (Hb) saturation (see Chapter 8), with the result that O_2 carriage is reduced.
- O_2 delivery becomes insufficient for the tissues to maintain their normal metabolic processes; that is, hypoxaemic hypoxia develops.

Saturated vapour pressure of water is unchanged by altitude (6.3 kPa at 37°C), so it has a proportionally greater effect on P_AO_2 at higher altitudes, when P_B is reduced.

How does the body adapt to survive at altitude?

Survival at altitude depends on a coordinated response by the respiratory, cardiovascular, haematological and renal systems. No physiological changes are seen below 2500 m in a healthy adult, probably because P_aO_2 is above the threshold for activation of the peripheral chemoreceptors (around 8 kPa).

The acute response to altitude produces a compensatory increase in P_aO_2 by hyperventilation, but its action is limited by the resulting respiratory alkalosis. This is followed by the chronic adaptive response, in which a further increase in ventilation is permitted as the kidney corrects the pH disturbance. System by system:

Respiratory system. Important aspects are:

- **Hyperventilation**. The peripheral chemoreceptors (but not the central chemoreceptors) are sensitive to changes in P_aO_2 (see Chapter 22). When P_aO_2 falls below 8 kPa, the peripheral chemoreceptors stimulate the respiratory centre in the medulla, resulting in increased $\dot{V}_A$. The consequent fall in P_aCO_2 leads to an increase in P_AO_2, according to the AGE (see above).

- **'Braking effect'.** The unwanted consequence of hyperventilation is an increase in arterial pH; that is, a respiratory alkalosis. Hypocapnoea is detected by the central chemoreceptors, whilst alkalosis is detected by the carotid bodies; both act to limit the increase in $\dot{V}_A$.[1]
- **Diffusion limitation.** Transfer of O_2 across the alveolar–capillary barrier may become diffusion limited at altitude (see Chapter 10), especially in association with exercise (where the pulmonary capillary transit time is reduced) and in patients with high-altitude pulmonary oedema (interstitial fluid thickens the alveolar–capillary barrier).

Cardiovascular system. Key features are:

- **Increased heart rate** (HR) as a result of increased sympathetic outflow triggered by the peripheral chemoreceptors.
- **Reduced plasma volume.** Haematocrit increases due to a 20% reduction in plasma volume. This is the combined result of a pressure diuresis (an increase in renal perfusion driven by the increase in sympathetic activity), increased fluid loss (hyperventilation and reduced relative humidity) and decreased oral intake (loss of appetite). Stroke volume falls as a result of the reduction in preload, but overall cardiac output remains the same owing to tachycardia.
- **Increased myocardial work.** The high haematocrit of the blood (up to 0.6 with chronic acclimatisation) increases the viscosity of the blood. The work required to move blood in the circulation (i.e. the left ventricular work) is increased.
- **Hypoxic pulmonary vasoconstriction** (HPV). The pulmonary arterioles vasoconstrict in response to low P_AO_2 (see Chapter 23). Normally,

HPV is a useful mechanism to optimise $\dot{V}/\dot{Q}$ matching when a region of the lung is hypoxic (e.g. due to a lobar pneumonia). However, the generalised hypoxia that occurs at altitude results in a potentially harmful global pulmonary arteriolar vasoconstriction. Pulmonary vascular resistance increases by 50–300%, resulting in pulmonary hypertension. The increase in pulmonary capillary hydrostatic pressure may cause fluid transudation, known as high-altitude pulmonary oedema (HAPE). In addition, the sudden onset of pulmonary hypertension may precipitate right heart failure in susceptible individuals.

Haematological system. The sigmoid shape of the oxyhaemoglobin dissociation curve is important: S_aO_2 remains >90% at elevations of up to 3000 m in normal patients. At higher altitudes, compensatory mechanisms occur:

- **Leftward shift of the oxyhaemoglobin dissociation curve.** Hyperventilation-induced alkalosis shifts the P_{50} of the oxyhaemoglobin dissociation curve to the left. This aids the loading of scarce O_2 onto the Hb molecule in the lungs, but prevents offloading of O_2 to the tissues (see Chapter 8).
- **Increased 2,3-diphosphoglycerate** (DPG). To compensate for the leftward shift of the oxyhaemoglobin dissociation curve, erythrocytes produce a greater amount of 2,3-DPG. This causes a rightward shift of the curve in order to facilitate O_2 offloading from Hb, returning the P_{50} to the normal sea-level position within a week.
- **Increased red cell mass.** The kidney responds to chronic hypoxaemia within hours of ascent by increasing the secretion of erythropoietin, which stimulates erythrocyte production by the bone marrow. Over time, red cell mass increases, restoring the blood's O_2-carrying capacity to near normal.
- **Increased risk of thrombotic events.** This is as a result of both the increase in haematocrit (which increases the viscosity of the blood) and the activation of platelets due to hypoxaemia.

Thermoregulation. Continuous exposure to a cold environment causes a number of metabolic changes:

---

[1] It was previously thought that over the following days the alkalaemia is partially corrected as a result of increased renal HCO_3^- excretion: the 'brakes' are then taken off, allowing a further increase in $\dot{V}_A$. However, more recent studies show that the braking effect is decreased before renal HCO_3^- excretion begins. This suggests that a faster central mechanism is involved in acclimatisation. This may be due to a decrease in cerebrospinal fluid HCO_3^- concentration, although the mechanism for this is not completely elucidated.

- **Heat conservation**. Mechanisms include peripheral vasoconstriction, decreased sweating and behavioural changes (e.g. wearing more clothes).
- **Heat generation**. Mechanisms include increasing basal metabolic rate, shivering and increased brown fat activity (in infants). All of the heat-generating mechanisms increase O_2 consumption at a time of relative hypoxaemia.

What is acute high-altitude illness?

Acute high-altitude illness is a maladaptive physiological response to altitude occurring in unacclimatised people who ascend too quickly. The rate of acclimatisation has significant interpatient variability: some people acclimatise much more slowly than others, making them more susceptible to acute high-altitude illness. Three high-altitude syndromes are classically described:

- **Acute mountain sickness** (AMS) is a neurological syndrome whose cardinal feature is headache, combined with a number of other non-specific features: nausea, anorexia, dizziness and insomnia. Symptoms usually improve after 3–4 days at the same altitude; that is, allowing additional time for acclimatisation.
- **High-altitude cerebral oedema** (HACE) is similar to AMS, but at the severe end of the disease spectrum. The cardinal features of HACE are headache combined with ataxia or cognitive impairment. This is a serious condition, which may progress to seizures, coma and death. The mechanism by which HACE develops is unknown.
- **HAPE** is thought to occur as a result of changes to the Starling forces in the alveolus following HPV. Early symptoms are exertional dyspnoea and a persistent dry cough; patients later develop haemoptysis and orthopnoea. HAPE is the most serious of the acute high-altitude illnesses, accounting for the majority of mortality.

The only definitive treatment for the acute high-altitude illnesses is descent. Other treatments buy time:

- *Supplemental O_2*: the fastest way to increase P_AO_2, thereby counteracting the most harmful effects of high altitude.
- *Hyperbaric chamber*: reduces the effective altitude of the patient, simulating descent. A portable hyperbaric chamber (the Gamow bag) is available.

- *A variety of pharmacological treatments*, including acetazolamide, dexamethasone and nifedipine.

Clinical relevance: anaesthesia at altitude

Whilst it is clearly inadvisable to perform a general anaesthetic at extreme altitude, many hospitals worldwide are located at moderate altitude (2000–3000 m above sea level). In addition to the physiological changes associated with high altitude and the risks of hypoxaemia, there are a number of other equipment-related issues for the anaesthetist:

- **Vaporisers**. Saturated vapour pressure is not affected by changes in P_B. Therefore, the partial pressure of a volatile agent within a plenum vaporiser is the same at high altitude as at sea level. At altitude, the lower atmospheric pressure results in a higher concentration of volatile agent being delivered to the patient than that 'dialled' (i.e. percentage when calibrated at sea level). However, it is the alveolar partial pressure of the agent that determines its clinical effect, and this remains constant. Therefore, an isoflurane vaporiser set at 1% will have the same clinical effect at high altitude as at sea level.
- **Flowmeters**. Variable-orifice flowmeters are calibrated at sea level and are under-read at high altitude owing to a reduction in gas density. However, since it is the number of molecules (e.g. of O_2) and not the volume of gas that matters clinically, flowmeters can be used as normal.
- **Venturi-type O_2 masks**. At altitude, these deliver a slightly higher percentage of O_2 than at sea level.
- **Cuff pressures**. Pressures within cuffed endotracheal tubes or laryngeal mask airways may increase significantly with rapid acute changes in altitude, such as may occur during an aeromedical transfer of a critically ill patient. Unchecked, the increased cuff pressure may cause ischaemic injury to the tracheal or pharyngeal mucosa.

Further reading

J. B. West, R. B. Schoene, A. M. Luks, J. S. Milledge. *High Altitude Medicine and Physiology, 5th edition*. Boca Raton, CRC Press, 2012.

J. P. R. Brown, M. P. W. Grocott. Humans at altitude: physiology and pathophysiology. *Continuing Educ Anaesth Crit Care Pain* 2013; **13**(1): 17–22.

K. B. Leissner, F. U. Mahmood. Physiology and pathophysiology at high altitude: considerations for the anaesthesiologist. *J Anesth* 2009; **23**(4): 543–53.

Diving

You may wonder what a chapter entitled 'diving' is doing in a book for anaesthetists – only the few who work in coastal areas will ever be required to anaesthetise patients with decompression sickness. However, the primitive diving reflex is of clinical interest, and the physiology and physics associated with descent are not infrequently tested in postgraduate examinations.

What is the diving reflex?

The diving reflex is a relic of human evolution from aquatic species. Exposure of the face, specifically the areas of trigeminal nerve distribution, to ice-cold water triggers a reflex that is designed to allow prolonged submersion underwater. There are three cardiopulmonary changes:

- **Apnoea.** Breathing stops, often with a gasp, which prevents the lungs filling with water.
- **Bradycardia.** In humans, the bradycardia is mild (in the region of 10–25%), but in some sea mammals heart rate falls by up to 90%.
- **Peripheral vasoconstriction.** Blood is diverted away from the peripheries to maximise heart and brain perfusion.

In humans, the diving reflex is strongest in neonates and infants – the diving reflex enables photographs of babies 'swimming' underwater to be taken without the baby drowning! Perhaps more relevant to anaesthetists is that:

- The bradycardia is mediated by the vagus nerve. In addition to reducing the frequency of sinoatrial node impulses, conduction through the atrioventricular node is also reduced. Immersing a patient's face in a bowl of ice-cold water can therefore be used to terminate a supraventricular tachycardia.
- People have survived prolonged immersion (20–30 min) in icy water (e.g. falling through ice

on a frozen lake) – this is in part due to the diving reflex maximising cerebral blood flow by intense peripheral vasoconstriction. Children are more likely to survive prolonged immersion than adults owing to:

- A stronger diving reflex;
- A greater surface area-to-bodyweight ratio, resulting in a faster fall in body temperature, which reduces cerebral metabolic rate and protects against cerebral ischaemia.

Which physiological changes occur during head-out immersion?

The physiology of a body immersed in water differs from normal physiology on land in a number of ways:

- *Venous pooling in the legs does not occur.* The effect of gravity is opposed by the external hydrostatic pressure of the surrounding water. The end result is the mobilisation of around 500 mL of blood back into the circulation. In the heart, increased blood volume stretches the atrial and ventricular walls, causing the release of atrial natriuretic peptide and brain natriuretic peptide, which produce a diuresis.
- *Increased work of breathing.* The hydrostatic pressure of the surrounding water also has implications for respiratory mechanics, increasing the work of breathing by 60%.

What happens to the air in the lungs during a breath-hold dive?

Ambient pressure increases underwater; pressure is measured in metres of seawater (msw). In fact, for every 10-m descent, ambient pressure increases by 100 kPa.

As a breath-hold diver descends, ambient pressure increases: the volume of air within the lungs decreases

(Boyle's law). With deeper dives, the volume of the lungs may fall below residual volume, risking negative-pressure pulmonary oedema.

As the breath-hold diver ascends, the air within the lungs re-expands. However, as metabolic processes continue during the course of the dive, alveolar O_2 will have been consumed and CO_2 produced. On reaching the water's surface, the lung volume will be reduced slightly due to O_2 consumption being slightly higher than CO_2 production (see Chapter 18). The fraction of O_2 within the lung will be decreased: rapid ascent from a deep-water dive therefore results in a rapid fall in the alveolar partial pressure of O_2, potentially resulting in cerebral hypoxia and unconsciousness.

How does breath-hold diving compare with SCUBA diving?

SCUBA stands for 'self-contained underwater breathing apparatus'. Compressed air is delivered at ambient pressure from a tank to the diver via a demand valve (bear in mind that the ambient pressure depends on underwater depth). Breathing air at ambient pressure avoids the problem of reduced lung volume experienced by breath-hold divers, but introduces a number of other complications:

- **Increased gas density**. As the diver descends, the partial pressure of the inspired air increases. The density of the inhaled gases is therefore also higher. Increased gas density results in an increase in turbulent gas flow (see Chapter 21), especially during inspiration, resulting in an increased work of breathing. N_2 in air can be replaced by the lower-density helium (He) in a mixture known as Heliox in order to counteract this problem.

- **Nitrogen narcosis**. Very high pressures of N_2 can directly affect the central nervous system (CNS), leading to a feeling of euphoria, incoordination, loss of concentration and eventually coma. Again, N_2 can be replaced by He, which has no effect on CNS function at equivalent pressures.

- **O_2 toxicity**. As discussed in Chapter 24, breathing O_2 at high partial pressures is potentially harmful, causing acute lung injury, seizures and loss of consciousness. The latter two have profound consequences in the context of diving. The risk of O_2 toxicity is prevented by limiting the O_2

exposure time: divers calculate their maximum time underwater based on the depth of the dive.

What is decompression sickness?

Decompression sickness is a consequence of breathing N_2 at high partial pressures. N_2 is usually poorly soluble in blood, with very little dissolved in the circulation at sea level. However, SCUBA divers breathing compressed air mixtures inhale higher partial pressures of N_2. According to Henry's law, the amount of N_2 dissolved in solution is proportional to the partial pressure of N_2 above the solution. Therefore, additional N_2 crosses the alveolar–capillary membrane into the circulation, where it deposits into the body's tissues.

The problem comes at ascent:

- Slow, staged ascent allows a steady reduction in the partial pressure of inspired N_2. Allowing time for equilibration facilitates N_2 removal from the body's tissues.

- During rapid ascent, the sudden change in ambient pressure causes N_2 to come out of solution, with N_2 bubbles forming in (amongst other organs):

  - *Joints*, causing pain ('the bends');
  - *The pulmonary circulation*, causing dyspnoea ('the chokes') and retrosternal pain;
  - *The arterial circulation*, resulting in gas embolism.

In addition to slow ascent, decompression sickness can be prevented by breathing O_2–He gas mixtures. Once symptoms of decompression sickness have developed, the most effective treatment is recompression in a hyperbaric chamber. This forces the N_2 bubbles back into solution. This is then followed by a slow, controlled decompression.

Further reading

A. O. Brubakk, T. S. Neuman. *Bennett and Elliotts' Physiology and Medicine of Diving, 5th edition.* Philadelphia, Saunders, 2002.

M. Castellini. Life under water: physiological adaptations to diving and living at sea. *Compr Physiol* 2012; **2:** 1889–919.

A. S. Blix, B. Folkow. Cardiovascular adjustments to diving in mammals and birds. *Compr Physiol* 2011; (Suppl. 8): 917–45.

Temperature Regulation

How is body temperature regulated?

Core body temperature is one of the most tightly controlled physiological parameters. Normal core body temperature ranges from 36.5 to 37.5°C. Peripheral body temperature, involving the skin and subcutaneous tissues of the trunk and limbs, is less well controlled – the difference between core and peripheral temperatures is usually around 2–3°C, but can be as much as 20°C in extreme circumstances.

Body temperature is determined by a balance of heat loss and production:

- Heat loss occurs due to radiation, convection, evaporation (sweat and respiration), conduction and loss in urine and faeces.
- Heat is produced by basal metabolic processes, exercise, shivering and non-shivering thermogenesis (in neonates and infants).

Temperature is regulated by both feedforward and negative-feedback loop control. Feedforward control is mediated by the central nervous system (CNS) involving interpretation and prediction of the external environment. If it is snowing, you are likely to put on a coat before going outside. This prevents any temperature change from occurring.

Negative-feedback control contains the usual elements for sensing and correcting the internal environment:

- **Temperature sensors**. These are a large family of temperature-gated ion channels known as transient receptor potential channels. Peripheral and core temperature sensors send information to the hypothalamus.
- **A control centre**. The hypothalamus analyses the afferent temperature signals, checks them against a set-point and controls the efferent response.
- **Effector system**.
    - *Temperature-losing mechanisms* involving sweating and skin vasodilatation are controlled by the anterior hypothalamus.

    - *Temperature-conserving and -generating mechanisms* involving vasoconstriction, shivering, non-shivering thermogenesis, behavioural changes (e.g. putting on more clothes or turning up the central heating) are controlled by the posterior hypothalamus.

Whilst basal metabolic rate (BMR) cannot be increased to boost heat production, shivering is extremely effective, producing up to a sixfold increase in heat production.

How does general anaesthesia disturb the normal thermoregulatory mechanisms?

Mild hypothermia (34.0–36.5°C) is common during general anaesthesia – the cause is often multifactorial:

- Patients may arrive at theatre cold; for example, following a prolonged wait in a cold preoperative ward whilst wearing a thin hospital gown.
- The hypothalamic set-point is lowered during general anaesthesia. Normally, the hypothalamus responds to a core temperature below 36.5°C with vasoconstriction, and shivering commences at 36.0°C. Under general anaesthesia, these threshold temperatures are lowered by 2–3°C.
- Behavioural changes are (obviously) lost under general anaesthesia. The patient is no longer able to put on additional layers of clothes.
- Muscle paralysis prevents shivering.
- Most anaesthetic drugs cause vasodilatation, counteracting the normal vasoconstriction response to hypothermia.

The reduction in core body temperature associated with general anaesthesia normally follows a triphasic pattern (Figure 89.1):

- **Redistribution phase**. A decrease in core temperature of 1.5–2.0°C over 30–45 min. This is

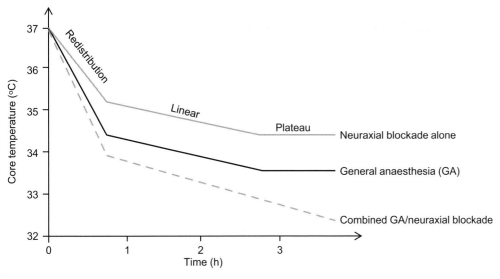

Figure 89.1 Characteristic pattern of intraoperative hypothermia.

a consequence of the administration of a vasodilator (e.g. a volatile anaesthetic) in combination with a reduction in the hypothalamic set-point for vasoconstriction.

- **Linear phase**. A more gradual fall of 1°C over the next 2–3 h due to radiation, convection and evaporation. The degree of evaporation depends on the type of surgery, being highest in open abdominal procedures.

- **Plateau phase**. When peripheral vasoconstriction becomes activated, core temperature reaches a plateau when the rate of heat loss is matched by basal metabolic heat production. However, in patients who have both general anaesthesia and neuraxial blockade, peripheral vasoconstriction is ineffective and core temperature continues to decline.

What are the adverse effects of hypothermia?

In addition to heat-conserving mechanisms such as peripheral vasoconstriction and shivering, hypothermia causes a number of other physiological changes:

- **Cardiovascular system**:
  - 'J'-waves may be seen on the electrocardiogram; they are thought to represent an increase in phase 1 repolarization.
  - Heart rate and blood pressure decrease with the severity of hypothermia; severe

bradycardia (<30 bpm) is very common below 28°C.
  - Arrhythmias are increasingly common. Below 28°C, spontaneous ventricular fibrillation (VF) can occur; more victims of the sinking of *RMS Titanic* died from hypothermia-induced VF than from drowning.
  - The oxyhaemoglobin dissociation curve is shifted to the left, increasing O_2 affinity and reducing O_2 offloading to the tissues.
  - Blood viscosity increases, which increases left ventricular work.
  - Myocardial ischaemia or infarction may be precipitated by the physiological changes above.

- **CNS**.
  - Confusion and irritability occur with mild hypothermia.
  - At a core temperature of 20°C, the electroencephalogram may be consistent with brain death.

- **Metabolic**.
  - BMR reduces by 6% for every 1°C drop in core temperature.
  - Hyperglycaemia occurs due to reduced cellular uptake of glucose.
  - Enzymatic reactions are slowed, including those of drug metabolism; the action of muscle relaxants is prolonged.

- **Renal**. Suppression of antidiuretic hormone secretion results in a 'cold diuresis'.
- **Haematological**. Hypothermia has been implicated in platelet and clotting dysfunction, but it is likely that these effects are only minor.

Clinical relevance: adverse effects of intraoperative hypothermia

There are a number of adverse effects associated with mild perioperative hypothermia:

- Myocardial ischaemia, infarction and arrhythmias;
- Increased intraoperative blood loss and increased requirement for transfusion;
- Increased incidence of post-operative wound infection;
- Prolonged post-operative recovery and prolonged hospital stay.

Common measures to prevent intraoperative hypothermia include:

- Active warming with forced-air warmers and heated mattresses;
- Warming of intravenous fluids and blood;
- Humidification of inspired gases.

Further reading

C. L. Tan, Z. A. Knight. Regulation of body temperature by the nervous system. *Neuron* 2018; **98**(1): 31–48.

B. Bindu, A. Bindra, G. Rath. Temperature management under general anesthesia: compulsion or option. *J Anaesthesiol Clin Pharmacol.* 2017; **33**(3): 306–16.

C. M. Harper, J. C. Andrzejowski, R. Alexander. NICE and warm. *Br J Anaesth* 2008; **101**(3): 293–5.

S. C. Kettner, C. Sitzwhol, M. Zimpfer, et al. The effect of graded hypothermia (36 °C–32 °C) on haemostasis in anaesthetized patients without surgical trauma. *Anesth Analg* 2003; **96**(6): 1772–6.

Index